Medical instrumentation

Application and design

Medical instrumentation
Application and design

John G. Webster, editor

Contributing authors

John W. Clark
Rice University

James E. Holden
University of Wisconsin–Madison

Michael R. Neuman
Case Western Reserve University

Walter H. Olson*
University of Illinois

Robert A. Peura
Worcester Polytechnic Institute

Frank P. Primiano, Jr.
University Hospitals of Cleveland

Melvin P. Siedband
University of Wisconsin–Madison

John G. Webster
University of Wisconsin–Madison

Lawrence A. Wheeler
Indiana University School of Medicine

* Currently with the Harvard – M.I.T. Division
  of Health Sciences and Technology

Houghton Mifflin Company   **Boston**
Dallas Geneva, Illinois
Hopewell, New Jersey Palo Alto London

Library of Congress Catalog Card Number: 77-76419

ISBN: 0-395-25411-6

Contents

Chapter three

Amplifiers and signal processing 103

John G. Webster

Chapter four

The origin of biopotentials 143

John W. Clark

Chapter five

Biopotential electrodes 215

Michael R. Neuman

Chapter six

Biopotential amplifiers 273

Michael R. Neuman

Chapter seven

Blood pressure and sound 336

Robert A. Peura

Chapter eight

Measurement of flow and volume of blood 385

John G. Webster

Chapter nine

Measurements of the respiratory system 434

Frank P. Primiano, Jr.

Preface

This book describes the principles, applications, and design of the medical instrumentation most commonly used in a hospital. Since equipment changes with time, we have stressed fundamental principles of operation and have avoided detailed descriptions and photographs of current equipment. Since biomedical engineering is an interdisciplinary field, requiring good communication with health-care personnel, we have provided some knowledge of the areas of application for each instrument. However, to keep the book to a reasonable length, we have omitted much of the physiology. We recommend the reading of background material from an inexpensive physiology text, such as *Review of Medical Physiology*, by W.F. Ganong, 8th edition, Los Altos, CA: Lange Medical Publications, 1977.

Chapter 1 covers general concepts that are applicable to all instrumentation systems. Chapter 2 describes basic transducers, while Chapter 3 presents the design of amplifiers for them. Chapters 4 – 6 deal with biopotentials, following the chain from origin, through electrodes, to the special amplifier design required. Chapters 7 and 8 cover the measurement of cardiovascular dynamics — pressure, sound, flow, and volume of blood. Chapter 9 presents the measurement of respiratory dynamics — pressure, flow, and concentration of gases. Chapter 10 describes that area in the hospital in which the greatest number of measurements are made — the clinical laboratory. Chapter 11 starts with general concepts of medical imaging and shows their application to x-ray, ultra-sound, and thermography. Chapter 12 deals with devices used in therapy, such as the pacemaker and defibrillator. Chapter 13 presents a guide to both electrical safety in the hospital and to minimization of hazards.

A feature of our book is its emphasis on *design*. A scientist or engineer with some background in electronics and instrumentation will gain enough information in many of the areas to be able to design medical instruments. This ability should be especially valuable in those frequently encountered situations that require special instruments that are not commercially available. The book provides both worked-out examples and homework problems, thus increasing its usefulness as a text. Rather than giving an exhaustive list of references, we have attempted to select a list of review articles and books that provide the key to organized further study on any given topic.

The book is written for a senior-to-graduate course in biomedical engineering. The typical student should have had chemistry, mathematics through differential equations, a strong background in physics, and courses in electrical circuits and electronics. However, readers without this background will gain much from the descriptive material, and should find it a valuable reference.

We have used the internationally recommended SI units throughout the book. In the case of units of pressure, we have presented both the commonly used millimeters of mercury and the SI unit pascal. To help the reader follow the trend toward SI units, the Appendix provides the most common conversion factors. The Appendix also provides a number of physical constants used in the book, and a list of abbreviations.

For their valuable assistance, we would like to thank the following individuals who reviewed this book during its developmental stages: David Arnett, Pennsylvania State University; Robert Northrup, University of Connecticut (Storrs); Kenneth C. Mylrea, University of Arizona; and Curran S. Swift, Iowa State University.

We are indebted to Albert M. Cook and James C. Hathaway, of the Department of Electrical and Electronic Engineering, California State University, Sacramento, California, for suggesting and providing material on the use of microcomputers in medical instrumentation. Section 3.16 gives an introduction to microcomputers, while Sections 6.9, 9.8, 10.2, and 12.5 give examples of applications, with references provided for further study.

The authors would welcome your suggestions for corrections and improvement of subsequent printings and editions.

John G. Webster
Department of Electrical and Computer Engineering
University of Wisconsin
Madison, Wisconsin 53706

List of symbols

This list gives single-letter symbols for quantities, without subscripts or modifiers. Symbols for physical constants are given in Appendix A.1, multiletter symbols in Appendix A.4, and chemical symbols in Appendix A.5.

Symbol	Quantity	Introduced in section
a	absorptivity	2.15
a	activity	5.2
a	coefficient	1.9
$\mathbf{a}$	lead vector	6.2
A	absorbance	2.15
A	area	2.2
A	coefficient	1.9
A	gain	3.1
A	percent	1.7
b	coefficient	1.9
b	intercept	1.7
B	coefficient	1.9
B	percent	1.7
B	viscous friction	1.9
$\mathbf{B}$	magnetic flux density	8.3
c	coefficient	7.13
c	specific heat	8.1
c	velocity of sound	8.4
C	capacitance	1.9
C	compilance	7.3
C	concentration	2.15
C	contrast	11.1
C	factor	11.7
d	derivative	1.9
d	diameter	1.9
d	distance	4.1
D	density	11.4
D	detector responsivity	2.17
D	d/dt	1.9
D	diameter	5.8
D	diffusing capacity	9.8

Symbol	Quantity	Introduced in section
D	distance	4.4
D	normalized detectivity	11.7
E	emf	2.7
E	energy	2.13
E	exposure	11.4
E	irradiance	2.17
E	modulus of elasticity	7.3
f	force	2.6
f	frequency	1.9
f	function	4.2
F	filter transmission	2.17
F	flow	7.3
F	force	2.2
F	fraction	11.1
F	molar fraction	9.3
g	conductance/area	4.1
G	conductance	2.9
G	form factor	2.4
G	gage factor	2.2
G	gain	1.5
h	height	7.13
H	feedback gain	1.6
i	current	2.6
I	current	3.7
I	intensity	11.10
j	$+(-1)^{1/2}$	1.7
J	number of standard deviations	11.1
k	constant	6.7
k	piezoelectric constant	2.6
K	constant	1.7
K	number	11.1
K	sensitivity	1.9
K	solubility product	5.3
K	spring constant	1.9
L	inductance	1.7
L	inertance	7.3
L	length	2.2
L	line-source response	11.8
m	average number	11.1
m	mass	7.3
m	slope	1.7
M	mass	1.9
M	measured values	11.2
$\overline{M}$	modulation	11.1
$\mathbf{M}$	cardiac vector	6.2
n	number	1.7

Symbol	Quantity	Introduced in section
n	refractive index	2.14
N	noise equivalent bandwidth	11.3
N	number	5.3
N	turns ratio	3.13
p	pressure	9.1
p	probability	11.1
P	power	1.7
P	pressure	7.3
P	projection	11.10
q	charge	2.6
q	rate of heat	8.1
q	volume flow	9.1
Q	heat content	8.2
Q	volume flow	9.1
r	radius	7.3
r	resistance/length	4.2
R	range	8.4
R	resistance	1.7
S	modulation transfer function	11.2
S	slew rate	3.11
S	source output	2.17
t	thickness	5.8
t	time	1.9
T	interval	1.9
T	temperature	2.8
T	transmittance	10.1
u	velocity	4.2
u	work function	11.6
$\dot{U}$	molar uptake	9.1
v	voltage	1.5
v	volume	9.1
V	voltage	1.5
V	volume	2.2
W	power	2.10
W	weight	2.15
W	weighting factor	11.10
x	constant	2.15
x	distance	2.4
x	input	1.5
X	chemical species	9.1
X	effort variable	1.7
y	constant	2.15
y	deflection	7.P
y	output	1.5
Y	admittance	1.7

Symbol	Quantity	Introduced in section
Y	flow variable	1.7
z	distance	4.1
Z	atomic number	11.6
Z	impedance	1.5

Greek letters

Symbol	Quantity	Introduced in section
α	ratio of specific heats	9.5
α	thermistor coefficient	2.9
α	thermoelectric sensitivity	2.8
β	thermistor constant	2.9
ϵ	emissivity	2.10
ϵ	dielectric constant	2.5
ζ	damping ratio	1.9
η	viscosity	7.3
θ	angle	2.2
Λ	logarithmic decrement	1.9
λ	wavelength	2.10
μ	attenuation coefficient	11.10
μ	mobility	5.2
μ	permeability	2.4
μ	Poisson's ratio	2.2
ν	frequency	2.13
ρ	density	7.3
ρ	mole density	9.1
ρ	resistivity	2.2
σ	conductance	12.4
σ	conductivity/distance	4.7
σ^2	variance	11.1
τ	time constant	1.9
ϕ	number of photons	11.6
ϕ	phase shift	1.9
ϕ	divergence	8.4
Φ	potential	4.6
ω	frequency	1.7

Chapter one

Basic concepts of instrumentation

Walter H. Olson

For centuries, without medical instruments, physicians were able to use only their five senses to acquire diagnostic information. Today's medical instruments use transducers, signal-processing devices, and displays to convert information about living systems to a form that human beings can perceive. Medical measurements are needed for diagnosis, monitoring, and research.

The accuracy required for each purpose influences the method of measurement and the complexity of the instrument. Instruments used for diagnosis and monitoring typically have lower requirements because the objective is to determine only whether a variable is within certain limits. All designers of medical instruments should strive *not* to alter the quantity being measured. They should also use fail-safe principles of design to ensure safety of patients and medical personnel.

This chapter will discuss basic characteristics that all medical instruments share, and will present a generalized set of specifications of instrumentation to guide you in the evaluation of instruments. For definitions of medical terminology, refer to Jacobson and Webster (1977) or *Dorland's Illustrated Medical Dictionary* (Anonymous, 1974).

1.1 Generalized instrumentation system

Every instrumentation system has at least some of the functional components shown in Figure 1.1. The primary flow of information is from left to right. Elements and relationships depicted by dashed lines are not essential. The major difference between this system of medical instrumentation and conventional instrumentation systems is that the source of the signals is living tissue or energy applied to living tissue.

Measurand

The physical quantity, property, or condition that the system measures is called the *measurand*. The accessibility of the measurand is important because it may be internal (blood pressure) or

1

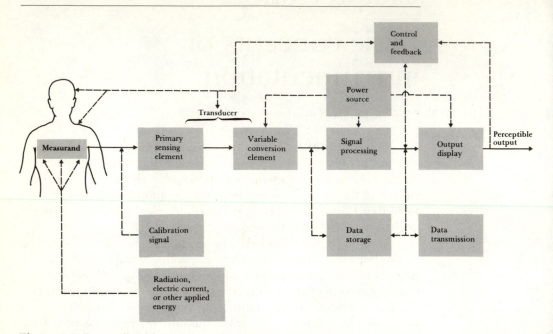

Figure 1.1 Generalized instrumentation system. The transducer converts energy or information from the measurand to another form (usually electrical). This signal is then processed and displayed so that humans can perceive the information. Elements and connections shown by dashed lines are optional for some applications.

on the body surface (bioelectric potentials) or it may emanate from the body (infrared radiation). Most medically important measurands can be grouped in the following categories: biopotential, pressure, flow, displacement (velocity, acceleration, and force), impedance, temperature, and chemical concentrations.

Transducer

Generally a transducer is defined as a device that converts one form of energy to another, usually electrical. The transducer should respond only to the form of energy present in the measurand, to the exclusion of all others. The transducer should interface with the living system in a way that minimizes the energy extracted, while being minimally invasive. Many transducers have a primary sensing element such as a diaphragm, which converts pressure to displacement. A variable-conversion element, such as a strain gage, then converts displacement to an electric voltage. Sometimes the sensitivity of the transducer can be adjusted over a wide range by changing the stiffness of the primary sensing element.

Many variable-conversion elements need external electric power to obtain a transducer output.

Signal conditioning

Usually the transducer output cannot be directly coupled to the display device. Simple signal conditioners may only amplify and filter the signal or merely match the impedance of the transducer to the display. Often transducer outputs are converted to digital form and then processed by specialized digital circuits or a general-purpose digital computer. For example, signal conditioning may compensate for undesirable transducer characteristics; it may also average repetitive signals to reduce noise; or it may convert information from the time domain to the frequency domain.

Output display

The results of the measurement process must be displayed in a form that can be perceived by the human operator. The best form for the display may be numerical or graphical, discrete or continuous, and permanent or temporary—depending on the particular measurand and the action to be taken by the operator. Although most displays rely on our visual sense, some information (Doppler ultrasound signals) is best perceived by other senses (auditory). The output may be compared directly with a standard, or some method of calibration may be employed.

Auxiliary elements

A calibration signal with the properties of the measurand should be applied to the transducer input. Both static and dynamic calibration signals are desirable. Many forms of control and feedback may be required to elicit the measurand, adjust the transducer and signal conditioner, and direct the flow of output for display, storage, or transmission. Control and feedback may be automatic or manual. Data may be stored briefly to meet the requirements of signal conditioning or to enable the investigator to examine data that precede alarm conditions. Or data may be stored before signal conditioning, so that different processing schemes can be utilized. Conventional principles of communications can often be used to transmit data to remote displays at nurses' stations, medical centers, or medical data-processing facilities.

1.2 Alternative operational modes

Direct-indirect modes

Often the desired measurand can be interfaced directly to a transducer because the measurand is readily accessible or acceptable invasive procedures are available. When the desired measurand is not accessible, then we can use either another measurand that bears a known relation to the desired one or some form of energy or material that interacts with the desired measurand to generate a new measurand that *is* accessible. Examples are cardiac output (volume of blood pumped per minute by the heart), determined from measurements of respiration and blood gas, or dye dilution; morphology of internal organs, determined from x-ray shadows; and pulmonary volumes, determined from variations in thoracic electrical impedance.

Sampling and continuous modes

Some measurands—such as body temperature and ion concentrations—change so slowly that they may be sampled infrequently. Other quantities—such as the electrocardiogram and respiratory gas flow—often require continuous monitoring. The frequency content of the measurand, the objective of the measurement, the condition of the patient, and the potential liability of the physician all influence temporal aspects of the acquisition of medical data. Many unused data are often collected.

Generating and modulating transducers

Generating transducers produce their signal output from energy taken from the measurand, while modulating transducers receive their energy from an external source and provide their output by varying this external energy according to the measurand. For example, a photovoltaic cell is a generating transducer because it provides an output voltage related to its illumination, without any additional external energy source. However, a photoconductive cell is a modulating transducer, since to measure its change in resistance with illumination, one must apply external energy to the transducer.

Analog and digital modes

Signals that carry measurement information are either *analog*, meaning continuous and able to take on any value, or *digital*, meaning discrete and able to take on only a finite number of different values. Most currently available transducers operate in the analog mode, although some inherently digital measuring devices have recently been developed. Increased use of digital signal processing has required concurrent use of analog-to-digital and digital-to-analog converters to interface computers with analog transducers and analog display devices. Researchers have developed indirect digital transducers that use analog primary sensing elements and digital variable-conversion elements (optical shaft encoders). Also quasi-digital transducers, such as quartz-crystal thermometers, give outputs with variable frequency, pulse rate, or pulse duration that are easily converted to digital signals.

Advantages of the digital mode of operation are greater accuracy, repeatability, reliability, and immunity to noise. Also periodic calibration is usually not required. Digital numerical displays are replacing many analog meter movements because of their greater accuracy and readability. Many clinicians, however, prefer analog displays when they are determining whether a physiological variable is within certain limits or when they are looking at a parameter that can quickly change, such as beat-to-beat heart rate. In the latter case, digital displays often change numbers so quickly that they are very difficult and annoying to observe.

Real-time and delayed-time modes

Of course transducers must acquire signals in real time as the signals actually occur. The output of the measurement system may not display the result immediately, however, since some types of signal processing, such as averaging and transformations, need considerable input before any results can be produced. Often such short delays are acceptable unless urgent feedback and control tasks depend on the output.

Deflection and null modes

For instruments that operate in the deflection mode, the output signal produces an effect that is opposed by a spring or similar device so that a displacement proportional to the quantity measured can be displayed. For example, the torque produced by current flowing through a D'Arsonval meter movement is opposed by a spring so that displacement of the needle is proportional to input current.

Instruments operating in the null mode utilize a detector of imbalance between the unknown quantity and a known calibrated opposing quantity. The output is read as the value of the opposing quantity for a balanced detector at maximum sensitivity. The null-type device is generally more accurate because the unknown is compared directly with a standard and the detector of imbalance can have high sensitivity because only a small range near zero need be covered. The null detector does not have to be calibrated, since it is used only to detect the presence or absence of a signal. The major disadvantage of null methods is the typically poor dynamic response, even when automatic balancing devices are used.

1.3 Medical measurement constraints

The medical instrumentation described throughout this book is designed to measure various medical and physiological parameters. The principal measurement and frequency ranges for each parameter are major factors that affect the design of all the instrument components shown in Figure 1.1. To get a brief overview of typical medical parameter measurement and frequency ranges, refer to Table 1.1. These are approximate ranges that may need to be expanded, depending on the purpose of the measurements. Most of the parameter measurement ranges are quite low compared with nonmedical parameters in most industries. Note for example that most voltages are in the microvolt range and that pressures are low (about 100 mm Hg = 1.93 psi = 13.3 kPa). Also note that all the signals listed are in the audiofrequency range or below and that many signals consist of dc and very low frequencies. These general properties of medical parameters limit the practical choices available to designers for all aspects of instrument design.

Many crucial variables in living systems are inaccessible because the proper measurand–transducer interface cannot be achieved. Unlike many complex physical systems, a biological system is of such a nature that it is not possible to turn it off and remove parts of it during the measurement procedure. Even if interference from other physiological systems can be avoided, the physical size of many transducers prohibits the formation of a proper interface. Either such inaccessible variables must be measured indirectly as just described, or corrections must be applied to data that are affected by the measurement process. The cardiac output is an important measurement that is obviously quite inaccessible.

Variables measured from the human body or from animals are seldom deterministic. Most measured quantities vary with time, even when all controllable factors are fixed. Many medical measurements vary widely among normal patients, even when conditions are similar. This inherent *variability* has been documented at the molecular and organ levels, and even for the whole body. There are many internal anatomical variations that accompany the obvious external differences between patients. Large tolerances on physiological measurements are partly the result of interactions between many physiological systems. Many feedback loops exist

Parameter or measuring technique	Principal measurement range of parameter	Signal frequency range, Hz	Standard transducer or method
Ballistocardiography (BCG)	0–7 mg	dc–40	Accelerometer, strain gage
	0–100 μm	dc–40	Displacement (LVDT)
Bladder pressure	1–100 cm H_2O	dc–10	Strain-gage manometer
Blood flow	1–300 ml/s	dc-20	Flowmeter (electro-magnetic or ultrasonic)
Blood pressure (arterial)			
Direct	10–400 mm Hg	dc–50	Strain-gage manometer
Indirect	25–400 mm Hg	dc–60	Cuff, auscultation
(Venous)	0–50 mm Hg	dc–50	Strain gage
Blood gases			
P_{O_2}	30–100 mm Hg	dc–2	Specific electrode, volumetric or manometric
P_{CO_2}	40–100 mm Hg	dc–2	Specific electrode, volumetric or manometric
P_{N_2}	1–3 mm Hg	dc–2	Specific electrode, volumetric or manometric
P_{CO}	0.1–0.4 mm Hg	dc–2	Specific electrode, volumetric or manometric
Blood pH	6.8–7.8 pH units	dc–2	Specific electrode
Cardiac output	4–25 liter/min	dc–20	Dye dilution, flowmeter
Electrocardiography (ECG)	0.5–4 mV	0.01–250	Skin electrodes
Electroencephalography (EEG)	5–300 μV	dc–150	Scalp electrodes
(Electrocorticography and brain depth)	10–5000 μV	dc–150	Brain-surface or depth electrodes
Electrogastrography	10–1000 μV	dc–1	Skin-surface electrodes
	0.5–80 mV	dc–1	Stomach-surface electrodes
Electromyography (EMG)	0.1–5 mV	dc–10,000	Needle electrodes
Eye potentials			
EOG	50–3500 μV	dc–50	Contact electrodes
ERG	0–900 μV	dc–50	Contact electrodes
Galvanic skin response (GSR)	1–500 kΩ	0.01–1	Skin electrodes
Gastric pH	3–13 pH units	dc–1	pH electrode; antimony electrode

Table 1.1 Medical and physiological parameters. (Revised from *Medical Engineering*, C.D. Ray (ed.). Copyright © 1974 by Year Book Medical Publishers, Inc., Chicago. Used by permission.)

Parameter or measuring technique	Principal measurement range of parameter	Signal frequency range, Hz	Standard transducer or method
Gastrointestinal pressure	0–100 cm H_2O	dc–10	Strain-gage manometer
Gastrointestinal forces	1–50 g	dc–1	Displacement system, LVDT
Nerve potentials	0.01–3 mV	dc–10,000	Surface or needle electrodes
Phonocardiography (PCG)	Dynamic range 80 dB, threshold about 10^{-4} Pa	5–2000	Microphone
Plethysmography (volume change)	Varies with organ measured	dc–30	Displacement chamber or impedance change
Circulatory	0–30 ml	dc–30	Displacement chamber or impedance change
Respiratory functions			
Pneumotachography (flow rate)	0–600 liter/min	dc–40	Pneumotachograph head and differential pressure
Respiratory rate	2–50 breaths/min	0.1–10	Strain gage on chest, impedance, nasal thermistor
Tidal volume	50–1000 ml/breath	0.1–10	Above methods
Temperature of body	32–40°C 90–104°F	dc–0.1	Thermistor, thermocouple

Table 1.1 (Continued)

between physiological systems and many of the interrelations are poorly understood. It is seldom feasible to control or neutralize the effects of these other systems on the measured variable. The most common method of coping with this variability is to assume empirical statistical and probabilistic distribution functions. Single measurements are then compared with these *norms*.

Nearly all biomedical measurements depend either on some form of energy being applied to the living tissue or on some energy being applied as an incidental consequence of transducer operation. X-ray and ultrasonic imaging techniques and electromagnetic or Doppler ultrasonic blood flowmeters all depend on externally applied energy interacting with living tissue. Safe levels of these various types of energy are difficult to establish because many mechanisms of interaction are not well understood. The heating of tissue is one effect that must be limited, because even reversible physiological changes can affect measurements. Damage to tissue at the molecular level has been demonstrated in some instances at surprisingly low energy levels.

Operation of instruments in the medical environment imposes important additional constraints. Equipment must be reliable, simple to operate, and capable of withstanding physical abuse and exposure to corrosive chemicals. Electronic equipment must be designed to minimize electric-shock hazards (Chapter 13). The safety of patients and medical personnel must be considered in all phases of design and testing of instruments. The Medical Device Amendments of 1976 (Public Law 94-295) amend the Federal Food, Drug, and Cosmetic Act to provide for the safety and effectiveness of medical devices intended for human use (Section 1.10).

1.4 Classifications of biomedical instruments

The study of biomedical instruments can be approached from at least four viewpoints. Techniques of biomedical measurement can be grouped according to the *quantity that is transduced,* such as pressure, flow, or temperature. One advantage of this classification is that different methods for measuring any quantity can be compared readily.

A second classification scheme uses the *principle of transduction,* such as resistive, inductive, capacitive, ultrasonic, or electrochemical. Different applications of each principle can be used to strengthen understanding of each concept; also new applications may be more apparent.

Measurement techniques can be studied separately for each *physiological system,* such as the cardiovascular, pulmonary, nervous, or endocrine systems. This approach isolates all important measurements for specialists who need to know only about a specific area, but it results in considerable overlap of principles of transduction.

Finally, biomedical instruments can be classified according to the *clinical medicine specialties,* such as pediatrics, obstetrics, cardiology, or radiology. This approach is valuable for medical personnel who are interested in specialized instruments. Certain measurements—such as blood pressure—are important to many different medical specialties.

1.5 Interfering and modifying inputs

A general block diagram for classifying desired and undesired inputs to instruments is shown in Figure 1.2 (Draper et al., 1955, p. 58; Doebelin, 1975, p. 19). *Desired inputs* are the measurands that the instrument is designed to isolate. *Interfering inputs* are quantities that inadvertently affect the instrument as a consequence of the principles used to acquire and process the desired inputs. If spatial or temporal isolation of the measurand is incomplete, the interfering input can be the same quantity as the desired input. *Modifying inputs* are undesired quantities that indirectly affect the output by altering the performance of the instrument itself. Modifying inputs can affect processing of either desired or interfering inputs. Some undesirable quantities can act as both a modifying input and an interfering input.

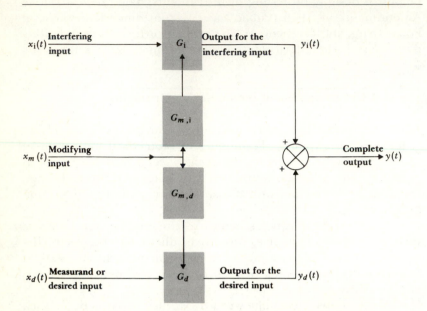

Figure 1.2 Generalized input-output diagram. The output is the sum of two components: the desired part, obtained by processing the desired input, and an unwanted part, obtained from undesired interfering inputs. Modifying inputs affect the processing of desired and interfering inputs. (Modified from *Measurement Systems: Application and Design,* by E.O. Doebelin. Copyright © 1975 by McGraw-Hill, Inc. Used with the permission of McGraw-Hill Book Co.)

The input-output relationship for desired inputs is given the symbol G_d in Figure 1.2. This symbol represents the mathematical operation required to obtain the desired output component from the measurand. The operation G_d may be (1) linear amplification (simple constant), (2) some nonlinear transducer or processor (nonlinear equation), (3) a dynamic relation that may even be time-varying (differential equations), or (4) a nondeterministic relationship with random or stochastic components (statistical distribution function).

The operation G_i, for relating interfering inputs and outputs may or may not be the same as G_d. The symbols $G_{m,d}$ and $G_{m,i}$ represent the mechanism of how modifying inputs affect the operations G_d and G_i, respectively. The cross inside the circle is the standard symbol for an instantaneous algebraic summing device. More than one interfering and/or modifying input are often present and some instrument systems may have multiple inputs and outputs. Interfering inputs often combine with desired inputs in front of G_d

and this combined input is processed by G_d. This is functionally the same as the diagram in Figure 1.2 if $G_i = G_d$ and the G's are linear. These are simple extensions of the configuration in Figure 1.2.

   A typical electrocardiographic recording system, shown in Figure 1.3, is used as an example to illustrate these concepts. The desired input is the electrocardiographic voltage v_{ecg} that appears between the two electrodes. One interfering input is 60-Hz noise voltage induced in the shaded loop by ac magnetic fields. The desired and the interfering voltages are in series and both components appear in the output. Also capacitively coupled displacement current flowing through the electrodes and the body to ground causes an interfering voltage to appear between the two electrodes.

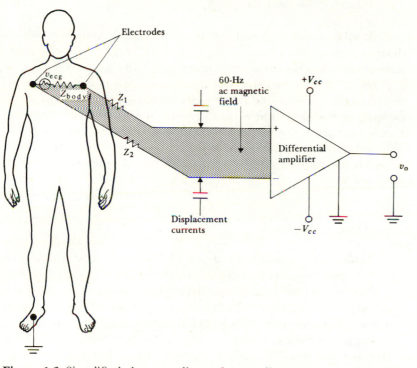

Figure 1.3 Simplified electrocardiograph recording system. Two possible interfering inputs are stray magnetic fields and capacitively coupled noise. Orientation of patient cables and changes in electrode-skin impedance are two possible modifying inputs.

   An example of a modifying input is the orientation of the patient cables. If the plane of the cables is parallel to the ac magnetic field, magnetic interference is zero. If the plane of the cables is perpendicular to the ac magnetic field, magnetic interference is maximum. Time-dependent changes in electrode impedance are an example of a modifying input that affects G_d.

1.6 Compensation techniques

The effects of most interfering and modifying inputs can be reduced or eliminated either by altering the design of essential instrument components or by adding new components designed to offset the undesired inputs. The former alternative is preferred when feasible because the result is usually simpler. Unfortunately, designers of instruments can only rarely eliminate the actual source of the undesired inputs. We shall discuss several compensation methods for eliminating the effects of interfering and modifying inputs.

Inherent insensitivity

If all instrument components are inherently sensitive only to desired inputs, then interfering and modifying inputs obviously have no effect. This amounts to making G_i and $G_{m,d}$ zero so that, as Figure 1.2 shows, the effects of interfering and modifying inputs are blocked. An example for the electrocardiograph system is the twisting of the electrode wires to reduce the number of magnetic flux lines that cut the shaded loop in Figure 1.3. The voltage of the induced noise is proportional to the area of that loop. The effects of electrode motion can be reduced by techniques described in Chapter 5.

Negative feedback

When G_d is altered by a modifying input that cannot be avoided, then improved instrument performance requires a strategy that makes the output less dependent on G_d. The feedback method, shown in Figure 1.4(a), takes a portion of the output at any instant of time and feeds it back to the input of the instrument. This output-dependent signal is subtracted from the input and the difference becomes the effective system input. For Figure 1.4(a), we can write

$$(x_d - H_f y)G_d = y \tag{1.1}$$

$$x_d G_d = y(1 + H_f G_d) \tag{1.2}$$

$$y = \frac{G_d}{1 + H_f G_d} x_d \tag{1.3}$$

If G_d includes amplification, then $H_f G_d \gg 1$ and $y \cong (1/H_f)(x_d)$. This well-known relationship shows that only the feedback element determines the output for a given input. Of course, this strategy fails if H_f is also affected by modifying inputs,

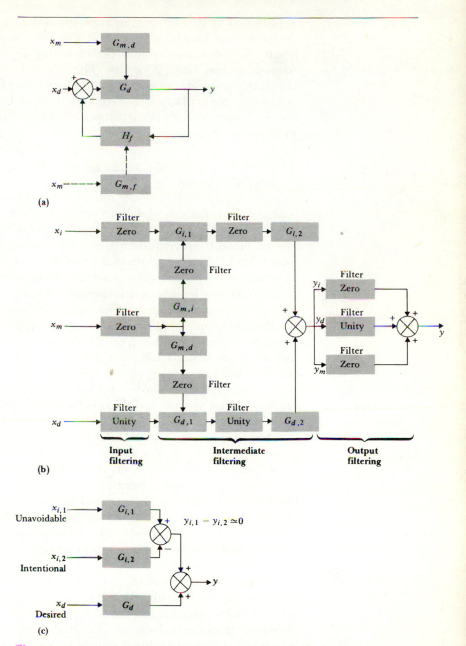

Figure 1.4 Methods of compensating errors due to interfering and modifying inputs. (a) Feedback. (b) Filtering: input, intermediate, output. (c) Opposing inputs. (Modified from *Measurement Systems: Application and Design*, by E.O. Doebelin. Copyright © 1975 by McGraw-Hill, Inc. Used with permission of McGraw-Hill Book Co.)

as indicated by dashed lines in Figure 1.4(a). Usually the feedback device carries less power, so it is generally more accurate and linear. Also less input-signal power is needed for this feedback scheme, so less loading occurs. The major hazard of using this feedback principle is that dynamic instability leading to oscillations can occur, particularly if G_d contains time delays. The study of feedback systems is a well-developed discipline that cannot be pursued further here (Kuo, 1975).

Signal filtering

A filter separates signals according to their frequencies. Most filters accomplish this by attenuating the part of the signal that is in one or more frequency bands. A more general definition for a filter is "a device or program that separates data, signals or material in accordance with specified criteria" (Anonymous, 1972).

Filters may be inserted at the instrument input, at some point within the instrument, or at the output of the instrument. In fact, the limitations of people's senses may be used to filter unwanted signal components coming from display devices. An example is the utilization of flicker fusion for rapidly changing images from a real-time ultrasonic scanner.

Input filtering is shown in Figure 1.4(b). Note that the filter blocks interfering and modifying inputs, but does not alter the desired input. The three filter elements shown may be distinct devices that block or pass all inputs, or they may be embodied in a single device that selectively blocks only undesired inputs. Many designers do not use input filters that are electric circuits, but instead use mechanical, pneumatic, thermal, or electromagnetic principles to block out undesired environmental inputs. For example, instruments are often shock-mounted to filter vibrations that affect sensitive instrument components. Electromagnetic shielding is often used to block interfering electric and magnetic fields, such as those indicated in Figure 1.3.

Electronic filters are often incorporated at some intermediate point within the instrument. To facilitate filtering based on differences in frequency, mixers and modulators are used to shift desired and/or undesired signals to another frequency range. Digital computers are used to filter signals based on template-matching techniques and various time-domain signal properties. These filters may even have time- or signal-dependent criteria for isolating the desired signal. Intermediate filtering is symbolically shown in Figure 1.4(b).

Output filtering is possible, though usually more difficult because desired and undesired output signals are superimposed. The selectivity needed may be easier to achieve with higher-level output signals, or maneuvers performed by G_i, $G_{m,i}$, $G_{m,d}$, or G_d may facilitate filtering at the output. The selectivity necessary for output filtering is evident in Figure 1.4(b).

Opposing inputs

When interfering and/or modifying inputs cannot be filtered, additional interfering inputs can be used to cancel undesired output components, as shown in Figure 1.4(c). These extra intentional inputs may be the same as the ones to be canceled, which implies that $G_{i,1} = G_{i,2}$. In general, the inputs and the operators G_i can be quite different, so long as the two output components are equal, so that cancelation results. The two outputs must cancel despite variations in all the unavoidable interfering inputs and variations in the desired inputs. The actual cancelation of undesired output components can be implemented either before or after the desired and undesired outputs are combined. Indeed, either the intentional or the unavoidable interfering input signal might be processed by G_d. The method of opposing inputs can also be used to cancel the effects of modifying inputs.

Automatic real-time corrections are implied for the method of opposing inputs just described. Actually, output corrections are often calculated manually or by computer methods and applied after data are collected. This requires quantitative knowledge of the interfering and/or modifying input at the time of the measurement and also of how these inputs affect the output. This method is usually cumbersome, loses real-time information, and is often used only for rather static interfering inputs, such as temperature and atmospheric pressure.

An example of the opposing-input method is to intentionally induce a voltage from the same 60-Hz magnetic field present in Figure 1.3 to be amplified and inverted until cancelation of the 60-Hz noise in the output is achieved. An obvious disadvantage of this method is that the amplifier gain has to be adjusted whenever the geometry of the shaded loop in Figure 1.3 changes. In electronic circuits that must operate over a wide temperature range, *thermistors* (temperature-dependent resistors) are often used to counteract unavoidable temperature-dependent changes in characteristics of active circuit elements, such as transistors and integrated circuits. This is an example of the correction of undesired modifying inputs by the method of opposing inputs.

1.7 Generalized static characteristics

To enable one to compare commercially available instruments and evaluate new instrument designs, quantitative criteria for the performance of instruments are needed. These criteria must clearly specify how well an instrument measures the desired input and how much the output depends on interfering and modifying inputs. Characteristics of instrument performance are usually subdivided into two classes, based on the frequency of the inputs.

Static characteristics describe performance of instruments for dc or very low-frequency inputs. The properties of the output for a wide range of constant inputs demonstrate the quality of the measurement, including nonlinear and statistical effects. Some transducers and instruments, such as piezoelectric devices, respond only to time-varying inputs and have no static characteristics.

Dynamic characteristics require the use of differential and/or integral equations to describe the quality of the measurements. Although dynamic characteristics usually depend on static characteristics, the nonlinearities and statistical variability are usually ignored for dynamic inputs because the differential equations become difficult to solve. Complete characteristics are approximated by the sum of static and dynamic characteristics. This necessary oversimplification is frequently responsible for differences between real and ideal instrument performance.

Accuracy

The *accuracy* of a single measured quantity is the true value minus the measured value, and this difference is divided by the true value. This ratio is usually expressed in percent. Since the true value is seldom available, the accepted true value or reference value should be traceable to the National Bureau of Standards.

The accuracy usually varies over the normal range of the quantity measured, usually decreases as the full-scale value of the quantity decreases on a multirange instrument, and also often varies with the frequency of desired, interfering, and modifying inputs. Accuracy is a measure of the total error without regard to the type or source of the error. The + and − accuracy are assumed equal. The accuracy can be expressed as percent of reading, percent of full scale, ± number of digits for digital readouts, or $\pm\frac{1}{2}$ the smallest analog scale division. Often the accuracy is expressed as a sum of these. For example, on a digital device: $\pm 0.01\%$ of reading $\pm 0.015\%$ of full scale ± 1 digit. If accuracy is expressed simply as a percentage, full scale is usually assumed. Some instrument manufacturers specify accuracy for a limited period of time.

Precision

The *precision* of a measurement expresses the number of distinguishable alternatives from which a given result is selected. For example, a meter that displays a reading of 2.434 V is more precise than one that displays a reading of 2.43 V. High-precision measurements do not imply high accuracy, however, because the former meter may be less accurate than the latter.

Resolution

The smallest incremental quantity that can be measured with certainty is the *resolution*. If the measured quantity starts from zero, the term threshold is synonomous with resolution. Resolution expresses the degree to which nearly equal values of a quantity can be discriminated.

Reproducibility

The ability of an instrument to give the same output for equal inputs applied over some period of time is called *reproducibility* or *repeatability*. Reproducibility does not imply accuracy. For example, an unplugged digital clock gives very reproducible values that are accurate only twice a day.

Statistical control

The accuracy of an instrument is not meaningful unless all factors, such as the environment and the method of use, are considered. Statistical control means that random variations in measured quantities that result from all factors that influence the measurement process are tolerable. Any systematic errors or bias can be removed by calibration and correction factors, but random variations pose a more difficult problem. The measurand and/or the instrument may introduce statistical variations that make outputs unreproducible. If the cause of this variability cannot be eliminated, then statistical analysis must be used to determine the error variation. The estimate of the true value can be improved by making multiple measurements and averaging the results.

Static sensitivity

A static calibration is performed by holding all inputs (desired, interfering, and modifying) constant except one. The one input is varied incrementally over the normal operating range, resulting in a range of incremental outputs. The static sensitivity of an instrument or system is the ratio of the incremental output quantity to the incremental input quantity. This ratio is the static component of G_d for inputs within the range of the incremental

inputs. The incremental slope can be obtained from either the se-
cant between two adjacent points or the tangent to one point on the
calibration curve. The static sensitivity may be constant for only
part of the normal operating range of the instrument, as shown in
Figure 1.5(a). For input-output data that indicate a straight-line calibration curve, the slope m and intercept b for the line with the
minimal sum of the squared differences between data points and
the line are given by the following equations:

$$m = \frac{n\Sigma x_d y - (\Sigma x_d)(\Sigma y)}{n\Sigma x_d^2 - (\Sigma x_d)^2} \tag{1.4}$$

$$b = \frac{(\Sigma y)(\Sigma x_d^2) - (\Sigma x_d y)(\Sigma x_d)}{n\Sigma x_d^2 - (\Sigma x_d)^2} \tag{1.5}$$

$$y = mx_d + b \tag{1.6}$$

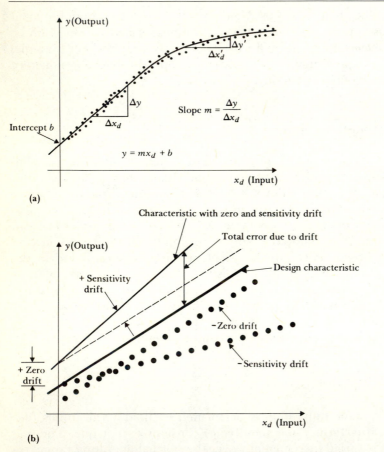

(a)

(b)

Figure 1.5 (a) Static sensitivity curve that relates desired input x_d to output
y. Static sensitivity may be constant for only a limited range of inputs. (b)
Static sensitivity: zero drift and sensitivity drift. Dotted lines indicate that
zero and sensitivity drift can be negative. [Part (b) modified from *Measure-
ment Systems: Application and Design*, by E.O. Doebelin. Copyright © 1975 by
McGraw-Hill, Inc. Used with permission of McGraw-Hill Book Co.]

where n is the total number of points and each sum is for all n points. Programmable calculators can be used to compute m and b. The static sensitivity for modulating transducers is usually given per volt of excitation because the output voltage is proportional to the excitation voltage. For example, the static sensitivity for a blood-pressure transducer containing a strain-gage bridge might be 50 $\mu V \cdot V^{-1} \cdot mm\ Hg^{-1}$.

Example 1.1 A variable-reluctance differential-pressure transducer contains two inductors. One inductance increases slightly $(+ \Delta L)$ as a function of pressure and the other inductance decreases slightly $(- \Delta L)$ by an equal amount. Two methods for placing these inductances in an ac bridge are shown in Figure 1.6. The bridge-completion resistors have the value $R = \omega L$. Find the *sensitivity* $(V_o/\Delta L)$ for the two methods and compare.

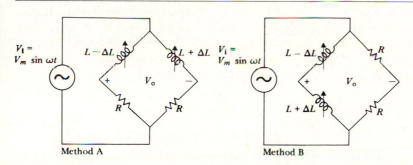

Figure 1.6 Example 1.1: Alternative methods of connecting a variable-reluctance pressure transducer (two inductors) to an ac bridge.

Answer
Method A:

$$V_o = \frac{R}{R + j\omega(L - \Delta L)} V_i - \frac{R}{R + j\omega(L + \Delta L)} V_i$$

$$= V_i R \left[\frac{R + j\omega(L + \Delta L) - R - j\omega(L - \Delta L)}{R^2 + j\omega R(2L + \Delta L - \Delta L) - \omega^2(L^2 - \Delta L^2)} \right]$$

$$\cong \frac{V_i R(j\omega 2 \Delta L)}{j\omega 2RL} = \frac{V_i \Delta L}{L}$$

$$\frac{V_o}{\Delta L} = \frac{V_i}{L}$$

Method B:

$$V_o = \frac{j\omega(L + \Delta L)V_i}{j\omega(2L + \Delta L - \Delta L)} - \frac{V_i R}{2R} = \frac{V_i \Delta L}{2L} + \frac{V_i L}{2L} - \frac{V_i R}{2R}$$

$$= \frac{V_i \Delta L}{2L}$$

$$\frac{V_o}{\Delta L} = \frac{V_i}{2L}$$

Method A has twice the sensitivity of method B.

Zero drift

Interfering and/or modifying inputs can affect the static calibration curve in Figure 1.5(a) several ways. Zero drift has occurred
when all output values increase or decrease by the same absolute
amount. The slope of the sensitivity curve is unchanged, but the
output-axis intercept increases or decreases as shown in Figure
1.5(b). The following factors can cause zero drift: manufacturing
misalignment, variations in ambient temperature, hysteresis, vibration, shock, and sensitivity to forces from undesired directions.
A change in the dc-offset voltage at the electrodes in the electrocardiograph example in Figure 1.3 is an example of zero drift.
Slow changes in the dc-offset voltage do not cause a problem, because the amplifier is ac-coupled. Fast changes due to motion of
the subject do cause zero drift to appear at the output.

Sensitivity drift

When the slope of the calibration curve changes as a result of
an interfering and/or modifying input, a drift in sensitivity results.
Sensitivity drift causes error that is proportional to the magnitude
of the input. The slope of the calibration curve can either increase
or decrease, as indicated in Figure 1.5(b). Sensitivity drift can result
from manufacturing tolerances, power-supply variations, nonlinearities, and changes in ambient temperature and pressure. Variations in the electrocardiograph-amplifier voltage gain as a result of
fluctuations in dc power-supply voltage or change in temperature
are examples of sensitivity drift.

Linearity

A system or element is linear if it has properties such that, if y_1
is the response to x_1 and y_2 is the response to x_2, then $y_1 + y_2$ is the
response to $x_1 + x_2$ and Ky_1 is the response to Kx_1 (Anonymous,
1972). These two requirements for system linearity are restated in
Figure 1.7(a). They are clearly satisfied for an instrument with a
calibration curve that is a straight line.

Keep in mind, however, that high accuracy does not necessarily imply linearity. In practice, no instrument has a perfect linear
response, so a measure of deviation from linearity is needed. *Inde-*

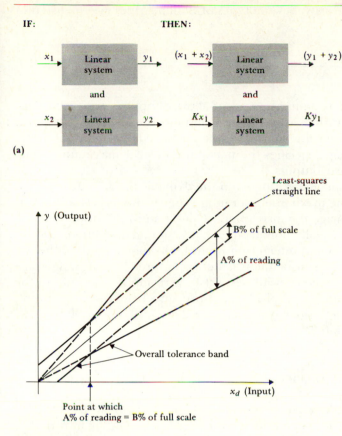

(a)

(b)

Figure 1.7 (a) Basic definition of linearity for a system or element. The same linear system or element is shown four times for different inputs. (b) A graphic illustration of independent nonlinearity equals $\pm A\%$ of the reading, or $\pm B\%$ of full scale, whichever is greater (that is, whichever permits the larger error). [Part (b) modified from *Measurement Systems: Application and Design,* by E. O. Doebelin. Copyright © 1975 by McGraw-Hill, Inc. Used with permission of McGraw-Hill Book Co.]

pendent nonlinearity expresses the maximum deviation of points from the least-squares fitted line as either $\pm A\%$ of the reading or $\pm B\%$ of full scale, whichever is greater (that is, whichever permits the larger error). This linearity specification is shown in Figure 1.7(b). For up-scale readings, the percent-of-reading figure is desirable because most errors are proportional to the reading. For small readings near zero, however, percentage of full scale is more realistic because it is not feasible to test for small percent-of-reading deviations near zero. All data points must fall inside the "funnel" in Figure 1.7(b). For most instruments that are essentially linear, if other sources of error are minimal, the accuracy is equal to the nonlinearity. Several types of nonlinearities are discussed in Section 1.8.

Input ranges

Several maximum ranges of allowed input quantities are applicable for various conditions. Minimum resolvable inputs put a lower bound on the quantity to be measured. The normal linear operating range specifies the maximum or near-maximum inputs that give linear outputs.

The static linear range and the dynamic linear range may be different. The maximum operating range is the largest input that does not damage the instrument. Operation in the upper part of this range is usually nonlinear. Finally, storage conditions specify environmental and interfering input limits that should not be exceeded when the instrument is not being used. These ranges are not always symmetric with respect to zero input, particularly for storage conditions. Typical blood-pressure transducer operating ranges have a positive bias such as $+200$ mm Hg to -60 mm Hg ($+26.6$ to -8.0 kPa).

Input impedance

Because biomedical transducers and instruments usually convert nonelectrical quantities into voltage or current, we introduce a generalized concept of input impedance. This is necessary to properly evaluate the degree to which instruments disturb the quantity being measured. For every desired input x_{d1} that we seek to measure, there is another implicit input quantity x_{d2}, such that the product $x_{d1} \cdot x_{d2}$ has the dimensions of power. This product represents the instantaneous rate at which energy is transferred across the tissue-transducer interface. The generalized input impedance is the ratio of the phasor equivalent of a steady-state sinusoidal *effort* input variable (voltage, force, pressure) to the phasor equivalent of a steady-state sinusoidal *flow* input variable (current, velocity, flow):

$$Z_x = \frac{X_{d1}}{X_{d2}} = \frac{\text{effort variable}}{\text{flow variable}} \tag{1.7}$$

The power is the time rate of energy transfer from the measurement medium:

$$P = X_{d1} \cdot X_{d2} = \frac{X_{d1}^2}{Z_x} = Z_x X_{d2}^2 \tag{1.8}$$

To minimize P, when measuring effort variables X_{d1}, the generalized input impedance should be as large as possible. This is usually achieved by minimizing the flow variable. However, most instruments function by measuring minute values of the flow variable, so the flow variable cannot be reduced to zero. Of course, when measuring flow variables X_{d2}, small input impedance is needed to minimize P. The loading caused by measuring devices depends on the magnitude of the input impedance $|Z_x|$ compared with the magnitude of the source impedance $|Z_s|$ for the desired input. Unfortunately, biological source impedances are usually unknown, variable, and difficult to measure and control. Thus the instrument designer must usually focus on maximizing the input impedance Z_x for effort-variable measurement. When the measurand is a flow variable instead of an effort variable, the admittance $Y_x = 1/Z_x$ is more convenient to use than the impedance.

1.8 Nonlinear static characteristics

In this section, we shall discuss several fundamental types of nonlinear input-output characteristics and give typical causes for nonlinear behavior. Any deviation of the input-output characteristic from a straight line is a nonlinearity. The basic nonlinearities illustrated in Figure 1.8 show abrupt departures from linearity. Nonlinear characteristics with smooth curves are simple extensions of these basic nonlinearities.

Saturation

All real instruments exhibit saturation if input magnitudes are large enough. The typical input-output characteristic for saturation is shown in Figure 1.8(a). The characteristic is linear for inputs up to some level. Additional increases in input give less-than-proportional rises in output, so the slope of the characteristic curve decreases and may become zero. The transition may be smooth or abrupt, depending on the cause of the nonlinearity. Saturation is probably the most common type of nonlinearity. It is often intentionally introduced to protect primary sensing elements from destruction by over-range input signals. Mechanical or electronic stops are frequently designed to protect transducers and instruments. Most transducers and instrumentation components also have inherently limited linear operating ranges. Amplifier output voltages saturate when the output approaches the dc power-supply voltage.

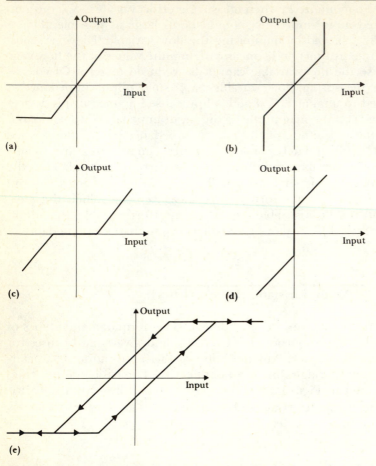

Figure 1.8 Basic nonlinear static characteristics. (a) Saturation, (b) break-down, (c) dead zone, (d) bang-bang, (e) hysteresis.

Breakdown

Occasionally the slope of a characteristic curve increases for large inputs, as shown in Figure 1.8(b). Some devices, such as Zener diodes, exhibit this type of nonlinearity without being destroyed. As the name "breakdown" implies, this type of nonlinearity may result from exceeding the elastic limit of instrument components, particularly primary sensing elements. The increased amplification indicated by this type of nonlinearity may lead to unstable operation in electronic instrumentation. Although this type of nonlinearity is obviously similar to saturation, breakdown is much less prevalent than saturation.

Dead zone

The output of some devices does not begin to increase until some threshold value of the input is reached. This threshold or dead-zone nonlinearity is shown in Figure 1.8(c). The dead-zone region need not be at zero output, and its width and symmetry are quite variable. Gears and nearly all mechanical linkages have dead zones, as do many diode circuits and devices affected by static friction. To minimize static friction, *dithering* (application of intermittent or oscillatory forces) is a useful technique.

Bang-bang

An abrupt change in the output when the sign of the input reverses—called bang-bang—is shown in Figure 1.8(d). This type of nonlinearity is encountered in some control systems and in thin-metal diaphragms connected to displacement transducers for measurement of pressure. You can observe this type of nonlinearity by pressing and releasing the bottom of an empty beverage can.

Hysteresis

Curves for some input-output characteristics are different for increasing inputs from those for decreasing inputs. Figure 1.8(e) shows a typical static hysteresis characteristic. Hysteresis results when some of the energy applied to the instrument for an increasing input is not recovered when the input decreases. The lost energy is usually dissipated as heat. Actually all instruments have some hysteresis because the second law of thermodynamics prohibits perfect reversibility. In practice some materials and devices have more internal friction than others. For example, inductive devices typically have considerable hysteresis if eddy currents are not minimized. Some materials, such as most plastics, show more hysteresis when stressed than others, such as metals. Hysteresis is often quite dependent on the rate of change of the input; it is often combined with saturation.

The nonlinear characteristics shown in Figure 1.8 are symmetric, and sharp transitions between linear and nonlinear behavior are evident. Unsymmetric and smoother nonlinearities are common, and many combinations of these basic nonlinearities are possible. Describing functions for 23 combinations of these nonlinearities are available (Gibson, 1963, p. 358).

1.9 Generalized dynamic characteristics

Only a few medical measurements, such as body temperature, are constant or slowly varying quantities. Most medical instruments must process signals that are functions of time. It is this time-varying property of medical signals that requires us to consider dynamic instrument characteristics. Differential or integral equations are required to relate dynamic inputs to dynamic outputs for continuous systems. Fortunately many engineering instruments can be described by ordinary linear differential equations with constant coefficients. The input $x(t)$ is related to the output $y(t)$ according to the following equation:

$$a_n \frac{d^n y}{dt^n} + \cdots + a_1 \frac{dy}{dt} + a_0 y(t)$$
$$= b_m \frac{d^m x}{dt^m} + \cdots + b_1 \frac{dx}{dt} + b_0 x(t) \quad (1.9)$$

where the constants $a_i (i = 0, 1, \ldots, n)$ and $b_j (j = 0, 1, \ldots, m)$ depend on the physical and electrical parameters of the system. By introducing the differential operator, $D^k \equiv d^k(\ )/dt^k$, we can write this equation as

$$(a_n D^n + \cdots + a_1 D + a_0) y(t)$$
$$= (b_m D^m + \cdots + b_1 D + b_0) x(t) \quad (1.10)$$

Readers familiar with Laplace transforms may recognize that D may be replaced by the Laplace parameter s to obtain the equation relating the transforms $Y(s)$ and $X(s)$. This is a *linear* differential equation because the linear properties stated in Figure 1.7(a) are assumed and the coefficients a_i and b_j are not functions of time or the input $x(t)$. The equation is *ordinary* because there is only one independent variable y. Essentially such properties mean that the instruments' methods of acquiring and analyzing the signals do not change as a function of time or the quantity of input. For example, an autoranging instrument may violate these conditions.

Most practical instruments are described by differential equations of zero, first, or second order; thus $n = 0, 1, 2$, and derivatives of the input are usually absent, so $m = 0$.

The input $x(t)$ can be classified as either transient, periodic, or random. No general restrictions are placed on $x(t)$, although, for particular applications, bounds on amplitude and frequency content can usually be assumed. Solutions for the differential equation depend on the input classifications previously given. The step function is the most common transient input for instrumentation. Sinusoids are the most common periodic function to use because, through the Fourier-series expansion, any periodic function can be approximated by a sum of sinusoids. Band-limited white noise (uniform-power spectral content) is a common random input because one can test instrument performance for all frequencies in a particular bandwidth.

Transfer functions

The transfer function for a linear instrument or system mathematically expresses the relationship between the input signal and the output signal. If the transfer function is known, the output can be predicted for any input. The *operational transfer function* is the ratio $y(D)/x(D)$ as a function of the differential operator D:

$$\frac{y(D)}{x(D)} = \frac{b_m D^m + \cdots + b_1 D + b_0}{a_n D^n + \cdots + a_1 D + a_0} \tag{1.11}$$

This form of the transfer function is particularly useful for transient inputs. For linear systems, the output for transient inputs, which occur only once and do not repeat, is usually expressed directly as the function of time, $y(t)$, which is the solution to the differential equation.

The *frequency transfer function* for a linear system is obtained by substituting $j\omega$ for D in (1.11):

$$\frac{Y(j\omega)}{X(j\omega)} = \frac{b_m(j\omega)^m + \cdots + b_1(j\omega) + b_0}{a_n(j\omega)^n + \cdots + a_1(j\omega) + a_0} \tag{1.12}$$

where $j = +\sqrt{-1}$ and ω is the angular frequency in radians per second. The input is usually given as $x(t) = A_x \sin(\omega t)$ and all transients are assumed to have died out. The output $y(t)$ is a sinusoid with the same frequency, but the amplitude and phase depend on ω, that is, $y(t) = B(\omega) \sin[\omega t + \phi(\omega)]$. The frequency transfer function is a complex quantity having a magnitude that is the ratio of the magnitude of the output to the magnitude of the input and a phase angle ϕ which is the phase of the output $y(t)$ minus the phase of the input $x(t)$. The phase angle for most instruments is negative. The output of the system is not usually expressed as $y(t)$ for each frequency because we know that it is just a sinusoid with a particular magnitude and phase. Instead, the amplitude ratio and the phase angle are given separately as functions of frequency.

The dynamic characteristics of instruments are illustrated below by examples of zero-, first-, and second-order linear instruments for step and sinusoidal inputs.

Zero-order instrument

The simplest nontrivial form of the differential equation results if all the a's and b's are zero except a_0 and b_0:

$$a_0 y(t) = b_0 x(t) \qquad (1.13)$$

This is an algebraic equation, so

$$\frac{y(D)}{x(D)} = \frac{Y(j\omega)}{X(j\omega)} = \frac{b_0}{a_0} = K = \text{static sensitivity} \qquad (1.14)$$

where the single constant K replaces the two constants a_0 and b_0. This zero-order instrument has ideal dynamic performance because the output is proportional to the input for all frequencies and there is no amplitude or phase distortion.

A linear potentiometer is a good example of a zero-order instrument. Figure 1.9 shows that if the potentiometer has pure uniform resistance, the output voltage $y(t)$ is directly proportional to the input displacement $x(t)$, with no time delay for any frequency of input. In practice, at high frequencies, some parasitic capacitance and inductance might cause slight distortion. Also low-resistance circuits connected to the output can load this simple zero-order instrument.

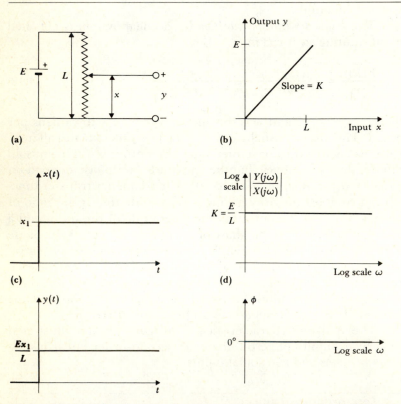

Figure 1.9 (a) A linear potentiometer, an example of a zero-order system. (b) Linear static characteristic for this system. (c) Step response is proportional to input. (d) Sinusoidal frequency response is constant with zero phase shift.

First-order instrument

If the instrument contains a single energy-storage element, then a first-order derivative of $y(t)$ is required in the differential equation:

$$a_1 \frac{dy(t)}{dt} + a_0 y(t) = b_0 x(t) \tag{1.15}$$

This equation can be written in terms of the differential operator D as

$$(\tau D + 1)y(t) = Kx(t) \tag{1.16}$$

where $K = b_0/a_0 =$ static sensitivity and $\tau = a_1/a_0 =$ time constant.

Exponential functions offer solutions to this equation if appropriate constants are chosen. The operational transfer function is

$$\frac{y(D)}{x(D)} = \frac{K}{1 + \tau D} \tag{1.17}$$

and the frequency transfer function is

$$\frac{Y(j\omega)}{X(j\omega)} = \frac{K}{1 + j\omega\tau} = \frac{K}{\sqrt{1 + \omega^2\tau^2}} \underline{/\phi = \arctan(-\omega\tau/1)} \tag{1.18}$$

The RC low-pass filter circuit shown in Fig. 1.10(a) is an example of a first-order instrument. The input is the voltage $x(t)$ and the output is the voltage $y(t)$ across the capacitor. The first-order differential equation for this circuit is $RC[dy(t)/dt] + y(t) = Kx(t)$. The static-sensitivity curve given in Fig. 1.10(b) shows that static outputs are equal to static inputs. This is verified by the differential equation because, for static conditions, $dy/dt = 0$. The step response in Fig. 1.10(c) is exponential with a time constant $\tau = RC$.

$$y(t) = K(1 - e^{-t/\tau}) \tag{1.19}$$

The smaller the time constant, the faster the output approaches the input. For sinusoids, (1.18) and Figure 1.10(d) show that the magnitude of the output decreases as frequency increases. For larger time constants, this decrease occurs at lower frequency.

When $\omega = 1/\tau$, the magnitude is $1/\sqrt{2}$ times smaller and the phase angle is $-45°$. This particular frequency ω is known as the *corner, cutoff,* or *break* frequency. Figure 1.10(d) verifies that this is a low-pass filter because low-frequency sinusoids are not severely attenuated, whereas high-frequency sinusoids produce very little output voltage. The ordinate of the frequency-response magnitude

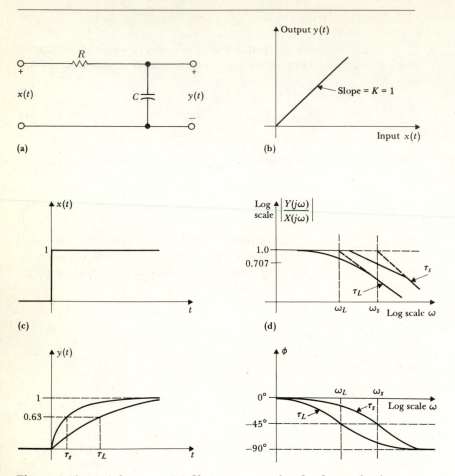

Figure 1.10 (a) A low-pass RC filter, an example of a first-order instrument. (b) Static sensitivity for constant inputs. (c) Step response for large time constants (τ_L) and small time constants (τ_S). (d) Sinusoidal frequency response for large and small time constants.

in Figure 1.10(d) is usually plotted on a log scale and may be given in units of decibels (dB), which are defined as dB $= 20\ \log_{10}$ $|Y(j\omega)/X(j\omega)|$. A mercury-in-glass thermometer is another example of a low-pass first-order instrument.

Example 1.2 A first-order low-pass instrument has a time constant of 20 ms. Find the maximum sinusoidal input frequency that will keep output error due to frequency response less than 5%. Find the phase angle at this frequency.

Answer

$$\frac{Y(j\omega)}{X(j\omega)} = \frac{K}{1 + j\omega\tau}$$

$$\left|\frac{K}{1 + j\omega\tau}\right| = \frac{K}{\sqrt{1 + \omega^2\tau^2}} = 0.95K$$

$$(\omega^2\tau^2 + 1)(0.95)^2 = 1$$

$$\omega^2 = \frac{1 - (0.95)^2}{(0.95)^2(20 \times 10^{-3})^2}$$

$$\omega = 16.4 \text{ rad/s}$$

$$f = \frac{\omega}{2\pi} = 2.62 \text{ Hz}$$

$$\phi = \tan^{-1}\left(\frac{-\omega\tau}{1}\right) = -18.2°$$

If R and C in Figure 1.10(a) are interchanged, the circuit becomes another first-order instrument, known as a *high-pass filter*. The static characteristic is zero for all values of input and the step response jumps immediately to the step voltage, but decays exponentially toward zero as time increases. Thus $y(t) = Ke^{-t/\tau}$. Low-frequency sinusoids are severely attenuated, whereas high-frequency sinusoids are little attenuated. The sinusoidal transfer function is $Y(j\omega)/X(j\omega) = j\omega\tau/(1 + j\omega\tau)$.

Second-order instrument

An instrument is second order if a second-order differential equation is required to describe its dynamic response.

$$a_2 \frac{d^2y(t)}{dt^2} + a_1 \frac{dy(t)}{dt} + a_0 y(t) = b_0 x(t) \tag{1.20}$$

Many medical instruments are second order or higher, and low pass. Furthermore, many higher-order instruments can be approximated by second-order characteristics if some simplifying assumptions can be made. The four constants in (1.20) can be reduced to three new ones that have physical significance:

$$\left[\frac{D^2}{\omega_n^2} + \frac{2\zeta D}{\omega_n} + 1\right] y(t) = Kx(t) \tag{1.21}$$

where

$$K = \frac{b_0}{a_0} = \text{static sensitivity, output units divided by input units}$$

$$\omega_n = \sqrt{\frac{a_0}{a_2}} = \text{undamped natural frequency, rad/s}$$

$$\zeta = \frac{a_1}{2\sqrt{a_0 a_2}} = \text{damping ratio, dimensionless}$$

Again exponential functions offer solutions to this equation, although the exact form of the solution varies as the damping ratio becomes greater than, equal to, or less than unity. The operational transfer function is

$$\frac{y(D)}{x(D)} = \frac{K}{\dfrac{D^2}{\omega_n^2} + \dfrac{2\zeta D}{\omega_n} + 1} \tag{1.22}$$

and the frequency transfer function is

$$\frac{Y(j\omega)}{X(j\omega)} = \frac{K}{(j\omega/\omega_n)^2 + (2\zeta j\omega/\omega_n) + 1}$$

$$= \frac{K}{\sqrt{[1 - (\omega/\omega_n)^2]^2 + 4\zeta^2\omega^2/\omega_n^2}} \bigg/ \phi = \arctan \frac{2\zeta}{\omega/\omega_n - \omega_n/\omega} \tag{1.23}$$

A mechanical force-measuring instrument illustrates the properties of a second-order instrument (Doebelin, 1975, p. 127). Mass, spring, and viscous-damping elements oppose the applied input force $x(t)$, and the output is the resulting displacement $y(t)$ of the movable mass attached to the spring [Figure 1.11(a)]. If the natural frequency of the spring is much greater than the frequency components in the input, the dynamic effect of the spring can be included by adding one-third of the spring's mass to the mass of the moving elements to obtain the equivalent total mass M. Hooke's law for linear springs is assumed, so the spring constant is K_s. Dry friction is neglected and perfect viscous friction is assumed, with constant B.

To eliminate gravitational force from the equation, we adjust the scale until $y = 0$ when $x = 0$. Then the sum of the forces equals the product of mass and acceleration.

$$x(t) - B\frac{dy(t)}{dt} - K_s y(t) = M\frac{d^2 y(t)}{dt^2} \tag{1.24}$$

This equation has the same form as (1.21) if the static sensitivity, undamped natural frequency, and damping ratio are defined in terms of K_s, B, and M, as follows:

$$K = 1/K_s \tag{1.25}$$

$$\omega_n = \sqrt{K_s/M} \tag{1.26}$$

$$\zeta = \frac{B}{2\sqrt{K_s M}} \tag{1.27}$$

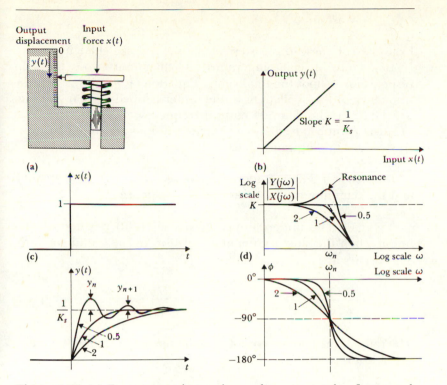

Figure 1.11 (a) Force-measuring spring scale, an example of a second-order instrument. (b) Static sensitivity. (c) Step response for overdamped case $\zeta = 2$, critically damped case $\zeta = 1$, underdamped case $\zeta = 0.5$. (d) Sinusoidal steady-state frequency response, $\zeta = 2$, $\zeta = 1$, $\zeta = 0.5$. [Part (a) modified from *Measurement Systems: Application and Design*, by E.O. Doebelin. Copyright © 1975 by McGraw-Hill, Inc. Used with permission of McGraw-Hill Book Co.]

The static response is $y(t) = Kx(t)$, as shown in Figure 1.11(b). The step response can have three forms, depending on the damping ratio. For a unit-step input, these three forms are:

Overdamped, $\zeta > 1$:

$$y(t) = -\frac{\zeta + \sqrt{\zeta^2 - 1}}{2\sqrt{\zeta^2 - 1}} K e^{(-\zeta + \sqrt{\zeta^2 - 1})\omega_n t}$$

$$+ \frac{\zeta - \sqrt{\zeta^2 - 1}}{2\sqrt{\zeta^2 - 1}} K e^{(-\zeta - \sqrt{\zeta^2 - 1})\omega_n t} + K \quad (1.28)$$

Critically damped, $\zeta = 1$:

$$y(t) = -(1 + \omega_n t)K e^{-\omega_n t} + K \quad (1.29)$$

Underdamped, $\zeta < 1$:

$$y(t) = -\frac{e^{-\zeta \omega_n t}}{\sqrt{1 - \zeta^2}} K \sin\left(\sqrt{1 - \zeta^2}\, \omega_n t + \phi\right) + K$$

$$\phi = \arcsin \sqrt{1 - \zeta^2} \tag{1.30}$$

Examples of these three step responses are sketched in Figure 1.11(c). Only for damping ratios less than unity does the step response overshoot the final value. Equation (1.30) shows that the frequency of the oscillations in the underdamped response in Figure 1.11(c) is the damped natural frequency $\omega_d = \omega_n\sqrt{1 - \zeta^2}$. A practical compromise between rapid rise time and minimal overshoot is a damping ratio of about 0.7.

Example 1.3 For underdamped second-order instruments, find the damping ratio ζ from the step response.

Answer The underdamped response (1.30) reaches a maximum when the sine argument equals $3\pi/2$, $7\pi/2$, and so forth. This occurs at

$$t_n = \frac{3\pi/2 - \phi}{\omega_n\sqrt{1 - \zeta^2}} \quad \text{and} \quad t_{n+1} = \frac{7\pi/2 - \phi}{\omega_n\sqrt{1 - \zeta^2}} \tag{1.31}$$

The ratio of the first overshoot y_n to the second overshoot y_{n+1} [Figure 1.11(c)] is

$$\frac{y_n}{y_{n+1}} = \frac{\left(\dfrac{K}{\sqrt{1 - \zeta^2}}\right)\left(\exp\left\{-\zeta\omega_n\left[\dfrac{(3\pi/2 - \phi)}{\omega_n\sqrt{1 - \zeta^2}}\right]\right\}\right)}{\left(\dfrac{K}{\sqrt{1 - \zeta^2}}\right)\left(\exp\left\{-\zeta\omega_n\left[\dfrac{(7\pi/2 - \phi)}{\omega_n\sqrt{1 - \zeta^2}}\right]\right\}\right)}$$

$$= \exp\left(\frac{2\pi\zeta}{\sqrt{1 - \zeta^2}}\right) \tag{1.32}$$

$$\ln\left(\frac{y_n}{y_{n+1}}\right) = \Lambda = \frac{2\pi\zeta}{\sqrt{1 - \zeta^2}}$$

where Λ is defined as *logarithmic decrement*. Solving for ζ yields

$$\zeta = \frac{\Lambda}{\sqrt{4\pi^2 + \Lambda^2}} \tag{1.33}$$

For sinusoidal steady-state responses, the frequency transfer function (1.23) and Figure 1.11(d) show that low-pass frequency responses result. The rate of decline in the amplitude frequency response is at twice the rate of decline for first-order instruments. Note that resonance phenomena can occur if the damping ratio is too small, and also that the output phase lag can be as much as 180°, whereas for single-order instruments, the maximum phase lag is 90°.

Figure 1.12 shows how an underdamped ($\zeta < 1$) second-order instrument can distort a blood-pressure waveform. A water-filled tube (catheter) is inserted into an artery and the other end is connected to a pressure transducer (details in Chapter 7). The length and internal diameter of the catheter determine the natural frequency ω_n and the damping ratio ζ. The input pressure wave in Figure 1.12(a) has frequency components as shown in Figure 7.4. All the catheters are 1 m long and catheter diameter is decreased from 5 to 0.3 mm. The instrument output in Figure 1.12(b) is undistorted because the very sharp resonant peak in the frequency response occurs at 352 Hz, where the frequency content of the signal is negligible.

As catheter diameter decreases [Figure 1.12(c) to (h)], the resonant frequency decreases and damping increases. Considerable distortion results because pressure-waveform frequencies near resonance are "amplified" and higher frequencies are attenuated. The low-frequency oscillations in Figure 1.12 (f) are sometimes erroneously attributed to the so-called catheter-whip phenomena (Section 7.7). Many other examples of second-order instruments are examined in this book.

Time delay

Instrument elements that give an output that is exactly the same as the input, except that it is delayed in time by τ_d, are defined as *time-delay elements*. The mathematical expression for these elements is

$$y(t) = Kx(t - \tau_d), \qquad t > \tau_d \tag{1.34}$$

These elements may also be called analog delay lines, transport lags, or dead times. Although first-order and second-order instruments have negative phase angles that imply time delays, the phase angle varies with frequency, so the delay is not constant for all frequencies. For time delays, Figure 1.13 gives the obvious static characteristic, the step response specified by (1.34), and the sinusoidal frequency response for magnitude and phase is

$$\frac{Y(j\omega)}{X(j\omega)} = Ke^{-j\omega\tau_d} \tag{1.35}$$

Time delays are present in transmission lines (electric, mechanical, hydraulic, and pneumatic), magnetic tape recorders, and some digital signal-processing schemes. Usually these time delays are to be avoided, especially in instruments or systems that involve feedback, because undesired oscillations may result.

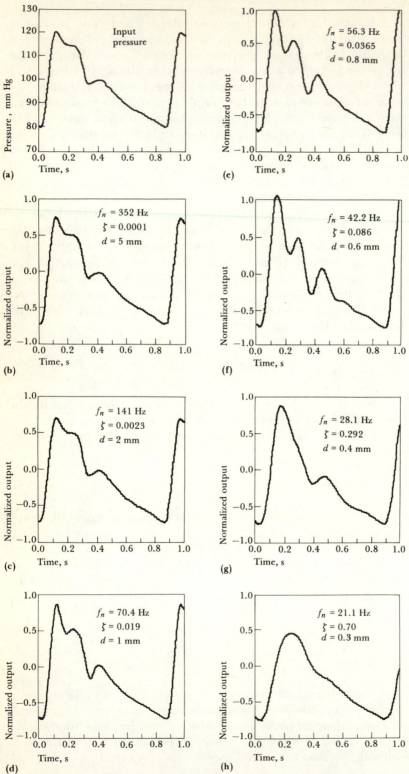

(a) — Input pressure

(b) $f_n = 352$ Hz, $\zeta = 0.0001$, $d = 5$ mm

(c) $f_n = 141$ Hz, $\zeta = 0.0023$, $d = 2$ mm

(d) $f_n = 70.4$ Hz, $\zeta = 0.019$, $d = 1$ mm

(e) $f_n = 56.3$ Hz, $\zeta = 0.0365$, $d = 0.8$ mm

(f) $f_n = 42.2$ Hz, $\zeta = 0.086$, $d = 0.6$ mm

(g) $f_n = 28.1$ Hz, $\zeta = 0.292$, $d = 0.4$ mm

(h) $f_n = 21.1$ Hz, $\zeta = 0.70$, $d = 0.3$ mm

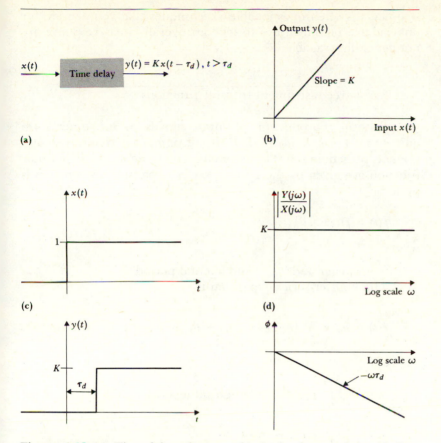

Figure 1.13 (a) Time-delay element. (b) Static characteristic. (c) Step response. (d) Sinusoidal frequency response.

Dynamic nonlinearities and errors

All the static nonlinearities discussed in Section 1.8 can also affect dynamic responses; the severity and even the type of nonlinearity may be frequency-dependent. In most useful instruments, the nonlinear effects are small and contribute only to the linearity specification defined in Section 1.7. Unfortunately, mathematical solutions for differential equations containing nonlinearities are complex even when they are obtainable with digital-computer algorithms. The usefulness of outputs from highly nonlinear in-

◀ **Figure 1.12** Blood-pressure waveforms disturbed by a second-order instrument that has progressively [(b) through (h)] decreasing frequency response. (a) Input blood-pressure waveform. (b) through (h) Instrument output for 100-cm-long catheters with internal diameters of 5 to 0.3 mm. Computer simulation of an ideal second-order instrument using backward Euler method of solution.

struments is often questionable. Techniques that compensate for unavoidable nonlinearities to give an overall linear response are not generally available.

Error-free instrument transfer functions

Faithful reproduction of input signals by instruments requires that $Y(j\omega)/X(j\omega) = K/\underline{0°}$ for all significant frequency components present in $x(t)$. The frequency components of any periodic function are given by the Fourier-series expansion. A function is periodic if

$$f(t) = f(t \pm nT) \tag{1.36}$$

where

n = integer and T = fundamental period.
The Fourier-series expansion is

$$f(t) = a_0 + \sum_{n=1}^{\infty} [a_n \cos (n\omega_0 t) + b_n \sin (n\omega_0 t)] \tag{1.37}$$

where

$$a_0 = \frac{1}{T} \int_0^T f(t)\ dt = \text{average value} \tag{1.38}$$

$$a_n = \frac{2}{T} \int_0^T f(t) \cos (n\omega_0 t)\ dt \tag{1.39}$$

$$b_n = \frac{2}{T} \int_0^T f(t) \sin (n\omega_0 t)\ dt \tag{1.40}$$

$$\omega_0 = 2\pi f_0 = \frac{2\pi}{T}$$

The Fourier series for a given periodic function is determined by evaluating the real coefficients a_n and b_n. This is done by inserting $f(t)$ in Equations (1.38) through (1.40) and performing the integrations indicated. There are several other equivalent ways to express the Fourier-series expansion, using only sine or only cosine terms (computing magnitude and phase instead of a_n and b_n), or using exponential functions (Kaplan, 1952). For periodic signals, the magnitude of the Fourier-series coefficients for the input signal determines the instrument's frequency-response needs.

Example 1.4 Find the Fourier series for the square-wave voltage in Figure 1.14.

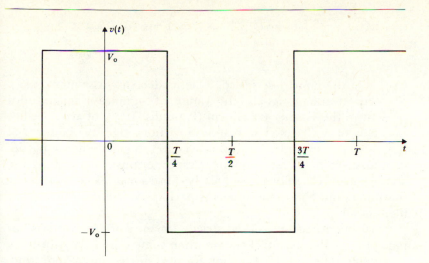

Figure 1.14 Example 1.4: Square-wave voltage for Fourier-series computation.

Answer

$$a_0 = 0$$

$$a_1 = \frac{2}{T} \left(V_o \int_0^{T/4} \cos(\omega_0 t)\, dt - V_o \int_{T/4}^{3T/4} \cos(\omega_0 t)\, dt \right.$$

$$\left. + V_o \int_{3T/4}^T \cos(\omega_0 t)\, dt \right)$$

$$= \frac{2V_o}{\omega_0 T} \left[\sin \frac{\omega_0 T}{4} - \left(\sin \frac{3\omega_0 T}{4} - \sin \frac{\omega_0 T}{4} \right) \right.$$

$$\left. + \left(\sin \omega_0 T - \sin \frac{3\omega_0 T}{4} \right) \right]$$

$$= \frac{V_o}{\pi} (1 + 2 + 1) = \frac{4V_o}{\pi} \qquad \text{since } \omega_0 T = 2\pi$$

Similarly,

$$a_n = +\frac{4V_o}{n\pi} \qquad \text{for } n = 1, 5, 9 \ldots$$

$$= -\frac{4V_o}{n\pi} \qquad \text{for } n = 3, 7, 11 \ldots$$

$$= 0 \qquad \text{for } n = 2, 4, 6 \ldots$$

$$b_n = 0 \qquad \text{all } n$$

Therefore the Fourier series is

$$v(t) = \frac{4V_0}{\pi} [\cos (\omega_0 t) - \tfrac{1}{3} \cos (3\omega_0 t) + \tfrac{1}{5} \cos (5\omega_0 t)$$

$$- \tfrac{1}{7} \cos (7\omega_0 t) + \cdots]$$

Note that the Fourier-series coefficients decrease as n increases.

For transient signals, the range of significant magnitudes present in the Fourier transform (Papoulis, 1962) of $x(t)$ specifies the necessary frequency response. Knowledge of biomedical signal-frequency content is thus crucial to rational design of particular instruments. The frequency response must be adequate for abnormal as well as normal signals, because a diagnostic instrument that filters out abnormal signals is perhaps worse than no instrument at all.

If the instrument is used strictly for measurement and is not part of a feedback-control system, then some time delay is usually acceptable. The transfer function for undistorted signal reproduction with time delay then becomes $Y(j\omega)/X(j\omega) = K/\underline{-\omega\tau_d}$. The transient response and the frequency response are shown in Figure 1.13. Our previous study of time-delay elements shows that the output magnitude is K times the input magnitude for all frequencies and the phase lag increases linearly with frequency.

The transfer-function requirements concern the *overall* instrument transfer function. The overall transfer function of linear elements connected in series is the product of the transfer functions for the individual elements. Many combinations of nonlinear elements can produce the overall linear transfer function required. Various forms of modulation and demodulation are used, and unavoidable transducer nonlinearities can sometimes be compensated for by other instrument elements.

1.10 Design criteria

As shown, many factors affect the design of biomedical instruments. The factors that impose constraints on the design are of course different for each type of instrument. However, some of the general requirements can be categorized into signal, environmental, medical, and economic factors. Figure 1.15 shows how these factors are incorporated into the initial design and development of an instrument (adapted from Cobbold, 1974, p. 54). The many steps required for commercial product development are not shown.

Note that the type of transducer selected usually stipulates the signal-processing equipment needed, so an instrument specification includes more than just deciding what type of transducer to use. To obtain a final design, some compromises in specifications are usually required. Actual tests on a prototype are always needed before final design decisions can be made. Often changes in per-

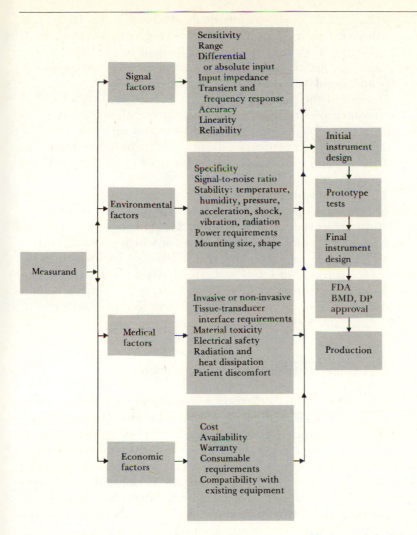

Figure 1.15 Design process for medical instruments. Choice and design of instruments are affected by signal factors, and also by environmental, medical, and economic factors. (Revised from *Transducers for Biomedical Measurements: Application and Design*, by R.S.C. Cobbold. Copyright © 1974, John Wiley and Sons, Inc. Used by permission of John Wiley and Sons, Inc.)

formance and interaction of the elements in a complex instrument require design modifications. Frequently good designs are the result of many compromises throughout the development of the instrument. In Chapter 2, we shall study basic methods of transducing biomedical quantities to ensure that all transducer design alternatives are carefully evaluated.

Anyone contemplating the design of a new medical instrument should examine the Medical Device Amendments of 1976

(Public Law 94-295) which amends the Federal Food, Drug, and Cosmetic Act to provide for the safety and effectiveness of medical devices intended for human use. The Bureau of Medical Devices and Diagnostic Products of the Food and Drug Administration will classify and regulate medical devices (Miller, 1977).

Devices in the lowest classification—*class I, general controls*—would require registration of manufacturers, adherence to good manufacturing procedures, record keeping and reporting; restriction of sale to certain professionals; possible banning; and notification of risks, along with repair, replacement, or refund of purchase price.

The next classification—*class II, performance standard*—would call for the development of standards to provide assurance of safety and effectiveness. The highest classification—*class III, premarket approval*—would apply to devices for which general controls and performance standards are not shown sufficient to provide reasonable assurance of safety and effectiveness for devices used in supporting or sustaining human life and preventing impairment of human health. It would also apply to devices that present a potential unreasonable risk of illness or injury.

1.11 Generalized instrument specifications

This final section of Chapter 1 is an attempt to set forth most of the technical specifications that should be given by instrument manufacturers and designers of new instruments. Of course, some specifications are not applicable to particular instruments and some instruments may need additional specialized specifications. The purpose of the following list is to facilitate evaluation of the completeness of specifications given by manufacturers and designers of new instruments. For convenience, the list is subdivided into the following categories: input and transducer specifications, signal-processing specifications, output specifications, errors and reliability, and physical and miscellaneous specifications.

Input and transducer specifications

1 Measurand A physical quantity, property, or condition that is measured. Directional specificity or other form of selectivity may be implicit.

2 Differential or absolute The input quantity may be the difference between two quantities or it may be measured with respect to an absolute reference.

3 Input common-mode rejection (Section 3.4) This is defined as differential gain divided by common-mode gain. The common-mode rejection ratio should be given for differential-input devices at a specified frequency or as a function of frequency for up to a given source-impedance imbalance.

4 Operating ranges The fixed or adjustable ranges of inputs for specifications operation. Adjustable transducers may require change of mechanical parts.

5 Overload ranges The range of inputs that can be tolerated without damage to the instrument.

6 Overload recovery time Time required for the device to return to the linear operating region following an overload.

7 Sensitivity The overall instrument output per unit input as a function of excitation for modulating transducers.

8 Input impedance Generalized input impedance is the ratio of the effort-input variable (voltage, force, pressure) to the flow-input variable (current, velocity, flow).

9 Transducer principle The principle of operation utilized by the transducer, e.g., resistive, piezoelectric, ultrasonic. May be expressed as a transfer function.

10 Transient response time The time constant may be given even if it is not a first-order instrument. The natural or resonant frequency may be given if it is a second- or higher-order instrument. Degree of damping or ringing for step inputs should be given.

11 Frequency response The magnitude and phase of the sinusoidal steady-state frequency response including the magnitude of the input.

12 Modulating transducer excitation The acceptable magnitude and frequency of modulating transducer power requirements. Usually an electrical quantity.

13 Isolation Electrical isolation or other methods of electric-shock protection (see Chapter 13) for instrument components that contact patients.

14 Physical dimensions The size and method of coupling the transducer primary sensing element to the medium that contains the measurand are often crucial parameters.

15 Special handling Some transducers are easily damaged if tapped against solid objects (large acceleration forces) and others may corrode if extended contact with tissue or body fluids is necessary.

Signal-processing specifications

1 Processing method The methods and theory of operation should be explained. The electronic circuitry and/or digital-signal analysis should be described in detail. May be expressed as a transfer function.

2 Compensation Nonlinear compensation of undesirable transducer characteristics may be necessary.

3 Zero suppression dc-amplifier offset adjustment to compensate for various sources of drift.

4 Filtering Electronic restrictions on the processor frequency response.

5 Interfacing Digital interfacing capability.

Output specifications

1 Output quantity Usually a voltage or current that drives a display device that may be a part of the instrument. Analog or digital.

2 Output range The range of linear output swing and the level of output saturation.

3 Output power Maximum average and/or peak output power that can be delivered to a load with a specified generalized impedance.

4 Output impedance Generalized output-effort variable divided by the output-flow variable.

5 Writing speed Some measure of the frequency response of the display device.

6 Output timing For noninstantaneous outputs: the time delay, averaging time interval, sampling, and/or display interval.

Errors and reliability

1 Overall accuracy The maximum difference between the measured and the true quantity without regard to the source of error.

2 Repeatability Overall variation of the output for constant input versus time.

3 Nonlinearity Deviation from linear operation that may be subdivided according to the type of nonlinearity: hysteresis, dead zone, threshold, and so forth.

4 Interfering signal susceptibility Sensitivity of the instrument to explicitly controlled interfering and modifying inputs.

5 Noise Maximum peak-to-peak electrical or nonelectrical noise referred to the input.

6 Signal-to-noise ratio The ratio of the value of the signal (peak or rms) to that of the noise (peak or rms, respectively) given as a fraction (SNR = $1000:1$, $100:1$, and so forth) in decibels (SNR (dB) = $20 \log_{10}$ [SNR (fraction)]) and usually dependent on the signal frequency and the noise bandwidth.

7 Stability Drift in the instrument output as a function of time, temperature, humidity, acceleration, shock, and vibration. Warm-up time.

8 Cycling life The minimum number of partial or complete output variations before the specifications are significantly altered.

9 Operating life The minimum continuous or intermittent operating time before the specifications are significantly altered.

10 Storage life The minimum time of exposure to specified environmental conditions before the specifications are significantly altered.

11 Reliability The reliability rating—mean time between failures (MTBF)—for individual components and the entire device are desirable, especially for implanted medical devices.

Physical and miscellaneous specifications

1 Power requirements Line voltage, line-voltage tolerance, frequency range, wattage consumed as a function of the input (if significant), battery voltage, battery capacity.

2 Circuit protection Fuses, diodes, isolation.

3 Codes and regulations UL-listed, FDA class and regulations.

4 Environmental requirements Usually different for operation and storage: temperature, humidity, altitudes, acceleration, radiation, and corrosive substances.

5 Mechanical and electrical connections Compatibility with other instruments; mechanical alignment.

6 Mounting Rack or bench-cabinet mounting, special mounting for portable use, and shock mounting.

7 Dimensions Height, width, and depth.

8 Weight Pounds and kilograms.

9 Construction materials Resistance to corrosion, nonglaze finishes.

10 Accessories and options Restrictions on multiple accessories.

11 Consumables Consumable-supplies requirements: paper, ultrasonic gel, disposable electrodes, electrode paste, chemicals.

12 Delivery Time, conditions, penalties, and shipping.

13 Warranty Time period and parts and/or labor.

14 Cost Bidding, quantity discounts, and minimum orders.

15 Service and parts Maintenance contracts, response time, and parts inventory.

Problems

1.1 The method of opposing input correction for an interfering input is illustrated in Figure 1.4(c). Construct a generalized block diagram that shows how the method of opposing inputs can be used to correct for an unavoidable *modifying* input that affects both G_i and G_d.

1.2 Find the independent nonlinearity as defined in Figure 1.7(b) for the following set of inputs and outputs from a nearly linear system. Instrument was designed for output = 2 × input. Full scale is 20.

Inputs	0.50	1.50	2.00	5.00	10.00
Outputs	0.90	3.05	4.00	9.90	20.50

1.3 Plot the output-versus-input static characteristic for the following combinations of two nonlinearities.
a Saturation and hysteresis
b Dead zone and hysteresis
c Breakdown and hysteresis

1.4 Derive the operational transfer function and the sinusoidal transfer function for an RC high-pass filter. Plot the step response and the complete frequency response (magnitude and phase).

1.5 A first-order low-pass instrument must measure hummingbird wing displacements (assume sinusoidal) with frequency content up to 100 Hz with an amplitude inaccuracy of less than 5%. What is the maximum allowable time constant for the instrument? What is the phase angle at 50 and 100 Hz?

1.6 A mercury thermometer has a cylindrical capillary tube with an internal diameter of 0.2 mm. If the thermometer and bulb volume are not affected by temperature, what volume must the bulb have if a sensitivity of 2 mm/°C is to be obtained? Assume operation near 24°C. Assume that the stem volume is negligible compared with the bulb internal volume. Differential expansion coefficient of Hg = 1.82×10^{-4} ml/(ml · °C).

1.7 Find the Fourier-series expansion for a 2 V p–p triangle waveform at 2 kHz. Let the minimum waveform value be 0 V. Assume that the positive peak is 2 V at $t = 0$.

1.8 For the spring scale in Fig. 1.11(a), find the transfer function when the mass is negligible.

1.9 Find the time constant from the following differential equation, given that x is the input, y is the output, and a through h are constants.

$$a \frac{dy}{dt} + bx + c + hy = e \frac{dy}{dt} + fx + g$$

1.10 A differential-capacitance displacement transducer consists of two variable capacitors with one plate in common. Displacement causes one capacitance to increase ($C + \Delta C$) and the other capacitance to decrease ($C - \Delta C$) by an equal amount. There are two ways to place these capacitors in an ac (1.59 kHz) bridge circuit (replace inductors with capacitors in Figure 1.6). Given that $C = 1000$ pF, find the value of the two equal resistors needed to make the impedances of all bridge arms equal for $\Delta C = 0$. Find and compare the sensitivities ($V_o/\Delta C$) of these two circuits.

1.11 A low-pass first-order instrument has a time constant of 20 ms. Find the frequency, in hertz, of the input at which the output will be 93% of the dc output. Find the phase angle at this frequency.

1.12 A second-order instrument has a damping ratio of 0.4 and an undamped natural frequency of 85 Hz. Sketch the step response and give numerical values for the amplitude and time of the first two maxima. Assume that the input goes from 0 to 1 and that the static sensitivity is 10.

1.13 Consider an underdamped second-order system with step response as shown in Figure 1.11(c). A different way to define logarithmic decrement is

$$\Gamma = \ln \frac{y_n}{y_{n+1}}$$

Here n refers not to the number of positive peaks shown in Figure 1.11(c), but to both positive and negative peaks. That is, n increases by 1 for each half-cycle. Derive an equation for the damping ratio ζ in terms of this different definition of logarithmic decrement.

References

Anonymous, *Dorland's illustrated medical dictionary*. 25th ed. Philadelphia: Saunders, 1974.

Anonymous, *IEEE standard dictionary of electrical and electronic terms*. New York: Wiley, 1972.

Anonymous, *Introduction to transducers for instrumentation*. Oxnard, CA: Statham Instruments, 1966.

Atherton, D.P., *Nonlinear control engineering*. New York: Van Nostrand, 1975.

Cobbold, R.S.C., *Transducers for biomedical measurements: Principles and applications*. New York: Wiley, 1974.

Cook, N.H., and E. Rabinowicz, *Physical measurement and analysis*. Reading, MA: Addison-Wesley, 1963.

Cromwell, L., F.J. Weibell, E.A. Pfeiffer, and L.B. Usselmann, *Biomedical instrumentation and measurements*. Englewood Cliffs, NJ: Prentice-Hall, 1973.

Cromwell, L., M. Arditti, F.J. Weibell, E.A. Pfeiffer, B. Steele, and J. Labok, *Medical instrumentation for health care*. Englewood Cliffs, NJ: Prentice-Hall, 1976.

Doebelin, E.O., *System dynamics: Modeling and response*. Columbus, OH: Merrill, 1972.

Doebelin, E.O., *Measurement systems: Application and design*, 2nd ed. New York: McGraw-Hill, 1975.

Draper, C.S., W. McKay, and S. Lees, *Instrument engineering.* Vol. III: *Applications of the engineering method.* Part 1, "Measurement systems." New York: McGraw-Hill, 1955.

Geddes, L.A., and L.E. Baker, *Principles of applied biomedical instrumentation,* 2nd ed. New York: Wiley, 1975.

Gibson, J.E., *Nonlinear automatic control.* New York: McGraw-Hill, 1963.

Harvey, G.F. (ed.) *Transducer compendium,* 2nd ed. New York: Plenum, 1969.

Herceg, E.E., *Handbook of measurement and control.* Pennsauken, NJ: Schaevitz Engineering, 1972.

Jacobson, B., and J.G. Webster, *Medicine and clinical engineering.* Englewood Cliffs, NJ: Prentice-Hall, 1977.

Kaplan, W., *Advanced calculus.* Reading, MA: Addison-Wesley, 1952.

Kuo, B., *Automatic control systems,* 3rd ed. Englewood Cliffs, NJ: Prentice-Hall, 1975.

Lion, K.S., *Elements of electrical and electronic instrumentation.* New York: McGraw-Hill, 1975.

Miller, M.J., "How medical-device legislation affects healthcare professionals." In C.A. Caceres (ed.), *The practice of clinical engineering.* New York: Academic, 1977.

Papoulis, A., *The Fourier integral and its applications.* New York: McGraw-Hill, 1962.

Ray, C.D. (ed.) *Medical engineering.* Chicago: Year Book, 1974.

Schenck, H., *Theories of engineering experimentation.* New York: McGraw-Hill, 1968.

Stein, P. K., *Measurement engineering.* Vol. I: *Basic principles.* Tempe, AZ: Stein Engineering Services, 1962.

Thomas, H.E., *Handbook of biomedical instrumentation and measurement.* Reston, VA: Reston, 1974.

Chapter two

Basic transducers and principles

Robert A. Peura and John G. Webster

Since the beginnings of medicine, physicians have been using their senses to determine various physical parameters of the patient, i.e., position of body organs, temperature of the body, color of the skin, etc. In an attempt to quantify the measurement of these and additional parameters from the living system, we have seen an increased application of technology to the areas of clinical and biomedical research. In many cases instruments were developed originally for the physical sciences and then adapted for specific medical applications.

This chapter deals with basic mechanisms and principles of transducers used in a number of medical instruments. A *transducer* is a device that converts energy from one form to another. An electrical output from the transducer is normally desirable because of the advantages it gives in further signal processing. Material in this chapter shows that there are many methods used to convert physiological events to electrical signals. Dimensional changes may be measured by variations in resistance, inductance, capacitance, and piezoelectric effect. Thermistors and thermocouples are employed to measure body temperatures. Electromagnetic-radiation transducers include thermal and photon detectors. In our discussion of the design of medical instruments in the following chapters, we shall use the principles described in this chapter.

2.1 Displacement measurements

The physician and biomedical researcher are interested in measuring the size, shape, and position of the organs and tissues of the body. Variations in these parameters are important in discriminating normal from abnormal function. Displacement transducers can be used in both direct and indirect systems of measurement. Direct measurements of displacement are used to determine the change in diameter of blood vessels and the changes in volume and shape of cardiac chambers.

Measurements of indirect displacement are used to quantify movements of liquids through heart valves. An example is the

49

movement of a microphone diaphragm that detects heart murmurs.

The following types of displacement-sensitive measurement methods are described in this section: resistive, inductive, capacitive, and piezoelectric.

2.2 Resistive transducers

Potentiometers

Figure 2.1 shows three types of potentiometric devices for measuring displacement. The potentiometer shown in Figure 2.1(a) measures translational displacements from 2 to 500 mm. Rotational displacements ranging from 10° to more than 50° are detected as shown in Figure 2.1(b) and (c). The resistance elements (composed of wire-wound, carbon-film, metal-film, conducting-plastic, or ceramic material) may be excited by either dc or ac voltages. These potentiometers produce a linear output (within 0.01% of full scale) as a function of displacement, provided that the potentiometer is not electrically loaded.

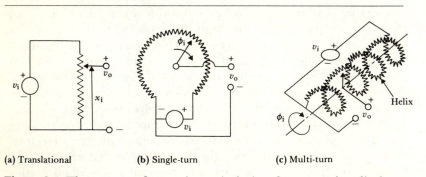

(a) Translational   (b) Single-turn   (c) Multi-turn

Figure 2.1 Three types of potentiometric devices for measuring displacements. (a) Translational. (b) Single-turn. (c) Multi-turn. (From *Measurement Systems: Application and Design*, by E.O. Doebelin. Copyright © 1975 by McGraw-Hill, Inc. Used with permission of McGraw-Hill Book Co.)

The resolution of these potentiometers is a function of the construction. A continuous stepless conversion of resistance is possible for low-resistance values up to 10 Ω by utilizing a straight piece of wire. For greater variations in resistance, from several ohms to several megohms, the resistance wire is wound on a mandrel or cord. The variation in resistance is thereby not continuous, but rather stepwise, because the wiper moves from one turn of wire to the next. The fundamental limitation of the resolution is a function of the wire spacing, which may be as small as 20 μm. The frictional and inertial components of these potentiometers should be low in order to minimize dynamic distortion of the system.

Strain gages

When a fine wire (25 μm) is strained within its elastic limit, the wire's resistance changes because of changes in the diameter, length, and resistivity. The resulting strain gages may be used to measure extremely small displacements, on the order of nanometers. The following derivation shows how each of these parameters influences the resistance change. The basic equation for the resistance R of a wire with resistivity ρ (ohms · meter), length L (meters), and cross-sectional area A (meters squared) is given by

$$R = \frac{\rho L}{A} \tag{2.1}$$

The differential change in R is found by taking the differential

$$dR = \frac{\rho \, dL}{A} - \rho A^{-2} L \, dA + L \frac{d\rho}{A} \tag{2.2}$$

We shall modify this expression so that it represents finite changes in the parameters and is also a function of standard mechanical coefficients. Thus dividing members of (2.2) by corresponding members of (2.1) and introducing incremental values gives

$$\frac{\Delta R}{R} = \frac{\Delta L}{L} - \frac{\Delta A}{A} + \frac{\Delta \rho}{\rho} \tag{2.3}$$

Poisson's ratio μ relates the change in diameter ΔD to the change in length, $\Delta D/D = - \mu \, \Delta L/L$. When this is substituted into the center term of (2.3), we get the following:

$$\frac{\Delta R}{R} = \underbrace{(1 + 2\mu) \frac{\Delta L}{L}}_{\substack{\text{Dimensional} \\ \text{effect}}} + \underbrace{\frac{\Delta \rho}{\rho}}_{\substack{\text{Piezoresistive} \\ \text{effect}}} \tag{2.4}$$

Note that the change in resistance is a function of changes in dimension—length ($\Delta L/L$) and area ($2\mu \, \Delta L/L$)—plus the change in resistivity due to strain-induced changes in the lattice structure of the material, $\Delta \rho/\rho$. The gage factor G, found by dividing (2.4) by $\Delta L/L$, is useful in comparing various strain-gage materials.

$$G = \frac{\Delta R/R}{\Delta L/L} = (1 + 2\mu) + \frac{\Delta \rho/\rho}{\Delta L/L} \tag{2.5}$$

Table 2.1 gives the gage factors and temperature coefficient of resistivity of various strain-gage materials. Note that the gage factor for semiconductor materials is approximately 50 to 70 times that of the metals. Also note that the gage factor for metals is primarily a function of dimensional effects. For most metals, $\mu = 0.3$ and thus G is at least 1.6; whereas, for semiconductors, the piezoresistive effect is dominant. The desirable feature of higher gage factors for semiconductor devices is offset by their greater resistivity-temperature coefficient.

Material	Composition (%)	Gage factor	Temperature coefficient of resistivity ($°C^{-1} - 10^{-5}$)
Constantan (advance)	Ni_{45}, Cu_{55}	2.1	± 2
Isoelastic	Ni_{36}, Cr_8 (Mn, Si, Mo)$_4$ Fe$_{52}$	3.52 to 3.6	$+17$
Karma	Ni_{74}, Cr_{20}, Fe_3 Cu$_3$	2.1	$+2$
Manganin	Cu_{84}, Mn_{12}, Ni_4	0.3 to 0.47	± 2
Alloy 479	Pt_{92}, W_8	3.6 to 4.4	$+24$
Nickel	Pure	-12 to -20	670
Nichrome V	Ni_{80}, Cr_{20}	2.1 to 2.63	10
Silicon	(p type)	100 to 170	70 to 700
Silicon	(n type)	-100 to -140	70 to 700
Germanium	(p type)	102	
Germanium	(n type)	-150	

Table 2.1 Properties of strain-gage materials (from R.S.C. Cobbold, *Transducers for biomedical measurements,* 1974, Wiley; used with permission of John Wiley and Sons, Inc., New York)

Designs for instruments that use semiconductor materials must incorporate temperature compensation.

Strain gages can be classified as either unbonded or bonded. An unbonded strain-gage unit is shown in Figure 2.2(a). The four sets of strain-sensitive wires are connected to form a Wheatstone bridge, as shown in Figure 2.2(b). These wires are mounted under stress between the frame F and the movable member M such that preload is greater than any expected external compressive load. This is necessary to avoid putting the wires in compression. This type of transducer may be used for rotational movements of M around pivot point P if the frame has a circular hole. A rectangular hole in the frame is used for translational measurements.

A bonded strain-gage element, consisting of a metallic wire, etched foil, vacuum-deposited film, or semiconductor bar, is cemented to the strained surface. Figure 2.3 shows typical bonded strain gages. The deviation from linearity is approximately 1%. One method of temperature compensation for the natural temperature sensitivity of bonded strain gages involves use of a second

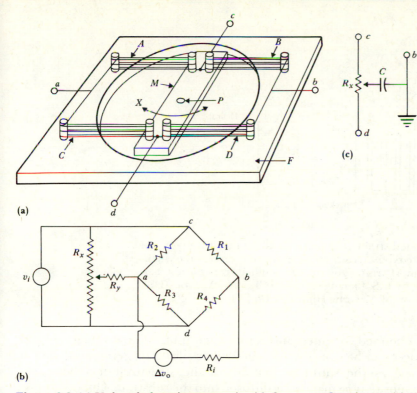

(a)

(b)

(c)

Figure 2.2 (a) Unbonded strain-gage unit with four sets of strain-sensitive wires (A, B, C, and D) mounted between a frame (F) and movable member (M). M may rotate about P in the hole in F to detect rotational motion. Translational motion is detected with a rectangular hole. (Modified from *Instrumentation in Scientific Research*, by K.S. Lion. Copyright © 1959 by McGraw-Hill, Inc. Used with permission of McGraw-Hill Book Co.) (b) Wheatstone bridge with four active elements. $R_1 = B$, $R_2 = A$, $R_3 = D$, and $R_4 = C$ when the unbonded strain gage is connected for translational motion. Resistor R_y and potentiometer R_x are used to initially balance the bridge. v_i is the applied voltage and Δv_o is the output voltage on a voltmeter or similar device with an internal resistance of R_i. (c) Balance circuit for ac-bridge operation.

strain gage as a dummy element that is also exposed to the temperature variation, but not to strain. When possible, the four-arm bridge shown in Figure 2.2 should be used, because it not only provides temperature compensation but also yields four times greater output if all four arms contain active gages.

Strain-gage technology advanced in the 1960s with the introduction of the semiconductor strain-gage element, which has the advantage of having a high gage factor, as shown in Table 2.1. However, it is more temperature-sensitive and inherently more nonlinear than metal strain gages because the piezoresistive effect varies with strain. Semiconductor elements can be used as bonded,

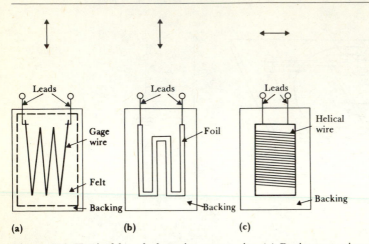

Figure 2.3 Typical bonded strain-gage units. (a) Resistance-wire type. (b) Foil type. (c) Helical-wire type. Arrows above units show direction of maximum sensitivity to strain. [Parts (a) and (b) are modified from *Instrumentation in Scientific Research*, by K.S. Lion. Copyright © 1959 by McGraw-Hill, Inc. Used with permission of McGraw-Hill Book Co.]

unbonded, or integrated strain-gage units. These integrated devices can be constructed using either silicon or germanium p or n type as the substrate that forms the structural member. The opposite-type material is diffused into the substrate. Opposite signs for the gage factor result for n- and p-type substrate gages. A large gage factor can be attained with lightly doped material. Figure 2.4 shows typical semiconductor strain-gage units.

The integrated-type transducer has an advantage in that a pressure transducer can be fabricated by using a silicon substrate for the structural member of the diaphragm. The gages are diffused directly onto the diaphragm. When pressure is applied to the diaphragm, a radial stress component occurs at the edge. The sign of this component is opposite to that of the tangential stress component near the center. The placement of the eight diffused strain-gage units shown in Figure 2.4(c) gives high sensitivity and good temperature compensation (Cobbold, 1974).

Elastic-resistance strain gages are extensively used in biomedical applications, especially in cardiovascular and respiratory dimensional and plethysmographic (volume-measuring) determinations. These systems normally consist of a narrow silicone-rubber tube (0.5 mm ID, 2 mm OD) from 3 to 25 cm long filled with mercury or with an electrolyte or conductive paste. The ends of the tube are sealed with electrodes (amalgamated copper, silver, or platinum). As the tube stretches, the diameter of the tube decreases and the length increases, causing the resistance to increase. The resistance per unit length of typical gages is approximately 0.02–2 Ω/cm. These units measure much higher displacements than other gages.

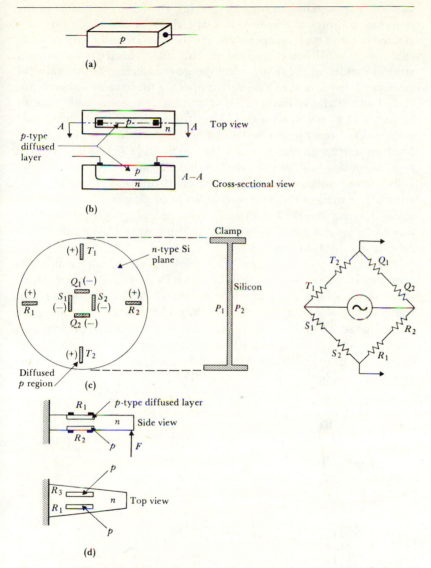

Figure 2.4 Typical semiconductor strain-gage units. (a) Unbonded, uniformly doped. (b) Diffused p-type gage. (c) Integrated pressure transducer. (d) Integrated cantilever-beam force transducer. (From *Transducers for Medical Measurements: Application and Design,* by R.S.C. Cobbold. Copyright © 1974, John Wiley and Sons, Inc. Reprinted by permission of John Wiley and Sons, Inc.)

The elastic strain gage is linear within 1% for 10% of maximum extension. As the extension is increased to 30% of maximum, the nonlinearity reaches 4% of full scale. The initial nonlinearity (dead band) is ascribed to slackness of the unit. Long-term creep is a property of the rubber tubing. This is not a problem for dynamic measurements.

Operational problems include: maintaining a good contact

between the mercury and the electrodes, ensuring continuity of the mercury column, and controlling the drift in resistance due to a relatively large gage temperature coefficient. In addition, accurate calibration is difficult because of the mass-elasticity and stress-strain relations of the tissue–strain-gage complex. The low value of resistance requires more power to operate these strain-gage units.

Lawton and Collins (1959) determined the static and dynamic response of elastic strain gages. They found that the amplitude and phase were constant up to 10 Hz. Significant distortion occurred for frequencies greater than 30 Hz. Cobbold (1974) indicated that a problem not fully appreciated is that the gage does not distend fully during pulsations when diameter of the vessel is being measured. The mass of the gage and its finite mechanical resistance can cause it to dig into the vessel wall as the vessel expands, thus giving a reading several times lower than that measured using ultrasonic or cineangiographic methods.

Hokanson *et al.* (1975) described an electrically calibrated mercury-in-rubber strain gage. Lead-wire errors are common with these devices because of the low resistance of the strain gage. In their design, the problem was eliminated by effectively placing the strain gage at the corners of the measurement bridge. A constant-current source causes an output that is linear for large changes in gage resistance. Figure 2.5 shows the device and its output when applied to the human calf.

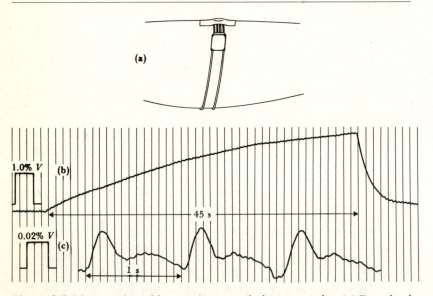

Figure 2.5 Mercury-in-rubber strain-gage plethysmography. (a) Four-lead gage applied to human calf. (b) Bridge output for venous-occlusion plethysmography. (c) Bridge output for arterial-pulse plethysmography. (Part (*a*) is based on D.E. Hokanson, D.S. Sumner, and D.E. Strandness, Jr., "An electrically calibrated plethysmograph for direct measurement of limb blood flow." 1975, BME-22, 25-29; used with permission of *IEEE Trans. Biomed. Eng.*, 1975, New York.)

2.3 Bridge circuits

The Wheatstone-bridge circuit is ideal for measuring small changes in resistance. Figure 2.2(b) shows a Wheatstone bridge with an applied dc voltage of v_i and a readout meter Δv_o with internal resistance R_i. It can be shown by the voltage-divider approach that Δv_o is zero, i.e., the bridge is balanced, when $R_1/R_2 = R_4/R_3$.

Resistance-type transducers may be connected in one or more arms of a bridge circuit. The variation in resistance can be detected by either null-balance or deflection-balance bridge circuits. The null-balance bridge results when the resistance change of the transducer is balanced out (zero output) by a variable resistance in an adjacent arm of the bridge. The calibrated adjustment required for the null is an indication of the change in resistance of the transducer. The deflection-balance method, on the other hand, utilizes the amount of bridge unbalance to determine the change in transducer resistance.

Assume that all values of resistance of the bridge are initially equal to R_o and that $R_o << R_i$. An increase in resistance, ΔR, of all resistances still results in a balanced bridge. However, if R_1 and R_3 increase by ΔR and R_2 and R_4 decrease by ΔR, then

$$\Delta v_o = \frac{\Delta R}{R_o} v_i \tag{2.6}$$

Because of the symmetry a similar expression results if R_2 and R_4 increase by ΔR and R_1 and R_3 decrease by ΔR. Note that (2.6), for the four-active-arm bridge, shows that Δv_o is linearly related to ΔR.

If the meter's internal resistance R_i is now included in the calculations, we get the following relationship for the four-active-arm bridge.

$$\Delta v_o = \frac{(\Delta R/R_o)v_i}{1 + (R_o/R_i)[1 + (\Delta R/R_o)^2]} \tag{2.7}$$

This relationship is linear provided that $R_o/R_i <<< 1$, a condition that also reduces (2.7) to (2.6).

A nonlinear relationship results when two opposite arms of the bridge circuit are changed equally:

$$\Delta v_o = \frac{(\Delta R/R_o)v_i}{2 + \Delta R/R_o + 2(R_o/R_i)(1 + \Delta R/R_o)} \tag{2.8}$$

A nonlinearity in $\Delta R/R_o$ is present even when $R_o/R_i = 0$.

It is common practice to incorporate a balancing scheme in the bridge circuit [see Fig. 2.2(b)]. Resistor R_y and potentiometer R_x are used to change the initial resistance of one or more arms. This arrangement brings the bridge into balance so that zero voltage output results from "zero" (or "base-level") input of the measured parameter.

To minimize loading effects, R_x is approximately 10 times the resistance of the bridge leg and R_y limits the maximum adjustment. Strain-gage applications normally use a value of $R_y = 25$ times the resistance of the bridge leg (Cook and Rabinowicz, 1963). Ac balancing circuits are more complicated because a reactive as well as resistive imbalance must be compensated. Figure 2.2(c) shows the additional circuit that could be connected in the bridge for this purpose.

Figure 2.5 shows an application of a mercury-in-rubber strain gage for the measurement of the circumference of the human calf. This device measures the changes in strain resistance in terms of bridge imbalance. Variation in dimensions are determined by means of the deflections in calibration shown.

Example 2.1 Show that $\Delta R/R_o = 2\Delta L/L + (\Delta L/L)^2$ for an elastic strain gage. Note that it is assumed that the volume of the liquid in the strain gage remains constant.

Answer The resistance of the mercury strain-gage unit is $R = \rho L/A$, where ρ = resistivity, L = length, and A = area of the mercury column. R_o denotes the unstretched and R_1 the stretched condition.

$$\Delta R = R_1 - R_o = \rho \left(\frac{L_1}{A_1} - \frac{L_o}{A_o} \right)$$

Since the volume V does not change,

$$V = A_o L_o = A_1 L_1$$

$$\frac{\Delta R}{R_o} = \frac{R_1}{R_o} - 1$$

$$\frac{\Delta R}{R_o} = \frac{\rho L_1/A_1}{\rho L_o/A_o} - 1$$

$$\frac{\Delta R}{R_o} = \frac{L_1 A_o}{L_o A_1} \frac{L_1 L_o}{L_1 L_o} - 1$$

Substituting in $V = A_o L_o$ and canceling the terms, we get

$$\frac{\Delta R}{R_o} = \frac{L_1^2}{L_o^2} - 1$$

We add and subtract like terms:

$$\frac{\Delta R}{R_o} = \frac{2L_1}{L_o} - 2 + \frac{L_1^2}{L_o^2} - \frac{2L_1}{L_o} + 1$$

Then

$$\frac{\Delta R}{R_o} = \frac{2(L_1 - L_o)}{L_o} + \left(\frac{L_1 - L_o}{L_o}\right)^2$$

or

$$\frac{\Delta R}{R_o} = \frac{2\Delta L}{L_o} + \left(\frac{\Delta L}{L_o}\right)^2$$

2.4 Inductive transducers

An inductance L can be used to measure displacement by varying any three of the coil parameters:

$$L = n^2 G \mu \tag{2.9}$$

where

n = number of turns of coil
G = geometric form factor
μ = effective permeability of the medium

Each of these parameters can be changed by mechanical means.

Figure 2.6(a) shows self-inductance; Figure 2.6(b), mutual-inductance; and Figure 2.6(c), differential transformer types of inductive displacement transducers. It is usually possible to convert a mutual-inductance system into a self-inductance system by series or parallel connections of the coils. Note in Figure 2.6 that the mutual-inductance device (b) becomes a self-inductance device (a) when terminals b–c are connected.

An inductive transducer has an advantage in not being affected by the dielectric properties of its environment. However, it may be affected by external magnetic fields due to the proximity of magnetic materials.

The variable-inductance method employing a single displaceable core is shown in Figure 2.6(a). This device works on the

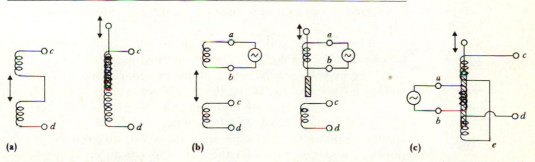

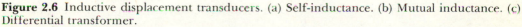

Figure 2.6 Inductive displacement transducers. (a) Self-inductance. (b) Mutual inductance. (c) Differential transformer.

principle that alterations in the self-inductance of a coil may be produced by changing the geometric form factor or the movement of a magnetic core within the coil. The change in inductance for this device is not linearly related to displacement. The fact that these devices have low power requirements and produce large variations in inductance makes them attractive for radiotelemetry applications. Allard (1962) used a single coil with a movable μ-metal core to measure the displacement of an intracardiac pressure transducer. Since this device has a frequency response that extends beyond 1 kHz, it may be used to measure both pressures and heart sounds. Chapter 7 discusses the principles involved in these measurements.

The mutual-inductance transducer employs two separate coils whose variation in mutual magnetic coupling is used to measure displacement [Fig. 2.6(b)]. Cobbold (1974) describes the application of these devices with respect to measuring cardiac dimensions, monitoring infant respiration, and ascertaining arterial diameters.

Van Citters (1966) provides a good description of applications of mutual-inductance transformers in measuring changes in dimension of internal organs (kidney, major blood vessels, and left ventricle). The induced voltage in the secondary coil is a function of the geometry of the coils (separation and axial alignment), the number of primary and secondary turns, and the frequency and amplitude of the excitation voltage. The induced voltage in the secondary coil is a nonlinear function of the separation of the coils. In order to maximize the output signal, a frequency is selected that causes the secondary coil (tuned circuit) to be in resonance. The output voltage is detected with standard demodulator and amplifier circuits.

The *linear variable differential transformer* (LVDT) is widely used in physiological research and clinical medicine to measure pressure, displacement, and force. As shown in Figure 2.6(c), the LVDT is composed of a primary coil (terminals a–b) and two secondary coils (c–e and d–e) connected in series. The coupling between these two coils is changed by the motion of a high-permeability alloy slug between them. The two secondary coils are connected in opposition in order to achieve a wider region of linearity.

The primary coil is sinusoidally excited, with a frequency between 60 Hz and 20 kHz. The alternating magnetic field induces nearly equal voltages v_{ce} and v_{de} in the secondary coils. The output voltage $v_{cd} = v_{ce} - v_{de}$. When the slug is symmetrically placed, the two secondary voltages are equal and the output signal is zero.

LVDT characteristics include: linearity over a large range; a change of phase by 180° when the core passes through the center position; and saturation on the ends. Specifications of commercially available LVDTs include: sensitivities on the order of 0.5–2

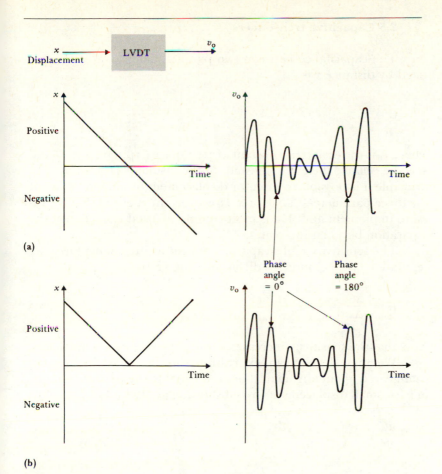

Figure 2.7 (a) As x moves through the null position, the phase changes 180°, while the magnitude of v_o is proportional to the magnitude of x. (b) An ordinary rectifier-demodulator cannot distinguish between (a) and (b), so a phase-sensitive demodulator is required.

mV for a displacement of 0.01 mm/V of primary voltage; full-scale displacement of 0.1–250 mm; and linearity of ±0.25%. Sensitivity for LVDTs is much higher than that for strain gages.

A disadvantage of the LVDT is that it requires more complex signal-processing instrumentation. Figure 2.7 shows that essentially the same magnitude of output voltage results with two very different input displacements. The direction of displacement may be determined by using the fact that there is a 180° phase shift when the core passes through the null position. A phase-sensitive demodulator is used for determining the direction of displacement. Figure 3.20 shows a ring-demodulator system that could be used with the LVDT.

2.5 Capacitive transducers

The capacitance between two parallel plates of area A separated by distance x is

$$C = \epsilon_0 \epsilon_r \frac{A}{x} \tag{2.10}$$

where ϵ_0 is the dielectric constant of free space (Appendix A.1) and ϵ_r is the relative dielectric constant of the insulator (1.0 for air). In principle it is possible to monitor displacement by changing any of the three parameters: ϵ_r, A, or x. However, the method that is easiest to implement and that is most commonly used is to change the separation between the plates.

The sensitivity K of a capacitive transducer to changes in plate separation, Δx, is found by differentiating (2.10):

$$K = \frac{\Delta C}{\Delta x} = - \epsilon_0 \epsilon_r \frac{A}{x^2} \tag{2.11}$$

Note that the sensitivity increases as the plate separation decreases.

We may develop an expression showing that the percent change in C about any neutral point is equal to the per-unit change in x for small displacements by substituting (2.10) into (2.11). Thus

$$\frac{dC}{dx} = \frac{-C}{x} \tag{2.12}$$

or

$$\frac{dC}{C} = \frac{-dx}{x} \tag{2.13}$$

The capacitance microphone shown in Figure 2.8 is an excellent example of a relatively simple method for detecting variation in capacitance (Doebelin, 1975, Cobbold, 1974). Since this is a dc-excited circuit, no current flows when the capacitor is stationary

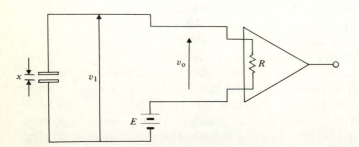

Figure 2.8 Capacitance transducer for measuring dynamic displacement changes.

(with separation x_0) and thus $v_1 = E$. A change in position $\Delta x = x_1 - x_0$ produces a voltage $v_o = v_1 - E$. The output voltage V_o is related to x_1 by

$$\frac{V_o(j\omega)}{X_1(j\omega)} = \frac{(E/x_0)j\omega\tau}{j\omega\tau + 1} \tag{2.14}$$

where $\tau = RC = R\epsilon_0\epsilon_r A/x_0$.

Typically, R is 1 MΩ or higher, and thus the readout device must have a high (10 MΩ or higher) input impedance.

For $\omega\tau \gg 1$, $V_o(j\omega)/X_1(j\omega) \cong E/x_0$, which is a constant. However, for low frequencies, the response drops off, and is zero when $\omega = 0$. Thus (2.14) describes a high-pass filter. This frequency response is quite adequate for a microphone that does not measure sound pressures at frequencies below 20 Hz. However, it is inadequate for measuring most physiological variables because of their low-frequency components.

The frequency response of the capacitance transducer may be extended to dc by means of an ingenious guarded parallel-plate capacitance transducer, shown in Figure 2.9(a) (Doebelin, 1975). In addition, this technique (employing a high-gain feedback amplifier) gives a linear relationship between displacement and capacitance. The displacement-varying capacitor is placed in the feedback loop of an operational amplifier circuit, as shown in Figure 2.9(b). The details of operational amplifier circuits are covered in Chapter 3.

The circuit gain of the inverting op-amp circuit shown in Figure 2.9 is given by the negative of the ratio of the feedback impedance to the input impedance; thus

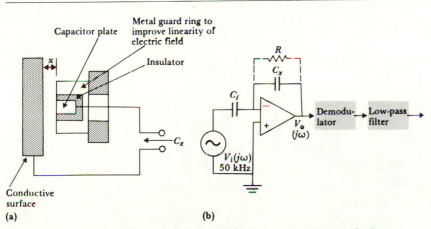

(a)   **(b)**

Figure 2.9 (a) Guarded parallel-plate displacement transducer. (b) Instrumentation system with output proportional to capacitance displacement. (Part (a) is from *Measurement Systems: Application and Design*, by E.O. Doebelin. Copyright © 1975 by McGraw-Hill, Inc. Used with permission of McGraw-Hill Book Co.)

$$\frac{V_o(j\omega)}{V_i(j\omega)} = \frac{-Z_f(j\omega)}{Z_i(j\omega)} \tag{2.15}$$

$$= -\frac{1/j\omega C_x}{1/j\omega C_i} \tag{2.16}$$

$$= -\frac{C_i}{C_x} \tag{2.17}$$

Substituting (2.10) in (2.17) yields

$$V_o(j\omega) = \frac{C_i x V_i(j\omega)}{\epsilon_0 \epsilon_r A} = Kx \tag{2.18}$$

Equation (2.18) shows that the output voltage is linearly related to the plate separation x. The source voltage $V_i(j\omega)$ is a high-frequency source (50 kHz). The output voltage $V_o(j\omega)$ is an amplitude-modulated signal and the mean value of $V_o(j\omega)$, proportional to x, is found by demodulation and low-pass filtering (10 kHz corner frequency). A discharge resistor R must be connected in parallel with C_x in order to provide bias current for the amplifier, which should be an FET op amp. The value of resistance selected is high with respect to the reactance of C_x.

Podolak *et al.* (1969) report the use of this device for re-

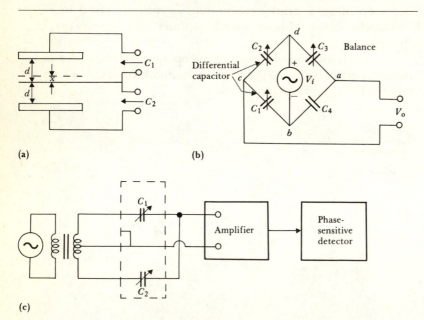

(a)   (b)   (c)

Figure 2.10 (a) Differential three terminal capacitor. (b) Capacitance-bridge circuit with output proportional to fractional difference in capacitance. (c) Transformer ratio-arm bridge. (From *Transducers for Medical Measurements: Application and Design,* by R.S.C. Cobbold. Copyright © 1974, John Wiley and Sons, Inc. Reprinted by permission of John Wiley and Sons, Inc.)

cordings of chest-wall motions, apex motion, heart sounds, and brachial and radial pulses. The advantages of the transducer are that it is noncontacting (skin is used as one side of the capacitor) and linear, and that it has a wide frequency response. Problems encountered with this transducer arise in connection with proper isolation of the patient from the high-amplitude ac-excitation voltages, mechanical positioning of the probe, and respiratory motions during the measuring process.

Differential-capacitor systems have the advantage of providing accurate measurements of displacement (Cobbold, 1974). Figure 2.10(a) shows a differential three-terminal capacitor that has the advantage of linearly relating displacement to $(C_1 - C_2)/(C_1 + C_2)$. This can be shown by letting d be the equilibrium displacement and x be the displacement with positive direction up. Then

$$C_1 = \frac{\epsilon_0 \epsilon_r A}{d - x} \quad \text{and} \quad C_2 = \frac{\epsilon_0 \epsilon_r A}{d + x} \tag{2.19}$$

and manipulation then gives

$$\frac{x}{d} = \frac{C_1 - C_2}{C_1 + C_2} \tag{2.20}$$

The bridge circuit shown in Figure 2.10(b) may be used to provide an output voltage proportional to the fractional difference in capacitance dictated by (2.20). Since the differential-capacitor values C_1 and C_2 are equal at the equilibrium position and C_3 is balanced to equal C_4, output voltage is given by

$$V_o = \frac{V_i}{2} \frac{C_1 - C_2}{C_1 + C_2} \tag{2.21}$$

or

$$V_o = \frac{V_i}{2d} x \tag{2.22}$$

Example 2.2 Show that the bridge circuit in Figure 2.10(b) provides an output voltage proportional to the fractional difference in capacitance.

Answer Using the voltage-divider relation, we get

$$V_{ab}(j\omega) = \frac{(1/j\omega C_4)V_i(j\omega)}{1/j\omega C_3 + 1/j\omega C_4} \tag{2.23}$$

$$V_{cb}(j\omega) = \frac{(1/j\omega C_1)V_i(j\omega)}{1/j\omega C_1 + 1/j\omega C_2}$$

$$V_o(j\omega) = V_{ab}(j\omega) + V_{bc}(j\omega)$$

$$= \left(\frac{C_3}{C_4 + C_3} - \frac{C_2}{C_1 + C_2} \right) V_i(j\omega)$$

C_3 is adjusted to equal C_4; then

$$V_o(j\omega) = \left(\frac{1}{2} - \frac{C_2}{C_1 + C_2} \right) V_i(j\omega)$$

$$= \frac{(C_1 - C_2)V_i(j\omega)}{2(C_1 + C_2)} \tag{2.24}$$

Because this relation does not change with frequency, (2.24) reduces to (2.22).

Figure 2.10(c) shows a transformer ratio-arm bridge that can also be used to solve (2.20). Amplifier current is directly related to the degree of bridge unbalance ($C_1 - C_2$) that may be found from (2.19):

$$C_1 - C_2 = \frac{2A\epsilon_0\epsilon_r x}{d^2 - x^2} \tag{2.25}$$

This expression is linear with x for the case $d \gg x$, which is the normal operating condition. This type of bridge circuit has high accuracy and sensitivity. Bridge balance is independent of the third terminal shield, which makes possible the measurement of capacitance at various distances from the bridge.

2.6 Piezoelectric transducers

Piezoelectric transducers are used to measure physiological displacements and record heart sounds. Piezoelectric materials generate an electrical potential when mechanically strained, and conversely an electrical potential can cause physical deformation of the material. The principle of operation is that, when an asymmetrical crystal lattice is distorted, a charge reorientation takes place, causing a relative displacement of negative and positive charges. The displaced internal charges induce surface charges of opposite polarity on opposite sides of the crystal. Surface charge can be determined by measuring the difference in voltage between electrodes attached to the surfaces.

The total induced charge q is directly proportional to the applied force f:

$$q = kf \tag{2.26}$$

where k = the piezoelectric constant, C/N. The change in voltage can be found by assuming that the system acts like a parallel-plate capacitor where the voltage v across the capacitor = charge q/capacitance C. Then by substitution of (2.10), we get

$$v = \frac{kf}{C} = \frac{kfx}{\epsilon_0 \epsilon_r A} \tag{2.27}$$

Tables of piezoelectric constants are given in the literature (Lion, 1959; and Cobbold, 1974).

Typical values for k are 2.3 pC/N for quartz and 140 pC/N for barium titanate. For a piezoelectric transducer of 1-cm^2 area and 1-mm thickness with an applied force due to a 10-g weight, the output voltage v is 0.23 and 14 mV for the quartz and barium titanate crystals, respectively.

There are various modes of operation of piezoelectric transducers, dependent on the material and the crystallographic orientation of the plate (Lion, 1959). These modes include: the thickness or longitudinal compression; transversal compression; thickness-shear action; and face-shear action.

Piezoelectric materials have a high but finite resistance. As a consequence, if a static deflection x is applied, the charge leaks through the leakage resistor (on the order of 100 GΩ). It is obviously quite important that the input impedance of the external voltage-measuring device be an order of magnitude higher than that of the piezoelectric transducer. It would be helpful to look at the equivalent circuit for the piezoelectric transducer [Figure 2.11(a)] in order to quantify its dynamic-response characteristics.

This circuit has a charge generator q defined by

$$q = Kx \tag{2.28}$$

where

K = proportionality constant, C/m, and x = deflection.

The circuit may be simplified by converting the charge generator to a current generator, i_t.

$$i_t = \frac{dq}{dt} = K \frac{dx}{dt} \tag{2.29}$$

The modified circuit is shown in Figure 2.11(b), where the resistances and capacitances have been combined. Assuming that the amplifier does not draw any current, we then have

$$i_t = i_c + i_R \tag{2.30}$$

$$v_o = v_c = \left(\frac{1}{C}\right) \int i_c \, dt \tag{2.31}$$

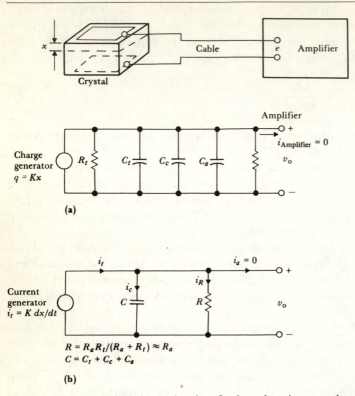

(a)

(b)

Figure 2.11 (a) Equivalent circuit of piezoelectric transducer, where R_t = transducer leakage resistance, C_t = transducer capacitance, C_c = cable capacitance, C_a = amplifier input capacitance, R_a = amplifier input resistance, and q = charge generator. (b) Modified equivalent circuit with current generator replacing charge generator. (From *Measurement Systems: Application and Design,* by E.O. Doebelin. Copyright © 1975 by McGraw-Hill, Inc. Used with permission of McGraw-Hill Book Co.)

$$i_t - i_R = C\left(\frac{dv_o}{dt}\right) = K\frac{dx}{dt} - \frac{v_o}{R} \tag{2.32}$$

or

$$\frac{V_o(j\omega)}{X(j\omega)} = \frac{K_s j\omega\tau}{j\omega\tau + 1} \tag{2.33}$$

where

$$K_s = K/C \text{ (sensitivity, V/m)}$$
$$\tau = RC \text{ (time constant)}$$

Example 2.3 A piezoelectric transducer has $C = 500$ pF. The amplifier input impedance is 5 MΩ. What is the low-corner frequency?

Answer We may use the modified equivalent circuit of the piezoelectric transducer given in Figure 2.11(b) for this calculation.

$$f_c = 1/2\pi RC = 1/2\pi(5 \times 10^6)(500 \times 10^{-12}) = 64 \text{ Hz}$$

Note that by increasing the input impedance of the amplifier by a factor of 100, we can lower the low-corner frequency to 0.64 Hz.

Another approach to improving the low-frequency response is the use of the charge amplifier described in Section 3.8.

Because of its mechanical resonance, the high-frequency equivalent circuit for a piezoelectric transducer is complex. This effect can be represented by adding a series *RLC* circuit in parallel with the transducer capacitance and leakage resistance. Figure 2.12 shows the high-frequency equivalent circuit and its frequency response. Note that in some applications the mechanical resonance is useful for accurate frequency control; for example, in the case of crystal filters.

Piezoelectric transducers are used quite extensively in cardiology for external (body-surface), and internal (intracardiac) phonocardiography. They are also used in the detection of Korot-

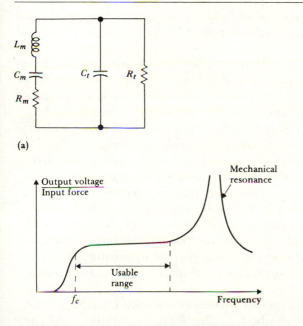

Figure 2.12 (a) High-frequency circuit model for piezoelectric transducer. R_t is the transducer leakage resistance and C_t the capacitance. L_m, C_m, and R_m represent the mechanical system. (b) Piezoelectric transducer frequency response. (From *Transducers for Medical Measurements: Application and Design*, by R.S.C. Cobbold. Copyright © 1974, John Wiley and Sons, Inc. Reprinted by permission of John Wiley and Sons, Inc.)

koff sounds in blood-pressure measurements (Chapter 7). Additional applications of piezoelectric transducers involve their use in measurements of physiological accelerations. Section 8.4 describes ultrasonic blood-flow meters in which the piezoelectric element operating at mechanical resonance emits and senses high-frequency sounds.

2.7 Temperature measurements

A patient's body temperature gives important information to the physician about the physiological state of the individual. External body temperature is one of many parameters used to evaluate patients in shock, since the reduced blood pressure of a person in circulatory shock results in low blood flow to the periphery. A drop in the big-toe temperature is a good early clinical warning of shock. Infections, on the other hand, are usually reflected by an increase in body temperature, with a hot flushed skin and loss of fluids. Increased respiration, perspiration, and blood flow to the skin result when high fevers destroy temperature-sensitive enzymes and proteins. Anesthesia decreases body temperature by depressing the thermal regulatory center. In fact, physicians routinely use the technique of inducing hypothermia in surgical cases in which they wish to decrease a patient's metabolic processes and blood circulation.

In pediatrics, special heated incubators are used for stabilizing the body temperature of infants. Accurate monitoring of temperature and regulatory control systems are used to maintain a desirable ambient temperature for the infant.

In the study of arthritis, physicians have shown that temperatures of joints are closely correlated with the amount of local inflammation. The increased blood flow due to arthritis and chronic inflammation can be detected by thermal measurements.

The specific site of body-temperature recording must be selected carefully so that it truly reflects the patient's temperature. Also, environmental changes and artifacts can cause misleading readings. For example, the skin and oral-mucosa temperature of a patient seldom reflects true body-core temperature. Robertson (1973) gives a good summary of clinical temperature measurements.

The following types of thermally sensitive methods of measurement will be described in the following sections: thermocouples, thermistors, and radiation and chemical detectors.

2.8 Thermocouples

Thermoelectric thermometry is based on the discovery of Seebeck in 1821. He observed that an *electromotive force* (emf) exists across a junction of two dissimilar metals. This phenomenon is due to the sum of two independent effects. The first effect, discovered by Peltier, is an emf due solely to the contact of two unlike metals and the junction temperature. The net Peltier emf is roughly proportional to the difference between the temperatures of the two junctions. The second effect, credited to Thomson (Lord Kelvin), is an emf due to the temperature gradients along each single conductor. The net Thomson emf is proportional to the difference between the squares of the absolute junction temperatures (T_1 and T_2). The magnitudes of the Peltier and Thomson emfs may be derived from thermodynamic principles (Anonymous, 1974) and either may predominate, depending on the metals chosen.

Knowledge of these two effects is not usually useful in practical applications, so empirical calibration data are usually curve-fitted with a power series expansion that yields the Seebeck voltage,

$$E = aT + \tfrac{1}{2}bT^2 + \cdots \tag{2.34}$$

where T is in degrees Celsius and the reference junction is maintained at 0°C.

Figure 2.13(a) is a thermocouple circuit with two dissimilar metals, A and B, at two different temperatures, T_1 and T_2. The net emf at terminals $c - d$ is a function of the difference between the temperatures at the two junctions and the properties of the two metals. In the practical situation, one junction is held at a constant known temperature (i.e., by an ice bath or controlled oven) for a reference in order to determine the desired or unknown temperature.

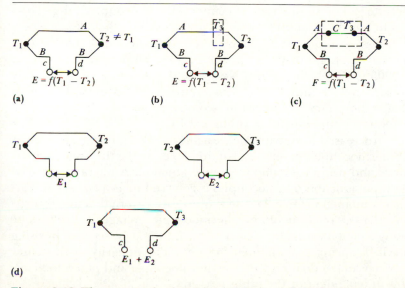

Figure 2.13 Thermocouple circuits. (a) Peltier emf. (b) Law of homogeneous circuits. (c) Law of intermediate metals. (d) Law of intermediate temperatures.

An understanding of the three empirical thermocouple laws leads to using them properly. The first law, *homogeneous circuits,* states that, in a circuit composed of a single homogeneous metal, one cannot maintain an electric current by the application of heat alone. In Fig. 2.13(b), the net emf at c–d is the same as in Figure 2.13(a) regardless of the fact that a temperature distribution (T_3) exists along one of the wires (A).

The second law, *intermediate metals,* states that the net emf in a circuit consisting of an interconnection of a number of unlike metals, maintained at the same temperature, is zero. The practical implication of this principle is that lead wires may be attached to the thermocouple without affecting the accuracy of the measured emf, provided that the newly formed junctions are at the same temperature [Figure 2.13(c)].

The third law, *successive* or *intermediate temperatures,* is illustrated in Figure 2.13(d), where emf E_1 is generated when two dissimilar metals have junctions at temperatures T_1 and T_2 and emf E_2 results for temperatures T_2 and T_3. It follows that an emf $E_1 + E_2$ results at c–d when the junctions are at temperatures T_1 and T_3. This principle makes it possible for calibration curves derived for a given reference-junction temperature to be used to determine the calibration curves for another reference temperature.

The *thermoelectric sensitivity* α (also called the thermoelectric power or the Seebeck coefficient) is found by differentiating (2.34) with respect to T. Then

$$\alpha = dE/dT = a + bT + \cdots \tag{2.35}$$

Note that α is not a constant, but varies (usually increases) with temperature. The sensitivities of common thermocouples range from 6.5 to 80 μV/°C at 20°C, with accuracies from $\frac{1}{4}\%$ to 1%.

For accurate readings, the reference junction should be kept in a triple-point-of-water device whose temperature is 0.01 $\pm$ 0.0005°C (Doebelin, 1975). Normally the accuracy of a properly constructed ice bath, 0.05°C with a reproducibility of 0.001°C, is all that is necessary. Temperature-controlled ovens can maintain a reference temperature to within $\pm$ 0.4°C.

Increased sensitivity may be achieved by connecting a number of thermocouples in series, all of them measuring the same temperature and using the same reference junction. An arrangement of multiple-junction thermocouples is referred to as a *thermopile.* Parallel combinations may be used to measure average temperature.

Direct readout of the thermocouple voltage is easily done using a digital voltmeter. Chart recordings may be secured by using a self-balancing potentiometer system. The linearity of this latter device is dependent only on the thermocouple and potentiometer; it is independent of the other circuitry.

Thermocouples have the following advantages: fast response

time (time constant as small as 1 ms), small size (down to 12 μm diameter), ease of fabrication, and long-term stability. Their disadvantages are: small output voltage, low sensitivity, and need for a reference temperature.

Numerous examples of the use of thermocouples in biomedical research are given in the literature (Hardy, 1962). Since thermocouples can be made small in size, they can be inserted into catheters and hypodermic needles.

2.9 Thermistors

Thermistors are semiconductors made of ceramic materials that are thermal resistors with a high negative temperature coefficient. These materials react to temperature changes in a way that is opposite to the way metals react to such changes. The resistance of thermistors decreases as temperature increases and increases as temperature decreases (Sachse, 1975).

Sapoff (1971) reviewed the various types of thermistors that have been found to be most suitable for biomedical use. The resistivity of thermistor semiconductors used for biomedical applications is between 0.1 to 100 $\Omega \cdot$ m. These devices are small in size (they can be made less than 0.5 mm in diameter), have a relatively large sensitivity to temperature changes (-3 to $-5\%/°C$), and have excellent long-term stability characteristics ($\pm 0.2\%$ of nominal resistance value per year).

Figure 2.14(a) shows a typical family of resistance-versus-temperature characteristics of thermistors. These properties are measured for the thermistor operated at a very small amount of power such that there is negligible self-heating. This resistance is commonly referred to as *zero-power resistance*. The empirical relationship between the thermistor resistance R_t and absolute temperature T in kelvins (K) (the SI unit *kelvin* does not use a degree sign) is

$$R_t = R_o e^{[\beta(T_o - T)/TT_o]} \tag{2.36}$$

where

β = material constant for thermistor, K
T_o = standard reference temperature, K

The value of β increases slightly with temperature. However, over the limited temperature spans for biomedical work (10–20 K), this does not present a problem. β, also known as the characteristic temperature, is in the range of 2500–5000 K. It is usually about 4000 K.

The temperature coefficient α can be found by differentiating (2.36) with respect to T and dividing by R_t. Thus

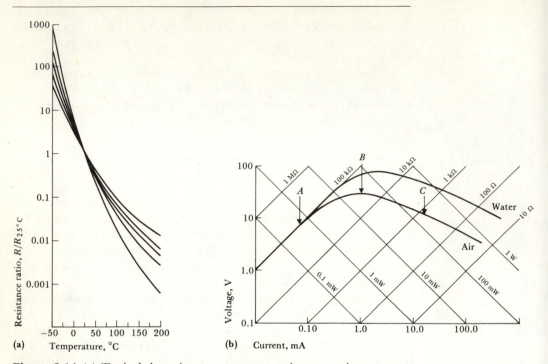

(a)   Temperature, °C

(b)   Current, mA

Figure 2.14 (a) Typical thermistor zero-power resistance ratio–temperature characteristics for various materials. (b) Thermistor voltage-versus-current characteristic for a thermistor in air and water. The diagonal lines with a positive slope give linear resistance values and show the degree of thermistor linearity at low currents. The intersection of the thermistor curves and the diagonal lines with negative slope give the device power dissipation. Point A is the maximum current value for no appreciable self-heat. Point B is the peak voltage. Point C is the maximum safe continuous current in air. [Part (b) is from *Thermistor Manual*, EMC-6, © 1974, Fenwal Electronics, Framingham, Mass.; used by permission.]

$$\alpha = \frac{1}{R_t}\frac{dR_t}{dT} = -\frac{\beta}{T^2} \quad (\%/\text{K}) \tag{2.37}$$

Note from (2.37) that α is a nonlinear function of temperature. This nonlinearity is also reflected in Figure 2.14(a).

The voltage-versus-current characteristics of thermistors, as shown in Figure 2.14(b), are linear up to the point at which self-heating becomes a problem. When there is large self-heating, the thermistor voltage drop decreases as the current increases. This portion of the curve displays a negative-resistance characteristic.

In the linear portion Ohm's law applies and the current is directly proportional to the applied voltage. The temperature of the thermistor is that of its surroundings. However, at higher currents a point is reached, because of increased current flow, at which the heat generated in the thermistor raises the temperature of the thermistor above ambient. At the peak of the v-i characteristics, the incremental resistance is zero, and for higher currents a negative-resistance relationship occurs. Operation in this region renders the device vulnerable to thermal destruction.

Figure 2.14(b) shows the difference in the self-heat regions for a thermistor in water and air due to the differences in thermal resistance of air and water. The principle of variation in thermal resistance can be used to measure blood velocity, as described in Section 8.5.

The current-time characteristics of a thermistor are important in any dynamic analysis of the system. When a step change in voltage is applied to a series circuit consisting of a resistor and a thermistor, a current flows. The time delay for the current to reach its maximum value is a function of the voltage applied, the mass of the thermistor, and the value of the series-circuit resistance. Time delays from milliseconds to several minutes are possible with thermistor circuits. Similar time delays occur when the temperature surrounding the thermistor is changed in a step fashion.

Various schemes for linearizing the resistance-versus-temperature characteristics of thermistors have been proposed (Beakley, 1951; Bryce, 1967; Cobbold, 1974; and Doebelin, 1975). The nonlinearity of a thermistor may be reduced by shunting the thermistor by a resistor R_p. Figure 2.15(a) shows the scheme for linearization and Figure 2.15(b) shows the plot of resistance versus temperature for the total resistance, with and without linearization.

In a similar way the conductance-temperature characteristics may be linearized by placing a resistance R_s in series with the thermistor [Figure 2.15(c)]. Figure 2.15(d) gives the conductance-versus-temperature characteristics with and without the series resistance. The linearization scheme of Figure 2.15(a) is employed when a constant-current source drives the current and the thermistor voltage is measured. That of Figure 2.15(c) is used when a constant voltage is applied and the current through the thermistor is measured.

Specific values of R_p and R_s can be found by calculation. In the first case, it is desirable to place the point of inflection of the linearized thermistor curve at the midscale of temperature variations. The parallel combination of R_p and R_t is

$$R = \frac{R_p R_t}{R_p + R_t} \tag{2.38}$$

The inflection point lies where the second derivative of R with respect to temperature is zero. From (2.36), this gives

$$R_p = R_{t,m} \frac{\beta - 2T_m}{\beta + 2T_m} \tag{2.39}$$

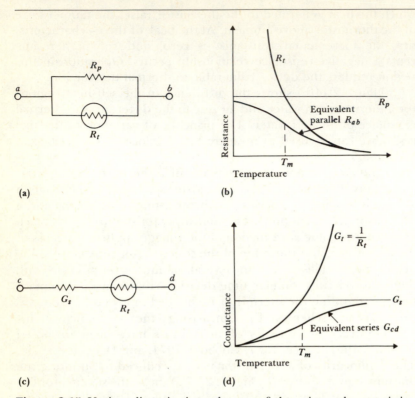

Figure 2.15 Various linearization schemes of thermistor characteristics. (a) Resistor R_p is connected in parallel with the thermistor R_t. (b) Resistance-versus-temperature characteristics for parallel compensation. (c) Conductance G_s is connected in series with the thermistor G_t. (d) Conductance-versus-temperature characteristics for series compensation. (From *Transducers for Medical Measurements: Application and Design*, by R.S.C. Cobbold. Copyright © 1974, John Wiley and Sons, Inc. Reprinted by permission of John Wiley and Sons, Inc.)

where $R_{t,m}$ is the thermistor resistance value at the midscale temperature T_m. The desired value of R_s for linearizing the conductance-versus-temperature curve may be found using the same approach. In this case,

$$G_s = \frac{1}{R_s} = G_{t,m}\frac{\beta - 2T_m}{\beta + 2T_m} \tag{2.40}$$

where $G_{t,m}$ is the thermistor conductance value at the midscale temperature.

A specific example with typical values illustrates the improvement in linearity (Beakley, 1951). If we assume that $\beta = 3000$ K and $T_m = 3000$ K, then $G_s = 1.5\,G_{300}$ [from (2.40)]. For a $\pm 10°$C variation in temperature, the deviation in linearity is less than $0.03°$C; whereas for a $\pm 15°$C change, it increases to $0.1°$C.

As with all improvements in circuit performance, there must

be a tradeoff in some other parameter of the system. In this case, the value of the temperature coefficient α is decreased in the parallel and series linearization circuits to

$$\alpha_{\text{parallel}} = + \frac{(\beta/T_m)^2}{R_{t,m}/R_p + 1} \tag{2.41}$$

and

$$\alpha_{\text{series}} = - \frac{(\beta/T_m)^2}{G_{t,m}/G_s + 1} \tag{2.42}$$

Using the same values as above, we find that α decreases from 3.3%/°C for the case with no series compensation to 2%/°C when an optimum value of resistance is inserted in series. More complex circuits may be used to linearize the thermistor characteristics over a wider temperature variation (Cobbold, 1974).

The circuitry used for thermistor readout is essentially the same as for conductive sensors, and many of the same techniques apply. Bridge circuits give high sensitivity and good accuracy. The bridge circuit shown in Figure 2.2(b) could be used with $R_3 = R_t$ and $R_4 = $ the thermistor resistance at the midscale value.

Very small differences in temperature can be found using a differential-temperature bridge. It is often necessary to measure such minute differences in biological work (Hardy, 1962). An example would be determining the difference in temperature of two organs or of multiple sites of the same organ.

The dc differential bridge shown in Figure 2.16(a) can achieve a linearity of better than 1% of full-scale output when bead thermistors matched to within ± 1% of each other at 25°C are used. The dc stability of this bridge is not normally a problem, since the output voltage of the bridge—even for temperature differences of 0.01%—is larger than the dc drift of good integrated-circuit operational amplifiers (Cobbold, 1974).

Nancollas and Hardy (1967) have designed an ac-excited differential bridge for use in *calorimetry* (the determination of the heats of reaction of components of cells). Figure 2.16(b) shows this bridge, which achieves a higher sensitivity than the dc version. A carrier frequency is selected such that the amplifier and thermistor noise is minimized. A phase-sensitive-demodulation system (Section 3.15) is used to detect the signal. The capacitive-reactance imbalance of the two thermistors can be nulled by placing a fixed capacitor across one of the thermistors and a variable capacitor across the other.

Operational-amplifier circuits may be used to measure the current in a thermistor as a function of temperature. In essence, this circuit applies a constant voltage to the thermistor and monitors its current with a current-to-voltage converter.

Various shapes of thermistors are available: beads, chips,

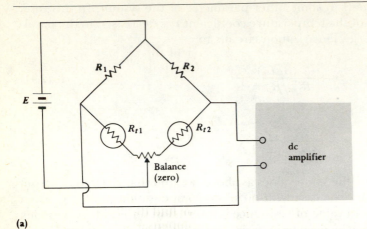

(a)

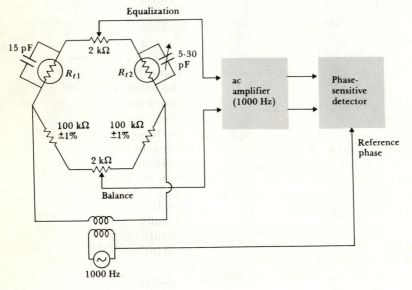

(b)

Figure 2.16 (a) dc differential-temperature bridge. (b) ac differential-temperature bridge. R_{t1} and R_{t2} are matched thermistors 100 kΩ ($\pm 1\%$). (From *Transducers for Medical Measurements: Application and Design*, by R.S.C. Cobbold. Copyright © 1974, John Wiley and Sons, Inc. Reprinted by permission of John Wiley and Sons, Inc.)

rods, and washers (Sapoff, 1971). The glass-encapsulated bead thermistor is the one most commonly used in biomedical applications. The glass coating protects the sensing element from the hostile environment of the body without significantly affecting the thermal response time of the system. The small size of these thermistors makes possible their placement at the tip of catheters or hypodermic needles. The thermodilution-catheter system discussed in Section 8.2 employs a four-lumen catheter with a thermistor located near the catheter tip.

An additional application of thermistors is in the clinical measurement of oral temperature. Thermistor probes with disposable sheaths are presently used. However, these systems have not been accepted as rapidly as some people expected them to. Many manufacturers are experimenting with completely disposable probes, hoping that this convenience feature will improve their acceptability in clinical use.

2.10 Radiation thermometry

The basis of *radiation thermometry* is that there is a known relationship between the surface temperature of an object and its radiant power. This principle makes it possible to measure the temperature of a body without physical contact with it. Medical thermography is a technique whereby the temperature distribution of the body is mapped with a sensitivity of a few tenths of a degree kelvin. It is based on the recognition that skin temperature can vary from place to place depending on the cellular or circulatory processes taking place in the body at each location. Thermography has been used successfully for the early detection of breast cancer, for determining the location and extent of arthritic disturbances, for gaging the depth of tissue destruction from frostbite and burns, and for detecting various peripheral circulatory disorders (venous thrombosis, carotid-artery occlusions, and so forth). Section 11.7 goes into specific details of this technique. Here we shall deal with the basic principles of thermal radiation and detector systems.

Every body that is above absolute zero radiates electromagnetic power, the amount being dependent on its temperature and physical properties. For room-temperature objects, the spectrum is predominantly in the far- and extreme-far-infrared regions.

A blackbody is an ideal thermal radiator; as such, it absorbs all incident radiation and emits the maximum possible thermal radiation. The radiation emitted from a body is given by Planck's law multiplied by emissivity ϵ. This expression relates the radiant flux per unit area per unit wavelength W_λ at a wavelength λ (μm), and is stated as

$$W_\lambda = \frac{\epsilon C_1}{\lambda^5 (e^{C_2/\lambda T} - 1)} \qquad (\text{W/cm}^2 \cdot \mu\text{m}) \qquad (2.43)$$

where

$C_1 = 3.74 \times 10^4 \qquad (\text{W} \cdot \mu\text{m}^4/\text{cm}^2)$
$C_2 = 1.44 \times 10^4 \qquad (\mu\text{m} \cdot \text{K})$
$T =$ blackbody temperature, K
$\epsilon =$ emissivity, the extent by which a surface deviates from a blackbody ($\epsilon = 1$)

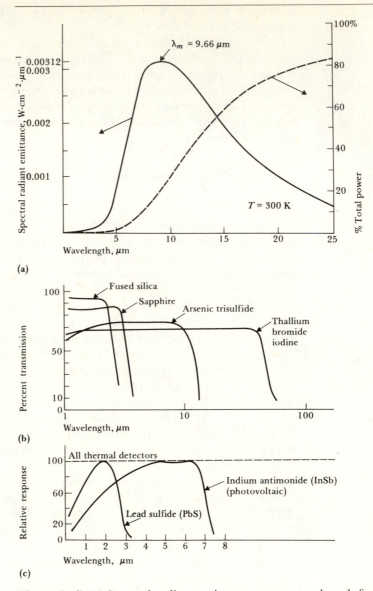

Figure 2.17 (a) Spectral radiant emittance versus wavelength for a black-body at 300 K on the left vertical axis; percentage of total energy on the right vertical axis. (b) Spectral transmission for a number of optical materials. (c) Spectral sensitivity of photon and thermal detectors. [Part (a) is from *Transducers for Medical Measurements: Application and Design,* by R.S.C. Cobbold. Copyright © 1974, John Wiley and Sons, Inc. Reprinted by permission of John Wiley and Sons, Inc. Parts (b) and (c) are from *Measurement Systems: Application and Design,* by E.O. Doebelin. Copyright © 1975 by McGraw-Hill, Inc. Used with permission of McGraw-Hill Book Co.]

Figure 2.17(a) shows a plot of (2.43), the spectral radiant emittance versus wavelength for a blackbody at 300 K.

Wien's displacement law gives the wavelength λ_m for which W_λ is a maximum. It can simply be found by differentiating (2.43) and setting this to zero.

$$\lambda_m = \frac{2898}{T} \quad (\mu m) \tag{2.44}$$

Figure 2.17(a) indicates $\lambda_m = 9.66$ μm ($T = 300$ K). Note from (2.43) that the maximum level of spectral emittance increases with T, and from (2.44) that λ_m is inversely related to T.

The total radiant power W_t can be found by integrating the area under the curve. This expression is known as the *Stefan-Boltzmann law*.

$$W_t = \epsilon \sigma T^4 \quad (W/cm^2) \tag{2.45}$$

where σ is the Stefan-Boltzmann constant (Appendix).

It is of interest to examine how the percentage of total radiant power varies with wavelength for room-temperature objects. This parameter, plotted in Figure 2.17(a), is found by dividing $\int_0^\lambda W_\lambda \, d\lambda$ by the total radiant power W_t (2.45). Note that approximately 80% of the total radiant power is found in the wavelength band from 4 to 25 μm.

Determining the effect of changes in surface emissivity with wavelength is important in order to accurately determine the temperature of a given source. It can be shown that, for $T = 300$ K and $\lambda = 3$ μm, a 5% change in ϵ is equivalent to a temperature change of approximately 1°C. Variations in ϵ with λ should be found in the case of absolute-temperature determinations, but are less significant if relative temperature is desired, provided that ϵ remains constant over the surface area being measured. The data relating the variation of ϵ with λ for human skin are not consistent and show variations as large as 5% from unity over the λ span from 2 to 6 μm (Cobbold, 1974).

The lenses used in infrared instruments must be carefully selected for their infrared spectral properties. Special materials must be chosen because standard glass used for the visible spectrum does not pass wavelengths longer than 2 μm. On the other hand, some materials (i.e., arsenic trisulfide) readily pass infrared and not visible light. Figure 2.17(b) shows the spectral transmission for a number of optical materials.

Infrared detectors and instrument systems must be designed with a high sensitivity because of the weak signals. These devices must have a short response time and appropriate wavelength-bandwidth requirements that match the radiation source. Thermal and photon detectors are used as infrared detectors. The detectors are of two types, both of which are described in Section 2.16. The thermal detector has low sensitivity and responds to all wavelengths, as shown in Figure 2.17(c), whereas quantum detectors respond only to a limited wavelength band.

Suitable instrumentation must be used to amplify, process, and display these weak signals from radiation detectors. Most radiometers make use of a beam-chopper system to interrupt the radiation at a fixed rate (several hundred hertz). This arrangement allows the use of high-gain ac amplifiers without the inherent problems of stability associated with dc amplifiers. In addition, comparison of reference sources and techniques of temperature compensation are more applicable to ac-instrumentation systems.

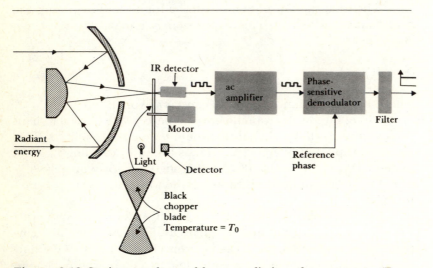

Figure 2.18 Stationary chopped-beam radiation thermometer. (From *Transducers for Medical Measurements: Application and Design*, by R.S.C. Cobbold. Copyright © 1974, John Wiley and Sons, Inc. Reprinted by permission of John Wiley and Sons, Inc.)

Figure 2.18 shows a typical chopped-beam radiation-thermometer system (Cobbold, 1974). A mirror focuses the radiation on the detector. However, a blackened chopper interrupts the radiation beam at a constant rate. The output of the detector circuit is a series of pulses with amplitude dependent on the strength of the radiation source. This ac signal is amplified, while the mean value, which is subject to drift, is blocked. A reference-phase signal, used to synchronize the phase-sensitive demodulator (Section 3.15), is generated in a special circuit consisting of a light source and detector. The signal is then filtered to provide a dc signal proportional to the target temperature. This signal can then be displayed or recorded. Infrared microscopes have also been designed using these techniques.

2.11 Chemical thermometry

A disposable clinical oral thermometer, recently introduced (Anonymous, 1975), operates on the principle that in certain substances there is a well-defined solid-liquid phase-transition temperature. The thermometer uses a substance whose melting point can be changed in increments of 0.2°F over the temperature range 96–104.8°F. It also uses a system that keeps the chemical action from starting until needed. Special dye-impregnated dots are not activated until the thermometer strip is pulled from the dispenser case. Body heat activates the chemicals and causes the appropriate white dots to turn to deep blue-green. A matrix of 45 elements provides a digital readout of the patient's temperature. Figure 2.19 shows the disposable thermometer with digital readout before and after use.

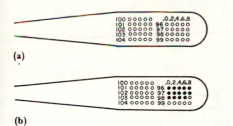

(a)

(b)

Figure 2.19 Digital-readout disposable thermometer. (a) When thermometer is taken from case, the 45 dots are white. (b) When exposed to body temperature, the dots turn green. In this example, the thermometer indicates 98.6°F. (From *DuPont Magazine*, Vol. 69, No. 5, p. 12, 1975; used with permission.)

2.12 Optical measurements

Optical systems are widely used in medical diagnosis. The most common use occurs in the clinical-chemistry lab, in which technicians analyze samples of blood and other tissues removed from the body. Optical instruments are also used during cardiac catheterization to measure the oxygen saturation of hemoglobin and to measure cardiac output.

Figure 2.20(a) shows that the usual optical instrument has a source, filter, and detector. Figure 2.20(b) shows a common arrangement of components. Figure 2.20(c) shows that in some cases, the function of source, filter, sample, and detector may be accomplished by solid-state components.

The remainder of this chapter is divided into parts, dealing with sources, geometrical optics, filters, detectors, and combinations of these.

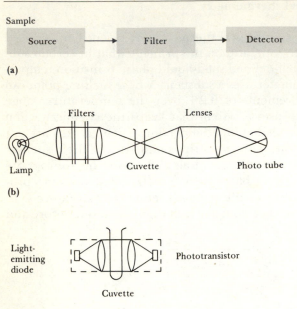

Sample

Source → Filter → Detector

(a)

Filters   Lenses

Lamp   Cuvette   Photo tube

(b)

Light-
emitting   Phototransistor
diode

Cuvette

(c)

Figure 2.20 (a) General block diagram of an optical instrument. (b) Highest efficiency is obtained by using an intense lamp, lenses to gather and focus the light on the sample in the cuvette, and a sensitive detector. (c) Solid-state lamps and detectors may simplify the system.

2.13 Radiation sources

Tungsten lamps

Incandescent tungsten-wire filament lamps are the most commonly used sources of radiation. Their radiant output varies with temperature and wavelength, as given by (2.43). For $\lambda < 1\ \mu m$, tungsten has an emissivity of about 0.4 and thus emits about 40% of what it would if the emissivity were 1.0. The relative-output spectrum shown in Figure 2.21(a) is only slightly altered. For higher temperatures, λ_m, the maximum wavelength of the radiant-output curves, shifts to a shorter wavelength, as given by (2.44) and as shown in Figure 2.21(a).

Thus low temperatures yield a reddish color (infrared lamps) while high temperatures yield a bluish color (photoflood lamps). The total radiation is given by (2.45). Hence the radiant output increases rapidly with temperature, as does the efficiency, the evaporation of tungsten and the blackening of the glass bulb. The life of the filament is thus drastically shortened by higher temperatures.

Filaments are usually coiled to increase their emissivity and efficiency (Laurin, 1974). For use in instruments, short linear coils may be arranged within a compact, nearly square area lying in a single plane. To produce a source of uniform radiant output over a substantial area, ribbon filaments may be used.

Tungsten-halogen lamps have iodine or bromine added to the gases normally used to fill the bulb. The small quartz bulbs operate at temperatures above 250°C and usually require cooling by a blower. The halogen combines with tungsten at the wall. The resulting gas migrates back to the filament, where it decomposes and deposits tungsten on the filament. As a result, these lamps maintain more than 90% of their initial radiant output throughout their life. The radiant output of a conventional lamp, on the other hand, declines as much as 50% over its lifetime.

Arc discharges

The fluorescent lamp is filled with a low-pressure Ar-Hg mixture. Electrons are accelerated and collide with the gas atoms, which are raised to an excited level. As a given atom's electron undergoes a transition from a higher level to a lower level, the atom emits a quantum of energy. The energy per quantum E is (Elenbaas, 1972):

$$E = h\nu = \frac{hc}{\lambda} \tag{2.46}$$

where

h = Planck's constant (Appendix)
ν = frequency
c = velocity of light (Appendix)
λ = wavelength

or

$$\lambda = \frac{hc}{E}$$

Example 2.4 Find the formula that relates wavelength λ in nanometers to quantum energy E_w in electron volts.

Answer 1 J = 1 C × 1 V. Because the charge on an electron is -1.602×10^{-19} C (Appendix), the energy of one electron volt is 1 eV = 1.602×10^{-19} J. Hence

$$\lambda = \frac{hc}{E_w} = \frac{(6.63 \times 10^{-34} \text{ J} \cdot \text{s})(3 \times 10^8 \text{ m/s})}{(E_w)(1.602 \times 10^{-19} \text{ J/eV})}$$

$$= \frac{1.24 \times 10^{-6}}{E_w} \text{ m}$$

$$= \frac{1240}{E_w} \text{ nm}$$

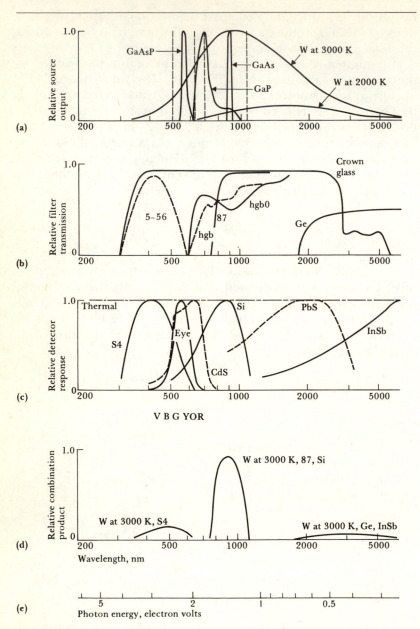

Figure 2.21 Spectral characteristics of sources, filters, detectors, and combinations of these. (a) Light sources. Tungsten (W) at 3000 K has a broad spectral output. At 2000 K output is lower at all wavelengths and peak output shifts to longer wavelengths. Light-emitting diodes yield a narrow spectral output with GaAs in the infrared, GaP in the red, and GaAsP in the green. Monochromatic outputs from common lasers are shown by dashed lines: Ar, 515 nm; HeNe, 633 nm; ruby, 693 nm; Nd, 1064 nm; CO_2 (not shown), 10,600 nm. (b) Filters. A Corning 5-56 glass filter passes a blue wavelength band. A Kodak 87 gelatin filter passes infrared and blocks visible wavelengths. Germanium lenses pass long wavelengths that cannot be passed by glass. Hemoglobin and oxyhemoglobin pass equally

Because the strongest transition of the mercury atom corresponds to about 5 eV, Figure 2.21(e) shows the resulting wavelength to be about 250 nm. A phosphor on the inside of the glass bulb absorbs this ultraviolet radiation and emits light of longer, visible wavelengths. The fluorescent lamp has low radiant output per unit area, so it is not used in optical instruments. However, it can be rapidly turned on and off in about 20 μs, so it is used in the *tachistoscope* (which presents brief stimuli to the eye) used in measurements of visual perception. Other low-pressure discharge lamps include the glowlamp (such as the neon lamp), the sodium-vapor lamp, and the laser.

High-pressure discharge lamps are more important for optical instruments because the arc is compact and the radiant output per unit area is high. The carbon arc has been in use for the longest time, but has largely been replaced by the mercury lamp (bluish-green color), the sodium lamp (yellow color), and the xenon lamp (white color). These lamps usually have a clear quartz bulb with electrodes at both ends of the spherical bulb. The zirconium arc lamp provides an intense point source.

Light-emitting diodes (LEDs)

LEDs are *p-n* junction devices that are optimized for radiant output (Gooch, 1973). The ordinary silicon *p-n* junction characteristic shown in Figure 2.22 emits radiant power when a current (typically 20 mA) passes in the forward direction. Spontaneous recombination of injected hole and electron pairs results in the emission of radiation. Because the silicon band gap is 1.1 eV, the wavelength is at about 1100 nm. The silicon device is not efficient. However, GaAs has a slightly higher band gap, as shown in Figure 2.22, and therefore radiates at 900 nm, as shown in Figure 2.21(a). Although the output is not visible, the efficiency is high and the GaAs device is widely used. It can be switched in less than 10 ns.

Figure 2.21(c) and (e) shows that, in order to produce visible light, the band gap of a *p-n* junction must exceed 1.9 eV. The GaP LED in Figure 2.22 has a band gap of 2.26 eV, requires a larger forward-bias voltage than silicon diodes, and is electroluminescent

at 805 nm and have maximum difference at 660 nm. (c) Detectors. The S4 response is a typical phototube response. The eye has a relatively narrow response, with colors indicated by VBGYOR. CdS plus a filter has a response that closely matches that of the eye. Si *p-n* junctions are widely used. PbS is a sensitive infrared detector. InSb is useful in far infrared. Note: These are only relative responses. Peak responses of different detectors differ by 10^7. (d) Combination. Indicated curves from (a), (b), and (c) are multiplied at each wavelength to yield (d), which shows how well source, filter, and detector are matched. (e) Photon energy: If it is less than 1 eV, it is too weak to cause current flow in Si *p-n* junctions.

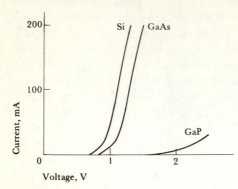

Figure 2.22 Forward characteristics for *p-n* junctions. Ordinary silicon diodes have a band gap of 1.1 eV and are inefficient radiators in the near-infrared. GaAs has a band gap of 1.44 eV and radiates at 900 nm. GaP has a band gap of 2.26 eV and radiates at 700 nm.

at 700 nm, as shown in Figure 2.21(a). It is an efficient visible LED and produces a bright red light. GaAsP LEDs make use of a special phosphor that absorbs two photons at one wavelength and emits a single photon at a shorter wavelength. GaAs is Si doped to emit radiation at 940 nm. Power at this wavelength is absorbed by the phosphor coating that emits green light at 540 nm, as shown in Figure 2.21(a). The decay time of the phosphor is about 1 ms.

LEDs are compact, rugged, economical, nearly monochromatic, and widely used in a variety of medical, transportation, and industrial circuits (Hertz, 1970).

Lasers

Laser (*Light Amplification by Stimulated Emission of Radiation*) action can occur in GaAs. The end faces perpendicular to the *p-n* junction are polished to serve as partial mirrors, thus forming a resonant optical cavity (Gooch, 1973). The forward current pumps a large population of the molecules to an excited energy level. Radiation incident on the molecules causes the production of additional radiation that is identical in character. This phenomenon is known as *stimulated emission*, and is produced by the feedback from the mirrors. Laser output is highly monochromatic, collimated (parallel), and phase-coherent. However, *p-n* junction lasers are not widely used because they operate in the infrared and require current densities of 10^3 A/cm^2 or more, thus requiring pulsed (10–100 ns) operation rather than CW (continuous wave).

The most common laser is the He-Ne laser that operates at 633 nm in the red region, as shown in Figure 2.21(a). The laser is operated by a low-pressure arc similar to a neon sign and provides up to 100 mW. Partially reflective mirrors at each end provide the resonant optical cavity and laser action.

Argon lasers provide the highest continuous-power levels (1–15 W) in the visible part of the spectrum at 515 nm [Figure 2.21(a)]. This high-power output permits photocoagulation of blood vessels in the eyes of patients suffering from diabetic retinopathy.

CO_2 lasers provide 50–500 W of CW output power and are used for cutting plastics, rubber, and metals up to 1 cm thick.

Two solid-state lasers—both usually operated in the pulsed mode—are widely used. The lasers are pumped by firing a flash tube that is wound around them. The ruby laser has a moderate (1 mJ) output in the red region of the spectrum at 693 nm, as shown in Figure 2.21(a). The neodymium in yttrium aluminum garnet (Nd:YAG) laser has a high (2 W/mm) output in the infrared region at 1064 nm, as shown in Figure 2.21(a).

The most important medical use of the laser has been to mend tears in the retina. A typical photocoagulator uses a pulsed ruby laser with a controllable output. It is focused on a tear in the retina. The heat dissipated by the pulse forms a burn which, on healing, develops scar tissue that mends the original tear (Smith, 1970). Section 12.8 provides further information on therapeutic applications of lasers.

Safety to the eye should be considered with respect to some light sources. It is safe to look at a 100-W frosted light bulb for long periods of time. However, looking at clear incandescent lamps, the sun, high-pressure arc sources, or lasers can cause burns on the retina. Protective eyewear worn by the physician to protect against lasers usually consists of a set of filters that attenuate at the specific wavelengths emitted by the laser, but transmit as much visible radiation as possible (Laurin, 1974).

2.14 Geometrical and fiber optics

Geometrical optics

There are a number of geometric factors that modify the power transmitted between the source and the detector. In Figure 2.20(b), the most obvious optical elements are the lenses. The lamp emits radiation in all directions. The first lens should have as small an *f number* (ratio of focal length to diameter) as practical. Thus it collects the largest practical solid angle of radiation from the lamp. The first lens is usually placed one focal length away from the lamp, so that the resulting radiation is *collimated* (that is, the rays are parallel). Thus, for a point source, the second lens can be placed at any distance without losing any radiation. Also some interference filters operate best in collimated rays.

The second lens focuses the radiation on a small area of sample in the cuvette. Since the radiation now diverges, third and fourth lenses are used to collect all the radiation and focus it on a detector. Some spectrophotometers [Fig. 2.20(c)] transmit collimated radiation through the sample section. The lenses may be coated with a coating that is a quarter-wavelength thick to prevent reflective losses at air–glass surfaces. Full mirrors may be used to fold the optical path to produce a compact instrument. Half-silvered mirrors enable users to split the beam into two beams for analysis or to combine two beams for analysis by a single detector. Curved mirrors may function as lenses for wavelengths that are absorbed by normal glass lenses.

Scattered radiation must be prevented from reaching the detector. Internal support structures and mechanical components of optical instruments are internally painted flat black to prevent scattered radiation. Stops (apertures that pass only the desired beam size) may be placed at several locations along the instrument's optical axis to trap scattered radiation.

Fiber optics

Fiber optics are an efficient way of transmitting radiation from one point to another (Allan, 1973). Transparent glass or plastic fiber with a refractive index n_1 is coated or surrounded by a second material of a lower refractive index n_2. By Snell's law,

$$n_2 \sin \theta_2 = n_1 \sin \theta_1 \tag{2.47}$$

where θ is the angle of incidence shown in Figure 2.23. Because $n_1 > n_2$, $\sin \theta_2 > \sin \theta_1$, so that $\sin \theta_2 = 1.0$ for a value of θ_1 that is less than 90°. For values of θ_1 greater than this, $\sin \theta_2$ is greater than unity, which is impossible, and the ray is internally reflected. The critical angle for reflection (θ_{ic}) is found by setting $\sin \theta_2 = 1.0$, which gives

$$\sin \theta_{ic} = \frac{n_2}{n_1} \tag{2.48}$$

A ray is internally reflected for all angles of incidence greater than θ_{ic}. Because rays entering the end of a fiber are usually refracted from air ($n = 1.0$) into glass ($n = 1.62$ for one type), a larger cone of radiation (θ_3) is accepted by a fiber than that indicated by calculations using $90° - \theta_{ic}$. Rays entering the end of the fiber at larger

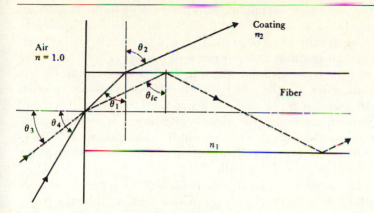

Figure 2.23 Fiber optics. The solid line shows refraction of rays that escape through the wall of the fiber. The dashed line shows total internal reflection within a fiber.

angles (θ_4) are not transmitted down the fiber; they escape through the walls.

Example 2.5 Find the angle θ_3 for the largest cone of light accepted from a medium of refractive index n that is totally reflected within a glass fiber of refractive index n_1 with a coating of refractive index n_2.

Answer At the interface of medium n and the glass, Snell's law (2.47) yields $n \sin \theta_3 = n_1 \sin (\theta_{ic} - 90°) = n_1 \cos \theta_{ic}$. Substituting this result into (2.48) yields

$$\frac{n_2}{n_1} = \sin \theta_{ic} = (1 - \cos^2 \theta_{ic})^{1/2} = \left(1 - \frac{n^2}{n_1^2} \sin^2 \theta_3\right)^{1/2}$$

$$\frac{n_2^2}{n_1^2} = 1 - \frac{n^2}{n_1^2} \sin^2 \theta_3$$

Rearranging and taking the square root,

$$\frac{n}{n_1} \sin \theta_3 = \frac{(n_1^2 - n_2^2)^{1/2}}{n_1}$$

yields

$$\sin \theta_3 = \frac{1}{n} (n_1^2 - n_2^2)^{1/2}$$

A 50-cm glass fiber exhibits a transmission exceeding 60% for wavelengths between 400 and 1200 nm. A 50-cm plastic fiber has a transmission exceeding 70% for wavelengths between 500 and 850 nm. Although a single fiber is useful for sampling incident radiation of a small area, most applications use flexible bundles of about 400 fibers. In *noncoherent bundles* (called *light guides*), the diameter of a fiber is typically 13 to 100 nm. There is no correlation between a fiber's spatial position at the input and output. These fibers are useful only for transmitting radiation. In one application, light is transmitted through the flexible bundle for viewing internal organs. In a second application, an instrument that measures blood oxygen saturation within the vessels alternately transmits radiation at two wavelengths down one bundle. The radiation is backscattered by the red-blood cells and returned to the instrument for analysis through a second bundle.

In *coherent-fiber bundles,* the fibers occupy the same relative position at both end faces. An image at one end is faithfully transmitted to the other end. The most important medical application of these fibers is in the *endoscope* (a tube for examining body cavities through natural openings). A typical endoscope is 1 m long and 1 cm in diameter and may be used for viewing the lining of the stomach, intestines, and so forth. A noncoherent bundle transmits light for illumination. A small lens focuses the image of the lining onto the end of a coherent bundle, which transmits the image in such a way that it may be viewed or photographed. External levers make it possible to steer the internal end of the optical-fiber device over a 360° range so that the examining physician may look at cavity walls and around corners.

Liquid crystals

Liquid crystals (Laurin, 1974) change their state in such a way that they modify passive scattering or absorption of light. As the crystals melt, the three-dimensional order becomes a two-dimensional or one-dimensional order. Layers or strands form that can be seen as a clarification of the previously turbid melt.

In one medical application, the patient's body is painted with a black water-soluble varnish, to show up the color of the liquid crystals better. Liquid crystals are painted over the varnish, and any inflammation causes a rise in temperature that is indicated by a color pattern. Liquid crystals are also used in measurement of oral temperatures, in the disposable thermometers discussed previously. They are also widely used in wristwatches because a low-voltage (1–15 V), low-power (1 μW/cm^2) electric field causes observable changes in digital-display elements (Gurtler, 1972).

2.15 Optical filters

Filters

Filters are frequently inserted in the optical system to control the distribution of radiant power or wavelength. To reduce radiant power only, neutral-density filters are used. When glass is partially silvered, most of the power is reflected and the desired fraction of the power is transmitted. When carbon particles are suspended in plastic, most of the power is absorbed and the desired fraction of the power is transmitted. Two Polaroid filters may also be used to attenuate the light. Each filter transmits only that portion of the light that is in a particular state of polarization. As one is rotated with respect to the other, the optical transmission of the combination varies.

Color filters transmit certain wavelengths and reject others. Gelatin filters are the most common type of absorption filters. An organic dye is dissolved in an aqueous gelatin solution and a thin film dried on a glass substrate. An example shown in Figure 2.21(b) is the infrared Kodak 87 Wratten filter. Glass filters, made by combining additives with the glass itself in its molten state, are extensively used. They provide rather broad passbands, as shown by the blue Corning 5-56 filter shown in Figure 2.21(b).

Interference filters are formed by depositing a reflective stack of layers on both sides of a thicker spacer layer. This sandwich construction provides multiple reflection and interference effects that yield sharp-edge high, low, and bandpass filters with bandwidths from 0.5 to 200 nm. Interference filters are usually used with collimated radiation and cost more than those just mentioned. Interference coatings are used on dichroic mirrors (cold mirrors), which reflect visible radiation from projection lamps. The nonuseful infrared radiation is transmitted through the coating and mirror to the outside of the optical system. This reduces heat within the optical system without sacrificing the useful light.

Diffraction gratings are widely used to produce a wavelength spectrum in the spectrometer. Plane gratings are formed by cutting thousands of closely spaced parallel grooves in a material. The grating is overcoated with aluminum, which reflects and disperses white light into a diffraction spectrum. A narrow slit selects a narrow band of wavelengths for use.

Although clear glass is not ordinarily thought of as a filter, Figure 2.21(b) shows that crown glass does not transmit below 300 nm (Mauro, 1963). For instruments that operate in the ultraviolet, fused quartz (silica glass) is used. Most glasses do not transmit well above 2600 nm, so instrument makers use either curved mirrors for infrared instruments or lenses made of Ge, Si, AsS_3, CaF_2, or Al_2O_3.

Oxygen saturation

The purpose of the optical instrument is usually to measure the concentration of a body substance placed in a cuvette. As an example, let us take the principle of an oximeter, which measures the fraction of hemoglobin (hgb) that is present in the form of oxyhemoglobin (hgbO). For *hemolyzed blood* (blood with red cells ruptured), Beer's law (Section 10.1) holds and the *absorbance* (optical density) at any wavelength is (Allan, 1973)

$$A(\lambda) = WL[a_o(\lambda)C_o + a_r(\lambda)C_r] \tag{2.49}$$

where

$$W = \text{weight of hemoglobin per unit volume}$$
$$L = \text{optical path length}$$
$$a_o \text{ and } a_r = \text{absorptivities of hgbO and hgb}$$
$$C_o \text{ and } C_r = \text{relative concentrations of hgbO and hgb}$$
$$(C_o + C_r = 1.0)$$

Figure 2.21(b) shows that a_o and a_r are equal at 805 nm, called the isobestic wavelength. If this wavelength is λ_2, then

$$WL = \frac{A(\lambda_2)}{2a(\lambda_2)} \tag{2.50}$$

where

$$a(\lambda_2) = a_o(\lambda_2) = a_r(\lambda_2) \tag{2.51}$$

Therefore

$$A(\lambda) = \frac{A(\lambda_2)}{2a(\lambda_2)} [a_o(\lambda)C_o + a_r(\lambda)C_r] \tag{2.52}$$

When absorbance is measured at a second wavelength λ_1, the oxygen saturation is given by

$$C_o = x + \frac{yA(\lambda_1)}{A(\lambda_2)} \tag{2.53}$$

where x and y are constants that depend only on the optical characteristics of blood. In practice λ_1 is chosen to be that wavelength at which the difference between a_o and a_r is a maximum, which occurs at 660 nm [see Figure 2.21(b)].

Oximeters may use interference filters in the form shown in Figure 2.20(b). They have been built as shown in Figure 2.20(c), using LEDs selected for proper wavelengths. One form uses fiber optics to transmit the wavelengths into and back from the blood within the vessels. Oximeters can be used to noninvasively measure %O_2 saturation by passing light through the pinna of the ear (Merrick and Hayes, 1976). Because of the complications caused by the light-absorbing characteristics of skin pigment and other absorbers, measurements are made at eight wavelengths and computer-processed. The ear is warmed to 41°C to stimulate arterial blood flow.

2.16 Radiation detectors

Radiation detectors may be classified into two general categories: thermal detectors and quantum detectors (Mauro, 1963).

Thermal detectors

The thermal detector absorbs radiation and transforms it into heat, thus causing a rise in temperature in the device. Typical detectors are the thermistor and the thermocouple. Sensitivity of a detector does not change with (is flat with) wavelength, and the detector has slow response [Figure 2.21(c)]. Changes in output due to changes in ambient temperature cannot be distinguished from changes in output due to the source, so a windmill-shaped mechanical chopper is frequently used to periodically interrupt the radiation from the source.

The *pyroelectric detector* (Laurin, 1974) absorbs radiation and converts it into heat. The resulting rise in temperature changes the polarization of the crystals, which produces a current proportional to the rate of change of temperature. As it is for the piezoelectric crystal, dc response is zero, so a chopper is required for dc measurements.

Quantum detectors

Quantum detectors absorb energy from individual photons and use it to release electrons from the detector material. Typical detectors are the eye, the phototube, the photodiode, and photographic emulsion. Detectors are sensitive over only a restricted band of wavelengths; most respond rapidly. Changes in ambient temperature cause only a second-order change in sensitivity of these devices.

Photoemissive detectors

These detectors—an example is the *phototube*—have photocathodes coated with alkali metals. If the energy of the photons of the incoming radiation is sufficient to overcome the work function of the photocathode, the forces that bind electrons to the photocathode are overcome, and it emits electrons. Electrons are attracted to a more positive anode and form a current that is measured by an external circuit. Photon energies below 1 eV are not large enough to overcome the work function, so wavelengths longer than 1200 nm cannot be detected. Figure 2.21(c) shows the spectral response of the most common photocathode, the S4, which has lower sensitivity in the ultraviolet region because of absorption of radiation in the glass envelope.

The *photomultiplier* shown in Figure 2.24 is a phototube combined with an electron multiplier (Lion, 1975). Each accelerated electron hits the first dynode with enough energy to liberate several electrons by secondary emission. These are accelerated to the second dynode, where the process is repeated, and so on. Time response is less than 10 ns. Photomultipliers are the most sensitive photodetectors. When they are cooled (to prevent electrons from being thermally generated), they can count individual photons. The eye is almost as sensitive; under the most favorable conditions, it can detect six photons arriving in a small area within 100 ms.

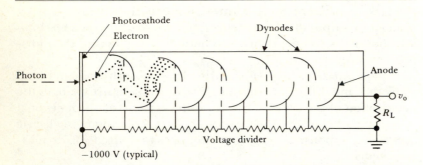

Figure 2.24 In the photomultiplier, an incoming photon strikes the photocathode and liberates an electron. This electron is accelerated toward the first dynode, which is 100 V more positive than the cathode. The impact liberates several electrons by secondary emission. They are accelerated toward the second dynode, which is 100 V more positive than the first dynode. This electron multiplication continues until the anode, where currents of about 1 μA flow through R_L.

Photoconductive cells

Photoresistors are the simplest solid-state photoelectric devices. A photosensitive crystalline material such as CdS or PbS [Figure 2.21(c)] is deposited on a ceramic substrate and ohmic electrodes are attached. If a photon of the incoming radiation has sufficient energy to jump the band gap, hole-electron pairs are produced because the electron is raised from the valence band to the conduction band. The presence of the electrons in the conduction band and the holes in the valence band increases the conductivity of the crystalline material so that the resistance decreases with input radiation. Photocurrent is linear at low levels of radiation, but nonlinear at levels that are normally used. It is independent of the polarity of applied voltage. After a step increase or decrease of radiation, the photocurrent response rises and decays with a time constant of from 10 to 0.01 s, depending on whether the radiation is low or high.

Photojunction devices

Photojunction devices are formed from p-n junctions and are usually made of silicon. If a photon has sufficient energy to jump the band gap, hole-electron pairs are produced that modify the junction characteristics, as shown in Figure 2.25. If the junction is reverse-biased, the reverse photocurrent increases linearly with an increase in radiation. The resulting photodiode responds in about 1 μs. In phototransistors, the base lead is not connected and the resulting radiation-generated base current is multiplied by the current gain (beta) of the transistor to yield a large current from collector to emitter. The radiation-current characteristics have a nonlinearity of about 2% because beta varies with collector current. The response time is about 10 μs. Silicon p-n junctions are also manufactured as photo Darlington transistors, photo FETs, photo unijunction transistors, and photo SCRs. Photon couplers are LED-photodiode combinations that are used for isolating electrical circuits. For example, they are used for breaking ground loops and for preventing dangerous levels of current from leaking out of equipment and entering the heart of a patient (Section 13.9).

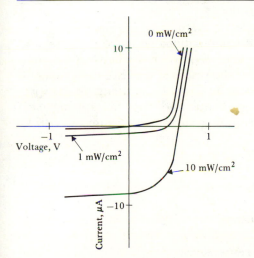

Figure 2.25 Voltage-current characteristics of irradiated silicon p-n junction. For 0 irradiance, both forward and reverse characteristics are normal. For 1 mW/cm², open-circuit voltage is 500 mV and short-circuit current is 0.8 μA. For 10 mW/cm², open-circuit voltage is 600 mV and short-circuit current is 8 μA.

Photovoltaic devices

The same silicon p-n junction can be used in the photovoltaic mode. Figure 2.25 shows that there is an open-circuit voltage when the junction receives radiation. The voltage rises logarithmically from 100 to 500 mV as the input radiation increases by a factor of 10^4. This is the principle of the solar cell that is used for the direct conversion of the sun's radiation into electric power.

Spectral response

All of the aforementioned silicon devices have the spectral response shown in Figure 2.21(c). There is no response above 1100 nm because the energy of the photons is too low to permit them to jump the band gap. For wavelengths shorter than 900 nm, the response drops off because there are fewer, more-energetic photons per watt. Each photon generates only one hole-electron pair.

Because none of the common detectors are capable of measuring the radiation emitted by the skin (300 K), which has a peak output at 9000 nm, special detectors have been developed, such as the InSb detector shown in Figure 2.21(c).

2.17 Optical combinations

In order to specify the combinations of sources, filters, and detectors, instrument designers require radiometric units that must be weighted according to the response curve of each element. E_e, the total effective irradiance, is found by breaking up the spectral curves into many narrow bands and then multiplying each together and adding the resulting increments (Stimson, 1974). Thus

$$E_e = \Sigma S_\lambda F_\lambda D_\lambda \ \Delta \lambda \tag{2.54}$$

where

S_λ = relative source output
F_λ = relative filter transmission
D_λ = relative detector responsivity

Figure 2.21(d) shows several results of this type of calculation. One of the examples shown is an efficient system capable of making measurements in the dark without stimulating the eye. Such a device can be used for tracking eye movements. It can be formed from a tungsten source, a Kodak 87 Wratten filter, and a silicon detector. If GaAs provides enough output, it can replace both the tungsten source and the Kodak 87 Wratten filter (Young and Sheena, 1975).

Problems

2.1 For Figure P2.1, plot the ratio of the output voltage to the input voltage v_o/v_i as a function of the displacement x_i of a potentiometer with a total displacement x_t for ranges of R_m, the input resistance of the meter. Show that the maximum error occurs in the neighborhood of $x_i/x_t = 0.67$. What is the value of this maximum error?

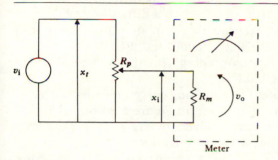

Meter

Figure P2.1

2.2 The practical limitation for wire spacing in potentiometer construction is between 20 and 40 turns/mm. Find the resolution limitation for a translational and a rotational potentiometer. Propose a way to increase the resolution of a rotational potentiometer.

2.3 Discuss some of the possible problems involved in elastic-resistance strain-gage units and their solutions.

2.4 Show that, for (2.8), the deviation from ideal linearity is $= \frac{1}{2}(\Delta R/R_0)$

2.5 Verify (2.25) for the transformer ratio-arm bridge.

2.6 The electromotive force E for a thermocouple is given by (2.34). Calculate and plot E for conditions in which the reference source is at 0°C and temperature varies from 0 to 50°C. The thermocouple material is copper constantan with $a = 38.7\ \mu V/°C$ and $b = 0.082\ \mu V/°C^2$. How significant is the second term in your calculations? Note that these calculated curves are not exactly satisfied in the practical situation. Thus an experimental calibration must be measured over the range of interest.

2.7 Using the results of Problem 2.6, calculate the sensitivity α at 37°C for the copper-constantan thermocouple.

2.8 Calculate the value of the thermistor temperature coefficient α for $T = 300$ K and $\beta = 4000$ K.

2.9 For the LVDT shown in Figure 2.6(c), sketch the voltages $c-e$, $d-e$, and $c-d$ as the core is displaced through its normal range.

2.10 For a 1-cm² capacitance transducer, R is 100 MΩ.

What is x, the plate spacing required to pass sound frequencies above 20 Hz?

2.11 What part of the circuit shown in Figure 2.9(b) is connected to the guard in Figure 2.9(a)? Sketch the resulting field lines.

2.12 For Example 2.3, what size shunting capacitor should be added to extend the low corner frequency to 0.05 Hz, as is required to detect pulse waveforms? How is the sensitivity changed?

2.13 Sketch typical thermistor v-i characteristics with and without a heat sink. Explain why there is a difference.

2.14 Calculate and sketch a curve for the radiant output of the skin at 300 K at 2000, 5000, 10,000, and 20,000 nm.

2.15 Calculate the photon energy for the peak wavelength given off by the skin at 300 K.

2.16 Sketch an optical system using curved mirrors instead of lenses that could replace that shown in Figure 2.20(b).

2.17 Oxygen saturation is given by $C_o = x + yA(\lambda_1)/A(\lambda_2)$. Solve for x and y in terms of known quantities.

2.18 Sketch the circuit for a photo Darlington transistor, which is two cascaded emitter-follower transistors. Estimate its linearity and response time.

2.19 For the solar cell shown in Figure 2.25, what value load resistor would receive the maximum power?

2.20 For the photomultiplier shown in Figure 2.24, when R_L is high enough for adequate sensitivity, the stray capacity–R_L product produces a time constant that is too long. Design a circuit that is ten times faster and has no loss in sensitivity.

2.21 For Figure 2.21(d), plot the relative combination product for GaP, hgbO, CdS.

References

Allan, W. B., *Fibre optics theory and practice*. New York: Plenum, 1973.

Allard, E.M. "Sound and pressure signals obtained from a single intracardiac transducer." *IRE Trans. Bio-Med. Electron.*, 1962, BME-9, 74–77.

Anonymous, *Manual on the use of thermocouples in temperature measurement*. Publication 470A. Philadelphia: American Society for Testing and Materials, 1974.

Anonymous, "A matter of degrees." *DuPont Magazine*, 1975, 69(5), 12–13.

Beakley, W.R., "The design of thermistor thermometers with linear calibration." *J. Sci. Instrum.*, 1951, 28, 176–179.

Bryce, C.H., and V.H.R. Hole, "Measurement and control by thermistors." *Ind. Electron.*, 1967, 5(1), 294–296; 1967, 5(2), 358–363.

Cobbold, R.S.C., *Transducers for biomedical measurements*. New York: Wiley, 1974.

Cook, N.H., and E. Rabinowicz, *Physical measurement and analysis*. Reading, MA: Addison-Wesley, 1963.

Doebelin, E.O., *Measurement systems: Application and design*, 2nd ed. New York: McGraw-Hill, 1975.

Elenbaas, L., *Light sources*. New York: Crane, Russak, 1972.

Geddes, L.A., and L.E. Baker, *Principles of applied biomedical instrumentation*, 2nd ed. New York: Wiley, 1975.

Gooch, C.H., *Injection electroluminescent devices*. New York: Wiley, 1973.

Gurtler, R.W., and C. Maze, "Liquid crystal displays." *IEEE Spectrum*, Nov. 1972, 25–29.

Hardy, J.D. (ed.), *Biology and medicine*, in C.M. Herzfeld (ed.), *Temperature: Its measurement and control in science and industry*. New York: Reinhold, 1962, vol. III, part 3.

Hertz, L.M., *Solid state lamps theory and characteristics manual*. Cleveland, OH: General Electric Co., 1970.

Hokanson, D.E., D.S. Sumner, and D.E. Strandness, Jr., "An electrically calibrated plethysmograph for direct measurement of limb blood flow." *IEEE Trans. Biomed. Eng.*, 1975, BME-22, 25–29.

Laurin, T.C. (ed.), *The optical industry and systems directory*, 21st ed. Pittsfield, MA: Optical Publishing Co., 1974, vol. 2.

Lawton, R.W., and C.C. Collins, "Calibration of an aortic circumference gauge." *J. Appl. Physiol.*, 1959, 14, 465–467.

Lion, K.S., *Elements of electronic and electrical instrumentation*. New York: McGraw-Hill, 1975.

Lion, K.S., *Instrumentation in scientific research*. New York: McGraw-Hill, Inc., 1959.

Mauro, J.A. (ed.), *Optical engineering handbook*. Scranton, PA: General Electric Co., 1963.

Merrick, E.B., and T.J. Hayes, "Continuous, non-invasive measurements of arterial blood oxygen levels." *Hewlett-Packard Journal*, Oct. 1976, 28(2), 2–9.

Nancollas, G.H., and J.A. Hardy, "A thermistor bridge for use in calorimetry." *J. Sci. Instrum.*, 1967, 45, 290–292.

Neubert, H.K.P., *Instrument transducers*, 2nd ed. Oxford: Clarendon, 1975.

Norton, H.N., *Handbook of transducers for electronic measuring systems*. Englewood Cliffs, NJ: Prentice-Hall, 1969.

Podolak, E., J.B. Kinn, and E.E. Westura, "Biomedical applications of a commercial capacitance transducer." *IEEE Trans. Bio-Med. Eng.*, 1969, BME-16(1), 40–44.

Robertson, T. L., "Temperature measurement." *Med. Electron. Data*, 4(2), March 1973, 86–95.

Sachse, H.B., *Semiconducting temperature sensors and their applications*. New York: Wiley, 1975.

Sapoff, M., *Thermistors for biomedical use*. Fifth Symposium on

Temperature, Proceedings. Washington, D.C.: Instrument Society of America, 1971, 2109–2121.

Smith, W.V., *Laser applications*. Dedham, MA: Artech House, 1970.

Stimson, A., *Photometry and radiometry for engineers*. New York: Wiley, 1974.

van Citters, R.L., *Mutual inductance transducers,* in R.F. Rushmer (ed.), *Methods in medical research,* Vol. XI, Chicago: Year Book, 1966, 26–30.

Wolfe, W.L., *Handbook of military infrared technology*. Washington, D.C.: Office of Naval Research, 1965.

Young, L.R., and D. Sheena, "Survey of eye movement recording techniques." *Behav. Res. Methodol. Instrum.,* 1975, 7, 397–429.

Chapter three

Amplifiers and signal processing

John G. Webster

Most bioelectric signals are small, and require amplification. Amplifiers are also used for interfacing transducers that sense body motions, temperature, and chemical concentrations. In addition to simple amplification, the amplifier may also modify the signal to produce frequency filtering or nonlinear effects. This chapter emphasizes the *operational amplifier* (op amp), which has revolutionized electronic circuit design. Most circuit design was formerly performed with discrete components, requiring laborious calculations, many components, and large expense. Now a 50-cent op amp, a few resistors, and a knowledge of Ohm's law are all that is needed.

3.1 Ideal op amps

An *op amp* is a high-gain dc differential amplifier. It is normally used in circuits that have characteristics determined by external negative-feedback networks.

The best way to approach the design of a circuit that uses op amps is first to assume that the op amp is ideal. After the initial design, the circuit is checked to determine whether the nonideal characteristics of the op amp are important. If they are not, the design is complete; if they are, another design check is made, which may require additional components.

Ideal characteristics

Figure 3.1 shows the equivalent circuit for a nonideal op amp. It is a dc differential amplifier, which means that any differential voltage, $v_d = (v_2 - v_1)$, is multiplied by the very high gain A to produce the output voltage v_o. To simplify calculations, we assume the following characteristics for an ideal op amp:

1 $A = \infty$ (gain is infinity)
2 $v_o = 0$ when $v_1 = v_2$ (no offset voltage)

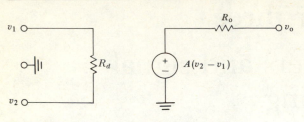

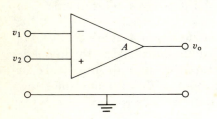

Figure 3.1 Op-amp equivalent circuit. The two inputs are v_1 and v_2. A differential voltage between them causes current flow through the differential resistance, R_d. The differential voltage is multiplied by A, the gain of the op amp, to generate the output-voltage source. Any current flowing to the output terminal v_0 must pass through the output resistance R_0.

3 $R_d = \infty$ (input impedance is infinity)
4 $R_0 = 0$ (output impedance is zero)
5 Bandwidth $= \infty$ (no frequency-response limitations) and no phase shift.

Later in the chapter we shall examine the effect on the circuit of characteristics that are not ideal.

Figure 3.2 shows the op-amp circuit symbol, which includes two differential input terminals and one output terminal. All these voltages are measured with respect to the ground shown. Power supplies, usually ± 15 V, must be connected to terminals indicated on the manufacturer's specification sheet (Anonymous, 1973).

Figure 3.2 Op-amp circuit symbol. A voltage at v_1, the inverting input, is greatly amplified and inverted to yield v_0. A voltage at v_2, the noninverting input, is greatly amplified to yield an in-phase output at v_0.

Two basic rules

Throughout this chapter we shall use two basic rules (or input terminal restrictions) that are very helpful in designing op-amp circuits.

Rule 1 When the op-amp output is in its linear range, the two input terminals are at the same voltage.

This is true because if the two input terminals were not at the same voltage, the differential input voltage would be multiplied by the infinite gain to yield an infinite output voltage. This is absurd, since op amps use a power supply of ± 15 V; therefore v_o is restricted to this range. Actually the op-amp specifications guarantee a linear output range of only ± 10 V, although most saturate at about ± 12 V.

Rule 2 No current flows into either input terminal of the op amp.

This is true because we assume that the input impedance is infinity, and no current flows into an infinite impedance. Even if the input impedance were finite, Rule 1 tells us that there is no voltage drop across R_d, so therefore no current flows.

3.2 Inverters

Circuit

Figure 3.3(a) shows the basic inverter circuit. It is widely used in analog computers as well as for instrumentation. Note that a portion of v_o is fed back via R_f to the negative input of the op amp. This provides the inverting amplifier with the many advantages associated with the use of negative feedback—increased bandwidth, lower output impedance, and so forth. If v_o is ever fed back to the positive input of the op amp, examine the circuit carefully. Either there is a mistake, or the circuit is one of the rare ones in which a regenerative action is desired.

Equation

Note that the positive input of the op amp is at 0 V. Therefore, by Rule 1, the negative input of the op amp is also at 0 V. Thus no matter what happens to the rest of the circuit, the negative input of the op amp remains at 0 V, a condition known as a *virtual ground*.

Since the right side of R_i is at 0 V and the left side is v_i, by Ohm's law, the current i through R_i is $i = v_i/R_i$. By Rule 2, no current can enter the op amp; therefore i must also flow through R_f. This produces a voltage drop across R_f of iR_f. Since the left end of R_f is at 0 V, the right end must be

$$v_o = -iR_f = -v_i \frac{R_f}{R_i} \qquad \text{or} \qquad \frac{v_o}{v_i} = \frac{-R_f}{R_i} \qquad (3.1)$$

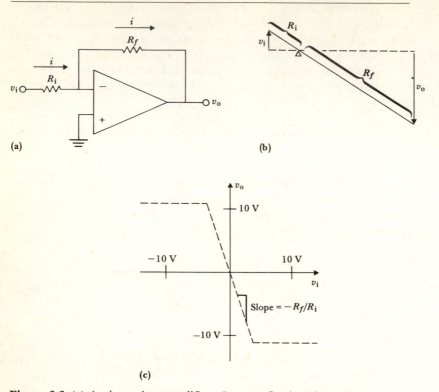

(a)

(b)

(c)

Figure 3.3 (a) An inverting amplifier. Current flowing through the input resistor R_i also flows through the feedback resistor R_f. (b) A lever with arm lengths proportional to resistance values enables the viewer to visualize the input-output characteristics easily. (c) The input-output plot shows a slope of $-R_f/R_i$ in the central portion, but the output saturates at about ± 12 V.

Thus the circuit inverts, and the *inverting-amplifier* gain (not the op-amp gain) is given by the ratio of R_f to R_i.

Lever analogy

Figure 3.3(b) shows an easy way to visualize the circuit's behavior. A lever is formed with arm lengths proportional to resistance values. Since the negative input is at 0 V, the fulcrum is placed at 0 V, as shown. If R_f is three times R_i, as shown, any variation of v_i results in a three-times-bigger variation of v_o.

Input-output characteristic

Figure 3.3(c) shows that the circuit is linear only over a limited range of v_i. When v_o exceeds about ± 12 V, it *saturates* (limits), and further increases in v_i produce no change in the output. The linear swing of v_0 is about 6 V less than the difference in power-supply voltages. Although op amps usually have power-supply voltages set at ± 15 V, reduced power-supply voltages may be used, with a corresponding reduction in the saturation voltages and the linear swing of v_0.

Summer

The inverter may be extended to form a circuit that yields the weighted sum of several input voltages. Each input voltage v_{i1}, $v_{i2}, \ldots, v_{ik}$ is connected to the negative input of the op amp by an individual resistor whose conductance $(1/R_{ik})$ is proportional to the desired weighting.

Example 3.1 The output of a biopotential preamplifier that measures the electro-oculogram (Section 4.7) is an undesired dc voltage of $+5$ V due to electrode half-cell potentials (Section 5.1), with a desired signal of ± 1 V superimposed. Design a circuit that will buck the dc voltage to zero and provide a gain of -10 for the desired signal without saturating the op amp.

Answer Figure E3.1(a) shows the design. We assume that v_b, the bucking voltage available from the 5-kΩ potentiometer, is ± 10 V. The undesired voltage at $v_i = 5$ V. For $v_0 = 0$, the current through R_f is zero. Therefore the sum of the currents through R_i and R_b is zero:

$$\frac{v_i}{R_i} + \frac{v_b}{R_b} = 0$$

$$R_b = \frac{-R_i v_b}{v_i} = \frac{-10^4(-10)}{5} = 2 \times 10^4 \ \Omega$$

For a gain of -10, (3.1) requires $R_f/R_i = 10$, or $R_f = 100$ kΩ. The circuit equation is

$$v_0 = -R_f \left(\frac{v_i}{R_i} + \frac{v_b}{R_b} \right)$$

$$v_0 = -10^5 \left(\frac{v_i}{10^4} + \frac{v_b}{2 \times 10^4} \right)$$

$$v_0 = -10 \left(v_i + \frac{v_b}{2} \right)$$

The potentiometer can buck out any undesired voltage in the range ± 5 V, as shown by Figure E3.1(b).

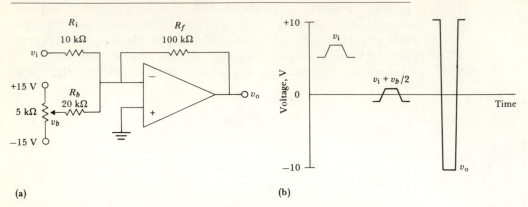

(a)   (b)

Figure E3.1 (a) This circuit sums the input voltage v_i plus one-half of the bucking voltage v_b. Thus the output voltage v_o can be set to zero even when v_i has a nonzero dc component. (b) The three waveforms show v_i, the input voltage; $(v_i + v_b/2)$, the bucked-out voltage; and v_o, the amplified output voltage. If v_i were directly amplified, the op amp would saturate.

3.3 Followers

Voltage follower

Figure 3.4(a) shows the circuit for a unity-gain follower. Since v_i exists at the positive input of the op amp, by Rule 1, v_i must also exist at the negative input. But v_o is also connected to the negative input. Therefore $v_o = v_i$, or the output voltage follows the input voltage. At first glance it seems as if nothing is gained by using this circuit, since the output is the same as the input. However, the circuit is very useful as a buffer, to prevent a high source resistance from being loaded down by a low-resistance load. By Rule 2, no current flows into the positive input, and therefore the source resistance in the external circuit is not loaded at all.

Follower with gain

Figure 3.4(b) shows how the follower circuit can be modified to produce gain. By Rule 1, v_i appears at the negative input of the op amp. This causes current $i = v_i/R_i$ to flow to ground. By Rule 2, none of i can come from the negative input; therefore all must flow through R_f. We can then calculate $v_o = i(R_f + R_i)$ and solve for the gain.

$$\frac{v_o}{v_i} = \frac{i(R_f + R_i)}{iR_i} = \frac{R_f + R_i}{R_i} \tag{3.2}$$

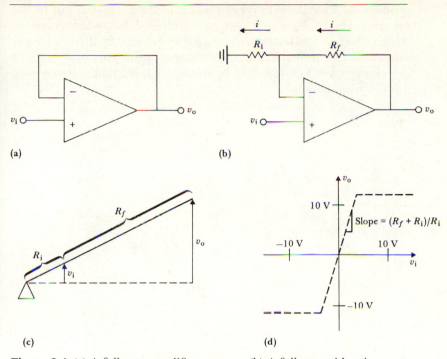

Figure 3.4 (a) A follower amplifier, $v_o = v_i$. (b) A follower with gain, v_i appears across R_i, which also flows through R_f. (c) A lever with arm lengths proportional to resistance values makes possible an easy visualization of input-output characteristics. (d) The input-output plot shows a positive slope of $(R_f + R_i)/R_i$ in the central portion, but the output saturates at about ± 12 V.

We note that the circuit gain (not the op-amp gain) is positive, always ≥ 1; and that if $R_i = \infty$ (open circuit), the circuit reduces to Figure 3.4(a).

Figure 3.4(c) shows how a lever makes possible an easy visualization of the input-output characteristics. The fulcrum is placed at the left end, since R_i is grounded at the left end. Because v_i appears between the two resistors, it provides an input at the central part of the diagram. v_o travels through an output excursion determined by the lever arms.

Figure 3.4(d), the input-output characteristic, shows that a one-op-amp circuit can have a positive amplifier gain. Again saturation is evident.

3.4 Differential amplifiers

One-op-amp differential amplifier

The right side of Figure 3.5(a) shows a simple one-op-amp differential amplifier. Current flows from v_4 through R_3 and R_4 to ground. By Rule 2, no current flows into the positive input of the op amp. Hence R_3 and R_4 act as a simple voltage-divider atten-uator, which is unaffected by having the op amp attached or by any other changes in the circuit. The voltages in this part of the circuit are visualized in Figure 3.5(b) by the single lever that is attached to the fulcrum (ground).

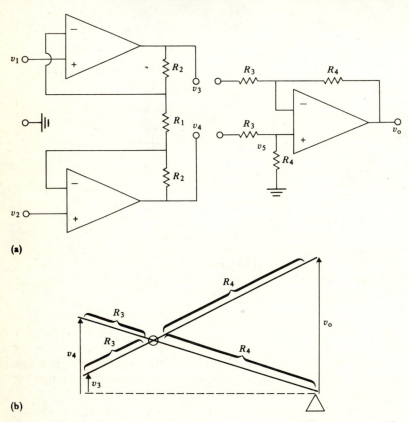

(a)

(b)

Figure 3.5 (a) The right side shows a one-op-amp differential amplifier, but it has low input impedance. The left side shows how two additional op amps can provide high input impedance and gain. (b) For the one-op-amp differential amplifier, two levers with arm lengths proportional to resistance values make possible an easy visualization of input-output characteristics.

By Rule 1, whatever voltage appears at the positive input also appears at the negative input. Once this voltage is fixed, the top half of the circuit behaves like an inverter. For example, if v_4 is 0 V, the positive input of the op amp is 0 V and the v_3-v_o circuit behaves exactly like an inverter. For other values of v_4, an inverting relation is obtained about some voltage intermediate between v_4 and 0 V. The relationship can be visualized in Figure 3.5(b) by noting that the two levers behave like a pair of scissors. The thumb and finger holes are v_4 and v_3 and the points are at v_o and 0 V.

We solve for the gain by finding v_5:

$$v_5 = \frac{v_4 R_4}{R_3 + R_4} \tag{3.3}$$

Then, solving for the current in the top half, we get

$$i = \frac{v_3 - v_5}{R_3} = \frac{v_5 - v_o}{R_4} \tag{3.4}$$

Substitution of (3.3) into (3.4) yields

$$v_o = \frac{(v_4 - v_3)R_4}{R_3} \tag{3.5}$$

This is the equation for a differential amplifier. If the two inputs are hooked together and driven by a common source, with respect to ground, then the *common-mode voltage* (CMV) is $v_3 = v_4$. Equation (3.5) shows that the output is 0. The differential amplifier circuit (not op amp) *common-mode gain* (CMG) is 0. In Figure 3.5(b), imagine the scissors to be closed. No matter how the inputs are varied, $v_o = 0$.

If on the other hand $v_3 \neq v_4$, then the differential voltage $(v_4 - v_3)$ produces an amplifier-circuit (not op-amp) *differential gain* (DG), that from (3.5) is equal to R_4/R_3. This result can be visualized in Figure 3.5(b) by noting that as the scissors open, v_o is geometrically related to $(v_4 - v_3)$ in the same ratio as the lever arms, R_4/R_3.

No differential amplifier perfectly rejects the common-mode voltage. To quantify this imperfection, we use the term *common-mode rejection ratio* (CMRR) that is defined as

$$\text{CMRR} = \frac{\text{DG}}{\text{CMG}} \tag{3.6}$$

This factor may be lower than 100 for some oscilloscope differential amplifiers and higher than 10,000 for a high-quality biopotential amplifier.

Three-op-amp differential amplifier

The one-op-amp differential amplifier is quite satisfactory for low-resistance sources, such as strain-gage Wheatstone bridges (Section 2.3). But the input resistance is too low for high-resistance sources. A first possibility is to add the simple follower shown in Figure 3.4(a) to each input. This provides the required buffering.

Since this solution uses two additional op amps, we may also obtain gain from these buffering amplifiers by using a follower with gain, as shown in Figure 3.4(b). However, this solution amplifies the common-mode voltage, as well as the differential voltage, so there is no improvement in CMRR.

A superior solution is achieved by hooking together the two R_i's of the followers with gain and eliminating the connection to ground. The result is shown on the left side of Figure 3.5(a). To examine the effects of common-mode voltage, assume that $v_1 = v_2$. By Rule 1, v_1 appears at both negative inputs to the op amps. This places the same voltage at both ends of R_1. Hence current through R_1 is 0. By Rule 2, no current can flow from the op-amp inputs. Hence the current through both R_2's is 0. So v_1 appears at both op-amp outputs and the CMG is 1.

To examine the effects when $v_1 \neq v_2$, we note that $v_1 - v_2$ appears across R_1. This causes a current to flow through R_1 that also flows through the resistor string R_2, R_1, R_2. Hence the output voltage

$$v_3 - v_4 = i(R_2 + R_1 + R_2)$$

while the input voltage

$$v_1 - v_2 = iR_1$$

The differential gain is then

$$\text{DG} = \frac{v_3 - v_4}{v_1 - v_2} = \frac{2R_2 + R_1}{R_1} \tag{3.7}$$

Since the CMG is 1, the CMRR is equal to the DG, which is usually much greater than 1. When the left and right halves of Figure 3.5(a) are combined, the resulting three-op-amp amplifier circuit is frequently called an *instrumentation amplifier*. It has high input impedance, high CMRR, and a gain that can be changed by adjusting R_1. This circuit finds wide use in measuring biopotentials (Section 6.7), since it rejects the large 60-Hz common-mode voltage that exists on the body.

3.5 Comparators

Simple

A comparator is a circuit that compares the input voltage with some reference voltage. The comparator's output flips from one saturation limit to the other, as the negative input of the op amp passes through 0 V. For v_i greater than the comparison level, the $v_o = -12$ V. For v_i less than the comparison level, $v_o = +12$ V. Thus this circuit performs the same function as a *Schmitt trigger*, which detects an analog voltage level and yields a logic level output. The simplest comparator is the op amp itself, as shown in Figure 3.2. If a reference voltage is connected to the positive input and v_i is connected to the negative input, the circuit is complete. The inputs may be interchanged to invert the output. The input circuit may be expanded by adding the two R_1 resistors shown in Figure 3.6(a). This provides a known input resistance for the circuit and minimizes overdriving the op-amp input. Figure 3.6(b) shows that the comparator flips when $v_i = -v_{ref}$. To avoid building a separate power supply for v_{ref}, one may connect v_{ref} to the -15-V power supply and adjust the values of the input resistors so that the negative input of the op amp is at 0 V when v_i is at the desired positive comparison level. When negative comparison levels are desired, v_{ref} is connected to the $+15$-V power supply.

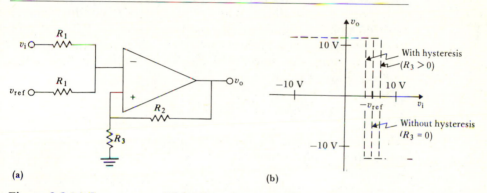

(a)   (b)

Figure 3.6 (a) Comparator. When $R_3 = 0$, v_o indicates whether $(v_i + v_{ref})$ is greater or less than 0 V. When R_3 is larger, the comparator has hysteresis, as shown in (b), the input-output characteristic

With hysteresis

For a simple comparator, if v_i is at the comparison level and there is noise on v_i, v_o fluctuates wildly. To prevent this, hysteresis may be added to the comparator, by adding R_2 and R_3, as shown in Figure 3.6(a). The effect of this positive feedback is illustrated by the input-output characteristics shown in Figure 3.6(b). To analyze this circuit, first assume that $v_{ref} = -5$ V and $v_i = +10$ V. Then, because the op amp inverts and saturates, $v_o = -12$ V. Divide v_o by R_2 and R_3, so that the positive input is at, say, -1 V. As v_i is lowered, the comparator does not flip until v_i reaches $+3$ V, which makes the negative input equal to the positive input, -1 V. At this point, v_o flips to $+12$ V, causing the positive input to change to $+1$

V. Noise on v_i cannot cause v_o to flip back, since the negative input must be raised to $+1$ V to cause the next flip. This requires v_i to be raised to $+7$ V, at which level the circuit can flip back to its original state. From this example, we see that the width of the hysteresis is four times as great as the magnitude of the voltage across R_3. The width of the hysteresis loop can be varied by replacing R_3 by a potentiometer.

Window comparator

Frequently we wish to know when v_i is between two comparison levels (that is, when it lies within a certain range). Such a *window comparator* (Tobey, 1971) could be formed from two simpler comparators, plus suitable logic, which would include an AND gate. But the window comparator shown in Figure 3.7(a) has several advantages. The center of the window can be set by a single voltage, v_{ref}. The width of the window can be set by a single voltage Δv. The circuit operates as follows. When $v_i + v_{ref} < 0$, D_2 conducts and D_1 is reverse-biased. Thus no current flows through $R/2$ and $R/4$, since the ends of these resistors are at 0 V. Since the other three resistors feeding the lower op amp are equal, it flips when $v_i + v_{ref} + \Delta v = 0$; or

$$v_i = -v_{ref} - \Delta v \tag{3.8}$$

When $v_i + v_{ref} > 0$, D_1 conducts and $v_1 = -(v_i + v_{ref})/2$. The lower op amp flips when

$$\frac{v_i}{R} + \frac{v_{ref}}{R} + \frac{\Delta v}{R} + \frac{-(v_i + v_{ref})/2}{R/4} = 0$$

or when

$$v_i = -v_{ref} + \Delta v \tag{3.9}$$

Figure 3.7(b) shows the input-output characteristics of the circuit, which is useful for pulse-height analysis (Section 11.8) and for measuring probability-density distributions.

Limiter

The output of the lower op amp in Figure 3.7(a) could have no feedback networks connected to it, as is done for the simple comparator. Instead we note a resistor-diode network. This is used to clamp the output to a limiting value, for example, to interface to digital-logic levels. When v_o is driven below -5 V, v_2 is driven below 0 V and the top diode conducts. The circuit then becomes an

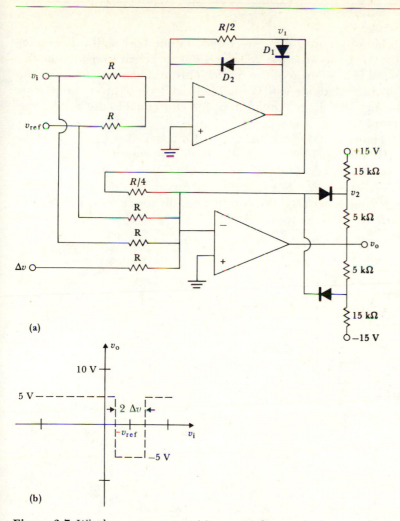

(a)

(b)

Figure 3.7 Window comparator. (a) v_{ref} sets the nominal comparison reference. If v_i is within $\pm \Delta v$ of v_{ref}, v_o is negative, as shown in (b), the input-output characteristic. The diode-resistor limiting network at the output clamps the output to ± 5 V. (From *Operational Amplifiers: Design and Application*, by Tobey *et al.* Copyright © 1971 by Burr-Brown Research Corporation. Used with permission of McGraw-Hill Book Co.)

inverter with a 5-kΩ feedback resistor. Provided that the input resistors are much greater than 5 kΩ, the gain is low, and $\Delta v_o / \Delta v_i$ has a low slope, effectively clamping v_o to -5 V. The bottom resistor-diode network clamps v_o to $+5$ V. This circuit can also be added to normal amplifiers to provide a normal gain over a desired range and a limited output beyond that. If needed, more effective clamping (lower $\Delta v_o / \Delta v_i$) can be achieved by replacing the diode with a transistor base-to-emitter junction; the transistor collector is connected to the power supply (Wait, 1975, p. 165).

3.6 Rectifiers

Simple resistor-diode rectifiers do not work well for voltages below 0.7 V, because the voltage is not sufficient to overcome the forward voltage drop of the diode. This problem can be overcome by placing the diode within the feedback loop of an op amp, thus reducing the voltage limitation by a factor equal to the gain of the op amp.

Figure 3.8(a) shows the circuit for a full-wave precision rectifier (Graeme, 1974b). For $v_i > 0$, D_2 and D_3 conduct, while D_1 and D_4 are backbiased. The top op amp is a follower with gain, with a gain of $1/x$, where x is a fraction corresponding to the potentiometer setting. Since D_4 is not conducting, the lower op amp does not contribute to the output.

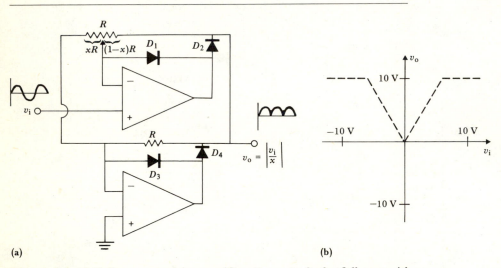

(a)   (b)

Figure 3.8 (a) Full-wave precision rectifier. For $v_i > 0$, the follower with gain at the top is active, making $v_o > 0$. For $v_i < 0$, the inverter at the bottom is active, making $v_o > 0$. Circuit gain may be adjusted with a single pot. (b) Input-output characteristics show saturation when $v_o > +12$ V. (Reprinted from *Electronics*, December 12, 1974; copyright © McGraw-Hill, Inc., 1974.)

For $v_i < 0$, D_1 and D_4 conduct, while D_2 and D_3 are backbiased. v_i, which appears at the potentiometer wiper, serves as the input to the lower op-amp inverter, which has a gain of $-1/x$. Since D_2 is not conducting, the upper op amp does not contribute to the output. And since the polarity of the gain switches with the polarity of v_i, $v_o = |v_i/x|$.

The advantage of this circuit over other full-wave rectifier circuits (Wait, 1975, p. 173) is that the gain can be varied with a single potentiometer and the input resistance is very high. If only a half-wave rectifier is needed, either the follower with gain or the inverter can be used separately, thus requiring only one op amp. The perfect rectifier is frequently used with an integrator to quantify the amplitude of electromyographic signals (Section 6.8).

3.7 Logarithmic amplifiers

The logarithmic amplifier makes use of the nonlinear volt-ampere relation of the silicon planar transistor (Jung, 1974):

$$V_{BE} = 0.060 \log \left(\frac{I_C}{I_0} \right) \tag{3.10}$$

where

V_{BE} = base-emitter voltage
I_C = collector current
I_0 = reverse saturation current, 10^{-13} A at 27°C

The transistor is placed in the *transdiode* configuration shown in Figure 3.9(a), in which $I_C = V_i/R$. Then the output $v_o = V_{BE}$ is logarithmically related to v_i as given by (3.10) over the approximate range 10^{-7} A $< I_C < 10^{-2}$ A. The approximate range of v_o is -0.36 to -0.66 V, so larger ranges of v_o are sometimes obtained by the alternate switch position shown in Figure 3.9(a). The resistor network feeds back only a fraction of v_o in order to boost v_o and uses the same principle as that used in the follower with gain. Figure 3.9(b) shows the input-output characteristics for each of these circuits.

Since semiconductors are temperature sensitive, accurate circuits require temperature compensation. Antilog (exponential) cir-

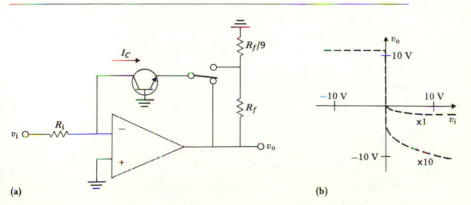

(a)   (b)

Figure 3.9 (a) A logarithmic amplifier makes use of the fact that a transistor's V_{BE} is related to the logarithm of its collector current. With the switch thrown in the alternate position, the circuit gain is increased by 10. (b) Input-output characteristics show that the logarithmic relation is obtained for only one polarity; ×1 and ×10 gains are indicated.

cuits are made by interchanging the resistor and semiconductor. These log and antilog circuits are used to multiply, divide, or raise a variable to a power, to compress large dynamic ranges into small ones, and to linearize the output of devices with logarithmic or exponential input-output relations. In the photometer (Section 10.1), the logarithmic converter can be used to convert transmittance to absorbance.

3.8 Integrators

So far in this chapter we have considered only circuits with a flat gain-versus-frequency characteristic. Now let us consider circuits that have a deliberate change in gain with frequency. The first such circuit is the *integrator*. Figure 3.10 shows the circuit for an integrator, which is obtained by closing switch S_1. The voltage across an initially uncharged capacitor is given by

$$v = \frac{1}{C} \int_0^{t_1} i \, dt \tag{3.11}$$

where i is the current through C and t_1 is the integration time. For the integrator, for v_i positive, the input current $i = v_i/R$ flows through C in a direction to cause v_0 to move in a negative direction. Thus

$$v_0 = -\frac{1}{RC} \int_0^{t_1} v_i \, dt + v_{ic} \tag{3.12}$$

This shows that v_0 is equal to the negative integral of v_i, scaled by the factor $1/RC$ and added to v_{ic}, the voltage due to the initial con-

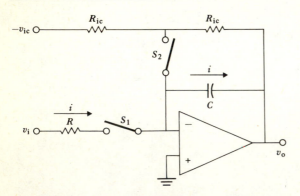

Figure 3.10 A three-mode integrator. With S_1 open and S_2 closed, the dc circuit behaves as an inverter. Thus $v_0 = v_{ic}$ and v_0 can be set to any desired initial condition. With S_1 closed and S_2 open, the circuit integrates. With both switches open, the circuit holds v_0 constant, making possible a leisurely readout.

dition. For $v_{ic} = 0$ and $v_i = $ constant, $v_o = -v_i$ after an integration time equal to RC. Since any real integrator eventually drifts into saturation, a means must be provided to restore v_o to any desired initial condition. If an initial condition of $v_o = 0$ V is desired, a simple switch to short out C is sufficient. For more versatility, S_1 is opened and S_2 closed. This dc circuit then acts as an inverter, which makes $v_o = v_{ic}$. During integration, S_1 is closed and S_2 open. After the integration, both switches may be opened to hold the output at the final calculated value, thus permitting time for a readout. The circuit is useful for computing the area under a curve, such as technicians do when they calculate cardiac output (Section 8.2). It is also the integrator circuit used in an analog computer.

The frequency response of an integrator is easily analyzed by realizing that the formula for the inverter gain (3.1) may be generalized to any input and feedback impedances. Thus for Figure 3.10, with S_1 closed,

$$\frac{V_o(j\omega)}{V_i(j\omega)} = -\frac{Z_f}{Z_i} = -\frac{1/j\omega C}{R}$$

$$= -\frac{1}{j\omega RC} = -\frac{1}{j\omega \tau} \tag{3.13}$$

where $\tau = RC$, $\omega = 2\pi f$, and $f = $ frequency. Equation (3.13) shows that the circuit gain decreases as f increases; Figure 3.11 shows the frequency response; and (3.13) shows that the circuit gain is 1 when $\omega\tau = 1$.

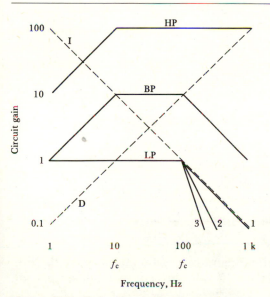

Figure 3.11 Bode plot (gain versus frequency) for various filters. Integrator (I); differentiator (D); low pass (LP), 1, 2, 3 section (pole); high pass (HP); bandpass (BP). Corner frequencies f_c for high-pass, low-pass, and bandpass filters.

Example 3.2 The output of the piezoelectric transducer shown in Figure 2.11(b) may be fed directly into the negative input of the integrator shown in Figure 3.10, as shown in Figure E3.2. Analyze the circuit of this charge amplifier and discuss its advantages.

Answer Because the FET-op-amp negative input is a virtual ground, $i_{tC} = i_{tR} = 0$. Hence long cables may be used without changing transducer sensitivity or time constant, as is the case with voltage amplifiers. From Figure E3.2, current generated by the transducer, $i_t = K \, dx/dt$, all flows into C, so, using (3.11), we find that v_o is

$$v_o = -v = -\frac{1}{C} \int_0^{t_1} \frac{K \, dx}{dt} \, dt = -\frac{Kx}{C}$$

which shows that v_o is proportional to x, even down to dc. Like the integrator, the charge amplifier slowly drifts with time, because of bias currents required by the op-amp input. A large feedback resistance R must therefore be added to prevent saturation. This causes the circuit to behave as a high-pass filter, with a time constant $\tau = RC$. It then responds only to frequencies above $f_c = 1/2\pi RC$ and has no frequency-response improvement over the voltage amplifier.

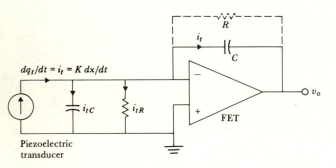

Figure E3.2 The charge amplifier transfers charge generated from a piezoelectric transducer to the op-amp feedback capacitor C.

3.9 Differentiator

By interchanging the integrator's R and C, we have the differentiator shown in Figure 3.12. The current through a capacitor is given by

$$i = C \frac{dv}{dt} \tag{3.14}$$

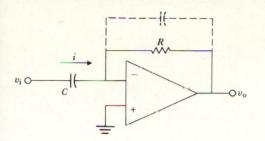

Figure 3.12 A differentiator. Dashed lines indicate that a small capacitor must usually be added across the feedback resistor to prevent oscillation.

If dv_i/dt is positive, i flows through R in a direction such that it yields a negative v_o. Thus

$$v_o = -RC\frac{dv_i}{dt}$$ (3.15)

The frequency response of a differentiator is given by the ratio of feedback to input impedance:

$$\frac{V_o(j\omega)}{V_i(j\omega)} = -\frac{Z_f}{Z_i} = -\frac{R}{1/j\omega C}$$

$$= -j\omega RC = -j\omega\tau$$ (3.16)

Equation (3.16) shows that the circuit gain increases as f increases, and is equal to unity when $\omega\tau = 1$. Figure 3.11 shows the frequency response.

Unless specific preventive steps are taken, the circuit tends to oscillate. The output also tends to be noisy, since the circuit emphasizes high frequencies. A differentiator followed by a comparator is useful for detecting an event whose slope exceeds a given value; for example, the detection of the R wave in an electrocardiogram.

3.10 Active filters

Low-pass filter

Figure 1.9(a) shows a low-pass filter that is useful for attenuating high-frequency noise. A low-pass active filter may be obtained by use of the one-op-amp circuit shown in Figure 3.13(a). The advantages of this circuit are that it is capable of gain and that it has a very low output impedance. The frequency response is given by the ratio of feedback to input impedance:

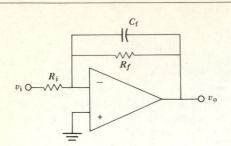

(a)

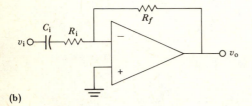

(b)

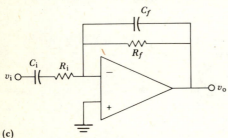

(c)

Figure 3.13 Active filters. (a) Low-pass filter attenuates high frequencies. (b) High-pass filter attenuates low frequencies and blocks dc. (c) Bandpass filter attenuates both low and high frequencies.

$$\frac{V_o(j\omega)}{V_i(j\omega)} = -\frac{Z_f}{Z_i} = -\frac{\dfrac{(R_f/j\omega C_f)}{[(1/j\omega C_f) + R_f]}}{R_i}$$

$$= -\frac{R_f}{(1 + j\omega R_f C_f)R_i} = -\frac{R_f}{R_i}\frac{1}{1 + j\omega\tau} \tag{3.17}$$

where $\tau = R_f C_f$. Note that (3.17) has the same form as (1.3). Figure 3.11 shows the frequency response, which is similar to that shown in Figure 1.9(d). For $\omega \ll 1/\tau$, the circuit behaves as an inverter (Figure 3.3), because the impedance of C_f is large compared with R_f. For $\omega \gg 1/\tau$, the circuit behaves as an integrator (Figure 3.10), because C_f is the dominant feedback impedance. The *corner frequency* f_c, which is defined by the intersection of the two asymptotes shown, is given by the relation $\omega\tau = 2\pi f_c\tau = 1$. When a designer wishes to limit the frequency of a wide-band amplifier, it is not necessary to add a separate stage, as shown in Figure 3.13(a), but only to add the correct size C_f to the existing wide-band amplifier.

High-pass filter

Figure 3.13(b) shows a one-op-amp high-pass filter. This is useful for amplifying a small ac voltage that rides on top of a large dc voltage, because C_i blocks the dc. The frequency-response equation is

$$\frac{V_o(j\omega)}{V_i(j\omega)} = -\frac{Z_f}{Z_i} = -\frac{R_f}{1/j\omega C_i + R_i}$$

$$= -\frac{j\omega R_f C_i}{1 + j\omega C_i R_i} = -\frac{R_f}{R_i}\frac{j\omega\tau}{1 + j\omega\tau} \tag{3.18}$$

where $\tau = R_i C_i$. Figure 3.11 shows the frequency response. For $\omega \ll 1/\tau$, the circuit behaves as a differentiator (Figure 3.12), because C_i is the dominant input impedance. For $\omega \gg 1/\tau$, the circuit behaves as an inverter, because the impedance of R_i is large compared with that of C_i. The corner frequency f_c, which is defined by the intersection of the two asymptotes shown, is given by the relation $\omega\tau = 2\pi f_c\tau = 1$.

Bandpass filter

A series combination of the low-pass filter and the high-pass filter results in a *bandpass filter,* which amplifies frequencies over a desired range and attenuates higher and lower frequencies. Figure 3.13(c) shows that the bandpass function can be achieved with a one-op-amp circuit. Figure 3.11 shows the frequency response. The corner frequencies are defined by the same relations as those for the low-pass and high-pass filters. This circuit is useful for amplifying a certain band of frequencies, such as those required for recording heart sounds or the electrocardiogram.

Higher-order filters

For filters with higher attenuation rates, we turn to higher-order filters. Figure 3.14 shows how a single op amp is used to design a low-pass *Butterworth filter.* Since the op amp is used as a follower, this configuration is known as a *VCVS* (voltage-controlled voltage-source) filter. The positive feedback through C_1 produces a flatter response in the passband than cascaded sections of one-section filters do. These filters are designed by choosing values

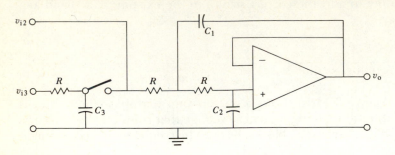

Figure 3.14 Low-pass VCVS filter. Two-section filter with switch open and input v_{i2}. Three-section filter with switch closed and input v_{i3}.

from the following table, assuming that all R's = 1 Ω, all C's are in farads, and $f_c = 1/2\pi$ Hz.

Sections	C_1	C_2	C_3
2	1.414	0.7071	—
3	1.392	0.2024	3.546

Since these C's are impractically large, larger values of R are first chosen to reduce the values of C. Then, for any desired f_c,

$$C_{\text{actual}} = \frac{C_{\text{table}}}{2\pi f_c R} \qquad (3.19)$$

Figure 3.11 shows the frequency responses obtained from two- and three-section low-pass filters.

High-pass filters are generated by interchanging the positions of all R's and C's in Figure 3.14. These filters are designed by choosing values from the following table (values are the reciprocal of those in the preceding table), assuming that all C's = 1 F, all R's are in ohms, and $f_c = 1/2\pi$ Hz.

Sections	R_1	R_2	R_3
2	0.707	1.414	—
3	0.718	4.941	0.282

Since these C's = 1 F are impractically large, smaller values of C are first chosen. Then for any desired f_c,

$$R_{\text{actual}} = \frac{R_{\text{table}}}{2\pi f_c C} \qquad (3.20)$$

Tables and formulas for designing VCVS filters of an order higher than 3 are found in Shepard (1969). Other types of active filters are found in Jung (1974).

3.11 Frequency response

Up until now, we found it useful to consider the op amp as ideal. Now we shall examine the effects of several nonideal characteristics, starting with that of frequency response.

Open-loop gain

Since the op amp requires very high gain, it has several stages. Each of these stages has stray or junction capacitance that limits its high-frequency response in the same way that a simple RC low-pass filter reduces high-frequency gain. At high frequencies, each stage has a -1 slope on a log-log plot of gain versus frequency, and has a $-90°$ phase shift. Thus a three-stage op amp, such as type 709, reaches a slope of -3, as shown by the dashed curve on Figure 3.15. The phase shift reaches $-270°$, which is quite satisfactory for a comparator, since feedback is not employed. For an amplifier, if the gain is > 1 when the phase shift $= -180°$ (the closed-loop condition for oscillation), there is undesirable oscillation.

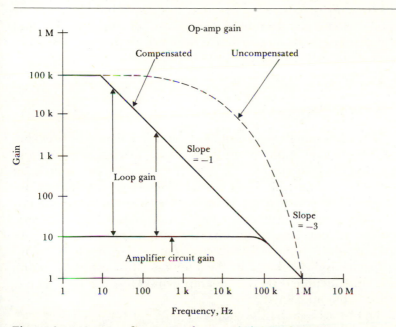

Figure 3.15 Op-amp frequency characteristics. Early op amps (such as the 709) were uncompensated, had a gain > 1 when the phase shift $= -180°$, and therefore oscillated unless compensation was added externally. A popular op amp, the 741, is compensated internally, so for a gain > 1, the phase shift is limited to $-90°$. When feedback resistors are added to build an amplifier circuit, the loop gain on this log-log plot is the difference between the op-amp gain and the amplifier-circuit gain.

Compensation

Adding an external capacitor to the terminals indicated on the specification sheet moves one of the RC filter corner frequencies to a very low frequency. This compensates the uncompensated op amp, resulting in a slope of -1 and a maximum phase shift of $-90°$. This is done with an internal capacitor in the 741, resulting in the solid curve, as shown in Figure 3.15. This op amp does not oscillate for any amplifier we have described. We note that this op amp has very high dc gain, but that the gain is progressively reduced at higher frequencies, until it is only 1 at 1 MHz.

Closed-loop gain

It might appear that the op amp has very poor frequency response, since its gain is reduced for frequencies above 10 Hz. However, an amplifier circuit is never built using the op-amp open loop, so we shall therefore discuss only the circuit closed-loop response. For example, if we build an amplifier circuit with a gain of 10, as shown in Figure 3.15, the frequency response is flat up to 100 kHz, and is reduced above that frequency only because the amplifier circuit gain can never exceed the op-amp gain. We find this an advantage of using negative feedback, in that the frequency response is greatly extended.

Loop gain

The loop gain for an amplifier circuit is obtained by breaking the feedback loop at any point in the loop, injecting a signal, and measuring the gain around the loop. For example, in a unity-gain follower [Fig. 3.4(a)] we break the feedback loop and then the injected signal enters the negative input, after which it is amplified by the op-amp gain. Therefore the loop gain equals the op-amp gain. To measure loop gain in an inverter with a gain of -1 [Figure 3.3(a)], assume that the amplifier-circuit input is grounded. The injected signal is divided by 2 by the attenuator formed of R_f and R_i, and is then amplified by the op-amp gain. Thus the loop gain is equal to (op-amp gain)/2.

Figure 3.15 shows the loop-gain concept for a follower with gain. The amplifier-circuit gain is 10. On the log-log plot, the difference between the op-amp gain and the amplifier-circuit gain is the loop gain. At low frequencies, the loop gain is high and the closed-loop amplifier-circuit characteristics are determined by the feedback resistors. At high frequencies, the loop gain is low and the amplifier-circuit characteristics follow the op-amp characteristics. High loop gain is good for accuracy and stability, since the feedback resistors can be made much more stable than the op-amp characteristics.

Gain-bandwidth product

The gain-bandwidth product of the op amp is equal to the product of gain and bandwidth at a particular frequency. Thus in Figure 3.15 the unity gain bandwidth product is 1 MHz, a typical value for op amps. Note that along the entire curve with a slope of -1, the gain-bandwidth product is still constant, at 1 MHz. Thus, for any amplifier circuit, we can obtain its bandwidth by dividing the gain-bandwidth product by the amplifier-circuit gain. For higher-frequency applications, op amps such as the 715 are available with gain-bandwidth products of 60 MHz.

Slew rate

Small-signal response follows the amplifier-circuit frequency response predicted by Figure 3.15. For large signals there is an additional limitation. When rapid changes in output are demanded, the capacitor added for compensation must be charged up from an internal source that has limited current capability I_{max}. The change in voltage across the capacitor is then limited, $dv/dt = I_{max}/C$, and dv_o/dt is limited to a maximum slew rate (0.6 V/μs for the 741). If this slew rate S_r is exceeded by a large-amplitude, high-frequency sine wave, distortion occurs. Thus there is a limitation on the sine-wave *full-power response,* or maximum frequency for rated output,

$$f_p = \frac{S_r}{2\pi V_{or}} \tag{3.21}$$

where V_{or} is the rated output voltage (usually 10 V). If the slew rate is too slow for fast switching of a comparator, an uncompensated op amp can be used, since comparators do not contain the negative-feedback path that may cause oscillations.

3.12 Offset voltage

Another nonideal characteristic is that of offset voltage. The two op-amp inputs drive the bases of transistors, and the base-to-emitter voltage drop may be slightly different for each. Thus, so that one can obtain $v_0 = 0$, the voltage $(v_1 - v_2)$ must be a few millivolts. This offset voltage is usually not important when v_i is 1–10 V.

But when v_i is on the order of millivolts, as when amplifying the output from thermocouples or strain gages, the offset voltage must be considered.

Nulling

The offset voltage may be reduced to zero by adding an external nulling pot to the terminals indicated on the specification sheet. Adjustment of this pot increases emitter current through one of the input transistors and lowers it through the other. This alters the base-to-emitter voltage of the two transistors until the offset voltage is reduced to zero.

Drift

Even though the offset voltage may be set to 0 at 25°C, it does not remain there if temperature is not constant. Temperature changes that affect the base-to-emitter voltages may be due to either environmental changes or to variations in the dissipation of power in the chip resulting from fluctuating output voltage. The effects of temperature may be specified as a maximum offset voltage change in volts per degree Celsius or a maximum offset voltage change over a given temperature range, say -25 to $+85°C$. If the drift of an inexpensive op amp is too high for a given application, tighter specifications (0.1 $\mu V/°C$) are available with temperature-controlled chips. An alternate technique modulates the dc as in chopper-stabilized and varactor op amps (Tobey, 1971).

Noise

All semiconductor junctions generate noise, which limits the detection of small signals. Op amps have transistor input junctions, which generate both noise-voltage sources and noise-current sources. These can be modeled as shown in Figure 3.16. For low source impedances, only the noise voltage v_n is important, since it is large compared with the $i_n R$ drop caused by the current noise i_n. The noise is random, but the amplitude varies with frequency. For example, at low frequencies the noise power density varies as $1/f$ (flicker noise), so a large amount of noise is present at low frequencies. At the midfrequencies, the noise is lower, and may be specified in rms units of $V \cdot Hz^{-1/2}$. In addition, some silicon planar-diffused bipolar integrated-circuit op amps exhibit bursts of noise, called *popcorn noise* (Wait, 1975).

3.13 Bias current

Since the two op-amp inputs drive transistors, base current must flow all the time to keep the transistors turned on. This is called *bias current,* which for the 741 is about 0.2 μA. This bias current must flow through the feedback network. It causes errors proportional to feedback-element resistances. To minimize these errors, low feedback resistors, such as those with resistances of 10 kΩ, are normally used. Lower values should be used only after a check to determine that the current flowing through the feedback resistor, plus the current flowing through all load resistors, does not exceed the op-amp output current rating (5 mA for the 741).

Differential bias current

The difference between the two input bias currents is much smaller than either of the bias currents alone. A degree of cancelation of the effects of bias current can be achieved by having each bias current flow through the same equivalent resistance. This is accomplished for the inverter and the follower with gain by adding, in series with the positive input, a compensation resistor whose value is equal to the parallel combination of R_i and R_f. There still is an error, but it is now determined by the difference in bias current.

Drift

Since the input bias currents are transistor base currents, they are temperature sensitive, because transistor gain varies with temperature. However, the changes in gain of the two transistors tend to track together, so the additional compensation resistor described above minimizes the problem.

Noise

Figure 3.16 shows how variations in bias current contribute to overall noise. The noise currents flow through the external equivalent resistances so that the total rms noise voltage is

$$v_t \cong \{[v_n^2 + (i_nR_1)^2 + (i_nR_2)^2 + 4\kappa TR_1 + 4\kappa TR_2]BW\}^{1/2}$$

$$(3.22)$$

where

R_1 and R_2 = equivalent source resistances

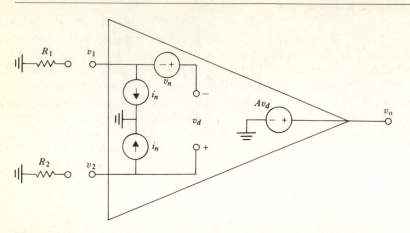

Figure 3.16 Noise sources in an op amp. The noise-voltage source v_n is in series with the input and cannot be reduced. The noise added by the noise-current sources i_n can be minimized by using small external resistances.

v_n = mean value of the rms noise voltage, in $V \cdot Hz^{-1/2}$, across the frequency range of interest

i_n = mean value of the rms noise current, in $A \cdot Hz^{-1/2}$, across the frequency range of interest

κ = Boltzmann's constant (Appendix)

T = temperature, K

BW = noise bandwidth, in Hz

The specification sheet provides values of v_n and i_n (sometimes v_n^2 and i_n^2), thus making it possible to compare different op amps. If the source resistances are 10 kΩ, bipolar-transistor op amps yield the lowest noise. For larger source resistances, low-input-current amplifiers such as the *field-effect transistor* (FET) input stage are best because of their lower current noise. Ary (1977) presents design factors and performance specifications for a low-noise amplifier.

For ac amplifiers, the lowest noise is obtained by calculating the characteristic noise resistance $R_n = v_n/i_n$ and setting it equal to the equivalent source resistance R_2 (for the follower with gain). This is accomplished by inserting a transformer with turns ratio $1:N$, where $N = (R_n/R_2)^{1/2}$, between the source and the op amp (Jung, 1974).

Example 3.3 Because the electromagnetic flowmeter (Section 8.3) produces a signal in the microvolt range, it requires a low-noise amplifier. Typical source resistance is 1 kΩ and bandwidth is 100 Hz. For the circuit shown in Figure E3.3, calculate the trans-

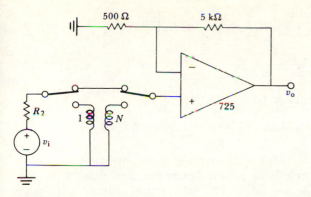

$R_1 = 500\ \Omega\ \|\ 5\ k\Omega$

500 Ω   5 kΩ

R_2 1   N   725 v_o v_i

Figure E3.3 The 725 is a low-noise op amp. For ac inputs, the noise obtained using a direct input (switches up) can be reduced by using an input transformer (switches down).

former turns ratio and also the noise voltage without and with the transformer.

Answer For 400 Hz, a typical electromagnetic flowmeter frequency, the specification sheet for the 625 gives $v_n^2 = 8 \times 10^{-17} \mathrm{V^2/Hz}$ and $i_n^2 = 2 \times 10^{-26} \mathrm{A^2/Hz}$. The characteristic noise resistance is

$$R_n = \frac{v_n}{i_n} = [(8 \times 10^{-17})/(2 \times 10^{-26})]^{1/2}$$

$$= 63\ k\Omega$$

The transformer turns ratio is

$$N = \left(\frac{R_n}{R_2}\right)^{1/2} = \left(\frac{63\ k\Omega}{1\ k\Omega}\right)^{1/2} = 8$$

For Figure E3.3, the R_1 of Figure 3.16 is much less than R_2, so we neglect noise originating in R_1. For the case without the transformer, (3.22) reduces to

$$v_t = \{[v_n^2 + (i_n R_2)^2 + 4\kappa T R_2]BW\}^{1/2}$$

$$= \{[(8 \times 10^{-17}) + (2 \times 10^{-26})(10^6)$$

$$+ 4(1.38 \times 10^{-23})(300)(10^3)]100\}^{1/2}$$

$$= \{[(8000 + 2 + 1700)10^{-20}]100\}^{1/2} = 98\ nV$$

Note that v_n dominates the other noise sources. When the transformer is added, v_i is multiplied by 8 prior to mixing with v_n, and the total noise referred to the input becomes

$$v_t' = \left\{\left[\left(\frac{v_n}{8}\right)^2 + (i_n R_2 8)^2 + 4\kappa T R_2\right] \text{BW}\right\}^{1/2}$$

$$= \left\{\left[\frac{8 \times 10^{-17}}{64} + (2 \times 10^{-26})(10^6)(64)\right.\right.$$

$$\left.\left. + 4(1.38 \times 10^{-23})(300)(10^3)\right] 100\right\}^{1/2}$$

$$= \{[(125 + 128 + 1700)10^{-20}]100\}^{1/2} = 43 \text{ nV}$$

Note that proper transformer matching of the source to the amplifier has made v_n negligible and reduced the total noise voltage to less than half its former value. The proper turns ratio can be incorporated into an existing transformer, as shown in Figure 8.6, thus eliminating the need for a separate transformer.

3.14 Input and output resistance

Input resistance

The op-amp differential-input resistance R_d is shown in Figures 3.1 and 3.17. For the typical op amp, it is about 0.5 MΩ which is comparable to the value of some feedback resistors used. However, we shall see that its value is usually not important, because of the benefits of feedback. Consider the follower shown in Figure 3.17. In order to calculate the amplifier-circuit input resistance, R_{ai}, assume a change in input voltage, v_i. Since this is a follower,

$$\Delta v_o = A \Delta v_d = A(\Delta v_i - \Delta v_o)$$

$$= \frac{A \Delta v_i}{A + 1}$$

$$\Delta i_i = \frac{\Delta v_d}{R_d} = \frac{\Delta v_i - \Delta v_o}{R_d} = \frac{\Delta v_i}{(A + 1)R_d}$$

$$R_{ai} = \frac{\Delta v_i}{\Delta i_i} = (A + 1)R_d \cong AR_d \tag{3.23}$$

Thus the amplifier-circuit input resistance R_{ai} is about $(10^5) \times$ (0.5 MΩ) = 50 GΩ. This value cannot be achieved in practice, because surface leakage paths in the op-amp socket lower it considerably. In general, all followers have a very high input resistance, which is equal to R_d times the loop gain. This is not to say that very high source resistances can be used, because usually the bias current causes much larger problems than the amplifier-circuit input impedance. For high source resistances, FET op amps such as the 3130 and 3140 are helpful.

The input resistance of an inverter is easy to determine. Since the negative input of the op amp is a virtual ground,

$$R_{ai} = \frac{\Delta v_i}{\Delta i_i} = R_i \qquad (3.24)$$

Thus the amplifier-circuit input resistance R_{ai} is equal to R_i, the input resistor. Since R_i is usually a low value, the inverter has low input resistance.

Output resistance

The op-amp output resistance R_o is shown in Figures 3.1 and 3.17. It is about 100 Ω for the typical op amp, which may seem high for some applications. However, its value is usually not important, because of the benefits of feedback. Consider the follower shown in Figure 3.17. In order to calculate the amplifier-circuit output resistance R_{ao}, assume that load resistor R_L is attached to the output, causing a change in output current Δi_o. Since i_o flows through R_o, there is an additional voltage drop $\Delta i_o R_o$.

$$-\Delta v_d = \Delta v_o = A \, \Delta v_d + \Delta i_o R_o = -A \, \Delta v_o + \Delta i_o R_o$$

$$(A + 1)\Delta v_o = \Delta i_o R_o$$

$$R_{ao} = \frac{\Delta v_o}{\Delta i_o} = \frac{R_o}{A + 1} \cong R_o/A \qquad (3.25)$$

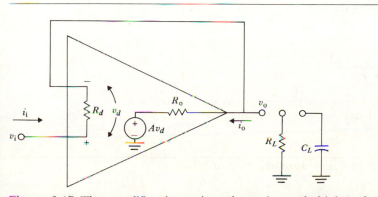

Figure 3.17 The amplifier input impedance is much higher than the op-amp input impedance R_d. The amplifier output impedance is much lower than the op-amp output impedance R_o.

Thus the amplifier-circuit output resistance R_{ao} is about $100/(10^5) = 0.001\ \Omega$, a value negligible in most circuits. In general, all followers and inverters have an output resistance that is equal to R_o divided by the loop gain. This is not to say that very low load resistances can be driven by the output. If R_L shown in Figure 3.17 is lower than 2 kΩ, the op amp saturates internally, since the maximum current output for a typical op amp is 5 mA. This maximum current output must also be considered when driving large capacitances C_L at a high slew rate. Then the output current

$$i_o = C_L \frac{dv_o}{dt} \tag{3.26}$$

The R_o–C_L combination also acts as a low-pass filter, which introduces additional phase shift around the loop and can cause oscillation. The cure is to add a small resistor between v_o and C_L, thus isolating C_L from the feedback loop.

To achieve higher current outputs, the *current booster* shown in Figure 3.18 is used. An ordinary op amp drives high-power transistors (on heat sinks if required). Then we can use the entire circuit as an op amp by connecting terminals v_1, v_2, and v_o to external feedback networks. This places the booster section within the feedback loop and keeps distortion low.

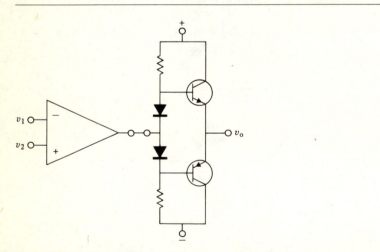

Figure 3.18 The complementary-symmetry output-current booster is a high-power transistor stage driven by an ordinary op amp.

3.15 Phase-sensitive demodulators

Figure 2.7 shows that a linear variable differential transformer requires a phase-sensitive demodulator to yield a useful output signal. A phase-sensitive demodulator does not measure phase, but yields a full-wave-rectified output of the in-phase component of a sine wave. Its output is proportional to the amplitude of the input, but it changes sign when the phase shifts by 180°.

Figure 3.19 shows the functional operation of a phase-sensitive demodulator. Figure 3.19(a) shows a switching function that is derived from a *carrier oscillator* and causes the double-pole double-throw switch in Figure 3.19(b) to be in the upper position for $+1$ and the lower position for -1. In effect, this multiplies the input signal v_i by the switching function shown in Figure 3.19(a). The in-phase sine wave in Figure 3.19(c) is demodulated by this switch to yield the full-wave-rectified positive signal in Figure 3.19(d). The sine wave in Figure 3.19(e) is 180° out of phase, so it yields the negative signal in Figure 3.19(f).

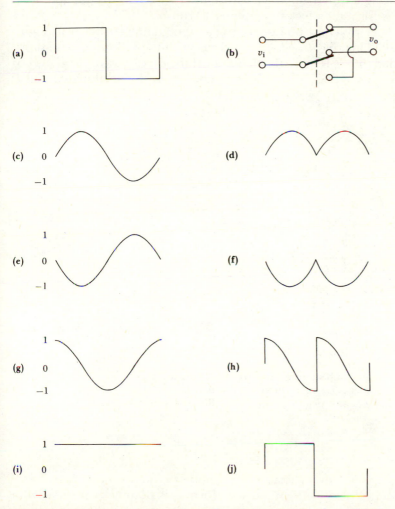

Figure 3.19 Functional operation of a phase-sensitive demodulator. (a) Switching function. (b) Switch. (c), (e), (g), (i) Several input voltages. (d), (f), (h), (j) Corresponding output voltages.

Amplifier stray capacitance may cause an undesirable *quadrature voltage* that is shifted 90°, as shown in Figure 3.19(g). The demodulated signal in Figure 3.19(h) averages to zero when passed through a low-pass filter and is rejected. The dc signal shown in Figure 3.19(i) is demodulated to the wave shown in Figure 3.19(j), and is rejected. Any frequency component not locked to the carrier frequency is similarly rejected. Because the phase-sensitive demodulator has excellent noise-rejection capabilities, it is frequently used to demodulate the suppressed-carrier waveforms obtained from LVDTs and the ac-excited strain-gage Wheatstone bridge (Section 2.3). A carrier system and phase-sensitive demodulator are also essential for operation of the electromagnetic blood flowmeter (Section 8.3). The noise-rejection capability may be improved by placing a tuned amplifier before the phase-sensitive demodulator, thus forming a lock-in amplifier (Aronson, 1977).

A practical phase-sensitive demodulator is shown in Figure 3.20. This *ring demodulator* operates with the following action, provided that v_c is more than twice v_i. If the carrier waveform v_c is positive at the black dot, diodes D_1 and D_2 are forward-biased and D_3

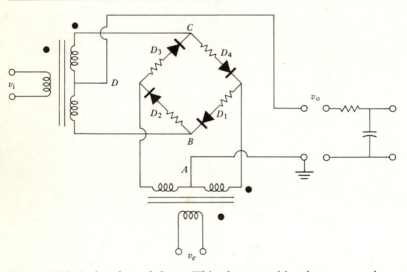

Figure 3.20 A ring demodulator. This phase-sensitive detector produces a full-wave-rectified output v_o that is positive when the input voltage v_i is in phase with the carrier voltage v_c and negative when v_i is 180° out of phase with v_c.

and D_4 are reverse-biased. By symmetry, points A and B are at the same voltage. If the input waveform v_i is positive at the black dot, this transforms to a voltage v_{DB}, that appears at v_o, as shown in the first half of Figure 3.19(d).

During the second half of the cycle, diodes D_3 and D_4 are forward-biased and D_1 and D_2 are reverse-biased. By symmetry, points A and C are at the same potential. v_i has reversed polarity, so v_{DC}, which appears at v_o, is positive. Thus v_o is a full-wave-rectified waveform. If v_i changes phase by 180°, as shown in Figure 3.19(e), v_o changes polarity. To eliminate ripple, the output is usually low-pass filtered by a filter whose corner frequency is about one-tenth of the carrier frequency.

The ring demodulator has the advantage of having no moving parts. Also v_i, v_c, and v_o can all be referenced to different dc levels, since transformer coupling is used. The availability of type 1596 solid-state double-balanced demodulators on a single chip (Fink, 1975) makes it possible to eliminate the bulky transformers, but requires more care in biasing v_i, v_c, and v_o at different dc levels.

3.16 Microcomputers in medical instrumentation

The electronic devices previously described in this chapter are useful for acquiring a medical signal and performing some initial processing such as filtering or demodulation. The generalized instrumentation system shown in Figure 1.1 also indicates additional signal processing, data storage, and control/feedback capability. Traditionally, this additional processing was handled either by using relatively simple digital-electronic circuits or, if a significant amount of processing was required, by connecting the instrument to a computer.

Microcomputers

The development of microcomputers has led to the combining of a medical instrument with a signal-processing capability sufficient to perform functions normally done by an operator or a computer. This computing function can certainly be implemented. But from the point of view of medical instrumentation, it is more instructive to view the microcomputer as a microcontroller. The use of a microcomputer generally results in fewer integrated-circuit packages. This reduced complexity, together with the capability for self-calibration and detection of errors, enhances the reliability of the instrument. The most useful applications of microcomputers for medical instrumentation involve this controller function. Microcomputers can provide self-calibration for measurement systems, automatic sequencing of events, and an easy method for entry of patient data such as height, weight, and sex for calculating expected or normal performance. All these functions are made possible by the basic structure of the microcomputer system shown in Figure 3.21.

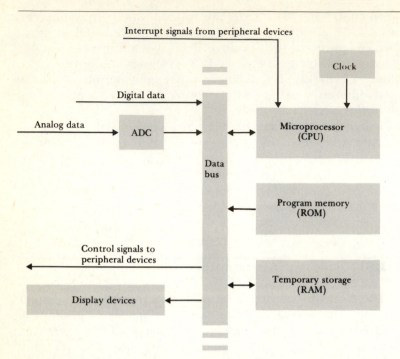

Figure 3.21 The microcomputer consists of the microprocessor chip (which frequently contains the CPU and its data) plus other chips that contain the clock, ROM, and RAM. (Copyright © by the Institute of Electrical and Electronics Engineers. Reprinted by permission from *IEEE Spectrum*, vol. 13, no. 4, April 1976, pp. 40–43.)

Data handling

Because most data are normally in the form of analog signals and the microcomputer can operate only on digital data, an *analog-to-digital converter* (ADC) is required. Sheingold (1972) gives an excellent discussion of the principles and practices of ADCs. The *microprocessor chip* is a *central processing unit* (CPU) capable of accepting data (input), outputting data, and carrying out some arithmetic operations (addition, subtraction, comparing, etc.), all under the direction of a *program*. In addition, the CPU chip has *registers* that store instructions (the program steps to be executed), keep track of the location of the next program step and temporarily store data (index registers).

Several other components are required for a functioning microcomputer. There must be a system *clock* (or clocks) to create a uniform operating cycle for all the elements of the system. There must also be a means of storing data and storing the program to be implemented—that is, a *memory*.

Two types of memory are used: *Random-access memory* (RAM)—read/write memory—provides for the temporary storage of data in a volatile form (if the power is turned off, the data are lost). Permanent storage of information (e.g., the program to be executed) is accomplished using a *read-only memory* (ROM). ROMs that may be programmed in the field are called PROMs, and those that are erasable (by ultraviolet light) are called EPROMs. Data and instructions (the program) are transferred to different units on a *bus*. The bus is simply a set (4, 8, or 16) of lines that carries a digital code (word). All the memories discussed have address lines and data lines. The RAM also has a read/write enable line.

Programming

It is instructive to think of the microcomputer as a flexible electronic device that may be reconfigured by using software (a program) rather than by rewiring. This flexibility means that the device can be performing one function at one time and a completely different function at a later time. This feature makes the microcomputer useful in medical-instrumentation systems for acquiring data, processing calculations, comparing results with the normal for that type of patient, and then displaying data. This flexibility is achieved through the use of instructions that are programmed into the PROM. The microprocessor executes each instruction in order, and the instrument performs a sequence of operations that do not involve the operator. Each microprocessor has a unique set of instructions, and Peatman (1977) provides an excellent description of how the major types operate.

Instructions fall into several categories: those that transfer data into or out of the CPU, those that operate on the data in the CPU (e.g., increment, decrement, compare, add, subtract, etc.), and those that cause the microprocessor to jump to a new part of the program. These *jump instructions* permit the use of the same subroutine (e.g., peak detection) at several different points in a program. They also provide the capability of changing the instrument operation based on either a calculation or an external (e.g., *data ready* from the ADC) or internal (e.g., a *high error rate*) condition.

In addition to this sequential processing of ordered instructions, many microprocessors also provide an *interrupt* capability. The interrupt allows external devices to stop the microprocessor program execution and then causes it to process data or control signals from that device. The interrupt is useful when a number of external devices are connected to the microcomputer, but each requires only brief periods of processing time.

Applications

A recently developed anesthesia-delivery system requires the entry of desired anesthesia-delivery rates, the updating of front-panel displays and alarms, and the setting of effectors to control the delivery of the anesthetic to the patient (Jurgen, 1976). The system is designed so that the microcomputer performs general processing (*background processing*) most of the time. It is interrupted by the front-panel controls, the effector transducers, or an external clock as necessary to carry out specific functions. This is especially useful in medical instrumentation, in which most signals contain low frequencies, and therefore require slow or infrequent processing.

These features are all useful in medical instrumentation because the microcomputer can carry out relatively complex functions in a predetermined sequence without the expense associated with a minicomputer system. Medically useful functions, which we shall see examples of in the following chapters, include: complex signal processing (an arrhythmia-detection system, Section 6.9); entry of patient parameters and calculation of responses as a percentage of normal (pulmonary-function analyzer, Section 9.8); self-calibration and sequencing of events (automated clinical-chemistry analyzer, Section 10.2); and monitoring of therapeutic instruments (ventilator-monitor system; Section 12.5).

Problems

3.1 (a) Design an inverter with an input resistance of 20 kΩ and a gain of -10. (b) Include a resistor to compensate for bias current. (c) Design a summer so that $v_o = -(10v_1 + 2v_2 + 0.5v_3)$.

3.2 Design a follower with gain having a gain of 10 and R_i of Figure 3.4(b) equal to 20 kΩ. Include a resistor to compensate for bias current.

3.3 An op-amp differential amplifier is built using four identical resistors, each having a tolerance of $\pm 5\%$. Calculate the worst possible CMRR.

3.4 Design a three-op-amp differential amplifier having a differential gain of 5 in the first stage and 6 in the second stage.

3.5 Design a comparator with hysteresis in which the hysteresis width extends from 0 to $+2$ V.

3.6 Design a window comparator that identifies voltages between $+5$ and $+7$ V and provides level outputs of 0 and -6 V.

3.7 For an inverting half-wave perfect rectifier, sketch the circuit. Plot the input-output characteristics for both the circuit output and the op-amp output, which are not the same point as in most op-amp circuits.

3.8 Using the principle shown in Figure 3.9, design a signal compressor for which an input-voltage range of ± 10 V yields an output-voltage range of ± 4 V.

3.9 Design an integrator with an input resistance of 1 MΩ.

Select the capacitor so that when $v_i = +10$ V, v_o travels from 0 to -10 V in 0.1 s.

3.10 In Problem 3.9, if $v_i = 0$ and offset voltage equals 5 mV, what is the current through R? How long will it take for v_o to drift from 0 V to saturation? Explain how to cure this drift problem.

3.11 In Problem 3.9, if bias current is 0.2 μA, how long will it take for v_o to drift from 0 V to saturation? Explain how to cure this drift problem.

3.12 Design a differentiator for which $v_o = -10$ V when $dv_i/dt = 100$ V/s.

3.13 Using 741 op amps, explain how an amplifier with a gain of 100 and a bandwidth of 100 kHz can be designed.

3.14 From Figure 3.15, if the amplifier gain is 1000, what is the loop gain at 100 Hz?

3.15 For Problem 3.14, calculate the amplifier input and output resistances at 100 Hz, for an inverter and a follower with gain.

3.16 For Figure 3.17, what is the maximum capacitive load C_L that can be connected to a 741 without degrading the normal slew rate (0.6 V/μs). at the maximum current output (5 mA).

3.17 (a) For Figure 3.20, assume that the carrier frequency is 3 kHz. Design the RC output low-pass filter to have a corner frequency of 20 Hz and a reasonable value capacitor (0.1 μF). Use (b) a one-section active filter, (c) a two-section active filter, and (d) a three-section active filter.

3.18 For Figure 3.20, if the forward drop of D_1 is 10% higher than that of the other diodes, what change occurs in v_o?

3.19 For the differentiator of Figure 3.12, ground the input, break the feedback loop at any point, and determine the phase shift in each section. Explain why the circuit tends to oscillate.

3.20 Find $V_o(j\omega)/V_i(j\omega)$ for the bandpass filter shown in Figure 3.13(c).

3.21 Design a one-section high-pass filter with a gain of 20 and a corner frequency of 0.05 Hz. Calculate its response to a step input of 1 mV.

3.22 Repeat Example 3.3 for the 741 op amp.

References

Anonymous, *μA741 frequency-compensated operational amplifier.* Mountain View, CA: Fairchild Semiconductor, 1973.

Aronson, M. H., "Lock-in and carrier amplifiers." *Med. Electron. Data,* 8(3), 1977, C1–C16.

Ary, J. P., "A head-mounted 24-channel evoked potential preamplifier employing low-noise operational amplifiers." *IEEE Trans. Biomed. Eng.,* BME-24, 1977, 293-297.

Fink, D.G. (ed.), *Electronic engineer's handbook.* New York: McGraw-Hill, 1975, pp. 14-14–14-15.

Graeme, J.G., *Applications of operational amplifiers*. New York: McGraw-Hill, 1974a.

Graeme, J.G., "Rectifying wide-range signals with precision, variable gain." *Electron.*, Dec. 12, 1974b, 45(25), 107–109.

Jung, W. G., *IC op-amp cookbook*. Indianapolis: Bobbs-Merrill, 1974.

Jurgen, R. K., "Software (and hardware) for the 'medics'." *IEEE Spectrum,* April 1976, 13(4), 40–43.

Peatman, J.B., *Microcomputer-based design*. New York: McGraw-Hill, 1977.

Sheingold, D.H. (ed.), *Analog-digital conversion handbook*. Norwood, MA: Analog Devices, 1972.

Shepard, R. R., "Active filters: Part 12, Short cuts to network design." *Electron.*, Aug. 18, 1969, 42(17), 82–92.

Stout, D.F., and M. Kaufman, *Handbook of operational amplifier circuit design*. New York: McGraw-Hill, 1976.

Tobey, G.E., J.G. Graeme, and L.P., Huelsman, *Operational amplifiers: Design and application*. New York: McGraw-Hill, 1971.

Wait, J.V., L.P., Huelsman, and G.A., Korn, *Introduction to operational amplifier theory and applications*. New York: McGraw-Hill, 1975.

Chapter four

The origin of biopotentials

John W. Clark, Jr.

This chapter deals with the genesis of various bioelectric signals that are recorded routinely in modern clinical practice. Given adequate monitoring equipment, the engineer of today can record many forms of bioelectric phenomena with relative ease. These phenomena include the electrocardiogram (ECG), electroencephalogram (EEG), electroneurogram (ENG), electromyogram (EMG), and electroretinogram (ERG).

Engineers generally have a good physical insight into the nature of electromagnetic fields produced by bioelectric sources, and, because of their comprehensive understanding of the physical problem, they may contribute to the solution of problems.

This chapter first explains bioelectric phenomena at the cellular level and then discusses volume conductor fields of simple as well as anatomically complex bioelectric sources. The volume-conductor-field problem serves as a necessary link between cellular activity and gross, externally recorded biological signals, such as the ECG. We shall describe the functional organization of the peripheral (outside the brain and spinal cord) nervous system and then examine the ENG and EMG. Finally, we shall discuss the ECG, ERG, and EEG.

4.1 Electrical activity of excitable cells

Bioelectric potentials are produced as a result of electrochemical activity of a certain class of cells, known as *excitable cells,* that are components of nervous, muscular, or glandular tissue. Electrically they exhibit a *resting potential,* and, when appropriately stimulated, an *action potential,* as we shall explain in the following paragraphs.

The resting state

The individual excitable cell maintains a steady electrical potential difference between its internal and external environments.

143

This resting potential of the internal medium lies in the range − 50 to − 100 mV, relative to the external medium.

Figure 4.1(a) shows how the resting potential is usually measured. A micromanipulator advances a microelectrode (see Section 5.8) close to the surface of an excitable cell and then, by small movements, pushes it through the cell membrane. For the membrane to seal properly around the penetrating tip, the diameter of the tip must be small relative to the size of the cell in which it is placed. Figure 4.1(b) shows a typical electrical recording from a

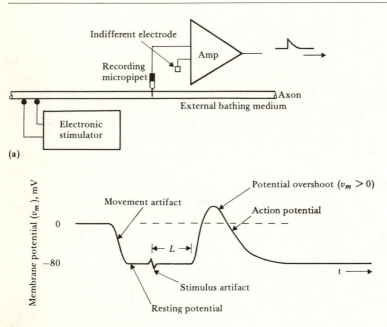

(a)

(b)

Figure 4.1 Recording of action potential of an invertebrate nerve axon. (a) An electronic stimulator supplies a brief pulse of current to the axon, strong enough to excite the axon. A recording of this activity is made at a downstream site via a penetrating micropipet. (b) Movement artifact is recorded as tip of micropipet drives through membrane to record resting potential. A short time later, an electrical stimulus is delivered to the axon; its field effect is recorded instantaneously at downstream measurement site as the stimulus artifact. The action potential proceeds along the axon at a constant propagation velocity. The time period L is the *latent period* or transmission time from stimulus to recording site.

single nerve fiber showing the dc offset potential (resting potential) that occurs upon penetration of the membrane. It also shows the transient disturbance of membrane potential (the action potential) when an adequate stimulus is given.

The cell membrane is a very thin (7−15 nm) lipoprotein complex that is essentially impermeable to intracellular protein and other organic anions (A⁻). The membrane in the resting state is moderately permeable to Na^+ and rather freely permeable to K^+ and Cl^-. The permeability of the resting membrane to potassium ion (P_K) is approximately 50–100 times larger than its permeability to sodium ion (P_{Na}). The reason for these differences in permeability of the membrane to various ionic species is as yet unknown, but it may be based on the size of pores in the membrane.

For frog skeletal muscle, the K^+ concentration of the internal media is 140 mmol/liter, while that of the external media is 2.5 mmol/liter. Thus there is a diffusion gradient that is directed outward across the membrane due to the concentration imbalance. The movement of the K^+ along this diffusion gradient (while the nondiffusible anion component stays within the cell) is in such a direction as to make the interior of the cell more negative relative to the outside of the cell (i.e., positive charge is removed from the interior). A transmembrane potential difference is thus established. The membrane may then be described electrically as a leaky capacitor. That is, it acts as a charge separator, yet it has a dielectric material (the lipoprotein complex of the membrane itself) that allows a leakage flow of ions across the membrane via pores. The electric field supported by the membrane capacitor is directed inward from positive to negative across the membrane, and tends to inhibit the outward flow of positively charged ions (such as K^+) and the inward flow of negatively charged ions (such as Cl^-). Thus the diffusional and electrical forces acting across the membrane are opposed to one another, and a steady state is ultimately achieved. The membrane potential at which this steady state exists (considering K^+ to be the main ionic species involved in the resting state, that is, $P_K \gg P_{Na}$) is called the *equilibrium potential* for potassium E_K. It is measured in volts, and is calculated from the Nernst equation

$$E_K = \frac{RT}{nF} \ln \frac{[K]_o}{[K]_i} = 0.0615 \log_{10} \frac{[K]_o}{[K]_i} \quad (V) \qquad (4.1)$$

at 37°C (body temperature). Here n is the valence of K^+; $[K]_i$ and $[K]_o$ are the intra- and extracellular concentrations of K^+ in moles per liter; R is the universal gas constant (Appendix); T is absolute temperature in K; and F is the Faraday constant (Appendix). Equation (4.1) gives a reasonably good approximation to the potential of the resting membrane, which indicates that the resting membrane is effectively a *potassium membrane*. A more accurate expression for the membrane equilibrium potential E that accounts for the influence of other ionic species in the internal and external media was first developed by Goldman (1943) and later modified by Hodgkin and Katz (1949), who assumed a constant electric field across the membrane:

$$E = \frac{RT}{F} \ln \left\{ \frac{P_K[K]_o + P_{Na}[Na]_o + P_{Cl}[Cl]_i}{P_K[K]_i + P_{Na}[Na]_i + P_{Cl}[Cl]_o} \right\} \qquad (4.2)$$

Here E is the equilibrium transmembrane resting potential when net current through the membrane is zero and P is the *permeability coefficient* of the membrane.

Example 4.1 For frog skeletal muscle, typical values for the intracellular and extracellular concentrations of the major ionic species (in millimoles per liter) are as follows.

Species	Intracellular	Extracellular
Na^+	12	145
K^+	155	4
Cl^-	4	120

Assuming room temperature (20°C) and typical values of permeability coefficient for frog skeletal muscle ($P_{Na} = 2 \times 10^{-8}$ cm/s, $P_K = 2 \times 10^{-6}$ cm/s, and $P_{Cl} = 4 \times 10^{-6}$ cm/s), calculate the resting equilibrium resting potential for this membrane, using the Goldman equation.

Answer From (4.2):

$$E = 0.0581 \log_{10} \left[\frac{P_K(4) + P_{Na}(145) + P_{Cl}(4)}{P_K(155) + P_{Na}(12) + P_{Cl}(120)} \right]$$

$$= 0.0581 \log_{10} \left(\frac{26.9 \times 10^{-6}}{790.24 \times 10^{-6}} \right) = -85.3 \text{ mV}$$

which is close to typical measured values for frog skeletal muscle.

Maintaining steady-state ionic imbalance between the internal and external media of the cell requires the continual active transport of ionic species diffusing out of and into the cell, according to their passive diffusion gradients. The active transport mechanism is located within the membrane, and is sometimes referred to as the *sodium-potassium pump*. It actively transports Na^+ out of the cell and K^+ into the cell. Energy for the pump is provided by a common source of cellular energy, adenosine triphosphate (ATP).

Thus the factors influencing the flow of ions across the membrane are (1) diffusion gradients, (2) the inwardly directed electric field, (3) membrane structure (availability of pores), and (4) active transport of ions against an established electrochemical gradient. The distribution of ions across the cell membrane and the structure of this membrane (P_K, P_{Na}, P_{Cl}) provide the explanation for the resting potential. Potassium ions diffuse out of the cell according to their concentration gradient, while the nondiffusible organic anion component remains within, creating a potential difference across the membrane. There is thus a slight excess of cations outside the membrane and a slight excess of anions within. The number of ions responsible for the membrane potential, however, is very small relative to the total number present in the internal and external media. The Na^+ influx does not compensate for the K^+ efflux because, in the resting state, $P_{Na} \ll P_K$. Chloride ion diffuses inward down its concentration gradient, but its movement is balanced by the electrical gradient.

Example 4.2 The giant axon of the squid is frequently used in electrophysiological investigations because of its size. It typically has a diameter of 1000 μm, a membrane thickness of 7.5 nm, a specific membrane capacity of 1 $\mu F/cm^2$, and a resting transmembrane potential (v_m) of 70 mV. If we assume a uniform electric field within the membrane, what is the magnitude and direction of the electric field intensity **E** within the membrane?

Answer The membrane is quite thin and serves as a charge separator. Based on what is known of its histological and electrophysiological behavior, we know that a unit area of membrane can be adequately represented by a parallel-plate capacitor with a separation distance d equal to 7.5 nm. In the space between the plates, **E** is constant and perpendicular to the two plates. Since $\mathbf{E} = -\nabla v(x)$, where x is distance measured outward through the membrane, and the gradient $\nabla v = dv/dx = -v_m/d$, the potential v varies linearly between the plates, and

$$\mathbf{E} = \frac{v_m}{d} = \frac{70 \times 10^{-3}}{7.5 \times 10^{-9}} = 9.33 \times 10^6 \text{ V/m}.$$

This vector-field quantity is directed inward through the membrane.

Calculate the relative dielectric constant ϵ_r of this parallel-plate capacitor. [*Hint:* $C_m = \epsilon_r \epsilon_0/d$ and ϵ_0 is given in the Appendix.] Answer: 8.47

The active state

Another property of an excitable cell is its ability to conduct an action potential [Fig. 4.1(b)] when adequately stimulated. An *adequate stimulus* is one that brings about a depolarization in a membrane that is sufficient to exceed the threshold potential of the membrane and thereby elicit an all-or-none action potential that travels in an unattenuated fashion at a constant conduction velocity along the membrane of the excitable cell. Because of the steady resting potential, the cell membrane is said to be *polarized*. A lessening of the magnitude of this polarization is called *depolarization*, while an increase in magnitude is referred to as *hyperpolarization*. The "all-or-none" property of the action potential means that the membrane potential goes through a very characteristic cycle: a change in potential from the resting level of a certain amount for a fixed duration of time; for a nerve fiber $\Delta v \cong 120$ mV and the duration is approximately 1 ms. Further increases in intensity or duration of stimulus beyond that required for exceeding the threshold level only produce the same result.

The origin of the action potential lies in the voltage and time-dependent nature of the membrane permeabilities (or equivalently, in electrical terms, membrane conductivities) to specific ions, notably sodium and potassium. As the membrane is depolarized, the permeability of the membrane to sodium P_{Na} (or, equivalently, the conductance of the membrane to sodium g_{Na}) is significantly increased. As a result, Na^+ rushes into the internal medium of the cell, bringing about further depolarization, which in turn brings about a further increase in g_{Na} (that is, g_{Na} is dependent on the voltage across the membrane). If the membrane threshold is exceeded, this process is self-regenerative and leads to *runaway* depolarization. Under these conditions, the membrane potential tends to approach the Nernst potential of sodium, E_{Na}, which has a value of about +60 mV.

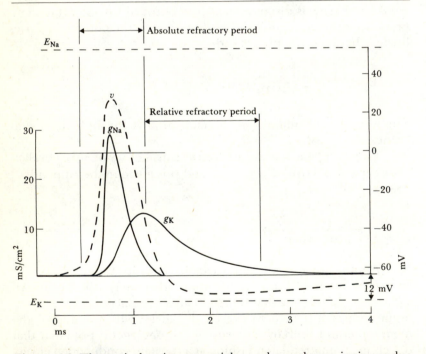

Figure 4.2 Theoretical action potential v and membrane ionic conductance changes for sodium (g_{Na}) and potassium (g_K) obtained by solving the differential equations developed by Hodgkin and Huxley for the giant axon of the squid at a bathing medium temperature of 18.5°C. E_{Na} and E_K are the Nernst equilibrium potentials for sodium and potassium across the membrane. Modified from A.L. Hodgkin and A.F. Huxley, "A Quantitative Description of Membrane Current and Its Application to Conduction and Excitation in Nerve," *J. Physiology* 1952, **117**, p. 530.

The membrane potential never achieves this level, however, because of two factors: (1) g_{Na} is not only voltage-dependent, but also time-dependent and (as shown in Figure 4.2) it is relatively short-lived compared with the duration of the action potential. (2) There is a delayed increase in g_K that acts as a hyperpolarizing influence, tending to return the membrane to resting levels (Figure 4.2). As the membrane potential ultimately returns to the resting level, g_K is still elevated with respect to its resting value and returns slowly along an exponential time course. Since potassium ions continue to leave the cell during this time, the membrane hyperpolarizes and an undershoot is produced in the transmembrane potential waveform (v_m).

The calculated g_{Na} and g_K waveforms of Figure 4.2 are based on *voltage-clamp* data from squid axon. In voltage-clamp experiments, voltage in a membrane is held at prescribed levels via a negative-feedback control circuit. Membrane currents in response to step changes in clamp voltages are studied in order to determine the voltage- and time-dependent nature of g_{Na} and g_K.

Figure 4.3 shows a network equivalent circuit describing the electrical behavior of a small increment of membrane. The entire nerve axon membrane could be characterized in a distributed fashion by utilizing an iterative structure of this same basic form.

When an excitable membrane has an action potential in

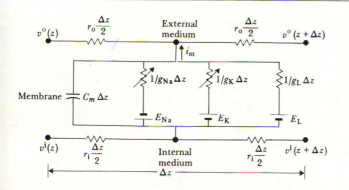

Figure 4.3 Diagram of network equivalent circuit of a small length (Δz) of nerve or muscle. The membrane proper is characterized by specific membrane capacitance C_m (μF/cm^2) and specific membrane conductances g_{Na}, g_K, and g_{Cl} in mS/cm^2 (mmho/cm^2). Here an average specific leakage conductance is included that corresponds to ionic current from sources other than Na$^+$ and K$^+$ (for example, Cl$^-$). This term is usually neglected. The cell cytoplasm is considered simply resistive, as is the external bathing medium; these media may thus be characterized by the resistance per unit length r_i and r_o (Ω/cm), respectively. Here i_m is the transmembrane current per unit length (A/cm) and v^i and v^o are the internal and external potentials v at point z, respectively. (Modified from A.L. Hodgkin and A.F. Huxley, "A Quantitative Description of Membrane Current and Its Application to Conduction and Excitation in Nerve," *Journal of Physiology*, 1952, **117**, p. 501.)

response to an adequate stimulus, the ability of the membrane to respond to a second stimulus of any sort is markedly altered. During the initial portion of the action potential, the membrane cannot respond to any stimulus, no matter how intense. This interval is referred to as the *absolute refractory period*. It is followed by the *relative refractory period*, wherein an action potential can be elicited by an intense superthreshold stimulus (Figure 4.2). The existence of the refractory period produces an upper limit to the frequency at which an excitable cell may be repetitively discharged. For example, a nerve axon has an absolute refractory period of 1 ms, and an upper limit of repetitive discharge of less than 1000 impulses/s.

For an action potential propagating along a single nerve fiber, the region of the fiber undergoing a transition into the active state (i.e., the *active region*) at an instant of time is usually small relative to the length of the fiber. Figure 4.4 schematically shows the charge distribution along the fiber in the vicinity of the active region. Here we see the direction of propagation of the action potential (considered frozen in time) and the membrane lying ahead of the active region is polarized, as in the resting state. A reversal of polarity is shown within the active region, due to depolarization of the membrane to positive values of potential. The membrane lying behind the active zone is repolarized membrane.

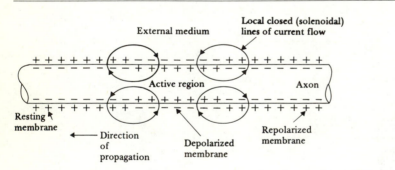

Figure 4.4 Charge distribution in vicinity of active region of fiber conducting an impulse.

From the indicated charge distribution, *solenoidal* (closed-path) current flows in the pattern shown in Figure 4.4. In the region ahead of the active zone, the ohmic potential drop across the membrane caused by this solenoidal current flowing outward through the membrane is of such a polarity as to reduce the magnitude of the transmembrane potential; that is, depolarize the membrane. When the membrane potential is depolarized to the threshold level (about 20 mV more positive than the resting potential), this region becomes activated as well. The same current pattern flowing behind the active region is ineffective in re-exciting the membrane, which is in the refractory state. The nature of this process is therefore self-excitatory, with each new increment of membrane being brought to the threshold level by lines of current from the active source region. The membrane stays in the active state for only a brief period of time and ultimately repolarizes completely. In this way, the action potential propagates down the length of the fiber in an unattenuated fashion, with the signal being built up at each point along the way.

4.2 Volume conductor fields

A fundamental problem in electrophysiology is the problem of the single active cell immersed in a volume conductor (a salt solution simulating the composition of body fluids). A study of this problem provides considerable insight into other more-complex volume-conductor-field problems, such as the ENG, EMG, ECG, and so forth.

The problem consists of two parts: (1) the bioelectric source and (2) its bathing medium or electrical load. The bioelectric source is the active cell that behaves approximately as a constant-current source, delivering its current to the bathing medium under a large range of loading conditions. The source considered for the present is the single active nerve fiber. The volume conductor is considered infinite in extent (that is, large relative to the extent of the electric field surrounding the nerve fiber). The lines of flow of the current emanating from the active fiber into the bathing medium of specific resistivity ρ are indicated schematically in Figure 4.4. This pattern of current flow is consistent with the charge distribution shown in Figure 4.4.

Since the action potential is assumed to be traveling down the fiber at a constant conduction velocity, a temporal waveform $v_m(t)$ may be easily converted to a spatial distribution $v_m(z)$, where z is the axial distance along the fiber. For a simple monophasic action potential, the associated potential waveform at the outer surface of the membrane is (1) triphasic in nature, (2) of greater spatial extent, and (3) much smaller in peak-to-peak magnitude than the action potential. Potentials in the extracellular medium of a single fiber fall off in magnitude with increasing radial distance from the fiber from about -70 μV at the surface to about -20 μV at a distance of 500 μm.

If, for the case of the infinite volume conductor, ρ is increased, the potential at the field point increases, as it would in the case in which the volume conductor is made smaller (the field point, of course, lies within the volume conductor). In each of these cases, the total extracellular resistance to current flow from the constant-current bioelectric source is greater. Therefore, from

Ohm's law applied to this passive cylindrical volume conductor, potential in the extracellular medium is increased.

If we consider the source to be, instead of the single fiber, an active nerve trunk with its thousands of component nerve fibers simultaneously activated, the extracellular field in an infinite homogeneous bathing medium appears quite similar to that of a single fiber, as shown in Figure 4.5. The extracellular field poten-

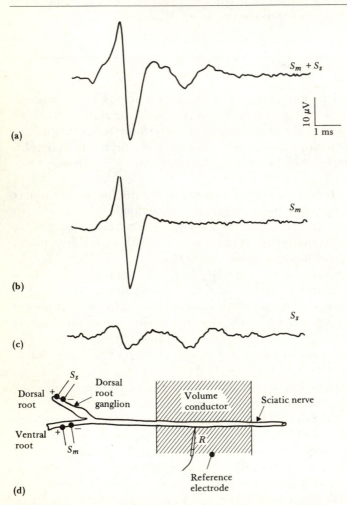

Figure 4.5 Extracellular field potentials (average of 128 responses) recorded at surface of an active (1-mm-diameter) frog sciatic nerve in an extensive volume conductor. Potential recorded with (a) both motor and sensory components excited ($S_m + S_s$), (b) only motor nerve components excited (S_m), and (c) only sensory nerve components excited (S_s).

tial is a signal formed from the contributions of the superimposed electric fields of the component sources within the trunk. The general form of the extracellular response of a nerve trunk to electrical stimulation is triphasic, and of an amplitude in the low-microvolt range. The potential loses amplitude and high-frequency content at larger radial distances from the nerve trunk.

The sciatic nerve utilized in this experiment is actually a rather complex bioelectric source. It consists of large motor fibers running from the spinal cord to the leg muscles, as well as large and small sensory fibers running from sensory receptors in the leg and skin to the spinal cord. In Figure 4.5(a), the entire nerve trunk (containing both motor and sensory fibers) was simultaneously excited using an intense suprathreshold electrical stimulus.

It is possible, however, to separately excite the motor and sensory components of the trunk by isolating the nerve trunk in the vicinity of the spinal cord. Here the nerve trunk divides into a sensory branch (the *dorsal root*) and a motor branch (the *ventral root*). The results of separate motor and sensory stimulation are shown in Figure 4.5(b) and (c). We observe that stimulation of the many large motor fibers in the trunk provides the largest extracellular response. We also observe that stimulation of the sensory root actually excites at least two groups of sensory fibers—a group of large fast fibers (group I) and a group of smaller, slower fibers (group II). Observing the extracellular waveform produced by combined stimulation [Figure 4.5(a)], we can see the approximate superposition of motor and sensory responses.

The load of the active nerve trunk may also be altered and made more complicated. A relatively simple variation is to increase the specific resistivity of the bathing medium or to decrease the radial extent of the volume conductor, or both. These alterations very predictably produce larger extracellular potentials.

The foregoing discussion may be considered as an explanation of the electrogenesis of the ENG, which is commonly recorded from the surface of an arm, a leg, or the face. Many of the concepts introduced here apply directly to the interpretation of other externally recorded bioelectric phenomena.

Example 4.3 An important topic in electrophysiology is the relationship between intracellular and extracellular potentials, especially for the case of an active elongated cell, such as a nerve or muscle fiber. This relationship is easily seen if we first assume that an action potential travels at a constant velocity along this long fiber, and therefore temporal and spatial events can be interchanged, since potentials must be of the form $f(z - ut)$, where z is axial distance along the fiber, t is time and u is the propagation velocity. Then, adopting an important result that follows from classical core conductor theory applied to the volume conductor problem [see, e.g., Clark and Plonsey (1968)], we state that the transmembrane current per unit length of fiber (i_m, A/cm) is given by the equation

$$i_m = \frac{1}{r_o + r_i} \frac{\partial^2 v_m(z)}{\partial z^2}$$

where v_m is the transmembrane potential and r_i and r_o are the intra- and extracellular resistances per unit length (Ω/cm), respectively. Since r_i and r_o are constants, i_m is directly proportional to the second derivative of v_m with respect to z (v_m is a function of z only). This means that the current flow out of the membrane into the volume conductor per unit length of fiber is proportional to the second spatial derivative of the action potential, as in Figure E4.1. Note that v_m is monophasic, while its second derivative is triphasic. The extracellular medium is simply resistive, and therefore the extracellular field potential is proportional to i_m. Hence it is proportional to $\partial^2 v_m / \partial z^2$.

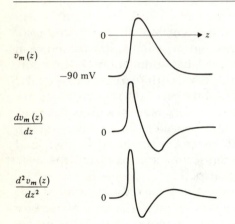

$v_m(z)$

-90 mV

$\dfrac{dv_m(z)}{dz}$

$\dfrac{d^2 v_m(z)}{dz^2}$

Figure E4.1 An action potential and its first and second derivatives. This concept enables the researcher to predict the waveshape of a volume conductor potential, given arbitrary data on action potential. It is only approximate for large-volume conductors, but becomes more accurate as the radial extent of the volume conductor decreases [Clark and Plonsey (1968).]

4.3 Functional organization of the peripheral nervous system

The reflex arc

The spinal nervous system is functionally organized on the basis of what is commonly called the *reflex arc* [Figure 4.6(a)]. The components of this arc are: (1) A *sense organ,* consisting of many individual sense receptors that respond preferentially to an environmental stimulus of a particular kind, such as pressure, temperature, touch, or pain. (2) A *sensory nerve,* containing many individual nerve fibers that perform the task of transmitting information (encoded in the form of action potential frequency) from a peripheral sense receptor to other cells lying within the central system (brain and spinal cord). (3) The *CNS,* which in this case serves as a central integrating station; here information is evaluated and, if warranted, a "motor" decision is implemented. That is, action potentials are initiated in motor-nerve fibers associated with the motor-nerve trunk. (4) A *motor nerve,* serving as a communication link between the CNS and peripheral muscle. (5) The *effector organ,* which consists, in this case, of skeletal muscle fibers that contract (shorten) in response to the driving stimuli (action potentials) conducted by motor-nerve fibers.

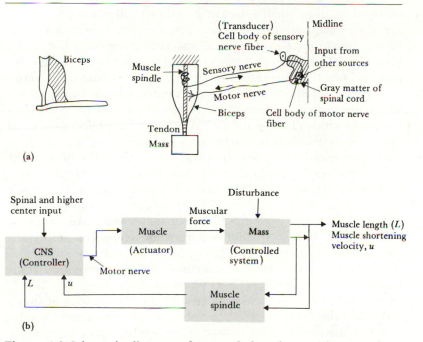

Figure 4.6 Schematic diagram of a muscle-length control system for a peripheral muscle (biceps). (a) Anatomical diagram of limb system, showing interconnections. (b) Block diagram of control system.

The simplest example of the behavior of the reflex arc is found in the knee-jerk reflex, in which the patellar tendon below the knee is given a slight tap that stretches specialized length receptors, called *muscle spindles,* within the muscle and subsequently excites them. This excitation results in action potentials which propagate along the sensory nerve that enters the spinal cord and communicates with CNS cells, specifically motoneurons. The resultant motor activity reflexly brings about contraction of the muscle that was initially stimulated, and the shortening muscle jerks the limb, producing the well-known knee-jerk response. Note that the initial stimulus to the muscle was a stretch, while the response was a contraction of the muscle. This simple reflex arc has many of the features of a negative-feedback loop, in which the control variable is muscle length [Figure 4.6(b)]. The CNS acts as the controller, the muscle spindle acts as a feedback length transducer, and the muscle-limb system as the process to be controlled. For an interesting, comprehensive description of this subject, see Mountcastle (1974, Chapters 20–25).

Junctional transmission

Within the reflex arc there are intercommunicating links between neurons (neuro–neuro junctions) called *synapses*. There are also communicating links between neurons and muscle fibers (*neuromuscular junctions*) at a small specialized region of the muscle fiber referred to as the *end-plate region*. The junctional transmission process in each of these cases is electrochemical in nature. There is a prejunctional fiber involved in the neuromuscular junction that, when depolarized, releases a neurotransmitter substance, *Acetylcholine* (Ach) which diffuses across a very small fluid-filled gap region approximately 20 nm in thickness. The fluid filling the gap is assumed to be ordinary interstitial body fluid. Once the neurotransmitter reaches the postjunctional membrane, it combines with a membrane receptor complex that ultimately leads to a relatively brief transient depolarization of the membrane and subsequent initiation of an action potential that propagates away from the junctional region. The electrochemical transmission process at the junction involves a time delay on the order of 0.5–1.0 ms. For a more complete description of interneuronal and neuromuscular transmission, see Mountcastle (1974, Chapters 5 and 6).

Another time delay associated with the neuromuscular system is the delay between electrical activation of the musculature and the onset of mechanical contraction. This is referred to as *excitation-contraction time*, and is a property of the muscle itself. When the muscle is repeatedly stimulated, the mechanical response summates. At high stimulation rates, the mechanical responses fuse into one continuous contraction, called a *tetanus* (or *tetanic contraction*).

4.4 The electroneurogram (ENG)

Conduction velocity in a peripheral nerve is measured by stimulating a motor nerve at two points a known distance apart along its course. Subtraction of the shorter latency from the longer latency (Figure 4.7) gives the conduction time along the segment of nerve between the stimulating electrodes. Knowing the separation distance, we can determine the conduction velocity of the nerve. The clinical value of knowing such velocity is that, following nerve

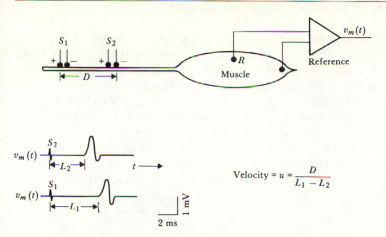

$$\text{Velocity} = u = \frac{D}{L_1 - L_2}$$

Figure 4.7 Measurement of neural conduction velocity via measurement of latency of evoked electrical response in muscle. Nerve stimulated at two different sites a known distance D apart.

injury, the conduction velocity in a regenerating nerve fiber is slowed (Berry *et al.*, 1944).

Although field potentials from nerves are of a much smaller amplitude than extracellular potentials from surrounding excitable muscle fibers, such potentials can be recorded, either with concentric needle electrodes or with surface electrodes. Nerve field potentials can be evoked by applying stimuli to "mixed" nerves that contain both motor and sensory components (such as the ulnar nerve), in which case the resultant field potentials are derived from both types of active fibers.

Neural field potentials can also be elicited from a purely sensory nerve (such as the sural nerve in the leg) or from sensory components of a mixed nerve, in which the stimulation is applied in a manner that does not excite the motor components of the nerve. The study of field potentials from sensory nerves in general has been shown to be of considerable value in diagnosing peripheral nerve disorders (Gilliatt and Sears, 1958).

Although conduction velocity and latency are the most generally useful parameters associated with peripheral nerve function, the characteristics of potential fields evoked in muscle supplied by the stimulated nerve are also important. When considering evoked muscle potentials, frequently the duration of the response is of interest, since a slowing of conduction in a few motor nerve fibers may, in fact, lead to late activation of a portion of the muscle, and the resultant field potential may be prolonged and polyphasic. When field potentials of the nerve are measured in such a case, temporal dispersion due to the slowed conduction in some of the fibers may lead to a significant decrease in the amplitude of the signal.

Field potentials of sensory nerves

Extracellular field responses from sensory nerves can be easily measured from the median or ulnar nerves of the arm by using ring-stimulating electrodes applied to the fingers (Figure 4.8). Recording at two sites along the course of the nerve a known distance apart enables one to compute the conduction velocity of the sensory nerve. In the case of the ulnar nerve (roughly speaking, it supplies the third and fourth fingers), evoked neural potentials can be recorded from different sites along the course of the nerve as high as the armpit. In the case of the median nerve (roughly speaking, it supplies the index and the second fingers), potentials can be recorded from the nerve at and above the elbow.

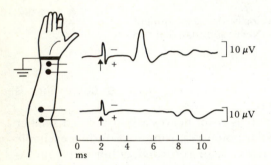

Figure 4.8 Sensory nerve action potentials evoked from median nerve of a healthy subject at elbow and wrist after stimulation of index finger with ring electrodes. Potential at the wrist is triphasic and of much larger magnitude than delayed potential recorded at the elbow. Considering the median nerve to be of the same size and shape at the elbow as at the wrist, we find that the difference in magnitude and waveshape of the potentials is due to the size of the volume conductor at each location and the radial distance of the measurement point from the neural source. (From J.A.R. Lenman and A.E. Ritchie, *Clinical Electromyography,* 2nd ed., Philadelphia: Lippincott, 1977; reproduced by permission of the authors.)

Long pulses cause muscle contractions, limb movement, and undesired signals (*artifacts*). These are easily avoided by positioning the limb in a comfortable relaxed posture and applying a brief, intense stimulus (square pulse of approximately 100-V amplitude with a duration of 100–300 μs). Such a stimulus excites the large, rapidly conducting sensory nerve fibers, but not small pain fibers or surrounding muscle. To minimize artifacts caused by stimuli, we use a stimulus isolation unit (isolation transformer, diode-bridge circuit, optical coupler, etc.) to isolate the bipolar stimulating electrodes from ground. A patient ground is placed at the wrist between the stimulating and recording electrodes to provide a ground point for the passive electric field coupling from the stimulating electrodes. The skin should be abraded under both the stimulating and recording electrodes (Section 5.5) to reduce skin resistance and ensure good contact.

Clinically, field potentials are recorded using high-gain, high-input-impedance differential preamplifiers with good common-mode rejection capability and low inherent amplifier noise (Section 6.5). Figure 4.8 shows that the measured ENGs are on the order of 10 μV and power-line interference is sometimes a problem even with good amplifier common-mode properties. The input leads should be properly twisted together and shielded. In addition, if warranted, the subject could be placed in an adequately shielded room or cage.

A further step we can use to enhance the signal-to-noise ratio in the presence of random noise (for the most part generated by the amplifier) is to use a *signal averager* (Section 6.8).

Motor-nerve conduction velocity

In vivo measurement of the conduction velocity of a motor nerve may be obtained as shown in Figure 4.7. For example, the peroneal nerve of the left leg may be stimulated first behind the knee and second behind the ankle. A muscular response is obtained from the side of the foot, using surface or needle electrodes.

Reflexly evoked field potentials

When a peripheral nerve is stimulated and an evoked field potential is recorded in the muscle it supplies, it is sometimes possible to record a second potential that occurs later than the initial response. The latency of the initial response decreases as the stimulus is brought closer to the muscle. However, the second response may exhibit a progressively greater latency as the stimulus is brought closer to the muscle. This behavior of the second response indicates that, to activate the muscle, the stimulus must travel along the nerve toward the central nervous system (i.e., proximally) for some distance before ultimately traveling in the opposite direction (i.e., distally). The latency of the second response is such that the activity could have traveled proximally along sensory nerves as far as the spinal cord to elicit a spinal reflex.

If the posterior tibial nerve in the leg is stimulated, a late potential can be evoked from the triceps sural muscle (Figure 4.9). This long latency response has a low threshold and appears at stimulus intensities that are well below the levels required to elicit the conventional (short-latency) *M wave*. This long-latency potential —known as the *H wave*—was discovered by Huffman (Figure 4.9). Its latency indicates that it is a spinal reflex. It is, in fact, the electrical homolog of the simple "ankle-jerk" reflex.

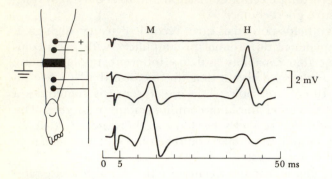

Figure 4.9 The H reflex. The four traces show potentials evoked by stimulation of the medial popliteal nerve with pulses of increasing magnitude (the stimulus artifact increases with stimulus magnitude). The later potential or H wave is a low-threshold response, maximally evoked by a stimulus too weak to evoke the muscular response (M wave). As the M wave increases in magnitude, the H wave diminishes. (From J.A.R. Lenman and A.E. Ritchie, *Clinical Electromyography,* 2nd ed., Philadelphia, Lippincott, 1977; reproduced by permission of the authors.)

Thus, when a mixed peripheral nerve such as the posterior tibial nerve is stimulated by a stimulus of low intensity, only fibers of large diameter are stimulated because they have the lowest threshold. These large fibers are sensory fibers from muscle spindles that conduct toward the CNS and ultimately connect with motor fibers in the spinal cord via a single synapse. The motoneurons discharge and produce a response in the gastrocnemius muscle of the leg (the *H* wave). With a stimulus of medium intensity, smaller motor fibers in the mixed nerve are stimulated in addition to the sensory fibers, producing a direct, short-latency muscle response, the *M* wave (Figure 4.9). With still stronger stimuli, impulses conducted centrally along the motor fibers may interfere with the production of the *H* wave (these excited motor fibers are in their refractory period) so that only an *M* wave is produced (Figure 4.9). The amplitude of the *H* response depends on the number of motoneurons discharged. Its amplitude is also somewhat variable, due to fluctuating background neural conditions within the spinal cord. These neural disturbances are provided by the activity of other spinal and higher center neurons impinging on the motoneuron(s) involved in the reflex.

4.5 The electromyogram (EMG)

Skeletal muscle is organized functionally on the basis of the *motor unit* (see Figure 4.10). The motor unit is the smallest unit that may be activated by a volitional effort, in which case all constituent muscle fibers are activated synchronously. The component fibers of the motor units extend lengthwise in loose bundles along the muscle. In cross section, however, the fibers of a given motor unit are interspersed with fibers of other motor units. Thus the component muscle fibers of the *single motor unit* (SMU) constitute a distributed, unit bioelectric source located in a volume conductor consisting of all other muscle fibers, both active and inactive. The evoked extracellular field potential from the active fibers of an SMU has a triphasic form of brief duration (3–15 ms) and an amplitude of 20–2000 μV depending on the size of the motor unit. The frequency of discharge usually varies from 6–30 per second.

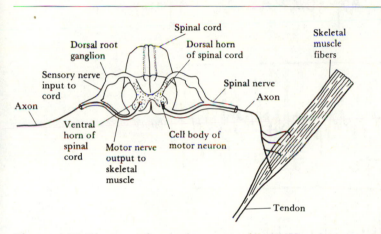

Figure 4.10 Diagram of a single motor unit (SMU), which consists of a single motoneuron and the group of skeletal muscle fibers that it innervates.

One of the disadvantages of recording the EMG using the convenient surface electrodes is that they can be used only with superficial muscles, and are sensitive to electrical activity over too wide an area. Various types of monopolar, bipolar, and multipolar insertion-type electrodes are commonly used in electromyography for recording from deep muscles and from SMUs. These types of electrodes generally record local activity from small regions within the muscle in which they are inserted. Often a simple fine-tipped monopolar needle electrode can be used to record SMU field potentials even during powerful voluntary contractions. Bipolar recordings are also employed. Various types of electrodes are discussed in Chapter 5.

Figure 4.11 shows motor unit potentials from the normal dorsal interosseus muscle under graded levels of contraction. At high levels of effort, many superimposed motor unit responses give rise to a complicated response (the *interference pattern*) in which individual units can no longer be distinguished. In interpreting Figure 4.11, note that when a muscle contracts progressively under

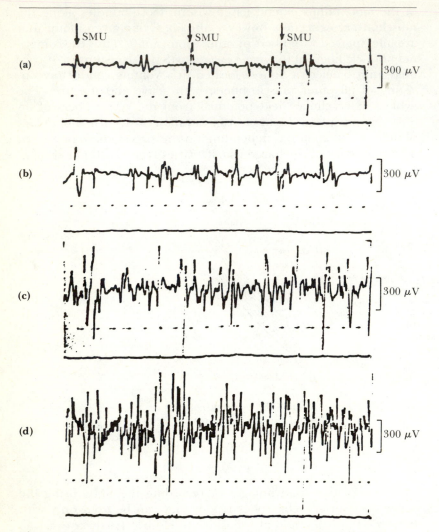

Figure 4.11 Motor unit action potentials from normal dorsal interosseus muscle during progressively more powerful contractions. In the interference pattern (c), individual units can no longer be clearly distinguished. (d) Interference pattern during very strong muscular contraction. Time scale is 10 ms per dot. (From J.A.R. Lenman and A.E. Ritchie, *Clinical Electromyography,* 2nd ed., Philadelphia: Lippincott, 1977; reproduced by permission of the authors.)

volition, active motor units increase their rate of firing and new (previously inactive) motor units are also recruited.

The shape of SMU potentials is considerably modified by disease. In peripheral neuropathies, partial denervation of the muscle frequently occurs and is followed by regeneration. Regenerating nerve fibers conduct more slowly than healthy axons. In addition, in many forms of peripheral neuropathy, the excitability of the neurons is changed and there is widespread slowing of the velocity of nerve conduction. One effect of this is that neural impulses are more difficult to initiate and take longer in transit to the muscle, generally causing scatter or desynchronization in the EMG pattern (Figure 4.12).

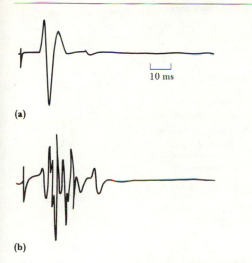

(a)

(b)

Figure 4.12 (a) Electromyographic response of normal subject recorded via concentric needle electrode in a muscle, when the muscle's nerve is stimulated. (b) Response of abnormal subject using same technique. In presence of pathology, both the excitability of neurons and the velocity of propagation along them may decrease or disappear, generally causing the desynchronization evident here.

4.6 The electrocardiogram (ECG)

Anatomy and function of the heart

The heart serves as a four-chambered pump for the circulatory system (Figure 4.13). The main pumping function is supplied by the ventricles, and the atria are merely antechambers to store blood during the time the ventricles are pumping. The resting or filling phase of the heart cycle is referred to as *diastole*. The contractile or pumping phase is called *systole*. The smooth, rhythmic contraction of the atria and ventricles has an underlying electrical precursor in the form of a well-coordinated series of electrical events that take place within the heart. That this set of electrical events is intrinsic to the heart itself is well demonstrated when the heart (particularly that of cold-blooded vertebrates such as the frog or turtle) is removed from the body and placed in a nutrient medium (e.g., glucose-Ringer solution). The heart continues to beat rhythmically for many hours. The coordinated contraction of the atria

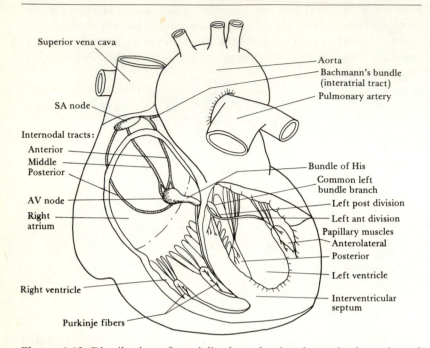

Figure 4.13 Distribution of specialized conductive tissues in the atria and ventricles, showing impulse-forming and conduction system of the heart. The rhythmic cardiac impulse originates in pacemaking cells in the sino-atrial (SA) node, located at junction of superior vena cava and right atrium. Note the three specialized pathways (anterior, middle, and posterior inter-nodal tracts) between the SA and atrioventricular (AV) nodes. Bachmann's bundle (interatrial tract) comes off the anterior internodal tract leading to the left atrium. Impulse passes from SA node in an organized manner through specialized conducting tracts in the atria to activate first the right and then the left atrium. Passage of the impulse is delayed at the AV node before it continues into the bundle of His, the right bundle branch, the common left bundle branch, the anterior and posterior divisions of the left bundle branch, and the Purkinje network. Right bundle branch runs along right side of interventricular septum to apex of right ventricle be-fore it gives off significant branches. Left common bundle crosses to left side of septum and splits into anterior division (which is thin and long and goes under the aortic valve in the outflow tract to the anterolateral papil-lary muscle) and posterior division (which is wide and short and goes to the posterior papillary muscle lying in the inflow tract). (From B.S. Lipman, E. Massie, and R.E. Kleiger, *Clinical scalar electrocardiography*. Copyright © 1972 by Yearbook Medical Publishers, Inc., Chicago. Used with permis-sion.)

and ventricles is set up by a specific pattern of electrical activation in the musculature of these structures. Moreover, the electrical ac-tivation patterns in the walls of the atria and ventricles are initiated by a coordinated series of events in the "specialized conduction system" of the heart (Figure 4.13).

In relation to the heart as a whole, the specialized conduction system is very small. It constitutes only a minute portion of the total mass of the heart. The wall of the left ventricle (Figure 4.13) is 2.5–3.0 times as thick as the wall of the right ventricle, while the intraventricular septum is nearly as thick as the left ventricular wall. The major portion of the muscle mass of the ventricle consists of the free walls of the right and left ventricles and the septum. Considering the heart as a bioelectric source, the strength of this source can be expected to be directly related to the mass of the active muscle (i.e., the number of active myocardial cells). Therefore the atria and the free walls and septum of the ventricles can be considered the major contributors to external potential fields from the heart.

Electrical behavior of cardiac cells

The heart is comprised of several different types of tissue (SA and AV nodal tissue; atrial, Purkinje, and ventricular tissue). Representative cells of each type of tissue differ anatomically to a considerable degree. They are all electrically excitable, with each type of cell exhibiting its own characteristic action potential (Figure 4.14).

The ventricular cell

The ventricular myocardium is composed of millions of individual cardiac cells (15 × 15 × 150 μm long). Figure 4.15 is a drawing of a small section of cardiac muscle as seen under light microscopy. The individual cells are relatively long and thin, and although they run generally parallel to one another, there is considerable branching and interconnecting (*anastamosing*). The cells are surrounded by a plasma membrane that makes end-to-end contact with adjacent cells at a dense structure known as the *intercalated disc* (Figure 4.15). Each fiber contains many contractile *myofibrils* that follow the axis of the cell from one end (intercalated disc) to the other. These myofibrils constitute the "contractile machinery" of the fiber. The component cells of cardiac tissue are in intimate contact at the intercalated discs, both electrically and mechanically, so that heart muscle functions as a unit (a *functional syncytium*) [Mountcastle, 1974, vol. 2].

Prior to excitation, the typical ventricular cell has a resting potential of approximately − 90 mV. The initial rapid depolarization phase has a rate of rise that is usually greater than 450 V/s. This phase is followed by an initial rapid repolarization that leads to a maintained depolarizing plateau region which lasts approximately 200–300 ms. A final repolarization phase follows that restores membrane potential to the resting level and is maintained for the remainder of the cardiac cycle. The duration of the action potential

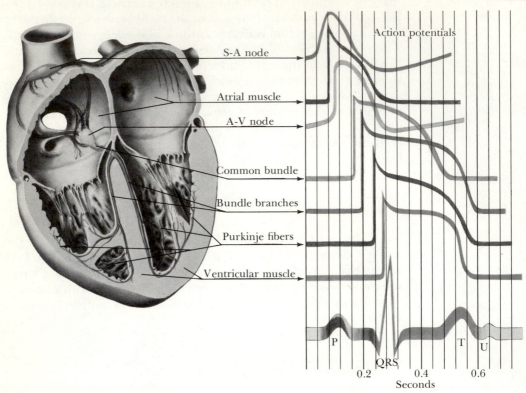

- S-A node
- Atrial muscle
- A-V node
- Common bundle
- Bundle branches
- Purkinje fibers
- Ventricular muscle

Action potentials

P QRS T U

0.2 0.4 0.6

Seconds

N8-65 Vol. 5/1 — Heart Physiology of Conduction System II — Dr. Brian Hoffman

Figure 4.14 Representative electrical activity from various regions of the heart. Bottom trace is scalar ECG. (© Copyright 1969 CIBA Pharmaceutical Company, Division of CIBA-GEIGY Corp. Reproduced, with permission, from *The Ciba Collection of Medical Illustrations,* by Frank H. Netter, M.D. All rights reserved.)

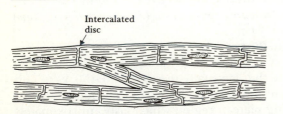

Intercalated disc

Figure 4.15 The cellular architecture of myocardial fibers. Note centroid nuclei and transverse intercalated discs between cells.

waveform is collectively referred to as *electrical systole;* the resting phase is referred to as *electrical diastole.*

Ventricular activation

Studies of ventricular activation have been conducted on experimental animals using multiple "plunge-type" electrodes inserted into many sites in the heart. The time of arrival of electrical activation is noted and *isochronous* (synchronously excited) excitation surfaces can be mapped. Figure 4.16 shows a plot of isochronous lines of activation for the perfused heart of a human who had died from a noncardiac condition. Note that activation first takes place on the septal surface of the left ventricle (5 ms into the QRS complex) and the activity spreads with increasing time in a direction from left to right across the septum. At 20 ms, several regions of the right and left ventricles are simultaneously active. As time increases, excitation spreads and tends to become more confluent. For example, at 30 ms a nearly closed activation surface is seen. Excitation then proceeds in a relatively uniform fashion in an

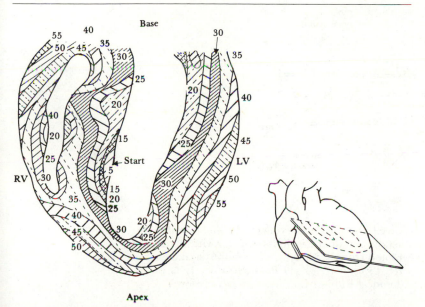

Figure 4.16 Isochronous lines of ventricular activation of the human heart. Note nearly closed activation surface at 30 ms into the QRS complex. (Modified from "The Biophysical Basis for Electrocardiography," by R. Plonsey, in *CRC Critical Reviews in Bioengineering,* **1,** 1, p. 5, 1971, © The Chemical Rubber Co., 1971. Used by permission of The Chemical Rubber Co. Based on data by D. Durrer *et al.,* "Total Excitation of the Isolated Human Heart," 1970, *Circulation,* **41,** by permission of the American Heart Association, Inc.)

epicardial (outside the heart) direction. The apex of the heart is activated roughly in the period 30–40 ms, along with other sites on the right and left ventricular walls where "breakthrough" of activation has occurred. From both Figure 4.16 and data taken in other planes, we can see that the posterior-basal region of the heart is the last region activated.

The isochronous electromotive surface propagates through the myocardium in an outward direction from the *endocardium* (the inside of the heart). The seat of this electromotive surface is, of course, the individual cardiac cell. In a localized region of the heart, however, many of these cells are active simultaneously, due to the high degree of electrical interaction between cells. The anatomical substrate for this electrical interaction is the high degree of branching of individual cardiac cells and the low resistance of the intercalated discs at the junctions between cells (Barr *et al.*, 1965). Thus the electrophysiological behavior within a small segment of the myocardial wall could be represented as in Figure 4.17. Here the electrical activity of the activation wavefront is represented by the spatial distribution of the ventricular action potential $\Phi_m(z)$,

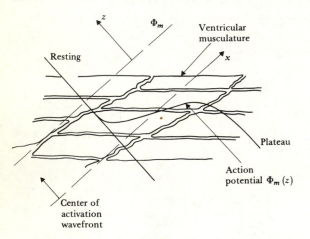

Figure 4.17 Activation wave passing through ventricular musculature. No variation is assumed in action potential distribution $\Phi_m(z)$ with distance x along the wavefront. (Adapted from R. Plonsey, "The biophysical basis for electrocardiography," *CRC Critical Reviews in Bioengineering*, **1**, 1, p. 10, October 1971, © The Chemical Rubber Co.; used by permission.)

where z is the direction of propagation. The wavefront proceeds at a constant propagation velocity, so that spatial and temporal events can be interchanged, because potentials must be of the form $f(z - ut)$, where u is the conduction velocity. The potential difference $\Delta\Phi$ measured by a sequential pair of closely spaced electrodes oriented in the direction of propagation of the wavefront is given by

$$\Delta \Phi \cong \frac{d\Phi_m(z)}{dz} \Delta z$$

where Δz is the small electrode spacing (< 1 mm). The form of the recorded waveform $\Delta \Phi$ is therefore proportional to $d\Phi_m(z)/dz$. The functional form of this electromotive surface is approximately that of an error function [that is, $d\Phi_m(z)/dz \cong \text{erfc}(z)$]. For a more comprehensive treatment of this subject, see Plonsey (1971a).

Body-surface potentials

The preceding section dealt with the sequence of events involved in electrical activation of the ventricle. This activation sequence leads to the production of closed-line action currents that flow in the thoracic volume conductor (considered to be a purely passive medium containing no electrical sources or sinks). Potentials measured at the outer surface of this medium—that is, on the body surface—are referred to as *electrocardiograms*, or ECGs.

In the electrocardiographic problem, the heart is viewed as an electrical equivalent generator. A common assumption is that, at each instant of time in the sequence of ventricular activation, the electrical activity of the heart can be represented by a net equivalent current dipole located at a point that we call the *electrical center* of the heart. This center is assumed to lie within the anatomical boundaries of the heart.

Of course, several regions of both ventricles may be simultaneously active (as in Figure 4.16). In this case, the electrical activity of each region at any instant of time could be thought of as being represented by a current dipole and a net dipolar contribution from all active areas determined at the electrical center. The thoracic medium can be considered the resistive load of this equivalent cardiac generator. There is attenuation of the field with increasing distance from the source, as well as ohmic potential drops measured between surface points (e.g., between points *A* and *B* in Figure 4.18), or between a single surface point and an assigned reference point. The general volume conductor problem is illustrated in a highly schematic fashion in Figure 4.18.

A scalar lead gives the magnitude of a single body-surface potential difference plotted versus time. A typical scalar electrocardiographic lead is shown in Figure 4.14 (bottom), where the significant features of the waveform are the P, Q, R, S, and T waves, the durations of each wave, and certain time intervals such as the P–R, S–T, and Q–T intervals. Figure 4.14 also shows the temporal relationship between single transmembrane cellular activities in various regions of the heart (atria, ventricles, and specialized conduction system) and this typical ECG waveform.

Clearly the P wave is produced by atrial depolarization, the

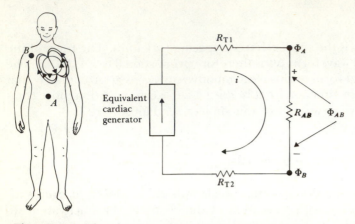

Figure 4.18 The electrocardiographic problem. Points *A* and *B* are arbitrary observation points on the torso, R_{AB} is the resistance between them, and R_{T1}, R_{T2} are lumped thoracic medium resistances. The bipolar ECG scalar lead voltage is $\Phi_A - \Phi_B$, where these voltages are both measured with respect to an indifferent reference potential.

QRS complex primarily by ventricular depolarization, and the T wave by ventricular repolarization. The manifestations of atrial repolarization are normally masked by the QRS complex. The P–R and S–T intervals are normally at zero potential, with the P–R interval being caused mainly by conduction delay in the AV node. The S–T segment is related to the average duration of the plateau regions of individual ventricular cells. A small additional wave, called the U wave, is sometimes recorded temporally after the T wave. It is an inconstant finding, believed to be due to slow repolarization of ventricular papillary muscles.

Section 6.2 describes the 12 standard leads that constitute a diagnostic ECG, so they will not be considered further here.

Normal and abnormal cardiac rhythms

The origin of each heartbeat of the normal human heart is in the SA node. The normal heart rate is approximately 70 beats per minute (bpm). The rate is slowed (*bradycardia*) during sleep and accelerated (*tachycardia*) by emotion, exercise, and fever, as well as many other stimuli. Detailed aspects of the control that the nervous system has over heart rate are beyond the scope of this book; the reader interested in further discussion is referred to Levy and Berne (1967) and Randall (1963). Since many parts of the heart possess an inherent rhythmicity (e.g., nodal tissue, Purkinje fibers of the specialized conduction system, and atrial tissues), any part under abnormal conditions can become the dominant cardiac pacemaker. This can happen when the activity of the SA node is depressed, when the bundle of His is interrupted or damaged, or when an abnormal (ectopic) focus or site in the atria or in specialized conduction-system tissue in the ventricles discharges at a rate faster than the SA node.

A simple experiment performed with hearts of cold-blooded animals such as frogs and turtles demonstrates the hierarchy of pacemakers in the heart. (The hearts of cold-blooded animals beat easily and rhythmically when they are totally removed from the body and placed in an appropriate bathing medium.) In these animals the heartbeat originates in a separate cardiac chamber, called the *sinus venosus,* instead of the SA node. If a ligature is tied around the junction of the sinus venosus and the right atrium, conduction from the sinus to the rest of the heart is prevented. The atria and ventricles stop for a moment and then resume beating at a slower rate, as a focus in the atrium becomes the pacemaker for the portion of the heart below the ligature. If a second ligature is tied between the atria and ventricles, the ventricles stop and then resume beating at an even slower rate than the atria. With both ligatures in place, there are three separate regions of the heart beating at three distinct rates.

It is not possible to perform this experiment in mammals because the SA node is embedded in the atrial wall. Tying a ligature between the atria and ventricles interrupts the coronary circulation, usually causing *ventricular fibrillation* (a feeble, uncoordinated twitching of the ventricles). In the frog or turtle there is no coronary circulation: The heart receives oxygen by diffusion from blood in the cardiac chambers. However, laboratory experiments on mammals involving the destruction of the SA and AV nodes, as well as electrophysiological studies of patients with diseased nodal tissue show that the same pacemaker hierarchy prevails.

When the bundle of His is interrupted completely, the ventricles beat at their own slow inherent rate (the *idioventricular rhythm*). The atria continue to beat independently at the normal sinus rate and complete or third-degree block is said to occur [Figure 4.19(a)]. The idioventricular rate in human beings is approximately 30 to 45 beats/min.

When the His bundle is not completely interrupted, incomplete heart block is present. In the case of *first-degree heart block,* all atrial impulses reach the ventricles, but the P–R interval is abnormally prolonged due to an increase in transmission time through the affected region [Figure 4.19(b)]. In the case of *second-degree heart block,* not all atrial impulses are conducted to the ventricles. There may be, for example, one ventricular beat every second or third atrial beat (2:1 block, 3:1 block, etc.).

In another form of incomplete heart block involving the AV node, the P–R interval progressively lengthens until the atrial impulse fails to conduct to the ventricle (*Wenckebach phenomenon*). The

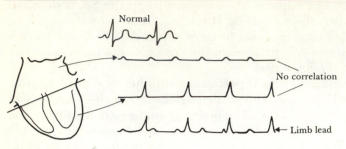

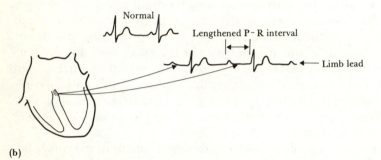

Complete heart block

(a)

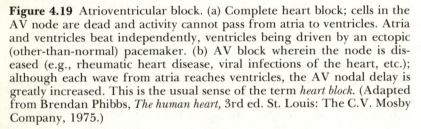

(b)

Figure 4.19 Atrioventricular block. (a) Complete heart block; cells in the AV node are dead and activity cannot pass from atria to ventricles. Atria and ventricles beat independently, ventricles being driven by an ectopic (other-than-normal) pacemaker. (b) AV block wherein the node is diseased (e.g., rheumatic heart disease, viral infections of the heart, etc.); although each wave from atria reaches ventricles, the AV nodal delay is greatly increased. This is the usual sense of the term *heart block*. (Adapted from Brendan Phibbs, *The human heart,* 3rd ed. St. Louis: The C.V. Mosby Company, 1975.)

first conducted beat after the pause (or dropped beat) has a shorter P–R interval (sometimes of normal length) than any subsequent P–R interval. Then the process of the lengthening of the P–R interval begins anew, progressing over several cardiac cycles until another beat is dropped. The electrocardiographic sequence starting with the ventricular pause and ending with the next blocked atrial beat constitutes a *Wenckebach period*. The ratio of the number of P waves to QRS complexes determines the block (for example, 6:5, 5:4, etc., Wenckebach periods).

When one branch of the bundle of His is interrupted, causing right- or left-bundle-branch block, excitation proceeds normally down the intact bundle and then sweeps back through the musculature to activate the ventricle on the blocked side. The ventricular rate is normal, but the QRS complexes are prolonged and deformed.

Arrhythmias

A portion of the myocardium (or the AV node or specialized conduction system) sometimes becomes "irritable" and discharges independently. This site is then referred to as an *ectopic focus*. If the focus discharges only once, the result is a beat that occurs before the next expected normal beat and the cardiac rhythm is therefore transiently interrupted. (With respect to atrial, nodal, or ventricular *ectopic beat*, see Figure 4.20.) If the focus discharges repetitively at a rate that exceeds that of the SA node, it produces rapid regular ta- chycardia. [With respect to atrial, nodal, or ventricular paroxysmal tachycardia or atrial flutter, see Figure 4.21(a) and (b).] A rapidly and irregularly discharging focus or, more likely, a group of foci in the atria or ventricles may be the underlying mechanism responsi- ble for atrial or ventricular fibrillation [Figure 4.22(a) and (b)].

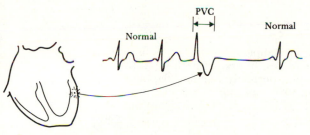

Ectopic beat

Figure 4.20 Normal ECG followed by an ectopic beat. An irritable focus or *ectopic pacemaker* within the ventricle or specialized conduction system may discharge, producing an extra beat or *extrasystole* that interrupts the normal rhythm. This extrasystole is also referred to as a preventricular contraction (PVC). (Adapted from Brendan Phibbs, *The human heart,* 3rd ed., St. Louis: The C.V. Mosby Company, 1975.)

Rhythm disturbances can arise from sources other than ec- topic foci or competing pacemakers. A feasible alternative is a *circus re-excitation* or *re-entrant* mechanism (Allessie *et al.,* 1973). This con- cept assumes a region of depressed conductivity within the atrium, Purkinje system, or ventricle. It therefore is *ischemic* (deficient in its blood supply) relative to surrounding normal tissue. This brings about pronounced electrophysiological changes in the ischemic zone and a decreased velocity of conduction (see Figure 4.23).

Propagation in this area is slow enough to permit other areas to recover from initial excitation and be re-entered by the slowly emerging impulse. The re-entrant impulse may in turn re-excite the area of slow conduction to complete a circus-movement loop. Intermittent establishment of a re-entrant circuit would result in occasional ectopic beats (or *extrasystoles*), and continuous propaga-

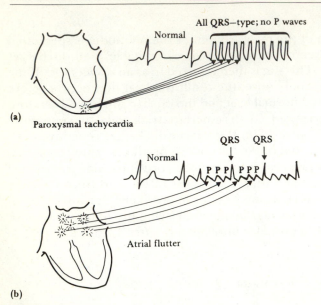

Figure 4.21 (a) Paroxysmal tachycardia; an ectopic focus may repetitively discharge at a rapid regular rate for minutes, hours, or even days. (b) Atrial flutter; the atria begin a very rapid, perfectly regular "flapping" movement, beating at rates of 200 to 300 beats/min. (Adapted from Brendan Phibbs, *The human heart*, 3rd ed., St. Louis: The C.V. Mosby Company, 1975.)

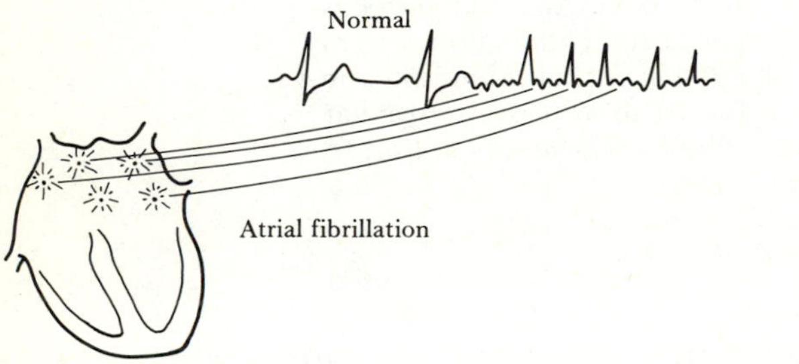

Figure 4.22 (a) Atrial fibrillation; the atria stop their regular beat and begin a feeble, uncoordinated twitching. Concomitantly, low-amplitude, irregular waves appear in the ECG, as shown. This type of recording can be clearly distinguished from the very regular ECG waveform containing atrial flutter. (b) Ventricular fibrillation; mechanically the ventricles twitch in a feeble, uncoordinated fashion with no blood being pumped from the heart. The ECG is likewise very uncoordinated, as shown. (Adapted from Brendan Phibbs, *The human heart*, 3rd ed., St. Louis: The C.V. Mosby Company, 1975.)

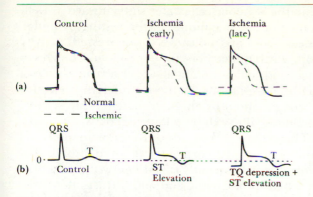

Figure 4.23 (a) Action potentials recorded from normal (solid lines) and ischemic (dashed lines) myocardium in dog. Control is before coronary occlusion. (b) During control period prior to coronary occlusion, there is no ECG S-T segment shift; after ischemia, there is such a shift. (From Andrew G. Wallace, "Electrophysiology of the Myocardium," in *Clinical Cardiopulmonary Physiology*, 3rd ed. New York: Grune & Stratton, 1969; used with permission of Grune & Stratton. Based on data by W.E. Sampson and H.M. Scher, "Mechanism of S-T Segment Alteration During Acute Myocardial Injury," 1960, *Circulation Research*, **8**, by permission of The American Heart Association.)

tion of impulses in the established circuit would underlie an episode of tachyarrhythmia.

Alteration of potential waveforms in ischemia

Of particular interest in Figure 4.23 is the change in the intra- and extracellular potential waveforms in ischemia. Note particularly that in late ischemia (i.e., ischemia that occurs several minutes after induced coronary occlusion), there are decreases in the magnitudes of the resting potential, the velocity of the upstroke, and the height and duration of the action potential. (The decrease in the velocity of the upstroke is indicative of a lowered velocity of conduction of the action-potential wavefront through this ischemic region.) The slope of the potential during the plateau region of the action potential is also altered in ischemia. These changes in the action-potential waveform bring about changes in the extracellular potential fields produced by individual cardiac cells. The field contributions of these, as well as other normal cells, superimpose in the linear volume-conductor medium to bring about altered forms of the ventricular portion of the ECG (for example, the QRS complex, S–T segment, and T wave, as shown in Figures 4.14 and 4.23).

It is now well known that occlusion of the blood supply to a given myocardial region brings about relatively rapid electrolytic adjustments in this region. Specifically, there is a loss of K^+ and an uptake of Na^+ within the ischemic cell (water shifts inward as well) resulting in a lessening of the magnitude of the resting potential. The shifts of the electrolytes are indicative of "depressed" activity of the Na^+-K^+ pump, which is metabolically dependent. Changes in the resting potential and action-potential waveform in ischemia are simply external manifestations of these underlying electrochemical changes brought about by an inadequate oxygen supply.

Cells in the ischemic zone exhibit a lowered, or "depressed," resting potential. Thus there is a steady difference in potential between the ischemic zone and its normal tissue surroundings that results in the flow of what is frequently called *injury current* at rest. Na^+ leaks into the cell at the ischemic end and diffuses down the length of the cell to the normal end, where it is pumped out by the Na^+-K^+ pump. Na^+ moving external to the cell to complete the closed-line current paths produces voltage drops in the external medium. Other charge carriers are also involved. This results in the electrocardiographic baseline shift seen in Figure 4.23.

During electrical systole (activity of the ventricle), the potential difference between the normal and ischemic regions tends to disappear, as shown qualitatively by the plateau regions of unit action potentials from each zone (Figure 4.23). The potential difference that does exist between the plateau potentials is usually smaller in magnitude than the potential difference observed at rest, and it is also of opposite polarity. This tends to produce an apparent upward (positive) shift of the S–T segment, as shown in Figure 4.23. This shift of the S–T segment is of great diagnostic value in evaluating the myocardial infarction that results from coronary occlusion.

Example 4.4 A condition seen in some otherwise-normal individuals who are susceptible to attacks of paroxysmal atrial arrhythmia is accelerated AV conduction [Wolff-Parkinson-White (WPW) syndrome]. Normally, the only conducting pathway between the atria and ventricles is the AV node. However, individuals with WPW syndrome probably have an additional aberrant muscular- or nodal-tissue connection between the atria and ventricles that conducts more rapidly than the slowly conducting AV node, and one ventricle is excited early. What changes from the normal ECG pattern would you expect to observe?

Answer One of the major changes observed would of course be a pronounced shortening of the P–R interval due to the shunt conduction pathway around the AV node, with resultant early activation of one ventricle. The slightly aberrant course taken by the ventricular activating signal would bring about changes in the QRS waveform. Notably it would be of greater duration and would have a slurred appearance due to unequal times of activation of the ventricles. Also, since this is merely a pre-excitation phenomenon, one would expect that the time interval between the start of the P wave and the end of the QRS complex would be the same as the interval in normal beats.

4.7 The electroretinogram

Anatomy of vision

The normal eye is an approximately spherical organ about 24 mm in diameter (Figure 4.24). The retina, located at the back of the eye, is the sensory portion of the eye.

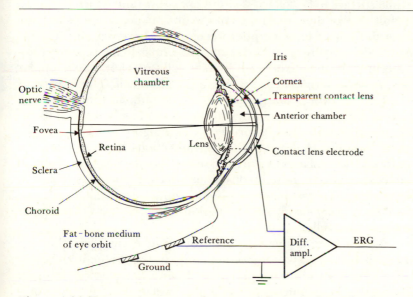

Figure 4.24 Transparent contact lens containing one electrode, shown on horizontal section of right eye. Reference electrode is placed on right temple.

The light-transmitting parts of the eye are the cornea, anterior chamber, lens, and vitreous chamber, named in the order in which these structures are traversed by light. A transparent fluid, the *aqueous humor*, is found in the anterior chamber. The vitreous chamber is filled by a transparent gel, the *vitreous body*. The aqueous humor provides a nutrient transport medium, but it is also of further optical significance inasmuch as it is normally maintained at a pressure (20–25 mm Hg) that is adequate to inflate the eye against its resistive outer coats (the sclera and choroid). This makes possible the precise geometrical configuration of the retina and the optical pathway that is necessary to ensure formation of a clear visual image. In addition, the aqueous humor is the essential link between the circulatory system and the lens and cornea, which themselves lack blood vessels. To satisfy the respiratory and nutritive requirements of these two structures, there is a continual movement of fluid and solute material between the aqueous humor and contiguous blood vessels. Interference with this flow, in pathological conditions, not only leads to damage of the lens and cornea, but may result in the development of pressures within the eye that are high enough to injure the retina. *Glaucoma* is the term applied to this high-pressure condition.

In considering the neural organization of the retina, only five types of nerve cells need occupy our attention: *photoreceptors* and *bipolar, horizontal, amacrine,* and *ganglion* cells. The ganglion cells, whose axons produce the nerve fibers sweeping across the inner retinal surface to be collected at the optic disc (and which form the greater bulk of the nerve fibers of the optic nerve) are substantially fewer in number than the photoreceptors. There is a convergence in the neural pathways of the retina as a whole. [That is, many photoreceptors terminate on each bipolar cell (*n*: 1) and many bipolar cells, in turn, terminate on a single ganglion cell. The degree of convergence varies considerably, being greater in the peripheral parts of the retina and minimal at the fovea (Figure 4.24). That is, the neural chain from photoreceptor to ganglion cell is 1 : 1 in the foveal region.] The synaptic interconnections between photoreceptors and bipolar cells and between bipolar cells and ganglion cells occur in two well-defined regions. The *external plexiform layer* is the region of contact between photoreceptor and bipolar cells and the *internal plexiform layer* is the region of contact between bipolar and ganglion cells.

Lateral connections are also found in both layers. For example, horizontal cells interconnect rods and cones (defined below) at the level of the external plexiform layer and amacrine cells provide a second horizontal network at the level of the inner plexiform layer. The retina may thus be considered functionally organized into two parts: an outer sensory layer containing the photoelectric transducers (photoreceptors) and an inner layer responsible for organizing and relaying electrical impulses generated in the photoreceptor layer to the brain.

Two types of photoreceptors occur in the human retina: *rods* (the agents of vision in dim light) and *cones* (the mediators of color vision in brighter light). Both rods and cones are differentiated into outer and inner segments. The inner segments are the major sites of metabolism and contain all the synaptic terminals. Outer segments—typically cylindrical and thin in rods and stout and conical in cones—are the sites of visual excitation. The first stage in the transduction of light to neural messages is in the absorption of photons by photopigments localized in the outer segments of the retina's photoreceptors (Dartnall, 1962). The photopigment localized in the compact membrane infoldings of the rod's external segment is *rhodopsin*. It is easily isolated and has been extensively studied (Wald, 1959). The cones in human beings contain one of three photopigments with photospectral absorption characteristics that differ from one another and from the rod pigment rhodopsin. The cone pigments are very difficult to isolate in humans and other vertebrates and their spectral characteristics have usually had to be measured by indirect means, e.g., via reflection densitometry (Rushton, 1963). All the pigments are *photolabile;* that is, events initiated by light absorption result eventually in breakdown or "bleaching" of the photopigment. The exact process of transduction is not entirely known, but the bleaching of the rhodopsin probably releases transmitter ions that cause a change in graded membrane potentials. These in turn result in ganglion-cell action potentials that are transmitted down the optic nerve.

Electrophysiology of the eye

When the retina is stimulated with a brief flash of light, a characteristic temporal sequence of potential changes can be recorded between an exploring electrode—placed either on the inner surface of the retina or on the cornea and an indifferent electrode placed elsewhere on the body (usually the temple, forehead, or earlobe). These potential changes are collectively known as the *electroretinogram* (ERG); and they are clinically recorded with the aid of an Ag-AgCl electrode embedded in a special contact lens used as the exploring electrode. (See, for example, Strong, 1973.) The saline-filled contact lens is in good contact with the cornea, which is very thin and in intimate contact with the aqueous humor and passive fluid medium of the inner eye. With the eye considered as a fluid-filled sphere and the retina as a thin sheetlike bioelectric source attached to the posterior pole of the sphere (Figure 4.24), we can easily visualize the volume-conductor problem in electroretinography.

The ERG, like the ECG, is an external potential waveform from a rather complex, distributed bioelectric source, a by-product of ongoing electrical activity in the retina. Figure 4.25 shows a typical vertebrate ERG waveform in response to a 2-s light flash. The four most commonly identified components of the ERG waveform (the a, b, c, and d waves) are common to most vertebrates, including humans.

As in the case of the ECG, research conducted on the ERG has determined the retinal locations responsible for the generation of the various components of the ERG. This has been done by probing the several layers of the retina with microelectrodes and relating the anatomical position of the electrode tip within the retina to the electrical activity recorded at that point (Wiesel and Brown, 1961). Both the a and c waves are largest in the deepest

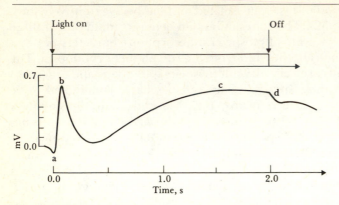

Figure 4.25 Vertebrate electroretinogram.

part of the retina (toward the posterior). The c wave most probably originates from the pigment epithelium layer beyond the photoreceptors (i.e., it is extraretinal in origin) because this response disappears when that layer is selectively poisoned and rendered nonfunctional, and also when the retina is removed from the eyecup. Research has also shown that the a wave can come only from the photoreceptive layer. The b wave has been shown to derive largely from the region of the bipolar cells. For example, the b wave can be selectively eliminated in vertebrate eyes by clamping the retinal artery that supplies the inner layers of the retina. The a wave remains, since the receptor layer is maintained by a separate set of vessels in the choroid layer of the eye beyond the photoreceptors, thus making it possible to study the a wave in isolation (Brown *et al.,* 1965).

The first part of the response to a brief light flash is the *early-receptor potential* (ERP) generated by the initial light-induced changes in the photopigment molecules. The second component, with a latency of 1–5 ms, is the *late-receptor potential* (LRP), which has been found to be maximal near the synaptic endings of the photoreceptors and therefore reflects the outputs of the receptors. Normally the ERP and LRP form the leading edge of the a wave. However, in the absence of the b wave, their entire time course can be studied. The ERP is linear with light intensity, while the LRP is already markedly nonlinear, varying approximately logarithmically with intensity. In the human ERG, the a and b waves have rod- and cone-related parts, and the latter are faster. The d wave recorded at the offset of the light stimulus is largely associated with the off responses of the a and b components.

Thus the ERP appears almost instantaneously with the occurrence of light stimulation, and the LRP leading to the a wave reflects activity at the synaptic endings of the photoreceptors and other cells at the level of the outer plexiform layer. The majority of

the b wave is contributed by bipolar-cell activity, but it can be shown
that ganglion cells are also active during the b wave. They are less
numerous than the bipolar cells, due to general retinal convergence. All the cells of the retina—with the exception of the
ganglion cells—respond to their appropriate stimuli with graded
potentials of a nonpropagating nature (in a sense, generator potentials), while depolarization of the cell body of a retinal ganglion
cell produces a propagated action potential that travels along the
axonal process to the brain. Further information on the processing of visual information within the retina is found in Ratliff
(1974), Granit (1962), and Brown (1968).

The volume-conductor problem in electroretinography

The eye is an approximately spherical conducting medium
with a layered, sheetlike bioelectric source at one pole on the optic
axis. At the corneal pole of the eye, the boundary is essentially with
air, whereas for the remainder of the eye, the bounding medium
adjacent to the sclera is the fat-bone medium of the orbit of the eye.
In all cases, the eye is bounded by a highly resistive medium with
little or no flow of current outward through the scleral coat. The
saline-filled lens is in contact with the fluid medium bathing the
outer surface of the cornea and can therefore be considered a mac-
roelectrode roughly covering the corneal pole of the spherical eye.
The indifferent electrode is effectively behind the eye and may be
considered to be uninfluenced by fields from the retinal source.
The potential $\Phi^0(r, \theta, \phi)$, expressed in spherical coordinates, at any
field point within the spherical inner-eye medium is given as the solution to the equation

$$\nabla^2 \Phi^0 = \frac{-i_{ret}}{\sigma_0}$$

where σ_0 is the specific conductivity (S/cm) of the inner-eye
medium and i_{ret} is the impressed flux source density (A/cm³) from
the retina. (The equation is a volume-conductor analog of Poisson's
equation in electrostatics.)

It would be desirable in electroretinography to identify the
retinal source (i.e., to discover the nature of i_{ret} in the equation
above). The retinal source is quite complicated, however. It is obviously layered, and even considering the most elementary form of
lumping (for example, an outer photoreceptor layer and an inner
neural processing layer), there are problems. One major problem is
the nonuniformity of the retina with regard to photoreceptor distribution. In the retina of a primate, the receptors in the fovea are
almost exclusively cones, whereas the rods are most numerous
some 15–20° from the fovea. Also, the fovea has virtually no

bipolar- or ganglion-cell layer. This does not imply a functional lack of these units, only that they have been moved to the sides of the foveal pit. The neural-convergence problem also contributes to the nonuniformity of the neural layer of the retina, in that convergence is greater (since there are fewer bipolar and ganglion cells relative to receptors) in the peripheral regions of the retina. In fact, the relative numbers of cell types and their lateral ramifications make it obvious that there is a considerable overlapping of pathways in the retina. In a human retina there are altogether about 6.5 million cones, 120 million rods, and only 1 million ganglion cells.

With this degree of complexity in mind, we suggest that a possible simple model of the retina for mimicking the potentials recorded in the clinical ERG (that still accounts for the spatial inhomogeneity of the retinal source) is a two-layer retinal mosaic model in which the retinal layers are divided into segmental volumes and a dipole source per unit volume is positioned at the center of each segment. For a fixed light input, dipole strengths are weighted spatially and the dipole source varies with time in a predetermined manner (dipole strength must also be graduated with light intensity). With a choice of model parameters based on electrophysiological and histological information, we can determine the potential field based on a superposition of dipole sources in a spherical volume conductor representing the body of the eye. For an interesting and detailed treatment of the theoretical and experimental aspects of electroretinography in the rabbit eye, consult Krakow (1958).

Spatial properties of the ERG

It is possible to record ERGs from localized areas of the retina in addition to the classical response that we have described in previous sections. [This conventional response is usually elicited from the dark-adapted eye via a brief light flash (flash ERG)]. Brindley (1956) was able to show that in a frog, the sum of the ERGs produced by several retinal regions is equal to the single ERG produced when all these regions are stimulated simultaneously.

The spatial properties of the human ERG have also been established in research that includes that of Brindley and Westheimer (1965) and Aiba *et al.* (1967). Linear superposition of ERG responses has likewise been confirmed in humans. In applying localized light stimuli to portions of the human retina, we must take precautions to prevent light scattered within the eye from stimulating a much larger area of retina than that intended. Thus relatively high steady background illumination is supplied that illuminates most of the retina, and a localized stimulus is superimposed. The background illumination light adapts the retina and renders it much less sensitive to light scattered from the stimulus region. In general, relatively high-background and low-stimulus intensities are preferred, making these locally generated ERG potentials low in amplitude and detectable only with average response calculations involving large numbers of responses. Without these special precautions, the resultant ERG represents the overall retinal response to light stimulation. Little is known about the actual nature of the light input to a particular retinal locus in the photoreceptive layer.

Despite the anatomical complexities of the retina, the problems of obtaining good records from untrained subjects and the need for employing averaging techniques in obtaining spatially localized ERGs, the ERG has potential importance in assessing functional retinal behavior. For an example of the application of modern systems theory and techniques of computer analysis to the clinical ERG, see Troelstra and Garcia (1975).

The electro-oculogram (EOG)

In addition to the transient potential recorded as the ERG, there is a steady corneal-retinal potential. This steady dipole may be used to measure eye position by placing surface electrodes to the left and right of the eye, on the nose and the temple. When the gaze is straight ahead, the steady dipole is symmetrically placed between the two electrodes and the EOG output is zero. When the gaze is shifted to the left, the positive cornea becomes closer to the left electrode, which becomes more positive. There is an almost linear relation between horizontal angle of gaze and EOG output up to approximately $\pm 30°$ of arc. Electrodes may also be placed above and below the eye to record vertical eye movements.

The EOG, unlike other bipotentials, requires a dc amplifier. The output is in the microvolt region, so recessed Ag-AgCl electrodes are required to prevent drift. It is necessary to abrade the skin to short out changes in the potential that exists between the inside and the outside of the skin. A noise is present that is compounded of effects from EEG, EMG, and the recording equipment, and is equivalent to approximately 1° of eye movement. Thus EOG data suffer from a lack of accuracy at the extremes. Specifically eye movements of less than 1 or 2° are difficult to record, whereas large eye movements (for example, $>30°$ of arc) do not produce bioelectric amplitudes that are strictly proportional to eye position. For an analysis of the accuracy and precision of electro-oculographic recording, consult North (1965) and Kris (1960).

The EOG is frequently the method of choice for recording eye movements in sleep and dream research, in recording eye movements from infants and children, and in evaluating reading ability and visual fatigue. For a practical clinical EOG setup, see Dement (1964), who employs EOG recordings to monitor eye movements during sleep.

4.8 The electroencephalogram

The background electrical activity of the brain in unanesthetized animals was described qualitatively in the nineteenth century, but it was first analyzed in a systematic manner by the German psychiatrist Hans Berger, who introduced the term *electroencephalogram* (EEG) to denote the potential fluctuations recorded from the brain. Conventionally, the electrical activity of the brain is recorded with three types of electrodes—scalp, cortical, and depth electrodes. When electrodes are placed on the exposed surface (cortex) of the brain, the recording is called an *electrocorticogram* (ECoG). Thin insulated needle electrodes of various designs may also be advanced into the neural tissue of the brain, in which case the recording is referred to as a *depth recording*. (There is suprisingly little damage to the brain tissue when electrodes of appropriate size are employed.) Whether obtained from the scalp, cortex, or depths of the brain, the recorded fluctuating potentials represent a superposition of the volume-conductor fields produced by a variety of active neuronal current generators. Unlike the relatively simple bioelectric source considered in Section 4.2 (i.e., the nerve trunk with its enclosed bundles of circular cylindrical nerve axons), the sources generating the field potentials recorded here are aggregates of neuronal elements with complex interconnections. The neuronal elements mentioned previously are the dendrites, cell bodies (somata), and axons of nerve cells. Moreover, the architecture of the neuronal brain tissue is not uniform from one location to another in the brain. Therefore, prior to undertaking any detailed study of electroencephalography, we must first discuss necessary background information regarding (1) the gross anatomy and function of the brain, (2) the ultrastructure of the cerebral cortex, (3) the potential fields of single neurons leading to an interpretation of extracellular potentials recorded in the cerebral cortex, and (4) typical clinical EEG waveforms recorded via scalp electrodes. We shall next focus on the general volume-conductor problem in electroencephalography, and then briefly discuss abnormal EEG waveforms.

Introduction to the anatomy and function of the brain

The central nervous system (CNS) consists of the spinal cord lying within the bony vertebral column and its continuation, the brain, lying within the skull [Figure 4.26(a)]. The brain is the

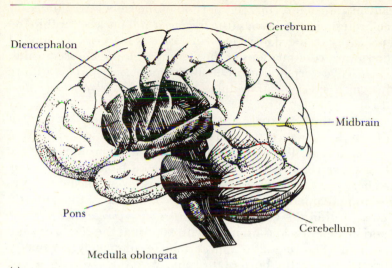

(a)

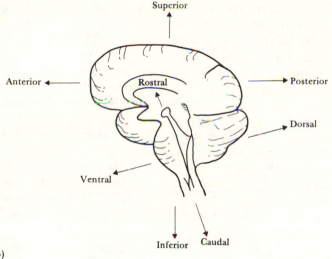

(b)

Figure 4.26 (a) Anatomical relation of brainstem structures (medulla oblongata, pons, midbrain, and diencephalon) to cerebrum and cerebellum. (b) General anatomic directions of orientation in the central nervous system. Here the directions rostral (toward head), caudal (toward tail), dorsal (back) and ventral (front) are associated with the brainstem; remaining terms are associated with the cerebrum. The terms medial and lateral imply nearness and remoteness, respectively, to central midline axis of brain. [Part (a) from Harry E. Thomas, *Handbook of Biomedical Instrumentation and Measurement*, 1974, p. 254. Reprinted with permission of Reston Publishing Company, Inc., a Prentice-Hall company, 11480 Sunset Hills Road, Reston, VA 22090.]

greatly modified and enlarged portion of the CNS, surrounded by three protective membranes (the *meninges*) and enclosed within the cranial cavity of the skull. The spinal cord is likewise surrounded by downward continuations of the meninges, and is encased within the protective vertebral column. Both brain and spinal cord are bathed in a special extracellular fluid called *cerebral spinal fluid* (CSF).

Within the CNS there are *ascending* (*sensory*) nerve tracts that run from the spinal cord to various areas of the brain, conveying information regarding changes in the external environment of the body that are reported by various peripheral biological transducers. There is a variety of such sensory transducers, including ones for sensing temperature, pain, fine touch, pressure, and so forth. Likewise, within the CNS there are *descending* (*motor*) nerve tracts that originate in various brain structures such as the cerebrum and cerebellum (Figure 4.26) and terminate ultimately on motor neurons in the ventral horn of the spinal cord (Figure 4.10). These motoneurons, in turn, control the contractile activity of the skeletal musculature.

Thus there exist two-way communication links between the brain and spinal cord that allow higher centers in the brain to control or modify the behavior of the elemental spinal reflex arc at a given spinal level. By means of such two-way communication links, the brain not only is informed of a peripheral event, but can modify the response of the spinal reflex to that environmental stimulus. Information is transmitted to the brain by means of a frequency-modulated train of nerve impulses that—upon reaching specific areas of the brain—stimulates the activity of other neurons there. Similarly, the decision to implement a motor action in response to the initial stimulus is manifested in the activity of cortical neurons from various areas of the brain, depending on the particular motor action to be taken. Such cortical activity is reflected in changes in the volume-conductor field potentials recorded from the brain as EEGs.

Division of the brain into three main parts—*cerebrum, brainstem,* and *cerebellum*—provides a useful basis for the study of brain localization and function. Phylogenetically, the brainstem is the oldest part of the brain. Its size and functions have changed very little with the evolution of the vertebrates. It is actually a short extension of the spinal cord, and serves three major functions: (1) It is a connecting link between the cerebral cortex, the spinal cord, and the cerebellum. (2) It is a center of integration for several visceral functions, such as control of heart rate and respiratory frequency. (3) It is an integration center for various motor reflexes.

The cerebellum is a coordinator in the voluntary (somatic) muscle system and acts in conjunction with the brainstem and cerebral cortex to maintain balance and provide harmonious muscle movements. The cerebrum occupies a special dominant position in the central nervous system, and within the cerebrum are localized the conscious functions of the nervous system.

The cerebrum

The cerebrum is a paired structure, with right and left cerebral hemispheres, each relating to the opposite side of the body. That is, voluntary movements of the right hand are "willed" by the left cerebral hemisphere. The surface layer of the hemisphere is called the *cortex;* it receives sensory information from skin, eyes, ears, and other receptors located generally on the opposite side of the body. This information is compared with previous experience and produces movements in response to these stimuli.

Each hemisphere consists of several layers. The outer layer is a dense collection of nerve cells that appear gray in color when examined in a fresh state. It is consequently called gray matter. This outer layer, roughly 1 cm thick, is called the *cerebral cortex*. It has a highly convoluted surface consisting of *gyri* (ridges) and *sulci* (valleys), the deeper sulci being termed *fissures*. The deeper layers of the hemisphere (i.e., beneath the cortex) consist of *axons* (or white matter) and collections of cell bodies, termed *nuclei*. Some of the integrative functions of the cerebrum can be localized within certain regions of the cortex, while others are more diffusely distributed.

A major dividing landmark of the cerebral cortex is the lateral fissure (Figure 4.27), which runs on the lateral (side) surface of the brain from the open end in front, posteriorly and dorsally (backward and upward). The lateral fissure defines a side lobe of cortex inferior to (below) it, called the *temporal lobe* (Figure 4.27). The superior (upper) part of this lobe contains the primary auditory cortex, which is the part of the cortex that receives auditory impulses via neural pathways leading from the auditory receptors in the inner ear. When a recording electrode is placed on this location at the time of neurosurgery, a large and characteristic electrical response follows when noise is played into the patient's ear. Furthermore, if a weak current is passed into a stimulating electrode in this same location, the conscious patient reports "hearing" tones or noises. For most individuals, the left temporal lobe surrounding the transverse temporal gyrus is involved in the more complex interpretation of auditory signals. If cells in this area are damaged and die, the subject is not able to interpret sound as words. This general cortical area surrounding the prime auditory reception area (primary auditory cortex) thus serves as an area of auditory association or interpretation.

The visual system is another example of the projection of the senses onto the cerebral cortex. The *occipital lobe* at the back of the head is the primary visual cortex. Light flashed into the eye

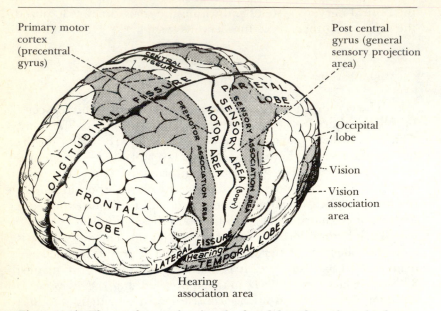

Primary motor
cortex
(precentral
gyrus)

Post central
gyrus (general
sensory projection
area)

Occipital
lobe

Vision

Vision
association
area

Hearing
association area

Figure 4.27 The cerebrum, showing the four lobes (frontal, parietal, temporal, and occipital), the lateral and longitudinal fissures, and the central sulcus. (From A.B. McNaught and R. Callander, *Illustrated Physiology,* 3rd ed., 1975. Edinburgh: Churchill Livingstone. Used with permission of Churchill Livingstone.)

evokes large electrical potentials from electrodes placed over this area of the cortex.

The ability of the visual system to detect spatial organization of the visual scene—that is, to detect the forms of objects, brightness of the individual parts of objects, shading, etc.—depends on the function of the primary visual cortex. Responses from either eye are projected onto this primary reception area. The area is also well organized in a spatial sense. The area of maximum visual acuity around the fovea occupies a major portion of the cortical volume associated with the primary visual cortex. Specific points on the retina connect with specific points of the visual cortex. The right halves of the two respective retinas connect with the right visual cortex and the left halves connect with the left visual cortex. Areas of visual association surround the primary reception area.

Another major landmark of the cerebral cortex is the central sulcus (Figure 4.27). However, it is not as prominent and unvarying an anatomical landmark as the lateral fissure. The central sulcus runs from the medial surface (surface along the midline of the brain) over the convexity of the hemisphere to the lateral fissure. The central sulcus also represents the posterior border of the frontal lobe. The gyrus lying just anterior (forward) to the central sulcus is the *precentral gyrus,* which functions as the primary motor cortex. From this gyrus, nerve signals run down through the brainstem to the spinal cord for control of skeletal muscles via neural control of motoneurons in the ventral horn of the spinal cord (Figure 4.10). Lesions (destruction) of part of the precentral gyrus cause partial paralysis on the opposite side of the body.

Proceeding more anteriorly from the central sulcus, we encounter an area called the *premotor cortex*. Here more complex motor movements such as speech are organized. The anterior and inferior portions of the frontal lobe are involved in the control of emotional behavior. For years this part of the cortex has been considered the locus of the higher intellect of the human being, largely because the main difference between the brains of monkey and of man is the great prominence of man's prefrontal lobes. However, efforts to demonstrate that the prefrontal cortex is more important to higher intellectual functions than other portions of the cortex have not been entirely successful.

Immediately behind the central sulcus lies the *parietal lobe*. Its anterior border is the central sulcus, its ventral boundary is the lateral fissure or a line continuing in the same direction, and its posterior boundary is rather ill defined on the lateral surface. Several component areas of the parietal lobe may be distinguished. Immediately posterior to the central sulcus is the primary *somatosensory cortex*, the *postcentral gyrus*. This region receives impulses from all the general sense receptors from the skin (e.g., pressure, touch, and pain receptors). Each little area along this gyrus is related to a particular part of the body. For example, the legs on the medial end, the hand in the center, and the face on the end next to the lateral fissure. If a recording electrode is placed appropriately during a neurosurgical procedure, a cortical response can be evoked by tactile stimuli delivered to the *contralateral* (opposite) hand. Likewise, if a stimulus is applied through the same electrode, the subject reports a tingling sensation in his contralateral hand. Higher-order sensory discrimination, such as the ability to recognize a number drawn on the palm of the hand, is organized solely in the parietal lobe. Destruction of this lobe results in a loss of this discriminative ability. For example, a subject may still know that he or she is being touched, but cannot tell where or what is being drawn on the palm of the hand. The parietal lobe is also responsible for a person's awareness of the general position of the body and its limbs in space. A subject with a lesion in the posterior portion of the parietal lobe may, for example, often forget to put the contralateral arm into a shirt sleeve.

The brain stem

The brainstem is composed of four regions, each of which has distinct functions: the *medulla oblongata*, the *pons*, the *midbrain*, and the *diencephalon* [Fig. 4.26(a)] Each contains groupings of cell bodies (nuclei) and bundles of nerve axons (tracts) that are intermingled. At the upper border of the medulla is a distinctive bulge, the pons. The medulla contains fiber tracts—as does the spinal cord—as well as motor and sensory nuclei for receiving sensory information from and controlling muscles in the mouth, neck, and throat. It also hosts centers for the reflex control of the respiratory and cardiovascular systems.

The nerves that connect directly to the brain are called *cranial nerves*. There are twelve pairs of cranial nerves, eleven of which enter the brainstem. (The olfactory nerve from the nose enters the cerebrum.)

The pons contains cranial nerve nuclei associated with sensory input and motor output to the face.

The midbrain contains the major nuclei controlling eye movement—blinking and startle reflexes and the pupillary light reflex. It also contains rather large tracts carrying signals down from the cerebral hemispheres, as well as sensory tracts arising from various sources (the spinal cord, auditory system, etc.) and continuing through the midbrain to higher centers.

The diencephalon is the most superior portion of the brainstem; its chief component and largest structure is the *thalamus*. The thalamus serves as a major relay station and integration center for all of the general and special sensory systems sending information to their respective cortical reception areas. It serves as a gateway to the cerebrum.

The cerebellum

The cerebellum [Figure 4.26(a)] receives information from the spinal cord regarding the position of the trunk and limbs in space. It receives information that has originated in the cerebral cortex. (Fibers descend from the cortex to nuclei in the pons, synapses occur, and postsynaptic fibers carry information to the cerebellum.) There is also a major outflow tract of the cerebellum. In a simplistic sense, the spinal cord sends the cerebellum feedback information about where the limbs are in space. The cortex sends the cerebellum a command about where they should be. The cerebellum compares information and sends commands to spinal motor neurons. The cerebellum receives a strong input from the vestibular system and is heavily involved in the continual adjustment of muscles to maintain the body's posture under a variety of operating conditions.

The reticular formation

Throughout the entire extent of the brainstem, there is a diffuse collection of neurons and nuclei collectively known as the reticular formation. Interspersed in the reticular formation are many special small nuclei, some motor and some sensory in function. A few of the motor nuclei operate in close association with the diffuse reticular neurons to stimulate many of the subconscious motor activities of the body. Most of the reticular formation is excitatory in function. Diffuse stimulation in this facilitory area produces a general increase in muscle tone. In the lower part of the reticular formation, there is a small area that has mainly inhibitory functions, since diffuse stimulation produces a general decrease in muscle tone.

If the facilitory area were not inhibited by signals from other parts of the nervous system, it would tend to fire impulses continually. Thus, when the facilitory portion of the reticular formation is uninhibited by signals from other sources, it transmits repetitive impulses to skeletal muscles throughout the body. In the normal animal, inhibitory signals impinging on this center from the cerebral cortex and other centers keep the facilitory area from becoming overactive.

In addition to the motor activity described above, the facilitory area provides input to the *reticular activating system* (RAS). The stimulation of this very important system causes a sleeping animal to awaken instantaneously. The reticular activating system may be considered essential for arousing us from sleep, keeping us awake, alerting or focusing our attention, and directing our perceptual association. Anesthesia and comatose states cause impairment of its function. In sleep this system is dormant; yet almost any type of sensory input signal—auditory, visual, pain, or even visceral sensation from the gut—can cause sudden activation of the RAS, producing arousal. When this happens, there is a concomitant change in typical EEG recordings from a sleeping to a waking pattern of activity.

The RAS is a complex polysynaptic pathway. Collateral nerve branches funnel into it not only from the long ascending sensory nerve tracts running from the spinal cord to the thalamus and cortex, but also from sensory nerve input from the face, as well as the auditory, visual, and olfactory systems. The complexity of the neuron network and the degree of convergence in it abolish any specificity with regard to sensory modality. Thus most reticular neurons of this system are activated with equal facility by different sensory stimuli. The system is therefore *nonspecific,* in contrast to the classical ascending sensory neural pathways to the thalamus and cortex, which are *specific,* in that the component nerve fibers are activated by only one particular type of sensory stimulation (e.g., temperature, pain, touch, and so forth). Activity in the RAS percolates upward, and part of it bypasses the thalamus to project in a diffuse manner to the cerebral cortex at large. Another part of the RAS ends in various nuclei of the thalamus, and from them it is projected diffusely to the cortex. These nonspecific nerve fibers terminate mostly in the superficial portions of the cortex. The importance of RAS in influencing the electrical activity of the cortex cannot be emphasized too strongly.

Ultrastructure of the cerebral cortex

The functional part of the cerebrum is the cerebral cortex, a relatively thin layer of gray matter (1.5–4.0 mm in thickness) covering the outer surface of the cerebrum, including its intricate convolutions. Since it is the most recent phylogenetic acquisition of the brain, the cerebral cortex has undergone a relatively greater development than other parts of the brain. The greatest advance in relative growth has been the neocortex, which is present on the superior and lateral aspects of the cerebral hemispheres. The distinctly different type of cortex located on the medial surface and base of the brain is known as the *paleocortex*. We shall use the term *cortex* in this chapter to refer specifically to the neocortex.

There are many types of cortical neurons and they are not randomly distributed along the axis normal to the cortical surface. They show an orderliness, in fact, that affects both the distribution of cell types and their packing density. Relative segregation by depth produces a stratification; each stratum is called a *cortical layer*. The cortex is generally arranged in six layers [Figure 4.28(a)], consisting mainly of pyramidal cells and granule cells (many subtypes of these neurons have been identified). Note in Figure 4.28(a) that there are a large number of horizontally oriented layers of nerve fibers that extend between adjacent areas of the cortex, as well as vertical bundles of nerve fibers that extend to and from the cortex to lower areas of the brainstem, or to much more distant regions of the cerebral cortex.

Figure 4.28(a) also shows a typical cortical pyramidal cell. The bodies of this type of cell are commonly triangular in shape, with the base down and the apex directed toward the cortical surface, (Pyramidal cell bodies vary greatly in size, from axial dimensions of 15×10 μm up to 120×90 μm or more for the giant pyramids of the motor cortex, called *Betz cells* after their discoverer.) These cells usually consist of: (1) A long apical dendrite (up to 2 mm in length) that ascends from the apex of the cell body through the overlaying cellular layers and that frequently reaches and branches terminally within the outermost layer of the cortex. (2) A basilar dendritic arborization that ramifies in the immediate vicinity of the cell body, largely horizontally. Axons of pyramidal cells emerge from the cortex as projection fibers to other areas of the cortex or to other structures such as the thalamus, cerebellum, or spinal cord. Frequently these axons send recurrent collateral (feedback) branches back on the cellular regions from which they sprang. Axons of some pyramidal cells turn back toward the cortical surface (never leaving the gray matter) to end via their many branches on the dendrites of other cells.

Stellate or granule cells differ remarkably from pyramidal cells. Their cell bodies are small and dendrites spring from them in all directions to ramify in the immediate vicinity of the cell. The axon may arise from a large dendrite and commonly divides repeatedly to terminate on the cell bodies and dendrites of immediately adjacent cells. The axons of other granular cells may turn upward toward the cortical surface, or may leave the cortex (though this is not common).

Figure 4.28(d) indicates, in a highly schematic fashion, typical neuronal connections in the neocortex. Note the extensive dendritic processes of the cells, especially those in the deep layers. On the left are afferent fibers from the thalamus. Afferents from the specific sensory nuclei of the thalamus terminate primarily in cortical layer IV and lower III, whereas the nonspecific afferents associated with the RAS are distributed to all cortical layers.

For a detailed exposition of the various cells, layers, cellular interconnections, inputs, and outputs of the neocortex, see Curtis, Jacobson, and Marcus (1972, Chapter 20).

Electrical potentials from the brain

When we make records of electrical potential differences between an exploring electrode resting on the cortical surface and a distant reference electrode, we are in effect recording the resultant field potential at a boundary of a large conductile medium containing an array of active elements. It is evident from what is now known of the electrophysiology of the cortex (information derived from depth and microelectrode recordings) that under normal circumstances, conducted action potentials in axons contribute little to surface cortical records, since they usually occur asynchronously in time in large numbers of axons, which run in many directions relative to the surface. Thus their net influence on potential at the surface is negligible.

An exception occurs, of course, in the case of a response evoked by the simultaneous stimulation of a cortical input, as in the case of direct stimulation of thalamic nuclei or their afferent pathways, which project directly to the cortex via thalamocortical axons. Electrophysiologists have shown that surface records obtained under other circumstances signal principally the net effect of local postsynaptic potentials of cortical cells. These may be of either sign (excitatory or inhibitory) and may occur directly underneath the electrode or at some distance from it. A potential change recorded at the surface is a measure of the net potential (current resistance iR) drop between the surface site and the distant refer-

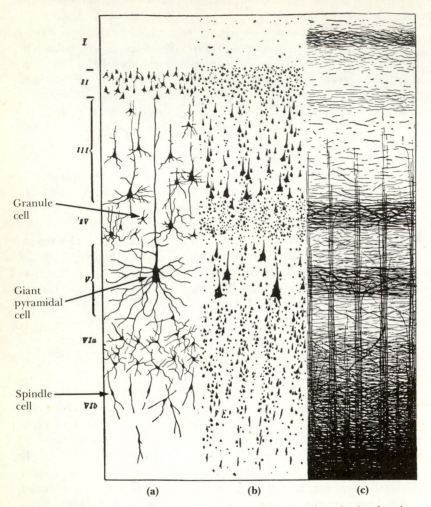

Figure 4.28 Structure of the cerebral cortex. Results obtained using different specific histological stains specific for cell bodies, dendritic and axonal processes, and myelin sheath are shown in (a) Golgi stain, (b) Nissl cellular stain, and (c) myelin sheath stain. The six layers of the cortex are also demonstrated: I = molecular layer, II = external granular layer, III = external pyramidal layer, IV = internal granular layer, V = large or giant pyramidal layer (ganglionic layer), VI = fusiform layer. (From

ence electrode. It is obvious, however, that if all the cell bodies and dendrites of cortical cells were randomly arranged in the cortical matrix, the net influence of synaptic currents would be zero. Any electrical change recorded at the surface must be due to the orderly and symmetric arrangement of some class of cells within the cortex.

Based on the anatomy of the cortex presented in the previous section, we might think that the vertically oriented pyramidal cells with their long apical dendrites running parallel to one another

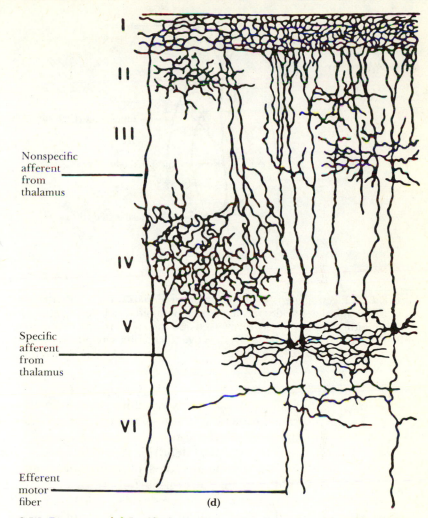

I

II

III

Nonspecific
afferent
from
thalamus

IV

V

Specific
afferent
from
thalamus

VI

Efferent
motor
fiber

(d)

S.W. Ranson and S.L. Clark, *Anatomy of the Nervous System,* Philadelphia: W.B. Saunders Co., 1959; used with permission.) (d) Neuronal connections in the neocortex. (Reproduced, with permission, from W.F. Ganong, *Review of Medical Physiology,* 8th edition, Lange Medical Publications, 1977. Based on drawing of Lorente de Nó, in Fulton, *Physiology of the Nervous System,* Oxford University Press, 1943.)

would be likely candidates. Potential changes in one part of the cell relative to another create "open" potential fields in which current may flow and potential differences can be measured at the cortical surface. Figure 4.29 illustrates this concept in diagrammatic fashion. Synaptic inputs to the apical dendritic tree cause depolarization of the dendritic membrane. As a result, subthreshold current flows in a closed path through the cytoplasmic core of the dendrites and cell body of the pyramidal cell, returning ultimately to the syn-

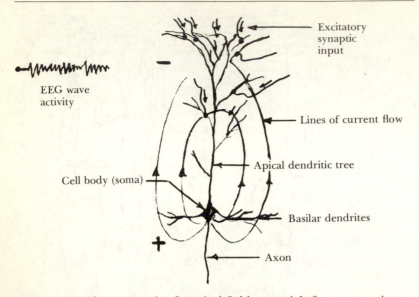

Excitatory synaptic input

EEG wave activity

Lines of current flow

Apical dendritic tree

Cell body (soma)

Basilar dendrites

Axon

Figure 4.29 Electrogenesis of cortical field potentials for a net excitatory input to the apical dendritic tree of a typical pyramidal cell. For the case of a net inhibitory input, polarity is reversed and the apical region becomes a source (+). Current flow to and from active fluctuating synaptic knobs on the dendrites produces wave activity.

aptic sites via the extracellular bathing medium. From the indicated direction of the lines of current flow, the extracellular medium about the soma behaves as a *source* (+), while the upper part of the apical dendritic tree behaves as a *sink* (−).

The influence of a particular dendritic *postsynaptic potential* (PSP) on the cortical surface recording depends on its sign—excitatory (−) or inhibitory (+)—orientation, and location relative to the measurement site. The effect of each PSP may be regarded as creating a radially oriented dipole. Therefore continuing synaptic input creates a series of potential dipoles and resulting current flows that are staggered, but overlapped in space and time. Surface potentials of any form can be generated by one population of presynaptic fibers and the cells on which they terminate, depending on the proportion that are inhibitory or excitatory, the level of the postsynaptic cells in the cortex, and so forth.

Granular cells in the neocortex, on the other hand, are unlikely to contribute substantially to surface records. Their spatially restricted dendritic trees are radially arranged around their cell bodies, so that charge differences between the dendrites and the cell body produce fields of current flow that sum to zero when viewed from a relatively great distance on the cortical surface.

Thus, to summarize, the apical dendrites of pyramidal cells are a forest of similarly oriented, densely packed units in the superficial layers of the cortex. As excitatory and inhibitory synaptic endings on the dendrites of each cell become active, current flows into and out of these current sinks and sources from the rest of the dendritic processes and the cell body. The cell–dendrite relationship is therefore one of a constantly shifting current dipole, and variations in orientation and strength of the dipole produce wavelike fluctuations in a volume conductor (Figure 4.29). When the sum of dendritic activity is negative relative to the cell, the cell is depolarized and quite excitable. When it is positive, the cell is hyperpolarized and less excitable.

Resting rhythms of the brain

Electrical recordings from the exposed surface of the brain or from the outer surface of the head demonstrate continuous oscillating electrical activity within the brain. Both the intensity and patterns of this electrical activity are determined to a great extent by the overall excitation of the brain resulting from functions in the RAS. The undulations in the recorded electrical potentials (Figure 4.30) are called *brain waves* and the entire record is called an *electroencephalogram* (EEG).

The intensities of the brain waves on the surface of the brain (recorded relative to an indifferent electrode such as the earlobe) may be as large as 10 mV, whereas those recorded from the scalp have a smaller amplitude of approximately 100 μV. The frequencies of these brain waves range from 0.5–100 Hz and their character is highly dependent on the degree of activity of the cerebral cortex. For example, the waves change markedly between states of wakefulness and sleep. Much of the time, the brain waves are irregular and no general pattern can be observed. Yet at other times, distinct patterns do occur. Some of these are characteristic of specific abnormalities of the brain, such as epilepsy (discussed later). Others occur in normal persons and may be classified as belonging to one of four wave groups (*alpha, beta, theta,* and *delta*), which are shown in Figure 4.30(a).

Alpha waves are rhythmic waves occurring at a frequency between 8 and 13 Hz. They are found in EEGs of almost all normal persons when they are awake in a quiet, resting state of cerebration. These waves occur most intensely in the occipital region, but can also be recorded at times from the parietal and frontal regions of the scalp. Their voltage is approximately 20–200 μV. When the subject is asleep, the alpha waves disappear completely. When the awake subject's attention is directed to some specific type of mental activity, the alpha waves are replaced by asynchronous waves of higher frequency, but lower amplitude. Figure 4.30(b) demonstrates the effect on the alpha waves of simply opening the eyes in bright light and then closing them again. Note that the visual sensa-

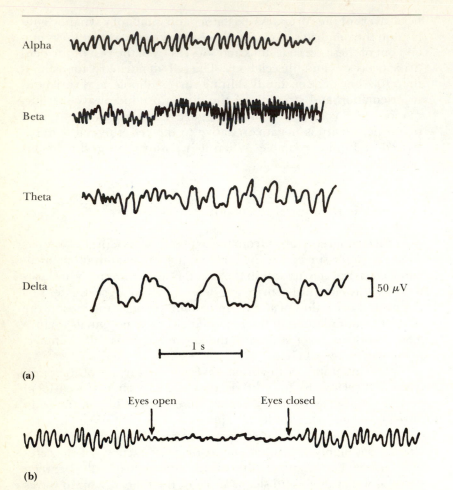

Figure 4.30 (a) Different types of normal EEG waves. (b) Replacement of alpha rhythm by an asynchronous discharge when patient opens eyes. (c) Representative abnormal EEG waveforms in different types of epilepsy.

tions cause immediate cessation of the alpha waves; these are replaced by low-voltage, asynchronous waves.

Beta waves normally occur in the frequency range of 14 to 30 Hz, and sometimes—particularly during intense mental activity—as high as 50 Hz. These are most frequently recorded from the parietal and frontal regions of the scalp. They can be divided into two major types: beta I and beta II. The beta I waves have a frequency about twice that of the alpha waves; and are affected by mental activity in much the same way as the alpha waves (i.e., they disappear and in their place appears an asynchronous, low-voltage recording). The beta II waves, on the other hand, appear during intense activation of the central nervous system or during tension. Thus one type of beta activity is elicited by mental activity, while the other is inhibited by it.

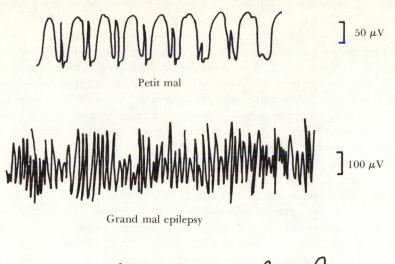

Petit mal

] 50 μV

Grand mal epilepsy

] 100 μV

Psychomotor

] 50 μV

(c)

(From A.C. Guyton, *Structure and Function of the Nervous System*, 2nd ed., Philadelphia: W.B. Saunders, 1972; used with permission.)

Theta waves have frequencies between 4 and 7 Hz. These occur mainly in the parietal and temporal regions in children, but they also occur during emotional stress in some adults, particularly during periods of disappointment and frustration. For example, they can often be brought about in the EEG of a frustrated person by allowing the person to enjoy some pleasant experience and then suddenly removing the element of pleasure. This causes approximately 20 s of theta waves.

Delta waves include all the waves in the EEG below 3.5 Hz. Sometimes these waves occur only once every 2 or 3 s. They occur in deep sleep, in infancy, and in serious organic brain disease. They can also be recorded from the brains of experimental animals that have had subcortical transections that produce a functional separation of the cerebral cortex from the reticular activating system. Delta waves can thus occur solely within the cortex, independent of activities in lower regions of the brain.

A single cortical cell can give rise only to small extracellular current, and therefore large numbers of neurons must be synchronously active to give rise to the potentials recorded from the cerebral surface. The individual waves of the EEG are of long duration (for example, 30 to 500 ms) and one might well ask how they are produced. They can be long-lasting depolarizations of the cell membranes—e.g., of the apical dendrites of pyramidal cells—or a summation of a number of shorter responses. In any event, a sufficiently large number of neurons must discharge together to give rise to these cortical potentials. The term *synchronization* is used to describe the underlying process that acts to bring a group of neurons into unified action. Synaptic interconnections are generally thought to bring about synchronization, although extracellular field interaction between cells has been proposed as a possible mechanism. For example, it has been shown that rhythmically firing neurons are very sensitive to voltage gradients in their surrounding medium (Terzuolo and Bullock, 1956).

Besides the synchronization required for each wave of resting EEG, the series of repeated waves suggests a rhythmic and a trigger or pacemaker process that initiates such rhythmic action. By means of knife cuts below the intact connective-tissue covering (*meningeal layer* or *pia matter*) of the brain, one may prepare *chronic islands* of cortex—with all neuronal connections cut, but with the blood supply via surface vessels intact (Kristiansen and Courtois, 1949). These investigators found only a low level of EEG activity remaining in such islands. Though the isolated islands of cortex may not show spontaneous EEG activity, they still have the ability to respond rhythmically. This can be readily demonstrated by the rhythmic responses that are elicited by applying a single electrical stimulus. The inference is that various regions of the cortex, although capable of exhibiting rhythmic activity, require trigger inputs to excite rhythmicity. The RAS, mentioned earlier, appears to provide this pacemaker function.

The clinical EEG

The system most often used to place electrodes for monitoring the clinical EEG is the International Federation 10–20 system shown in Fig. 4.31. This system uses certain anatomical landmarks to standardize placement of EEG electrodes. Three types of electrode connections are used: (1) Between each of a pair (bipolar), (2) between one monopolar lead and a distant reference electrode (usually attached to one or both earlobes), and (3) between one monopolar lead and the average of all. In the average reference mode, the system reference is formed by connecting all scalp-recording locations through equal high resistances to a common point. In the bipolar system, differential measurements are made between successive pairs of electrodes. The advantage of using a differential recording between closely spaced electrodes (e.g., between successive pairs in the standard system) is cancelation of far-field activity common to both electrodes, and thereby ob-

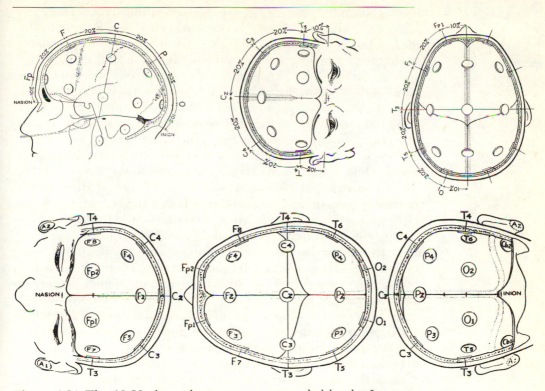

Figure 4.31 The 10-20 electrode system recommended by the International Federation of EEG Societies. (From H.H. Jasper, "The Ten-Twenty Electrode System of the International Federation in Electroencephalography and Clinical Neurophysiology," *EEG Journal*, 1958, **10** (Appendix), 371–375.)

taining sharp localization of the response. Although the same electrical events are recorded in each of the three ways, they appear in a different format in each case. The potential changes that occur are amplified by high-gain, differential, capacitively coupled amplifiers. The output signals are usually displayed via ink-writing strip-chart recorders, a method that usually limits the frequency response to the range of 0.5 to 80 Hz.

In the routine recording of clinical EEGs, the input electrodes are a problem. They must be small, easily affixed to the scalp with minimum disturbance of the hair, they must cause no discomfort, and they must remain in place for extended periods of time. Technicians prepare the surface of the scalp, degrease the recording area by cleaning it with alcohol, apply a conducting paste, and glue nonpolarizable Ag-AgCl electrodes to the scalp with collodion or hold them in place with rubber straps.

The EEG is usually recorded with the subject awake, but resting recumbent on a bed with eyes closed. With the patient relaxed in such a manner, artifacts from electrode-lead movement are significantly reduced, as are contaminating signals from the scalp. Muscle activity from the face, neck, ears, etc., is perhaps the most subtle contaminant of EEG records in the recording of both spontaneous ongoing activity in the brain and activity evoked by a sensory stimulus (*evoked response*). For example, the frequency spectrum of the field produced by mildly contracted facial muscles contains frequency components well within the nominal EEG range (0.5–100 Hz). After technicians have achieved resting, quiescent conditions in the normal adult subject, the subject's scalp recordings show a dominant alpha rhythm in the parietal-occipital areas, while in the frontal areas, in addition to the alpha rhythm, there is also a low-amplitude, higher-frequency beta rhythm. In the normal subject there is a symmetry between the recordings of the right and left hemisphere. To appreciate the wide range of EEG measurement artifacts, see Hill and Parr (1963).

In general there is a relationship between the degree of cerebral activity and the average frequency of the EEG rhythm, the frequency increasing progressively with higher and higher degrees of activity. For example, delta waves are frequently found in stupor, surgical anesthesia, and sleep; theta waves in infants; alpha waves during relaxed states; and beta waves during intense mental activity. However, during periods of mental activity, the waves usually become asynchronous rather than synchronous, so that the magnitude of the summed surface potential recording decreases despite increased cortical activity.

Sleep patterns

When an individual in a relaxed, inattentive state becomes drowsy and falls asleep, the alpha rhythm is replaced by slower, larger waves (Figure 4.32). In deep sleep, very large, somewhat irregular delta waves are observed. Interspersed with these waves—during moderately deep sleep—are bursts of alphalike activity, called *sleep spindles*. The alpha rhythm and the patterns of the drowsy and sleeping subject are *synchronized,* in contrast with the low-voltage *desynchronized,* irregular activity seen in the subject who is in an alert state.

The high-amplitude, slow waves seen in the EEG of a subject who is asleep are sometimes replaced by rapid, low-voltage irregular activity which resembles that obtained in alert subjects. However, the sleep of a subject with this irregular pattern is not interrupted; in fact, the threshold for arousal by sensory stimuli is elevated. This condition has therefore come to be called *paradoxical sleep.* During paradoxical sleep, the subject exhibits rapid, roving eye movements. For this reason, it is also called *rapid-eye-movement* or REM sleep. Conversely, *spindle* or synchronized sleep is frequently called *nonrapid-eye-movement,* NREM, or slow-wave

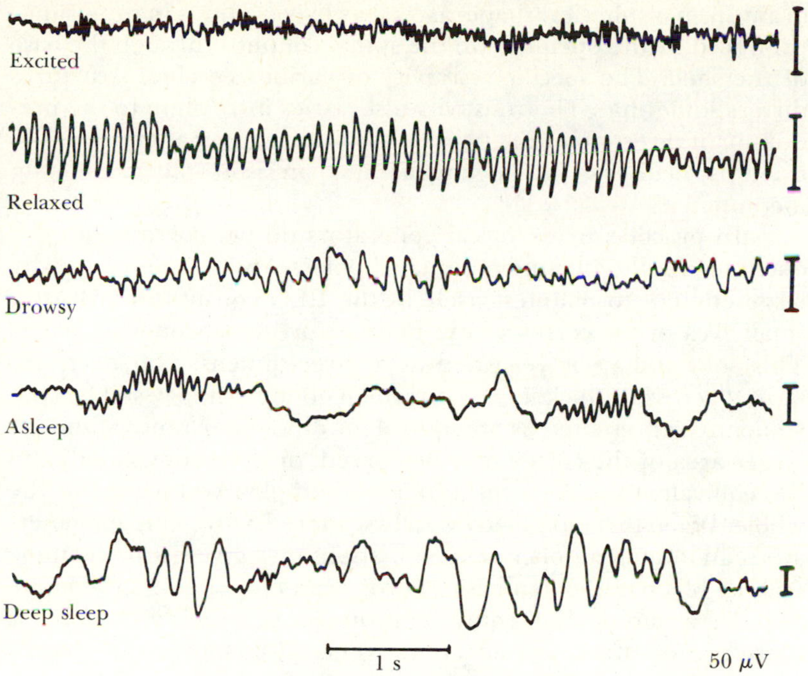

Figure 4.32 The electroencephalographic changes that occur as a human subject goes to sleep. The calibration marks on the right represent 50 μV. (From H.H. Jasper, "Electroencephalography," in *Epilepsy and Cerebral Localization*, edited by W.G. Penfield and T.C. Erickson. Springfield, Ill.: Charles C. Thomas, 1941.)

sleep. Human subjects aroused at a time when their EEG exhibits a paradoxical (REM) sleep pattern generally report that they were dreaming, whereas individuals wakened from spindle sleep do not. This observation and other evidence indicate that REM sleep and dreaming are closely associated. It is interesting that, during REM sleep, there is a marked reduction in muscle tone, despite the rapid eye movements.

The volume-conductor problem in electroencephalography

Geometrically speaking, the brain approximates a sphere surrounded by concentric shells that differ in impedance, and are comprised of the *meninges* (connective tissue coverings of the brain), cerebral spinal fluid, skull, and scalp. This model is inaccurate to the extent that the brain is not really a true sphere, and its coverings are irregular in shape and thickness. Such irregularities are insignificant for the upper half of the brain, but complications are introduced by the marked departure of the lower parts of the brain from a spherical shape, as well as by variations in impedance produced by the openings (to the spinal column) through the base of the shell. The specific resistivity of various cerebral structures differs somewhat. The resistivity also varies in relation to the predominant direction of the fibers within the white matter. Thus the brain is neither a homogeneous nor an isotropic conducting medium.

In practice, neurological generators do not correspond precisely to simple, one-dimensional dipoles. Any source of activity large enough to manifest itself in the EEG constitutes at least a small area of the cortex whose neurons are synchronously active. This source may be regarded as a three-dimensional sheet, polarized across its thickness. If it is small enough, it may still be conveniently represented as an equivalent dipole per unit volume. A larger area of the cortex may be curved, or even convoluted, and the equivalent dipole then becomes a complex vector sum of the whole. When there are many widely scattered active-current generators, an infinite number of combinations may give rise to the same pattern of surface potentials (see, for example, Plonsey, 1963a, b).

Determining the equivalent dipole of cerebral activity is therefore of practical value only when EEG sources are highly "focal". Fortunately, this condition occurs frequently in the brain's response to sensory stimulation, as well as in pathological conditions. Accordingly, there is some practical value in developing techniques for establishing the anatomical locus of focal generators, since there is the possibility of thereby achieving an analysis of more complex states. For example, a common technique for analyzing a problem of this type is as follows: (1) Assume a model (e.g., the eccentrically located dipole in a uniform, homogeneous spherical conducting medium; assume that the electric field is quasistatic). (2) After obtaining a solution to the associated boundary-value problem, produce model-generated potential values at measurement points on the cortical surface. (3) Compare these theoretical potential values with particular discrete-time values of EEG waveforms measured at the same surface sites and form a general least-squares reconstruction error function, wherein the error is defined as the difference between predicted and measured potential at several selected cortical measurement sites. (4) Iteratively adjust the EEG dipolar source parameters at each discrete-time instant so as to obtain the best fit to sampled EEG waveforms in a least-squares sense. You thus assume that the optimum dipole location is the dipole location that is obtained when the reconstruction error function is so minimized.

The influence of anisotropy on various EEG phenomena has been studied by a number of investigators, including Rush and Driscoll (1968, 1969) and Henderson, Butler, and Glass (1975). These investigations, together with various *in vivo* studies, substantially agree that the presence of tissue anisotropy tends to attenuate and smear the pattern of scalp-recorded EEGs. This type of degradation apparently does not affect the model's ability to predict the locus of the EEG equivalent-dipole generator (although the dipole moment might be underestimated). This is important in the sense that one of the major objectives of electroencephalography is the determination of the sources of cerebral activity—for localized or focal activity—because in evoked cortical potentials and deep-brain pathologies, this concept of the equivalent-dipole generator is of clinical value.

The abnormal EEG

One of the more important clinical uses of the EEG is in the diagnosis of different types of epilepsy and in the location of the focus in the brain causing the epilepsy. Epilepsy is characterized by uncontrolled excessive activity by either a part or all of the central nervous system. A person predisposed to epilepsy has attacks when the basal level of excitability of all or part of his nervous system rises above a certain critical threshold. However, as long as the degree of excitability is held below this threshold, no attack occurs.

There are two basic types of epilepsy: *generalized epilepsy* and *partial epilepsy*. Generalized epilepsy involves the entire brain at once, whereas partial epilepsy involves a portion of the brain—sometimes only a minute focal spot and at other times a fair amount of the brain. Generalized epilepsy is further divided into *grand mal* and *petit mal* epilepsy.

Grand mal epilepsy is characterized by extreme discharges of neurons originating in the brainstem portion of the RAS. These then spread out throughout the cortex, to the deeper parts of the brain, and even to the spinal cord to cause generalized tonic convulsions of the entire body. They are followed near the end of the attack by alternating muscular contractions, called *clonic convulsions*. The grand mal seizure lasts from a few seconds to as long as 3–4 min, and is characterized by post-seizure depression of the entire nervous system. The subject may remain in a stupor for 1 min to as long as a day or more after the attack is over.

The middle recording in Figure 4.30(c) shows a typical EEG during a grand mal attack. This response can be recorded from almost any region of the cortex. The recorded potential is of a high magnitude, and the response is synchronous, with the same periodicity as normal alpha waves. The same type of discharge occurs on both sides of the brain at the same time, indicating that the origin of the abnormality is in the lower centers of the brain that control the activity of the cerebral cortex, and not in the cortex itself. Electrical recordings from the thalamus and reticular formation of experimental animals during an induced grand mal attack indicate typical high-voltage synchronous activity in these areas, similar to that recorded from the cerebral cortex. Experiments on animals have further shown that a grand mal attack is caused by intrinsic hyperexcitability of the neurons comprising the RAS structures, or by some abnormality of the local neural pathways of this system.

Petit mal epilepsy is closely allied to grand mal epilepsy. It occurs in two forms: the *myoclonic* and the *absence* form. In the myoclonic form, a burst of neuronal discharges, lasting a fraction of a second, occurs throughout the nervous system. These are similar to those occurring at the beginning of a grand mal attack. The person exhibits a single violent muscular jerk involving arms or head. The entire process stops immediately, however, and the attack is over before the subject loses consciousness or stops what he or she is doing. This type of attack often becomes progressively more severe until the subject experiences a grand mal attack. Thus the myoclonic form of petit mal is similar to a grand mal attack, except that some form of inhibitory influence promptly stops it.

The absence type of petit mal epilepsy is characterized by 5–20 s of unconsciousness, during which the subject has several twitchlike contractions of the muscles, usually in the head region. There is a pronounced blinking of the eyes, followed by a return to consciousness and continuation of previous activities. This type of epilepsy is also closely allied to grand mal epilepsy. In rare instances, it can initiate a grand mal attack.

Figure 4.30(c) shows a typical *spike-and-dome* pattern that is recorded during absence-type petit mal epilepsy. The spike portion of the record is almost identical to the spikes occurring in grand mal epilepsy, but the dome portion is distinctly different. The spike-and-dome pattern can be recorded over the entire cortex, illustrating again that the seizure originates in the RAS.

Partial epilepsy can involve almost any part of the brain, either localized regions of the cerebral cortex or deeper structures of both the cerebrum and brainstem. Partial epilepsy almost always results from some organic lesion of the brain, such as a scar that pulls on the neuronal tissue, a tumor that compresses an area of the brain, or a destroyed region of the brain tissue. Lesions such as these can cause local neurons to fire very rapid discharges. When the rate exceeds approximately 1000 per second, synchronous waves begin spreading over adjacent cortical regions. These waves presumably result from the activity of localized reverberating neuronal circuits that gradually recruit adjacent areas of the cortex into the "discharge," or firing, zone. The process spreads to adjacent areas at rates as slow as a few millimeters per minute to as fast as several centimeters per minute. When such a wave of excitation spreads over the motor cortex, it causes a progressive "march" of muscular contractions throughout the opposite side of the body, beginning perhaps in the leg region and marching progressively upward to the head region, or at other times marching in the opposite direction. This is called Jacksonian epilepsy, or *Jacksonian march*.

Another type of partial epilepsy is the so-called *psychomotor seizure*, which may cause (1) a short period of amnesia, (2) an attack of abnormal rage, (3) sudden anxiety or fear, (4) a moment of incoherent speech or mumbling, (5) a motor act of rubbing the face with the hand, attacking someone, and so forth. Sometimes the person does not remember his or her activities during the attack; at other times the person is completely aware, but unable to control his or her behavior. The bottom tracing of Figure 4.30(c) shows a typical EEG during a psychomotor seizure showing a low-frequency rectangular-wave response with a frequency between 2 and 4 Hz with superimposed 14-Hz waves.

The EEG can frequently be used to locate tumors and also abnormal spiking waves originating in diseased brain tissue that might predispose to epileptic attacks. Once such a focal point is found, surgical excision of the focus often prevents future epileptic seizures.

For more detailed treatments of the anatomical and electrophysiological detail associated with the EEG, see the texts of Curtis, Jacobson, and Marcus (1972) and Guyton (1972). For a basic introduction to the EEG, see Lindsley and Wicke (1974). For basic current-generator characterization, see Rush and Driscoll (1968), Schneider (1972, 1974), and Vaughn (1974).

Problems

4.1 What are the four main factors involved in the movement of ions across the cell membrane in the steady-state condition?

4.2 An excitable cell is impaled by a micropipet and a second extracellular electrode is placed close by at the outer-membrane surface. Brief pulses of current are then passed between these electrodes, which may or may not cause it to conduct an action potential. Explain how the polarity of the stimulating pair influences membrane potential, and subsequently activity, of the excitable cell.

4.3 Explain the subthreshold-membrane potential changes that would occur in the immediate vicinity of each of two extracellular stimulating electrodes placed at the outer-membrane surface of an excitable cell. (See Figure P4.1.) Assume that membrane potential is determined by impaling the cell at various points in the vicinity of the stimulating electrodes with a micropipet and recording the potential with respect to an indifferent extracellular electrode.

4.4 Refer to Problem 4.3. Suppose that the electrical properties of an elongated excitable cell of cylindrical geometry (such as a nerve or skeletal muscle fiber) can be modeled fairly accurately

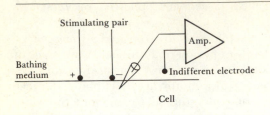

Figure P4.1

with a distributed parameter "cable" model such as that of Figure 4.3. What should the temporal-membrane potential response to brief square pulses of stimulating current look like at some fixed distance from a particular stimulating electrode? As the separation distance between the particular stimulating electrode and the exploring micropipet is progressively increased, in what manner should the amplitude of the subthreshold response change?

4.5 If a stimulus of adequate strength is supplied to the stimulating pair of Problem 4.3, an action potential is generated. Explain by means of the concept of "local-circuit" current flow how the action potential is able to propagate in an unattenuated fashion down the fiber and away from the site of stimulation.

4.6 If an elongated fiber is stimulated in the middle (as opposed to either end), is an action potential propagated in both directions along the fiber? If so, would you expect any differences in the action-potential response measured at equal distances on either side of the stimulation site?

4.7 Define the following terms: (a) absolute refractory period, (b) relative refractory period, (c) compound nerve-action potential, (d) synapse, (e) neuro-myo junction, (f) motor unit, (g) reflex arc.

4.8 An excised, active nerve trunk serves as a bioelectric source located on the axis of a circular cylindrical volume conductor. Field potentials are recorded at various radial distances from the nerve trunk from an appropriate electrode assembly connected to an amplifier. (a) Describe the behavior of the field potential with increasing radial distance from the nerve (angle and axial distance are fixed). (b) Describe the effect of increasing the specific resistivity ρ of the bathing medium on the magnitude of the field potential, and explain how this change in ρ might be accomplished experimentally. (c) In what manner would changing the radius of the surrounding volume conductor affect the magnitude and waveshape of the extracellular field potential? (d) When can a volume conductor of finite dimensions be considered an essentially "infinite" volume conductor?

4.9 The experimental situation posed in Problem 4.8 is roughly analogous to the problem of recording either surface or intramuscular potentials from the arm of a human subject whose ulnar or median nerve has been stimulated (e.g., Figure 4.8). Explain in terms of changes in specific resistivity and geometry why potential waveforms recorded at the wrist may differ considerably from those recorded at the level of the forearm (see Figure 4.8).

4.10 Define the *M* wave and the *H* reflex.

4.11 In many forms of peripheral neuropathies, the excitability of some neurons is changed and their conduction velocities are consequently altered. Describe the possible effect that this might have on an EMG recording and on muscular contraction.

4.12 A muscle is paralyzed if its neural connection to, or within, the CNS is interrupted. A disconnection at the level of the motor neuron is called a *lower motoneuron lesion*. A disconnection higher in the spinal cord or brain is called an *upper motoneuron lesion*. In both cases, the contractility of the peripheral skeletal muscle is initially preserved; but after a period of disuse, the muscle atrophies. (Atrophy, however, is much delayed in the case of an upper motoneuron lesion.) Consider Figure P4.2 to repre-

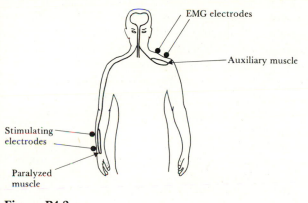

Figure P4.2

sent schematically a quadriplegic patient with paralyzed extremities as shown. Suggest a scheme for using the EMG from an auxiliary intact muscle (for example, the L. Trapezius m.) to aid in the control of the stimulation of the paralyzed limb. (The motor nerve supply to the trapezius muscle is assumed to lie above the site of spinal-cord lesion and is therefore under volitional control. Draw a block diagram of the suggested control system. Label the anatomical structures serving as the plant (or controlled system), the controller, the feedback pathway, the actuator, and so forth. [*Hint:* The EMG signal is usually amplified, rectified, and low-pass-filtered before it is used to modulate a stimulator. For further interesting discussions of the work in this area, see Vodovnik (1967).]

4.13 Conduct a search of the literature on the subject of the use of electromyography in the study of: (a) The function of ocular muscles. [The EMG yields valuable information regarding the synergistic action of the different ocular muscles, and is of value in the interpretation of paralytic squint (e.g., Breinin, 1962).] (b) Myasthenia gravis and other disorders of neuromuscular transmission (see, for example, Simpson, 1966a, b).

4.14 Define the following cardiac anatomical terms: (a) internodal tracts, (b) subendocardial layer, (c) intercalated disc, (d) bundle branches, (e) ventricular activation.

4.15 Draw a typical lead II electrocardiogram and label all waves (P, QRS, T) and intervals. Explain what is happening electrically within the heart during each wave or interval.

4.16 The electrical activity of the His bundle is normally not present in the typical ECG recorded at the body surface due to its relatively small tissue mass. However, clinical recordings of His bundle activity could be of considerable importance in the analysis of various disorders of the conduction system. The His bundle signal can be enhanced for such analyses by successive averaging of the surface electrocardiogram, or—better yet—by using an invasive technique wherein a small bipolar electrode is introduced into the right atrial chamber using conventional techniques of cardiac catherization (e.g., Siegel *et al.,* 1975). Conduct a search of the literature on the topics of noninvasive and invasive methods of recording His bundle activity, as well as the use of this signal in diagnosing various disorders of the conduction system.

4.17 Why is it necessary for the ventricular action potential to have a relatively long absolute refractory period?

4.18 Draw and label a block diagram of the retina considered as a photoelectric transducer. What is the output at the ganglion cell layer? At the photoreceptive layer?

4.19 Explain the components of the ERG in terms of retinal cell activity.

4.20 Discuss, in terms of volume-conductor theory, the production of an ERG signal at a point on the corneal surface of the eye when the retinal bioelectric source is considered an array of current dipole sources per unit volume. Consider the possibility of (experimentally) exciting each of the elements of retinal dipole array individually, one at a time, by applying a localized spot of light superimposed on a background illumination that partially adapts the retina. What special technical considerations are involved?

4.21 Discuss the use of the steady corneal-retinal potential of the eye to measure eye movements. How accurate is this technique? Discuss at least two applications of this method.

4.22 Explain the functional role played by the following CNS structures.

a The ascending pathways of the general sensory-nerve

fibers and the descending pathways of the motor-nerve fibers.

b The ascending reticular formation (RAS)

c The pre- and post-central gyri

d The primary auditory and visual cortices

e The specific and nonspecific thalamic neural fibers to the cortex

4.23 Relate EEG-wave activity recorded at the surface of the cortex to the underlying activity of cortical neurons.

4.24 Discuss in general terms the design of a spectrum analyzer for automatic analysis of EEG waves.

4.25 How might volume-conductor theory aid in the analysis of evoked cortical potentials produced by specific repetitive stimuli (auditory, visual, etc.)? [See, for example, Smith *et al.*, 1973.]

References

Aiba, T.S., *et al.*, "The electroretinogram evoked by the excitation of human foveal cones." *J. Physiol.*, 1967, 189, 43–62.

Allessie, M.A., *et al.*, "Circus movement in rabbit atrial muscle as a mechanism of tachycardia." *Circ. Res.*, 1973, 33, 54–62.

Barr, L., *et al.*, "Propagation of action potentials and the structure of the nexus in cardiac muscle." *J. Gen. Physiol.*, 1965, 48, 797–823.

Berry, C.M., *et al.*, "The electrical activity of regenerating nerves in the cat." *J. Neurophysiol.*, 1944, 7, 103–115.

Breinin, G. M., *The electrophysiology of extraocular muscle.* Toronto: University of Toronto Press, 1962.

Brindley, G.S., "The effect on the frog's electroretinogram of varying the amount of retina illuminated." *J. Physiol.*, 1956, 134, 353–359.

Brindley, G.S., and Westheimer, G., "The spatial properties of the human electroretinogram." *J. Physiol.*, 1965, 179, 518–537.

Brown, K.T., "The electroretinogram: Its components and their origins." *Vision Res.*, 1968, 8, 633–677.

Brown, K.T., K. Watanabe, and M. Murakami, "The early and late receptor potentials of monkey cones and rods." *Cold Spring Harbor Symp. Quant. Biol.*, 1965, 30, 457–482.

Clark, J.W., and R. Plonsey, "The extracellular potential field of the single active nerve fiber in a volume conductor." *Biophys. J.*, 1968, 8, 842–864.

Curtis, B.A., S. Jacobson, and E.M. Marcus, *An introduction to the neurosciences.* Philadelphia: Saunders, 1972.

Dartnall, H.J.A., "The photobiology of visual processes," in H. Dawson (ed.), *The eye,* 1st ed. New York: Academic Press, 1962, Vol. 2, pp. 321–533.

Dement, W.C., "Eye movements during sleep," in M.B.

Bender (ed.), *The oculomotor system*. New York: Harper, 1964, pp. 366–416.

Durrer, D., *et al.*, "Total excitation of the isolated human heart." *Circ.* 1970, 41, 899–912.

Gilliatt, R.W., and T.A. Sears, "Sensory nerve action potentials in patients with peripheral nerve lesions." *J. Neurol. Neurosurg. Psychiat.*, 1958, 21, 109–118.

Goldman, D.E., "Potential, impedance and rectification in membranes." *J. Gen. Physiol.*, 1943, 27, 37–60.

Granit, R., "The visual pathway," in H. Dawson (ed.), *The eye*, 1st ed. New York: Academic, 1962, Vol. 2, pp. 537–763.

Guyton, A.C., *Structure and function of the nervous system*. Philadelphia: Saunders, 1972.

Henderson, C.J., S.R. Butler, and A. Glass, "The localization of equivalent dipoles of EEG sources by the application of electric field theory," *Electroencephalog. Clin. Neurophysiol.*, 1975, 39, 117–130.

Hill, D., and G. Parr, *Encephalography*. London: MacDonald, 1963.

Hodgkin, A.L., and A.F. Huxley, "A quantitative description of membrane current and its application to conduction and excitation in nerve." *J. Physiol.*, 1952, 117, 500–544.

Hodgkin, A.L., and B. Katz, "The effect of sodium ions on the electrical activity of the giant axon of the squid." *J. Physiol.*, 1949, 108, 37–77.

Jasper, H.H. in W.G. Penfield and T.C. Erickson (eds.) *Epilepsy and cerebral localization*, Springfield, IL: Charles C. Thomas, 1941.

Jasper, H.H., "The ten-twenty electrode system of the International Federation." *Electroencephalog. Clin. Neurophysiol.*, 1958, 10 (Appendix), 371–375.

Krakow, C.E.T., "On the potential field of the rabbit electroretinogram," *Acta Ophthalmol.*, 1958, 36, 183–207.

Kris, C., "Electro-oculography," in O. Glasser (ed.), *Medical physics*, 1960, Vol. III, pp. 692–700.

Kristiansen, K., and B. Courtois, "Rhythmic electrical activity from the isolated cerebral cortex." *Electroencephalog. Clin. Neurophysiol.*, 1949, 1, 265–272.

Lenman, J.A.R., and A.E. Ritchie, *Clinical electromyography*. Philadelphia: Lippincott, 1970.

Levy, M.N., and R.M. Berne, *Cardiovascular physiology*. St. Louis: Mosby, 1967.

Lindsley, D. B., and J.D. Wicke, "The electroencephalogram: Autonomous electrical activity in man and animals," in R.F. Thompson and M.M. Patterson (eds.), *Bioelectric recording techniques,* New York: Academic, 1974, Part B.

Lipman, B.S., E. Massie, and R.E. Kleiger, *Clinical scalar electrocardiography*. Chicago: Year Book, 1972.

Lorente de Nó, R., in J.R. Fulton (ed.), *Physiology of the nervous system.* New York: Oxford, 1943.

McNaught, A.B., and R. Callender, *Illustrated physiology,* 3rd ed. New York: Churchill-Livingstone, 1975.

Mountcastle, V.B., *Medical physiology,* 13th ed. St. Louis: Mosby, 1974, Vols. 1 and 2.

Netter, F.H., *The Ciba collection of medical illustrations.* Vol. 5: *The heart.* Ciba Pharmaceutical Co., Div. of Ciba Corp., 1969.

North, A.W., "Accuracy and precision of electro-oculographic recording," *Invest. Ophthalmol.,* 1965, 4, 343–348.

Phibbs, B., *The human heart,* 3rd ed. St. Louis: Mosby, 1975.

Plonsey, R., "Current dipole images and reference potentials," *IEEE Trans. Biomed. Eng.,* 1963a, 10, 3–8.

Plonsey, R., "Reciprocity applied to volume conductors and the EEG," *IEEE Trans. Biomed. Eng.,* 1963b, 10, 9–12.

Plonsey, R., "The biophysical basis for electrocardiography," *Crit. Rev. Bioeng.,* 1971a, 1(1), 1–48.

Plonsey, R., "Determination of electrical sources in the mammalian heart from intracellular action potentials," *Circ. Res.,* 1971b, 29, 106–109.

Randall, W.C. (ed.), *Nervous control of the heart.* Baltimore: Williams & Wilkins, 1963.

Ranson, S.W. and S.L. Clark, *The anatomy of the nervous system.* Philadelphia: Saunders, 1959, p. 350.

Ratliff, F. (ed.), *Studies in excitation and inhibition in the retina.* London: Chapman and Hall, 1974.

Rush, S., and D.A. Driscoll, "Current distribution in the brain from surface electrode," *Anesth. Analg.* 1968, 47, 717–723.

Rush, S., and D.A. Driscoll, "EEG electrode sensitivity—An application of reciprocity," *IEEE Trans. Biomed. Eng.,* 1969, 16, 15–22.

Rushton, W.A.H., "A cone pigment in the protanope," *J. Physiol.,* 1963, 168, 345–359.

Schneider, M., "A multistage process for computing virtual dipolar sources of EEG discharges from surface information," *IEEE Trans. Biomed. Eng.,* 1972, 19, 1–12.

Schneider, M., "Effect of inhomogeneities on surface signals coming from a cerebral current-dipole source," *IEEE Trans. Biomed. Eng.,* 1974, 21, 52–54.

Siegel, L., *et al.,* "Conduction cardiograph bundle of His detector." *IEEE Trans. Biomed Eng.,* 1975, 22, 269–274.

Simpson, J.A., "Control of muscle in health and disease," in B. L. Andrew (ed.), *Control and innervation of skeletal muscle.* Edinburgh: Livingstone, 1966a, pp. 171–180.

Simpson, J.A., "Disorders of neuromuscular transmission." *Proc. Roy. Soc. Med.,* 1966b, 59, 993–998.

Smith, D.B., M.E. Lell, R.D. Sidman, and H. Mavor, "Nasopharyngeal phase reversal of cerebral evoked potentials and theoretical dipole implications." *Electroencephalog. Clin. Neurophysiol.*, 1973, 34, 654–658.

Strong, P., *Biophysical measurements*. Beaverton, OR: Tektronix, Inc., 1973.

Terzuolo, V.A., and T.H. Bullock, "Measurement of imposed voltage gradient adequate to modulate neuronal firing." *Proc. Nat. Acad. Sci.*, 1956, 42, 687.

Thomas, H.E., *Handbook of biomedical instrumentation and measurement*, Reston, VA: Reston, 1974.

Troelstra, A. and C.A. Garcia, "The electrical response of the human eye to sinusoidal light stimulation." *IEEE Trans. Biomed. Eng.*, 1975, 22, 369–378.

Vaughn, H.G., "The analysis of scalp recorded brain potentials," in R.F. Thompson and M.M. Patterson (eds.), *Bioelectric recording techniques*. New York: Academic, 1974, Part B.

Vodovnik, L., *et al.*, "Control of a skeletal joint by electrical stimulation of antagonists." *Med. Biol. Eng.*, 1967, 5, 97–109.

Wald, G., "The photoreceptor process in vision," in J. Field (ed.), *Handbook of physiology*, Vol. 1: *Neurophysiology*. Baltimore: Williams & Wilkins, 1959, Sec. 1, pp. 671–692.

Wallace, A.G., "Electrophysiology of the myocardium," in *Clinical Cardiopulmonary Physiology*, 3rd ed. B.L. Gordon, R.A. Carleton, and L.T. Faber, editors. New York: Grune and Stratton, 1969, pp. 171–185.

Wiesel, T.N., and K.T. Brown, "Localization of origins of electroretinogram components by intraretinal recording in the intact cat eye." *J. Physiol.*, 1961, 158, 257–280.

Chapter five

Biopotential electrodes

Michael R. Neuman

In order to measure and record potentials and, hence, currents in the body, it is necessary to provide some interface between the body and the electronic measuring apparatus. This interface function is carried out by biopotential electrodes. In any practical measurement of potentials, current flows in the measuring circuit for at least a fraction of the period of time over which the measurement is made. Ideally this current should be very small. However, in practical situations, it is never zero. Biopotential electrodes must therefore have the capability of conducting a current across the interface between the body and the electronic measuring circuit.

Our first impression is that this is a rather simple function to achieve, and that biopotential electrodes should be relatively straightforward. But when we consider the problem in more detail, we see that the electrode actually carries out a transducing function, because current is carried in the body by ions, while it is carried in the electrode and its lead wire by electrons. Thus the electrode must serve as a transducer to change an ionic current into an electronic current. This greatly complicates electrodes and places constraints on their operation. We shall briefly examine the basic mechanisms involved in the transduction process and look at how these affect electrode characteristics. We shall next examine the principal electrical characteristics of biopotential electrodes and discuss electrical equivalent circuits for electrodes based on these characteristics. We shall then cover some of the different forms that biopotential electrodes take in various types of medical instrumentation systems, and finally look at electrodes used for measuring the ECG, EEG, EMG, and intracellular potentials.

5.1 The electrode-electrolyte interface

The electrode-electrolyte interface is schematically illustrated in Figure 5.1. A net current that crosses the interface, passing from the electrode to the electrolyte, consists of (1) electrons moving in a direction opposite to that of the current in the electrode, (2) cations (denoted by C^+) moving in the same direction as the current, and (3) anions (denoted by A^-) moving in a direction opposite to that of the current in the electrolyte. For charge to cross the interface—since there are no free electrons in the electrolyte and no free cations or anions in the electrode—something must occur at the

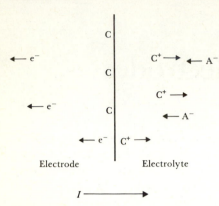

Electrode   Electrolyte

I —————→

Figure 5.1 Electrode-electrolyte interface with current crossing it from left to right. The electrode consists of metallic atoms C. The electrolyte is an aqueous solution containing cations of the electrode metal C^+ and anions A^-.

interface that transfers the charge between these carriers. What actually occurs are chemical reactions at the interface, which can be represented in general by the following equations:

$$C \rightleftharpoons C^{n+} + ne^- \tag{5.1}$$

$$A^{m-} \rightleftharpoons A + me^- \tag{5.2}$$

where n is the valence of C and m is the valence of A. Note that in (5.1) we are assuming that the electrode is made up of some atoms of the same material as the cations, and that this material in the electrode at the interface can become oxidized to form a cation and a free electron. The cation is discharged into the electrolyte, while the electron remains as a charge carrier in the electrode.

The reaction involving the anions is given in (5.2). In this case an anion coming to the electrode-electrolyte interface can be oxidized to a neutral atom, giving off one or more free electrons to the electrode.

Note that both reactions are often reversible, and that reduction reactions (going from right to left in the equations) can occur as well. As a matter of fact, when no current is crossing the electrode-electrolyte interface, these reactions often still occur. But the rate of oxidation reactions equals the rate of reduction reactions, so that the net transfer of charge across the interface is zero. When the current flow is from electrode to electrolyte, as indicated in Figure 5.1, the oxidation reactions dominate; and, when the current is in the opposite direction, the reduction reactions dominate.

To further understand the characteristics of the electrode-electrolyte interface, let us consider what happens when we place a piece of metal into a solution containing ions of that metal. These ions are cations, and the solution, if it is to maintain neutrality of charge, must have an equal number of anions. When the metal comes in contact with the solution, the reaction represented by (5.1) begins immediately. The reaction initially goes either predominantly to the left or to the right, depending on the concentration of cations in solution and the equilibrium conditions for that particular reaction. The local concentration of cations in the solution at the interface changes, which affects the anion concentration at this point as well. The net result is that neutrality of charge is not maintained in this region. Thus the electrolyte surrounding the metal is at a different electrical potential from the rest of the solution. A potential difference known as the *half-cell potential* is determined by the metal involved, the concentration of its ions in solution, and the temperature, as well as other second-order factors. Knowledge of the half-cell potential is important for understanding the behavior of biopotential electrodes.

The distribution of ions in the electrolyte in the immediate vicinity of the metal-electrolyte interface has been of great interest to electrochemists, and several theories have been developed to describe it. Geddes (1972) compares the charge and potential distributions for four of these theories, while Cobbold (1974), in a discussion of the half-cell potential, considers the Stern model. Rather than analyze these theories here, we shall accept their general conclusion. They concluded that some sort of separation of charges exists at the metal-electrolyte interface that results in an electrical double layer, wherein one type of charge is dominant on the surface of the metal and the opposite charge is distributed in excess in the immediately adjacent electrolyte.

It is not possible to measure the half-cell potential of an electrode because—unless we use a second electrode—we cannot provide a connection between the electrolyte and one terminal of the potential-measuring apparatus. Since this second electrode also has a half-cell potential, we merely end up measuring the difference between the half-cell potentials of the metal and the second electrode. There would of course be a very large number of combinations of pairs of electrodes. Therefore tabulations of such differential half-cell potentials would be extremely extensive. To avoid this problem, we shall adopt the standard convention that a particular electrode—the hydrogen electrode—is defined as having a half-cell potential of zero under conditions that are readily achievable in the laboratory. We can then measure the half-cell potentials of all other electrode materials with respect to this electrode.

Table 5.1 lists several common materials used for electrodes, and gives their half-cell potentials. The table also gives the oxidation-reduction reactions that occur at the surfaces of these

Metal and reaction	Potential E^0, V
$Al \longrightarrow Al^{3+} + 3e^-$	-1.706
$Zn \longrightarrow Zn^{2+} + 2e^-$	-0.763
$Cr \longrightarrow Cr^{3+} + 3e^-$	-0.744
$Fe \longrightarrow Fe^{2+} + 2e^-$	-0.409
$Cd \longrightarrow Cd^{2+} + 2e^-$	-0.401
$Ni \longrightarrow Ni^{2+} + 2e^-$	-0.230
$Pb \longrightarrow Pb^{2+} + 2e^-$	-0.126
$H_2 \longrightarrow 2H^+ + 2e^-$	0.000 by definition
$Ag + Cl^- \longrightarrow AgCl + e^-$	$+0.223$
$2Hg + 2Cl^- \longrightarrow Hg_2Cl_2 + 2e^-$	$+0.268$
$Cu \longrightarrow Cu^{2+} + 2e^-$	$+0.340$
$Cu \longrightarrow Cu^+ + e^-$	$+0.522$
$Ag \longrightarrow Ag^+ + e^-$	$+0.799$
$Au \longrightarrow Au^{3+} + 3e^-$	$+1.420$
$Au \longrightarrow Au^+ + e^-$	$+1.680$

Table 5.1 Half-cell potentials for common electrode materials at 25°C. The metal undergoing the reaction shown has the sign and potential E^0 when referenced to the hydrogen electrode. Data from *Handbook of Chemistry and Physics,* 55th edition, CRC Press, Cleveland, Ohio, 1974–1975, with permission.

electrodes to enable us to arrive at the potentials. The hydrogen electrode is based on the reaction

$$H_2 \rightleftharpoons 2H \rightleftharpoons 2H^+ + 2e^- \qquad (5.3)$$

where H_2 gas bubbled over a platinum electrode is the source of hydrogen molecules. Also the platinum serves as a catalyst for the reaction on the left-hand side of the equation and as an acceptor of the generated electrons.

Figure 5.2 gives the basic structure of the hydrogen electrode. A piece of platinum foil or wire is coated with finely divided metallic platinum, often referred to as *platinum black*. The granules are so small that they scatter diffusely and absorb the light falling on them, and thereby give the surface a black appearance. This treatment of a surface greatly increases the effective surface area available for chemical reactions. Platinum must be used because it is relatively inert. In addition, few, if any, platinum atoms are oxidized at the platinum-electrolyte interface. This platinum electrode is immersed in an electrolyte containing cations of the same material as the electrode whose half-cell potential is to be measured. A jet of H_2 gas is also placed in the electrolyte so that it produces small bubbles of H_2 which pass over the surface of the platinum electrode. Some of the hydrogen molecules are absorbed on the platinum surface and dissociate to hydrogen atoms. These hydrogen atoms can then become oxidized to hydrogen ions, which go into solution by giving up their electrons to the platinum electrode.

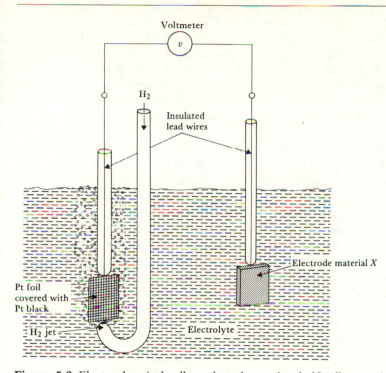

Figure 5.2 Electrochemical cell used to determine half-cell potential for material *X*. Left-hand electrode is a hydrogen electrode used as a reference electrode, since its half-cell potential is zero by definition. Voltmeter must have an infinite impedance to read true half-cell potential of *X*.

The remainder of the electrochemical cell consists of an electrode fabricated of the material of which the half-cell potential is to be measured. An *electrometer* (a very-high-input impedance voltmeter) connected between this electrode and the platinum of the hydrogen electrode reads the half-cell potential directly.

Other reference electrodes that are more convenient to use than the hydrogen electrode are described in Section 5.3.

5.2 Polarization

The half-cell potential of an electrode is described in Section 5.1 for conditions in which no electrical current exists between the electrode and the electrolyte. If, on the other hand, there is a current, the observed half-cell potential is often altered. The difference is due to polarization of the electrode. The difference in potential between the observed half-cell potential and the equilibrium zero-current half-cell potential is known as the *overvoltage*. There are three basic mechanisms that contribute to this phenomenon, and the overvoltage can be separated into three components: the ohmic, the concentration, and the activation overvoltages.

The *ohmic overvoltage* is a direct result of the resistance of the electrolyte. When a current passes between two electrodes immersed in an electrolyte, there is a voltage drop along the path of the current in the electrolyte, due to its resistance. This drop in voltage is proportional to the current and the resistivity of the electrolyte. The resistance between the electrodes can itself vary as a function of the current. Thus the ohmic overvoltage does not necessarily have to be linearly related to the current. This is especially true in electrolytes having low concentrations of ions. Thus, this situation does not necessarily follow Ohm's law.

The *concentration overpotential* results from changes in the distribution of ions in the electrolyte in the vicinity of the electrode-electrolyte interface. Recall that the equilibrium half-cell potential results from the distribution of ionic concentration in the vicinity of the electrode-electrolyte interface when no current flows between the electrode and the electrolyte. Under these conditions, reactions (5.1) and (5.2) reach equilibrium, so that the rates of oxidation and reduction at the interface are equal. When a current is established, this equality is no longer true. Thus it is reasonable to expect the concentration of ions to change. This change results in a different half-cell potential at the electrode. The difference between this and the equilibrium half-cell potential is the concentration overvoltage.

The third mechanism of polarization results in the *activation overvoltage*. The charge-transfer processes involved in the oxidation-reduction reaction (5.1) are not entirely reversible. In order for metal atoms to be oxidized to metal ions that are capable of going into solution, the atoms must overcome an energy barrier. This barrier, or *activation energy,* governs the kinetics of the reaction. The reverse reaction—in which a cation is reduced, thereby plating out an atom of the metal on the electrode—also involves an activation energy, but it does not necessarily have to be the same as that required for the oxidation reaction. When there is a current between the electrode and the electrolyte, either oxidation or reduction predominates, and hence the height of the energy barrier depends on the direction of the current. This difference in energy appears as a difference in voltage between the electrode and the electrolyte, which is known as the *activation overvoltage*.

These three mechanisms of polarization are additive. Thus the net overvoltage of an electrode is given by

$$V_p = V_r + V_c + V_a \tag{5.4}$$

where

V_p = total overvoltage, or polarization potential, of the electrode

V_r = ohmic overpotential
V_c = concentration overpotential
V_a = activation overpotential

When two aqueous ionic solutions of different concentration are separated by an ion-selective semipermeable membrane, an electrical potential exists across this membrane. It can be shown (Plonsey, 1969) that this potential is given by the Nernst equation

$$E = -\frac{RT}{nF} \ln\left(\frac{a_1}{a_2}\right)$$ (5.5)

where a_1 and a_2 are the activities of the ions on each side of the membrane. [Other terms are defined in (4.1) and the Appendix.] In dilute solutions, ionic activity is approximately equal to ionic concentration. When intermolecular effects become significant, which happens at high concentrations, the activity of the ions is less than their concentration.

The half-cell potentials listed in Table 5.1 are known as the standard half-cell potentials because they apply to standard conditions. When the electrode-electrolyte system no longer maintains this standard condition, half-cell potentials different from the standard half-cell potential are observed. The differences in potential are determined primarily by temperature and ionic activity in the electrolyte. *Ionic activity* can be defined as the availability of an ionic species in solution to enter into reaction.

The standard half-cell potential is determined at a standard temperature; the electrode is placed in an electrolyte containing cations of the electrode material having unity activity. As the activity changes from unity (due to changing concentration), the half-cell potential varies according to the Nernst equation

$$E = E^0 + \frac{RT}{nF} \ln(a_{c^{n+}})$$ (5.6)

where

E = half-cell potential
E^0 = standard half-cell potential
n = valence of electrode material
$a_{c^{n+}}$ = activity of cation C^{n+}

Equation (5.6) represents a specific application of the Nernst equation to the reaction of (5.1). The more general form of this equation can be written for a general oxidation-reduction reaction as

$$\alpha A + \beta B \rightleftharpoons \gamma C + \delta D + ne^-$$ (5.7)

where n electrons are transferred. The general Nernst equation for this situation is

$$E = E^0 + \frac{RT}{nF} \ln \left(\frac{a_C^\gamma a_D^\delta}{a_A^\alpha a_B^\beta} \right) \tag{5.8}$$

where the a's represent the activities of the various constituents of the reaction.

An electrode-electrolyte interface is not a necessary requirement for a potential difference to exist. If two electrolytic solutions are in contact and have different concentrations of ions with different ionic mobilities, a potential difference exists between them, known as a *liquid-junction potential*. For solutions of the same composition but different activities, its magnitude is given by

$$E_j = \frac{\mu_+ - \mu_-}{\mu_+ + \mu_-} \frac{RT}{nF} \ln \left(\frac{a'}{a''} \right) \tag{5.9}$$

where μ_+ and μ_- are the mobilities of the positive and negative ions, and a' and a'' are the activities of the two solutions. Though liquid-junction potentials are generally not as high as electrode-electrolyte potentials, they can easily be of the order of tens of millivolts. For example, two solutions of sodium chloride, at 25°C, with activities that vary by a factor of 10, have a potential difference of approximately 12 mV. Note that you can generate potentials of the order of some biological potentials by merely creating differences in concentration in an electrolyte. This is a factor to consider when you are examining actual electrode systems used for biopotential measurements.

Example 5.1 A Zn and an Ag electrode coated with AgCl are placed in a $1M$ ZnCl solution (activities of Zn^+ and Cl^- are approximately unity) to form an electrochemical cell. The solution is maintained at a temperature of 25°C.

    a What chemical reactions might you expect to see at these electrodes?

    b If a very-high-input impedance voltmeter were connected across these electrodes, what would it read?

    c If the lead wires from the electrodes were shorted together, would a current flow? How would this affect the reactions at the electrodes?

    d How would you expect the voltage between the electrodes to differ from the equilibrium open-circuit voltage of the cell immediately following removal of the short circuit?

Answer

    a Zn is much more chemically active than Ag, so the atoms on its surface oxidize to Zn^{++} ions according to the reaction

$$Zn \rightleftharpoons Zn^{++} + 2e^- \qquad (E5.1)$$

which, according to Table 5.1, has an E^0 of -0.763 V. At the Ag electrode, Ag can be oxidized to form Ag^+ ions according to the reaction

$$Ag + Cl^- \rightleftharpoons AgCl + 1\ e^- \qquad (E5.2)$$

This reaction has an E^0 of 0.223 V at 25°C.

   b When no current is drawn from or supplied to either electrode, the difference in voltage between the electrodes is the difference between the half-cell potentials.

$$V = E^0_{Zn} - E^0_{Ag} = -0.763 - 0.223 = -0.986 \text{ V} \qquad (E5.3)$$

Since the Zn oxidizes at a higher potential, the electrons remaining in it are at a higher energy than those in the Ag. Thus the Zn electrode has a negative voltage with respect to the Ag.

   c Since there is a potential difference between the two electrodes, when they are shorted together current flows. The flow of electrons is from the Zn to the Ag, since the Zn electrons are at a higher energy. Thus reaction (E5.1) goes from left to right and reaction (E5.2) goes from right to left.

   d When the electrodes are connected, they must be at the same potential at the point of connection. Thus the 0.986-V half-cell potential difference must be opposed by polarization overpotentials and ohmic losses in the electrodes and connecting wires. When the connection is broken and the current stops, the ohmic overpotential and electrode losses become zero, but the concentration overpotential remains until the gradient of the ionic concentration at the electrode surfaces returns to its equilibrium value for zero current. Thus the difference in voltage between the two electrodes is less than 0.986 V, but it rises to that value asymptotically with time.

5.3 Polarizable and nonpolarizable electrodes

   Theoretically two types of electrodes are possible: those that are perfectly polarizable and those that are perfectly nonpolarizable. This classification refers to what happens to an electrode when a current passes between it and the electrolyte. *Perfectly polarizable electrodes* are those in which no actual charge crosses the electrode-electrolyte interface when a current is applied. Of course, there has to be current across the interface, but this current is a displacement current, and the electrode behaves as if it were a capacitor. *Perfectly nonpolarizable electrodes* are those in which current passes freely across the electrode-electrolyte interface, requiring no energy to make the transition. Thus, for perfectly nonpolarizable electrodes there are no overvoltages.

Neither of these two electrodes can be fabricated; however, some practical electrodes can come close to acquiring their characteristics. Electrodes made of noble metal come closest to behaving as perfectly polarizable electrodes. Since the materials of these electrodes are relatively inert, it is difficult for them to oxidize and dissolve. Thus, current passing between the electrode and the electrolyte primarily changes the concentration of ions at the interface, so that a majority of the overvoltage seen from this type of electrode is a result of V_c, the concentration overvoltage. The electrical characteristics of such an electrode produce a strong capacitive effect.

The silver–silver chloride electrode

The silver–silver chloride (Ag-AgCl) electrode is a practical electrode that approaches the characteristics of a perfectly nonpolarizable electrode and can be easily fabricated in the laboratory. It is a member of a class of electrodes consisting of a metal coated with a layer of a slightly soluble ionic compound of that metal with a suitable anion. The whole structure is immersed in an electrolyte containing the anion in relatively high concentrations.

The structure is shown in Figure 5.3. A silver metal base with attached insulated lead wire is coated with a layer of the ionic compound AgCl. (This material—AgCl—is only very slightly soluble in water, so it remains stable.) The electrode is then immersed in an electrolyte bath in which the principal anion of the electrolyte is Cl^-. For best results, the electrolyte solution should also be saturated with AgCl so that there is no chance for any of the surface film on the electrode to dissolve.

The behavior of the Ag-AgCl electrode is governed by two chemical reactions. The first involves the oxidation of silver atoms on the electrode surface to silver ions in solution at the interface.

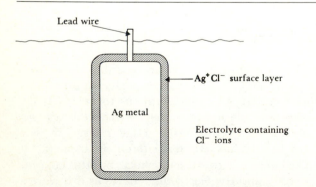

Lead wire

Ag^+Cl^- surface layer

Ag metal

Electrolyte containing Cl^- ions

Figure 5.3 A silver–silver chloride electrode, shown in cross section.

$$Ag \rightleftharpoons Ag^+ + e^- \tag{5.10}$$

$$Ag^+ + Cl^- \rightleftharpoons AgCl \downarrow \tag{5.11}$$

The second reaction occurs immediately after the formation of Ag^+ ions. These combine with Cl^- ions already in solution to form the ionic compound AgCl. As mentioned before, AgCl is only very slightly soluble in water, so most of it precipitates out of solution onto the silver electrode and contributes to the silver chloride deposit. Silver chloride's rate of precipitation and of returning to solution is a constant, K_s, known as the *solubility product*. Under equilibrium conditions the ionic activities of the Ag^+ and Cl^- ions must be such that their product is the solubility product.

$$a_{Ag^+} \times a_{Cl^-} = K_s \tag{5.12}$$

In biological fluids the concentration of Cl^- ions is relatively high, giving it an activity somewhat less than unity. The solubility product for AgCl, on the other hand, is of the order of 10^{-10}. This means that, when an Ag-AgCl electrode is in contact with biologic fluids, the activity of the Ag^+ ion must be very low and of the same order of magnitude as the solubility product.

We can determine the half-cell potential for the Ag-AgCl electrode by writing (5.6) for the reaction of (5.10).

$$E = E^0_{Ag} + \frac{RT}{nF} \ln (a_{Ag^+}) \tag{5.13}$$

By using (5.12), we can rewrite this as

$$E = E^0_{Ag} + \frac{RT}{nF} \ln \left(\frac{K_s}{a_{Cl^-}}\right) \tag{5.14}$$

or

$$E = E^0_{Ag} + \frac{RT}{nF} \ln (K_s) - \frac{RT}{nF} \ln (a_{Cl^-}) \tag{5.15}$$

The first and second terms on the right-hand side of (5.15) are constants; only the third term is determined by ionic activity. In this case it is the activity of the Cl^- ion, which is relatively large and not related to the oxidation of Ag, which is caused by the current through the electrode. The half-cell potential of this electrode is consequently quite stable when it is placed in an electrolyte containing Cl^- as the principal anion. Since this is the case in the body, we shall see in later sections of this chapter that the Ag-AgCl electrode is relatively stable in biologic applications.

There are several procedures, as reviewed by Janz and Ives (1968), that can be used to fabricate Ag-AgCl electrodes. Two of these are of particular importance in biomedical electrodes. Figure 5.4 illustrates the electrolytic process for forming Ag-AgCl electrodes. An electrochemical cell is made up in which the Ag electrode on which the AgCl layer is to be deposited serves as anode and another piece of Ag—having a surface area greater than that of the anode—serves as cathode. A 1.5-V battery serves as the energy source; and a series resistance limits the peak current, thereby controlling the maximum rate of reaction. A milliammeter can be placed in the circuit to observe the current, which is proportional to the rate of reaction.

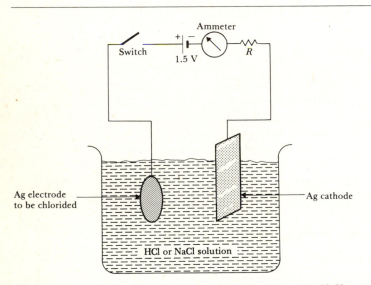

Figure 5.4 An electrochemical cell used to grow an AgCl film on surface of Ag electrode.

When the switch is closed, the reactions of (5.10) and (5.11) begin to occur and the current jumps to its maximum value. As the thickness of the deposited AgCl layer increases, the rate of reaction decreases and the current drops. This situation continues, and the current approaches zero asymptotically. Theoretically, the reaction is not complete until the current drops to zero. In practice this never occurs because of other processes going on which conduct a current. Therefore the reaction can be stopped after a few minutes, once the current has reached a relatively stable low value—of the order of 10 μA for most biologic electrodes.

Example 5.2 An AgCl surface is grown on an Ag electrode by the electrolytic process. The current passing through the cell is measured and recorded during the growth of the AgCl layer. The current is found to be given by the equation

$$I = 100 \text{ mA } e^{-t/10} \qquad \text{(E5.4)}$$

a Suppose that the reaction is allowed to run for a long period of time, so that the current at the end of this period is essentially zero. How much charge is removed from the battery driving this reaction?

b How many grams of AgCl are deposited on the electrode's surface by this reaction?

c The electrode is placed in a beaker containing 1 liter of 0.9 molar NaCl solution. How much of the AgCl is dissolved?

Answer

a The total charge crossing the electrode-electrolyte interface is

$$q = \int_0^\infty I\, dt = 100 \text{ mA} \int_0^\infty e^{-t/10}\, dt \qquad (E5.5)$$
$$= 1 \text{ C}$$

b One molecule of AgCl is deposited for each electron. The number of atoms deposited is

$$N = \frac{1 \text{ C}}{1.6 \times 10^{-19} \text{ C/atom}} = 6.25 \times 10^{18} \text{ atoms} \qquad (E5.6)$$

The number of moles can be found by dividing by Avogadro's number:

$$N = \frac{6.25 \times 10^{18}}{6.03 \times 10^{23}} = 1.036 \times 10^{-5} \text{ mol} \qquad (E5.7)$$

The molecular weight of AgCl is 142.3. Therefore the weight of AgCl formed is

$$142.3 \times 1.036 \times 10^{-5} = 1.47 \times 10^{-3} \text{ g}$$

c For AgCl, the solubility product $K_s = 1.56 \times 10^{-10}$ at 25°C. The activity and concentration are about the same at these low concentrations. Thus

$$[Ag^+][Cl^-] = 1.56 \times 10^{-10}$$
$$[Cl^-] = 0.9 \text{ mol/liter} \qquad (E5.8)$$
$$[Ag^+] = 1.73 \times 10^{-10} \text{ mol/liter}$$

Therefore 1.73×10^{-10} mol of AgCl must dissolve, or in terms of mass, this becomes

$$1.73 \times 10^{-10} \times 142.3 = 2.46 \times 10^{-8} \text{ g}$$

The second process for producing Ag-AgCl electrodes useful in medical instrumentation is a sintering process that forms pellet electrodes, as shown in Figure 5.5. The electrode consists of an Ag lead wire surrounded by a sintered Ag-AgCl cylinder. It is formed by placing the cleaned lead wire in a die that is then filled with a mixture of powdered Ag and AgCl. The die is compressed in an arbor press to form the powdered components into a pellet, which is then removed from the die and baked at 400°C for several hours. These electrodes tend to have a greater endurance than the electrolytically deposited AgCl electrodes, and are best applied when repeated usage is necessary. The electrolytically deposited AgCl has a tendency to flake off under mechanical stress, leaving portions of metallic Ag in contact with the electrolyte.

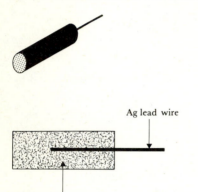

Ag lead wire

Sintered AgCl and Ag

Figure 5.5 A sintered Ag-AgCl electrode.

In addition to its nonpolarizable behavior, the Ag-AgCl electrode exhibits less electrical noise than the equivalent metallic Ag electrodes, as shown in Figure 5.6 [Geddes and Baker (1967)]. Pairs of 1.35-mm Ag spherical electrodes immersed in a normal saline solution were used to obtain the data in the figure. In Figure 5.6(a), all three sets of electrodes had an AgCl layer electrolytically grown on their surfaces using the technique shown in Figure 5.4. Following this recording, the electrodes were removed from the saline solution and the AgCl layer was scraped off all of them. They were then placed back in the solution and the recording in Figure 5.6(b) was obtained. An AgCl layer was again grown electrolytically on the electrodes and the recording of Figure 5.6(c) was made. It is clear from the data that the electrodes with the AgCl layer exhibited far less noise than was observed when the AgCl layer was removed. Also, a majority of the noise for the purely metallic electrodes was at low frequencies. This would provide the most serious interference for low-frequency recordings, such as the EEG.

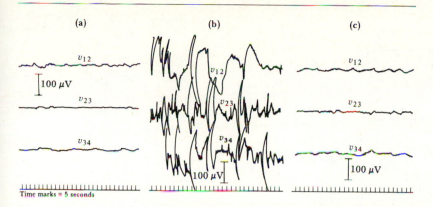

Figure 5.6 Spontaneous noise seen from pairs of electrodes immersed in a physiological saline solution: (a) from spherical metallic Ag electrodes coated with AgCl film, (b) from the two electrodes when AgCl film has been removed using emery paper, (c) from the electrodes when a new AgCl layer has been deposited. (From L.A. Geddes and L.E. Baker, "Chlorided Silver Electrodes," in *Medical Research Engineering*, 1967, 6(3), 33–34, © 1967 by Medical Research Engineering. Reprinted by permission.)

A second kind of electrode that has characteristics approaching those of the perfectly nonpolarizable electrode is the *calomel electrode*. It is used primarily as a reference electrode for electrochemical determinations and is frequently applied as the reference electrode when pH is measured (see Section 10.3). The calomel electrode is often constructed in the form shown in Figure 5.7. A glass tube with a porous glass plug at its base is filled with a paste of mercurous chloride or calomel (Hg_2Cl_2) mixed with a saturated potassium chloride (KCl) solution. As with AgCl, the Hg_2Cl_2 is only slightly soluble in water, so that most of it retains its solid form. A layer of elemental mercury is placed on top of the paste layer with an electrical lead wire within it. This entire assembly is then positioned in the center of a larger glass tube with a porous glass plug at its base. The tube is filled with a saturated KCl solution, so that the Hg_2Cl_2 layer of the inner tube is in contact with this electrolyte through the porous plug of the inner tube. We have a half-cell made up of Hg in intimate contact with an Hg_2Cl_2 layer, which is in contact with the saturated KCl electrolyte. The KCl solution makes contact with the solution in which the electrode is immersed through the porous plug at the bottom of the electrode assembly. This is actually a liquid-liquid junction that can result in a liquid-liquid junction potential, which will add to the electrode half-cell potential.

Using the same argument as that used for the Ag-AgCl electrode, we can show that the half-cell potential of this electrode is dependent on the Cl^- activity in the saturated KCl solution. This is stable at a given temperature, due to the fact that the solution is sat-

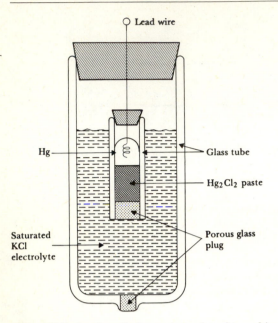

○ Lead wire

Hg

Glass tube

Hg$_2$Cl$_2$ paste

Saturated
KCl
electrolyte

Porous glass
plug

Figure 5.7 A calomel electrode such as is used in electrochemical determinations.

urated. In application, the tip of this electrode assembly containing the porous plug is dipped into the electrolytic solution which it is to contact. In pH measurements, a similar pH electrode is dipped into the solution, and the potential difference between the two electrodes is measured.

Example 5.3 To measure the potential across the rectal mucosa (inner surface of the rectum), a technique has been developed whereby an Ag-AgCl reference electrode is placed at some convenient point on the skin surface of the body away from the anal orifice. Another Ag-AgCl electrode is placed against the inner wall of the rectum about 8 cm up from the anus. The potential difference between these two electrodes is measured with a high-input impedance voltmeter, and the result recorded. The rectal electrode is then removed and immediately touched to the skin surrounding the anus, as close to it as possible. Another potential difference is measured, and again recorded. The difference between the two measurements is then determined. This is considered the true potential across the rectal mucosa.

At first glance, this appears to be a rather difficult way to make this simple measurement. We may wonder why we couldn't simply place one of the Ag-AgCl electrodes on the skin surrounding the anus and the other in the rectum and merely measure the potential difference between them. Explain why the bio-medical engineer who developed this procedure considered the latter case inadequate and chose the more complicated two-measurement technique.

Answer Although theoretically every Ag-AgCl electrode should have the same half-cell potential, there are usually differences from one to another. These differences should be quite small, of the order of millivolts. However, occasions can arise in which the difference can be as high as tens—or in extreme cases even hundreds—of millivolts. When we are measuring the potential difference between two Ag-AgCl electrodes, the difference between the half-cell potentials of each electrode enters into the measured value. When both half-cell potentials are equal, the difference cancels out. However, if the half-cell potentials are different, errors are introduced into the measurements. The engineer who designed this measurement knew that this was a possibility, and thus used a single electrode instead of two different Ag-AgCl electrodes, to measure the potential across the rectal mucosa. With this technique, the half-cell potential when the electrode is in the rectum and when it is on the perianal skin are identical, and thus cancel completely.

5.4 Electrode behavior and circuit models

The electrical characteristics of electrodes have been a subject of much study. Often the current-voltage characteristics of the electrode-electrolyte interface are found to be nonlinear, and, in turn, nonlinear elements are required for modeling electrode behavior. Specifically, the characteristics of an electrode are sensitive to the current passing through the electrode, and at relatively high current densities, the electrode characteristics can be considerably different from those at low current densities. The characteristics of electrodes are also waveform-dependent. When sinusoidal currents are used to measure the electrode's circuit behavior, the characteristics are also frequency dependent.

The characterization of electrode-electrolyte interfacial impedances has been well reviewed by Geddes (1972), Cobbold (1974), Ferris (1974), and Schwan (1963). It is only summarized here. For sinusoidal inputs, the terminal characteristics of an electrode have both a resistive and a reactive component. Over all but the lowest frequencies, this can be modeled as a series resistance and capacitance. We should not be surprised to see a capacitance entering into this model, since the half-cell potential described earlier was the result of the distribution of ionic charge at the electrode-electrolyte interface that had been considered as a dou-

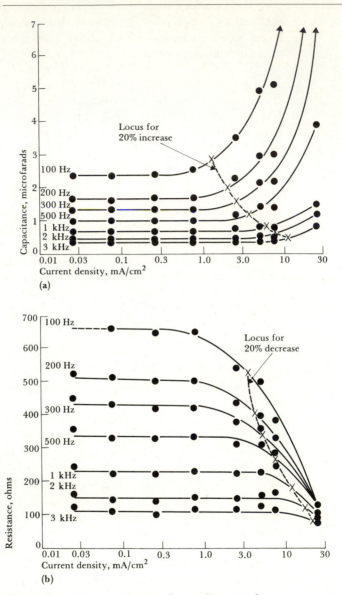

Figure 5.8 (a) Dependence of capacitance value on current density and frequency, given that the impedance of a stainless steel electrode in contact with physiologic saline is represented as a series *RC* circuit. (b) Relationship between series resistance, frequency, and current density for the electrode of part (a). (From L.A. Geddes, C.P. DaCosta, and G. Wise, "The Impedance of Stainless Steel Electrodes," *Medical and Biological Engineering,* 1971, **9,** pp. 511–521.)

ble layer of charge. This, of course, should behave as a capacitor—hence the capacitive reactance seen for real electrodes.

The simple series equivalent circuit, however, does not present the entire picture. The circuit elements are found to be frequency-dependent, and at higher electrode current densities, current-dependent as well. This dependence has been illustrated by Geddes (1972) in terms of the equivalent series capacitance and series resistance as a function of current density at the electrode, at frequencies ranging from 100 to 3000 Hz. Note from the curves reproduced in Figure 5.8 that increasing the frequency results in a decrease in both the series resistance and the series capacitance, whereas increasing the current density causes an increase in series capacitance and a decrease in series resistance, at current densities greater than approximately 1 mA/cm^2.

The series resistance-capacitance equivalent circuit breaks down at the lower frequencies, where this model would suggest an impedance going to infinity as the frequency approaches dc. To avoid this problem, we can convert this series RC circuit to a parallel RC circuit that has a purely resistive impedance at very low frequencies. If we combine this circuit with a voltage source representing the half-cell potential and a series resistance representing the resistance of the electrolyte, we can arrive at the biopotential electrode equivalent circuit model of Figure 5.9.

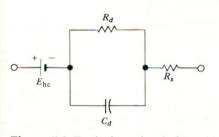

Figure 5.9 Equivalent circuit for a biopotential electrode in contact with an electrolyte. E_{hc} is the half-cell potential, R_d and C_d make up the impedance associated with electrode–electrolyte interface and polarization effects, and R_s is the total series resistance in the circuit due to resistance in electrolyte and electrode lead wire.

In this circuit, R_d and C_d represent the resistive and reactive components just discussed. These components are still frequency- and current-density-dependent. However, since this is a parallel RC circuit, the dependence is no longer as illustrated in Figure 5.8. In this configuration it is also possible to assign physical meaning to the components. C_d represents the capacitance across the double layer of charge at the electrode-electrolyte interface. The parallel resistance R_d represents the leakage resistance across this double layer. All the components of this equivalent circuit have values determined by the electrode material, and—to a lesser extent—the material of the electrolyte and its concentration.

The equivalent circuit of Figure 5.9 demonstrates that the electrode impedance is frequency-dependent. At high frequencies, where $1/\omega C \ll R_d$, the impedance is constant at R_s. At low frequencies, where $1/\omega C \gg R_d$, the impedance is again constant, but its value is larger, being $R_s + R_d$. At frequencies between these extremes, the electrode impedance is frequency-dependent.

The impedance of Ag-AgCl electrodes varies significantly from that of a pure silver electrode at frequencies under 100 Hz. This has been demonstrated by Geddes *et al.* (1969), whose data are reproduced in Figure 5.10.

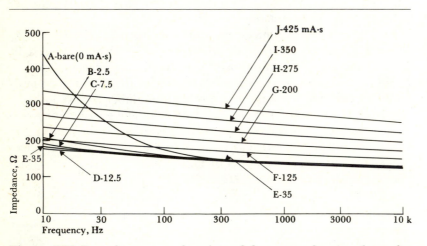

Figure 5.10 Impedance as a function of frequency for Ag electrodes coated with an electrolytically deposited AgCl layer. Electrode area is 0.25 cm². Numbers attached to curves indicate number of mA·s for each deposit. (From L.A. Geddes, L.E. Baker, and A.G. Moore, "Optimum Electrolytic Chloriding of Silver Electrodes," *Medical and Biological Engineering*, 1969, **7**, pp. 49–56.)

A metallic silver electrode having a surface area of 0.25 cm² had the impedance characteristic shown by curve *A*. At a frequency of 10 Hz, the magnitude of its impedance was almost three times the value at 300 Hz. This indicates a strong capacitive component to the equivalent circuit. Electrolytically depositing 2.5 mA·s of AgCl greatly reduced the low-frequency impedance, as depicted by curve *B*. Depositing thicker AgCl layers had minimal effects, until the charge deposited exceeded approximately 100 mA·s. The curves were then seen to shift to higher impedances in a parallel fashion as the amount of AgCl deposited increased. Geddes (1972) points out that depositing an AgCl layer using a charge of between 100 and 500 mA·s/cm² provides the lowest value of electrode impedance. If the current density is maintained at greater than 5 mA/cm², we can adjust current and time to provide the most convenient values for depositing the desired layer.

Example 5.4 We want to develop an electrical model for a specific biopotential electrode studied in the laboratory. The electrode is characterized by placing it in a physiologic saline bath in the laboratory along with an Ag-AgCl electrode having a much greater surface area and a known half-cell potential of 0.223 V. The dc voltage between the two electrodes is measured with a very-high-impedance voltmeter and found to be 0.572 V with the test electrode negative. The magnitude of the impedance between the two electrodes is measured as a function of frequency at very low currents, and found to be that given in Figure E5.1. From these data, determine a circuit model for the electrode.

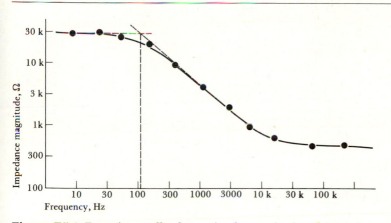

Figure E5.1 Experimentally determined magnitude of impedance as a function of frequency for electrode system of Example 5.4.

Answer The very large surface area of the Ag-AgCl reference electrode makes its impedance very small in comparison with the test electrode, so we can neglect it. We cannot, however, neglect its half-cell potential, which is unaffected by surface area. The half-cell potential of the test electrode is found by

$$0.572 \text{ V} = 0.223 \text{ V} - E_x^0$$
$$E_x^0 = -0.349 \text{ V} \tag{E5.9}$$

At frequencies above about 20 kHz, the electrode impedance is constant. From Figure 5.9 we see that the equivalent-circuit model for the electrode behaves in this way, since at high frequencies

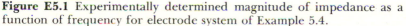

$$\frac{1}{\omega C_d} << R_s \quad \text{and} \quad \frac{1}{\omega C_d} << R_d \tag{E5.10}$$

making the net impedance equal R_s. Thus, from Figure E5.1, $R_s = 500 \ \Omega$.

At frequencies less than 50 Hz, the impedance is again seen to be a constant $R_s + R_d$, since at these frequencies

$$\frac{1}{\omega C_d} \gg R_d \qquad (E5.11)$$

to give the constant $|Z|$-versus-f characteristic. Therefore

$$R_d = 30 \text{ k}\Omega - 500 \ \Omega = 29.5 \text{ k}\Omega$$

We can get an approximate idea of the size of C_d by considering that $R_s \ll R_d$. The slope of the $|Z|$-versus-f characteristic should be approximately the same as that for the $R_d C_d$ parallel combination alone. The corner frequency, as determined from Figure E5.1, is 100 Hz. Thus

$$R_d C_d = \frac{1}{2\pi f}$$

$$C_d = \frac{1}{2\pi \times 10^2 \times 3 \times 10^4} = 5.3 \times 10^{-8} \text{ F} \qquad (E5.12)$$

This determines all the elements of the circuit of Figure 5.9, which can then be used to model the electrode.

5.5 The electrode-skin interface and motion artifact

In Section 5.1 we examined the electrode-electrolyte interface and saw how it influenced the electrical properties that are seen in practical electrodes. When biopotentials are recorded from the surface of the skin, we must consider an additional interface—the interface between the electrode-electrolyte and the skin—in order to understand the behavior of the electrodes. In coupling an electrode to the skin, we usually use an electrolyte paste containing Cl^- as the principal anion to maintain good contact. The interface between this paste and the electrode is an electrode-electrolyte interface, as described above. However, the interface between the electrolyte and the skin is different, and will require some explanation. Before we give this explanation, let us briefly review the structure of the skin.

Figure 5.11 shows a cross-sectional diagram of the skin. The skin consists of three principal layers that surround the body to protect it from its environment, and also serve as appropriate interfaces. The outermost layer, or *epidermis*, plays the most important role in the electrode-skin interface. This layer, which consists of three sublayers, is constantly renewing itself. Cells divide and grow in the deepest layer, the *stratum germinativum*, and are displaced outward as they grow by the newly forming cells underneath them. As they pass through the *stratum granulosum*, they begin to die and lose their nuclear material. As they continue their outward

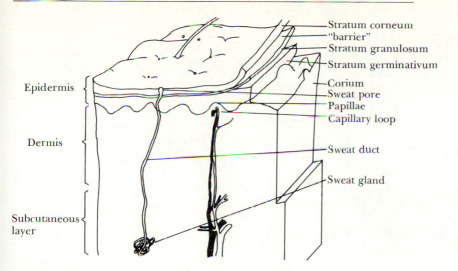

Epidermis

Dermis

Subcutaneous layer

Stratum corneum
"barrier"
Stratum granulosum
Stratum germinativum
Corium
Sweat pore
Papillae
Capillary loop
Sweat duct
Sweat gland

Figure 5.11 Magnified section of skin, showing the various layers. (Copyright © 1977 by The Institute of Electrical and Electronics Engineers. Reprinted, with permission, from *IEEE Trans. Biomed. Eng.*, March 1977, vol. BME-24, no. 2, pp. 134–139.)

journey, they degenerate further into layers of flat keratinous material which forms the *stratum corneum*, or horny layer of dead material on the skin's surface. These layers are constantly being worn off and replaced at the stratum granulosum by new cells. The epidermis is thus a constantly changing layer of the skin, the outer surface of which consists of dead material that has different electrical characteristics from live tissue.

The deeper layers of the skin contain the vascular and nervous components of the skin, as well as the sweat glands, sweat ducts, and hair follicles. These layers are similar to other tissues within the body and, with the exception of the sweat glands, do not ascribe any unique electrical characteristics to the skin.

When we consider the electrical connection between an electrode and the skin through the agency of electrolyte paste, our equivalent circuit of Figure 5.9 must be expanded, as shown in Figure 5.12. The electrode-electrolyte interface equivalent circuit is shown adjacent to the electrode-paste interface. The series resistance R_s is now the effective resistance of the paste between the electrode and the skin. We can consider the epidermis, or at least the stratum corneum, as a membrane that is semipermeable to ions, so that, if there is a difference in ionic concentration across this membrane, there is a potential difference, E_{se}, which is given by the Nernst equation. The epidermal layer is also found to have an electrical impedance that behaves as a parallel RC circuit, as shown. The dermis and the subcutaneous layer under it behave in general as pure resistances. They generate negligible dc potentials.

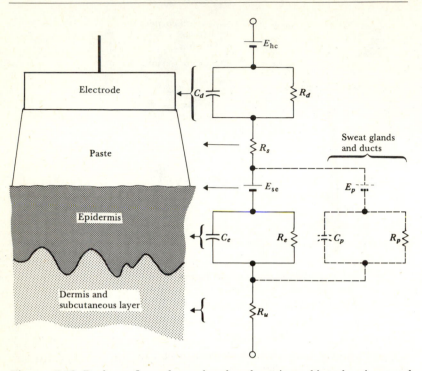

Figure 5.12 Body-surface electrode placed against skin, showing total electrical equivalent circuit obtained in this situation. Each circuit element on the right is at approximately the same level at which the physical process that it represents would be in the left-hand diagram.

Thus we see that—if the effect of the stratum corneum can be reduced—a more stable electrode will result. We can minimize the effect of the stratum corneum by removing it, or at least a part of it, from under the electrode. There are many ways to do this, ranging from vigorous rubbing with a pad soaked in acetone or abrasion with sandpaper to puncturing the stratum corneum with dental burrs or a lancet. In all cases, this process tends to short out E_{se}, C_e and R_e, as shown in Figure 5.12, thereby improving the stability of the signal.

A factor that is sometimes important when considering, for example, psychogenic electrodermal responses or the galvanic skin reflex (GSR), is the contribution from the sweat glands and sweat ducts. The fluid secreted by sweat glands contains Na^+, K^+, and Cl^- ions, whose concentrations differ from those in the extracellular fluid. Thus there is a potential difference between the lumen of the sweat duct and the dermis and subcutaneous layers. There also is a parallel $R_p C_p$ combination in series with this potential representing the wall of the sweat gland and duct, as shown by the broken lines in Figure 5.12. These components are often neglected in consider-

ing biopotential electrodes that are not used to measure electrodermal response or GSR.

When a polarizable electrode is in contact with an electrolyte,
a double layer of charge forms at the interface. If the electrode is
moved with respect to the electrolyte, this mechanically disturbs the
distribution of charge at the interface and results in a momentary
change of the half-cell potential until equilibrium can be reestab-
lished. If a pair of electrodes are in an electrolyte and one moves
while the other remains stationary, a potential difference appears
between the two electrodes during this movement. This potential is
known as *motion artifact* and can be a serious cause of interference
in the measurement of biopotentials.

Since motion artifact is primarily the result of mechanical disturbances of the distribution of charge at the electrode-electrolyte
interface, it is reasonable to expect that motion artifact is minimal
for nonpolarizable electrodes. This is demonstrated for the Ag-
AgCl electrode in Figure 5.13. A pair of Ag wire electrodes is immersed in physiological saline and the bath is agitated during the
intervals denoted by the heavy lines. An electrolytic film of AgCl is
then deposited on the two wires by connecting them and making
them the anode of a cell, as shown in Figure 5.4. The electrodes are
then placed in a similar saline solution; their response to mechanical agitation of the solution is as shown in Figure 5.13(b). We can
clearly see the reduction in motion artifact resulting from chloriding the electrodes.

From an observation of the motion-artifact signals in Figure
5.13, we see that a major component of this noise is at low frequencies. Section 6.6 and Figure 6.20 will show that different biopotential signals occupy different portions of the frequency spectrum. Figure 6.20 shows that low-frequency artifact does not affect
signals such as the EMG or axon action potential (AAP) nearly as
much as it does the ECG, EEG, and EOG. In the former case, filtering can be effectively used to minimize the contribution of motion artifact on the overall signal. But in the latter case, such filtering also distorts the signal. Consequently, it is important in these
applications to use a nonpolarizable electrode to minimize motion
artifact stemming from the electrode-electrolyte interface.

This interface, however, is not the only source of motion artifact encountered from biopotential electrodes when they are applied to the skin. The equivalent circuit in Figure 5.12 shows that,
in addition to the half-cell potential E_{hc}, there is the electrolyte
paste-skin potential E_{se} that can also cause motion artifact if it
varies with movement of the electrode. Tam and Webster (1977)
have demonstrated that variations of this potential indeed do represent a major source of motion artifact in Ag-AgCl skin electrodes. They have shown that this artifact can be significantly
reduced when the stratum corneum is removed by mechanical
abrasion with a fine abrasive paper. This method also helps to

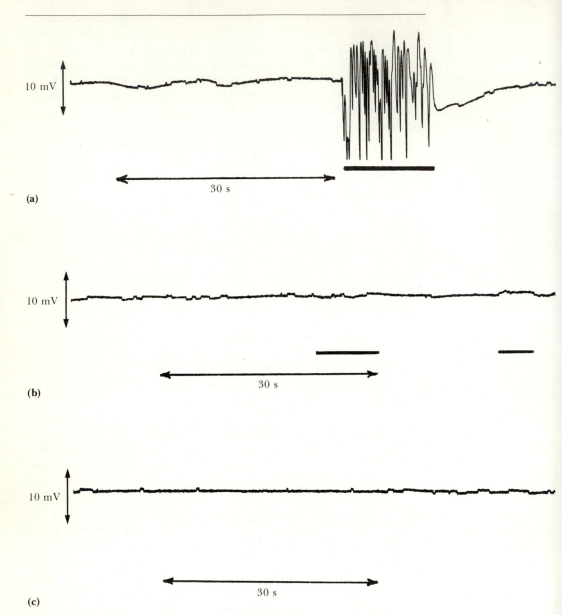

Figure 5.13 Motion artifact in Ag-AgCl electrodes. (a) Metallic Ag electrodes in agitated physiological saline solution. (b) Same electrodes with an AgCl surface film in agitated physiological saline solution. (c) Output from amplifier used for recordings when electrodes are replaced by a 1.5-kΩ resistor. Heavy lines under curves indicate periods of agitation of saline solution.

reduce the epidermal component of the skin impedance. Tam and Webster (1977) also point out, however, that the removal of the body's outer protective barrier makes that region of skin more susceptible to irritation from the electrolyte paste. Therefore the choice of a paste material is important. Remembering the dynamic nature of the epidermis, note that it is also important to realize that the stratum corneum can regenerate itself in as short a time as 24 hours, thereby renewing the source of motion artifact. This is a factor to be held in mind if the electrodes are to be used for chronic recording. Webster (1977) reviews the causes and cures for many types of motion artifact and interference in biopotential recording.

5.6 Body-surface recording electrodes

Over the years many different types of electrodes for recording various potentials on the body surface have been developed. This section describes the various types of these electrodes and gives an example of each. The reader who is interested in more extensive examples should consult Geddes (1972).

Metal-plate electrodes

One of the most frequently used forms of biopotential sensing electrodes is the metal-plate electrode. In its basic form it consists of a metallic conductor in contact with the skin. It uses an electrolyte paste to establish and maintain the contact.

Figure 5.14 shows several forms of this electrode. The one most commonly used for limb electrodes with the electrocardiograph is shown in Figure 5.14(a). It consists of a flat metal plate that has been bent into a cylindrical segment. A terminal is placed on its outside surface near one end; this terminal is used to attach the lead wire to the electrocardiograph. A post, placed on this same side near the center, is used to connect a rubber strap to the electrode to hold it in place on an arm or leg. The electrode is traditionally made of German silver (a nickel-silver alloy). Before it is attached to the body, its concave surface is covered with electrolyte paste. Similarly arranged flat metal disks are also used for this type of electrode.

A second common variety of metal-plate electrode is the metal disk illustrated in Figure 5.14(b). This electrode, which has a lead wire soldered or welded to the back surface, can be made of several different materials. Sometimes the connection between lead wire and electrode is protected by a layer of insulating material, such as epoxy or polyvinyl chloride. This device can be used as a chest electrode for recording the ECG. It is also frequently used in

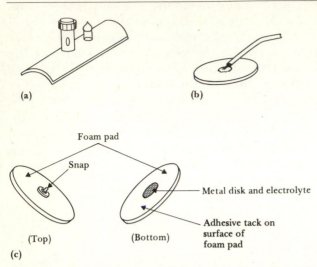

(a)

(b)

Foam pad

Snap

(Top)   (Bottom)

Metal disk and electrolyte

Adhesive tack on
surface of
foam pad

(c)

Figure 5.14 Body-surface biopotential electrodes. (a) Metal-plate electrode used for application to limbs. (b) Metal-disk electrode applied with surgical tape. (c) Disposable foam-pad electrodes, often used with electrocardiographic monitoring apparatus.

cardiac monitoring for long-term recordings. In these applications the electrode is frequently fabricated from a disk of Ag which may or may not have an electrolytically deposited layer of AgCl on its contacting surface. It is coated with electrolyte paste and then pressed against the patient's chest wall. It is maintained in place by a strip of surgical tape or a plastic foam disk with a layer of tack on one surface.

This style of electrode is also popular for surface recordings of EMG or EEG. In recording EMGs, investigators use stainless steel, platinum, or gold-plated disks to minimize the chance that the electrode will enter into chemical reactions with perspiration or the paste. And even though these materials produce polarizable electrodes, the motion artifact generated is usually not a problem because it can be removed by filtering. Electrodes used in monitoring EMGs or EEGs are generally smaller in diameter than those used in recording ECGs. Disk-shaped electrodes such as these have also been fabricated from metal foils, primarily silver foil, and are applied as single-use disposable electrodes. The thinness of the foil allows it to conform to the shape of the body surface. Also, because it is so thin, when it is discarded the user is not wasting appreciable amounts of silver.

In the operation of a modern hospital, economics plays an important part in determining materials and apparatus to be used in hospital administration and patient care. In choosing suitable cardiac electrodes for patient-monitoring applications, physicians are more and more turning to pregelled, disposable electrodes with the adhesive already in place, since these devices are ready to be applied to the patient and need not be cleaned for reuse. This minimizes the amount of time that personnel must devote to the use of these electrodes.

A popular type of electrode of this variety is illustrated in Figure 5.14(c). It consists of a relatively large disk of plastic foam material with a silver-plated disk on one side attached to a silver-plated snap similar to that used on clothing in the center of the other side. The silver-plated disk serves as the electrode and may be coated with an electrolytically deposited AgCl layer. A layer of electrolyte paste covers the disk. The electrode side of the foam material is covered with an adhesive material that is compatible with the skin. A protective cover or strip of release paper is placed over this side of the electrode and foam and is packaged in a foil envelope so that the water component of the paste will not evaporate. To apply the electrode to the patient, the technician has only to clean the area of skin on which the electrode is to be placed, open the electrode packet, remove the release paper from the tack, and press the electrode against the patient. A lead wire with the female portion of the snap is then snapped onto the electrode and connected to the monitoring apparatus. This procedure is quickly accomplished and requires no special technique to be learned, such as using the correct amount of paste or cutting strips of adhesive tape to hold the electrode in place.

Suction electrodes

A modification of the metal-plate electrode that requires no straps or adhesives for holding it in place is the suction electrode illustrated in Figure 5.15. This electrode is frequently used in electrocardiography as the *precordial* (chest) lead, since it can be placed at a particular location, used to take a recording, and then quickly moved to the next location. It consists of a hollow metallic cylindrical electrode that makes contact with the skin at its base. An appropriate terminal for the lead wire is attached to the metal cylinder and a rubber suction bulb fits over its other base. Electrolyte paste is placed over the contacting surface of the electrode, the bulb is squeezed, and the electrode is then placed on the chest wall. The bulb is released and applies suction against the skin, holding the electrode assembly in place. This electrode can be used only for short periods of time, since the suction and the pressure of the contact surface against the skin can cause serious irritation. Although the electrode itself is quite large, Figure 5.15 shows that the actual contacting area is relatively small. This electrode thus tends to have a higher source impedance than the relatively large-surface-area metal-plate electrodes used for ECG limb electrodes, as shown in Figure 5.14(a). Consequently, suction electrodes can produce more

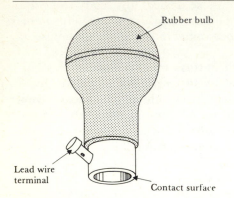

Rubber bulb

Lead wire
terminal

Contact surface

Figure 5.15 Metallic suction electrode, often used as a precordial electrode on clinical electrocardiographs.

distortion of the electrocardiogram when used with relatively low-input impedance amplifiers.

Floating electrodes

The previous section explained that one source of motion artifact in biopotential electrodes is a result of the double layer of charge at the electrode-electrolyte interface. The use of nonpolarizable electrodes, such as the Ag-AgCl electrode, can greatly diminish this artifact. But it still can be present, and efforts to stabilize the interface mechanically can further reduce it. *Floating electrodes* offer a suitable technique to do so.

Figure 5.16 shows examples of these devices. Figure 5.16(a) depicts a floating electrode, known as a top-hat electrode; its internal structure is illustrated in cross section in Figure 5.16(b). The principal feature of the electrode is that the actual electrode element or metal disk is recessed in a cavity so that it does not come in contact with the skin itself. Instead, the element is surrounded by electrolyte paste in the cavity. The cavity does not move with respect to the metal disk, and therefore does not produce any mechanical movement of the double layer of charge. In practice the electrode is filled with electrolyte paste and then attached to the skin surface by means of a double-sided adhesive-tape ring, as shown in Figure 5.16. The electrode element can be a disk made of a metal such as silver, and often it is coated with AgCl. Another frequently encountered form of the floating electrode uses—instead of a metal disk—a sintered Ag-AgCl pellet. These electrodes are found to be quite stable and suitable for multiple uses.

A single-use, disposable modification of the floating electrode is shown in cross section in Figure 5.16(c). Its structure is basically

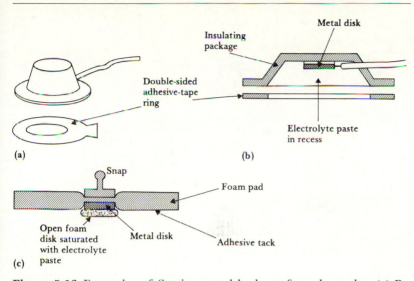

Figure 5.16 Examples of floating metal body-surface electrodes. (a) Recessed electrode with top-hat structure. (b) Cross-sectional view of electrode in (a). (c) Cross-sectional view of disposable recessed electrode of same general structure as in Fig. 5.14(c). Recess in this electrode is formed from an open foam disk, saturated with electrolyte paste, placed over metal electrode.

the same as that of the disposable metal-plate electrode of Figure 5.14(c), but it has one added component—a disk of thin open-cell foam saturated with electrolyte paste. The foam is firmly affixed to the metal-disk electrode, thereby providing an intermediate electrolyte-paste layer between the electrode and the skin. Because the foam is fixed to the metal disk, the paste contained within it at the disk interface is mechanically stable. The other surface of the foam that is placed against the skin is able to move with the skin, thereby diminishing motion artifact that sometimes results from differential movement between the skin and the electrolyte paste.

Flexible electrodes

The electrodes described so far are solid and either are flat or have a fixed curvature. The body surface, on the other hand, is irregularly shaped and can change its local curvature with movement. Solid electrodes cannot conform to this change in body-surface topography, which can result in additional motion artifact. To avoid such problems, *flexible electrodes* have been developed, examples of which are shown in Figure 5.17.

One of the more common forms of flexible electrodes has a mesh woven from fine silver wire attached to a lead wire and substi-

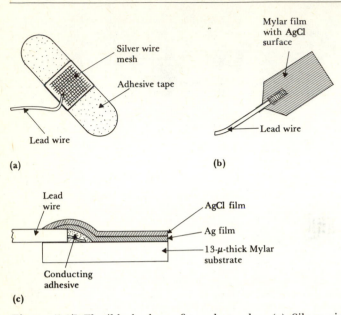

Mylar film
with **AgCl**
surface

Silver wire
mesh

Adhesive tape

Lead wire

(a)

Lead wire

(b)

Lead
wire

AgCl film

Ag film

13-μ-thick Mylar
substrate

Conducting
adhesive

(c)

Figure 5.17 Flexible body-surface electrodes. (a) Silver-wire-mesh electrode on an adhesive-tape bandage. (b) Flexible thin-film neonatal electrode (after Neuman, 1973). (c) Cross-sectional view of thin-film electrode in (b). [Parts (b) and (c) are from International Federation for Medical and Biological Engineering, *Digest of the 10th ICMBE*, 1973.]

tuted for the gauze-sponge portion of a small plastic bandage, as illustrated in Figure 5.17(a). Electrolyte paste is applied to the wire mesh and the electrode is applied as a small bandage.

Another technique employed to provide flexible electrodes is that of a carbon-filled silicone rubber compound in the form of a thin strip or disk being used as the active element of an electrode. A lead wire is attached and the electrode is used in the same way as a similar type of metal-plate electrode.

Flexible electrodes are especially important when premature infants are the patients to be monitored. Electrodes for detecting the ECG and respiration by the impedance technique are attached to the chest of premature infants, who usually weigh less than 2500 g. Conventional electrodes are not appropriate, since they cannot conform to the shape of the infant's chest and can cause severe skin ulceration at pressure points. They must also be removed when chest x rays are taken of the infant, since they are opaque and can obstruct the view of significant portions of the thoracic cavity. Neuman (1973) developed flexible, thin-film electrodes for use on newborn infants that minimize these problems. The basic electrode consists of a 13-μm-thick Mylar film on which an Ag and AgCl film have been deposited, as shown in Figure 5.17(b). The actual structure of the electrode is illustrated in cross section in Figure 5.17(c).

The flexible lead wire is attached to the flexible Mylar substrate using a conducting adhesive, and a silver film approximately 1 μm thick is deposited over this and the Mylar. An AgCl layer is then grown on the surface of the silver film, using the electrolytic process.

In addition to the advantage of being flexible and conforming to the shape of the newborn's chest, these electrodes have a layer of silver thin enough to be essentially x-ray-transparent, so that they need not be removed when chest x rays of the infant are taken. All that shows up on the x rays is the lead wire. Consequently, the infant's skin is also protected from the irritation caused by removing and reapplying the adhesive tape that holds the electrode in place. This has been demonstrated to reduce the occurrence of skin irritation significantly in nurseries in which this electrode has been used.

Dry electrodes

All the surface electrodes described so far require an electrolyte paste to establish and maintain contact between the electrode and the skin. Recent advances in solid-state electronic technology have made it possible to record surface biopotentials from electrodes that can be applied directly to the skin without an intermediate layer of electrolyte paste. The significant feature of these electrodes is a self-contained, very-high-input impedance amplifier. A metal electrode placed against the skin establishes some contact with the skin; and even though there is not a metal-electrolyte interface, an equivalent circuit similar to that of Figure 5.9 still exists. In this case the impedance is primarily resistive, but there is a capacitive component resulting from the metal plate contacting the stratum corneum. The stratum corneum has a relatively high electrical resistance, but the deeper layers of skin have a higher conductivity. Thus we have a capacitor with the electrode and dermis serving as plates and the stratum corneum serving as dielectric.

The spacing between the plates of this capacitor is much greater than it is for the double layer of charge of the electrode-electrolyte interface, so the capacitance is considerably lower than the capacitance (C_d) for wet electrodes. A resistance, which is much higher than for the electrode-electrolyte case, is in parallel with the capacitor due to the resistance of the stratum corneum. The series resistance R_s still represents the resistance through the body and is approximately the same value. In addition, if there is any moisture (such as perspiration) on the skin surface, it can establish a half-cell potential, although this is usually neglected. Thus the overall effect of this equivalent circuit is primarily a resistive one, with the resistance being several orders of magnitude higher than observed for wet electrodes. By putting an impedance-converting amplifier on the electrode, we can detect the biopotential, even though it has a very high source impedance, with minimal or no distortion. The input impedance of the amplifier on the electrode must be of the order of 1 GΩ for good results.

An example of a dry-electrode system developed by Ko and Hynecek (1974) is shown in Figure 5.18. The electrode itself consists of a 7-mm-diameter stainless steel disk. An integrated-circuit microelectronic impedance-converting amplifier is mounted on the back surface of the disk and its input is connected to the disk. Two lead wires connect this amplifier to a remotely located power supply, consisting of a constant-current source. The biopotential signal detected by the electrode appears on the power-supply line as a variation in voltage. The back surface of the stainless steel electrode containing the amplifier is encapsulated in epoxy to make the structure approximately 3 mm thick. A twisted pair of fine lead wires provides the connection to the power supply, where the signal is separated and amplified by a conventional biopotential amplifier.

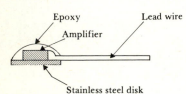

(a)

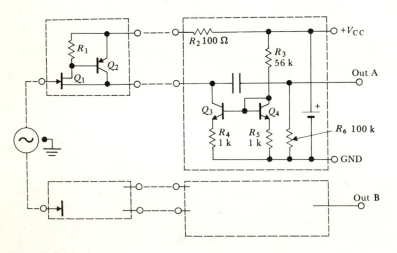

(b)

Figure 5.18 (a) Dry, active electrode and (b) its amplifier circuit. (From W.H. Ko and J. Hynecek, "Dry Electrodes and Electrode Amplifiers," in *Biomedical Electrode Technology,* by H.A. Miller and D.C. Harrison, editors. New York: Academic Press, 1974.)

Dry electrodes can also be made in the form of insulated electrodes where there is no metal-electrolyte interface at all. Richardson (1967) describes electrodes that are basically capacitors consisting of a metal electrode on which a surface oxide film of the metal has been grown. This is placed against the patient's skin so that the skin forms one plate of a parallel-plate capacitor and the metal the other, the oxide film being the dielectric. Such electrodes have a capacitance of from 1 to 5 nF between the metal and the body. They can be used to couple the biopotential signal capacitively to an amplifier. If the input impedance of the amplifier is sufficiently high, high-pass filter effects due to the RC circuit formed by the electrode and the amplifier input impedance are minimized. These electrodes require an amplifier having an input impedance of the order of 0.1 to 1 GΩ. As in the case of dry metal electrodes, we should locate these amplifiers as close to the electrode as possible to reduce noise from electrostatically detected signals.

In Richardson's electrode (1967), a disk of aluminum or tantalum had an appropriate oxide layer grown anodically on one surface. A source-follower impedance-converting amplifier circuit was mounted on the back of this electrode and the entire device appropriately packaged. Yon (1970) developed similar electrodes using semiconductor-grade, single crystal silicon (Si) with a high-purity SiO_2 layer grown thermally on its surface. The technology for growing highly uniform stable SiO_2 films is well known in the semiconductor industry. Yon applied the technique to his electrodes so that smaller-sized electrodes could be built by making thinner insulating films, thereby enabling the capacitance to remain of the order of 1 nF. A hybrid microelectronic source-follower amplifier in a small integrated circuit flat-pack package was then placed on the back of the electrode to complete the system.

Although dry electrodes offer the advantage of not requiring electrolyte paste, they embody certain disadvantages as well. For the metal-type dry electrodes, care must be taken so that any half-cell potentials that might exist do not saturate the amplifier. The capacitor dry electrodes, on the other hand, present a problem in that the electrode-skin capacitance can be less than the predicted value if the electrode is not in good contact with the skin, or if a layer of oil develops between the electrode and the skin surface. This can have two effects: The low-frequency response of the electrode can be compromised due to the diminished capacitance, or, if there is any charge on the capacitance (which is usually the case), the changing capacitance results in a changing voltage, and hence artifact.

Another serious source of artifact in dry electrodes is a result of the very-high-input impedance amplifier. Pickup of voltages from electric fields in the vicinity of the electrode and the amplifier input can produce unwanted interference. It is for this reason that it is so important for the amplifier to be located directly at the electrode, since a lead wire connecting the amplifier to the electrode is all the more susceptible to this kind of pickup. Static electricity generated in dry environments, especially when the subjects are in the vicinity of fabrics made from synthetic fibers, can produce serious artifacts with this type of electrode.

5.7 Internal electrodes

Electrodes may also be used within the body to detect biopotentials. They can take the form of either *transcutaneous electrodes,* in which the electrode itself or the lead wire crosses the skin, or they may be entirely *internal electrodes,* in which the connection is to an implanted electronic circuit such as a radio-telemetry transmitter. These electrodes differ from body-surface electrodes in that they do not have to contend with the electrolyte-skin interface and its associated limitations, as described in Section 5.5. Instead, the electrode behaves in the way dictated entirely by the electrode-electrolyte interface. No electrolyte paste is required to maintain this interface, since extracellular fluid is present.

There are many different designs for internal electrodes. An investigator studying a particular bioelectric phenomenon using internal electrodes frequently designs his or her own electrodes for the purpose. The following paragraphs describe some of the more common forms of these electrodes and give examples of their application.

Figure 5.19 shows different types of transcutaneous needle and wire electrodes. The basic needle electrode consists of a solid needle, usually made of stainless steel, with a sharp point. The shank of the needle is insulated with a coating such as an insulating varnish, with only the tip left exposed. A lead wire is attached to the other end of the needle and the joint is encapsulated in a plastic hub to protect it. This electrode, frequently used in electromyography, is shown in Figure 5.19(a). When it is placed in a particular muscle, it obtains an EMG from that muscle acutely and can then be removed.

A variation of this type of electrode is frequently used on patients undergoing surgery, to monitor the ECG continuously. The electrode consists of stainless steel hypodermic needles placed subcutaneously on each limb. Lead wires with special connectors that attach to the needle at the hub connect the electrodes to the cardioscope (Section 6.9). These electrodes remain in place as the patient is manipulated during the surgical procedure. They are away from the surgical field. Electrolyte paste is not necessary.

A shielded transcutaneous electrode can be fabricated in the form shown in Figure 5.19(b). It consists of a small-gage hypodermic needle that has been modified by running an insulated fine wire down the center of its lumen and filling the remainder of the

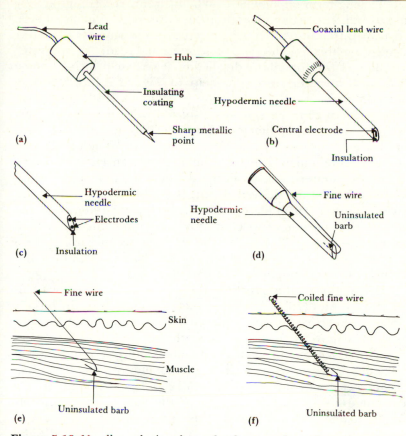

Figure 5.19 Needle and wire electrodes for transdermal measurement of biopotentials. (a) Insulated needle electrode, (b) coaxial needle electrode, (c) bipolar coaxial electrode. (d) Fine-wire electrode connected to hypodermic needle, before being inserted. (e) Cross-sectional view of skin and muscle, showing fine-wire electrode in place. (f) Cross-sectional view of skin and muscle, showing coiled fine-wire electrode in place.

lumen with an insulating material such as an epoxy resin. When the resin has set, the tip of the needle is filed to its original bevel, exposing an oblique cross section of the central wire, which serves as the active electrode. The needle itself is connected to ground through the shield of a coaxial cable, thereby extending the coaxial structure to its very tip.

Multiple electrodes in a single needle can be formed as shown in Figure 5.19(c). Here two wires are placed within the lumen of the needle and can be connected differentially so as to be sensitive to electrical activity only in the immediate vicinity of the electrode tip.

The needle electrodes just described are principally for acute measurements, since their stiffness and size make them uncomfortable for long-term implantation. When chronic recordings are required, transcutaneous wire electrodes are more suitable. There are many different types of wire electrodes and schemes for introducing them through the skin. (The interested reader should refer to Geddes (1972) for a more detailed review.) The principle can be illustrated, however, with the help of Figure 5.19(d). A fine wire—often made of Karma alloy or stainless steel ranging in diameter from 25 to 125 μm—is insulated with an insulating varnish to within a few millimeters of the tip. This noninsulated tip is bent back on itself to form a J-shaped structure. The tip is introduced into the lumen of the needle, as shown in Figure 5.19(d). The needle is inserted through the skin into the muscle at the desired location, to the desired depth. It is then slowly withdrawn, leaving the electrode in place, as shown in Figure 5.19(e). Note that the bent-over portion of wire serves as a barb holding the wire in place in the muscle. To remove the wire, the technician applies a mild uniform force to straighten out the barb and pulls it out through the wire's tract.

A variation on this basic structure has been described by Caldwell and Reswick (1975). Realizing that wire electrodes chronically implanted in active muscles undergo a great amount of flexing as the muscle moves (which can cause the wire to slip as it passes through the skin and increase the irritation and risk of infection at this point, or even cause the wire to break), they developed the helical spiral electrode shown in Figure 5.19(f). It, too, is made from a very fine insulated wire coiled into a tight helix of approximately 150 μm diameter that is placed in the lumen of the inserting needle. The uninsulated barb protrudes from the tip of the needle and is bent back along the needle before insertion. It holds the wire in place when the needle is removed from the muscle. Of course, the external end of the electrode now passes through the needle and the needle must be removed—or at least protected—before the electrode is connected to the recording apparatus.

Another group of transcutaneous electrodes are those used for monitoring fetal heartbeat. In this case it is desirable to get the electrocardiogram from the fetus during labor by direct connection to the presenting part (usually the head) through the uterine cervix (the mouth of the uterus). Since the fetus lies in a bath of amniotic fluid that contains ions and is conductive, surface electrodes generally do not provide an adequate ECG due to the shorting effect of the amniotic fluid. Thus electrodes used to obtain the fetal ECG must penetrate the skin of the fetus.

An example of a suction electrode that does this is shown in Figure 5.20(a). A sharp-pointed probe in the center of a suction cup can be applied to the fetal presenting part, as shown in Figure 5.20(b). When suction is applied to the cup after it has been placed against the fetal skin, the surface of the skin is drawn into the cup and the central electrode pierces the stratum corneum, contacting

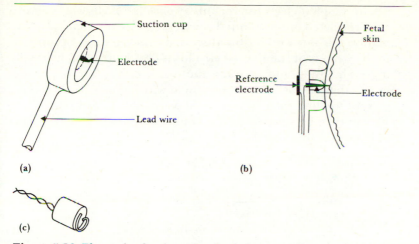

Suction cup

Electrode

Lead wire

(a)

Fetal skin

Reference electrode

Electrode

(b)

(c)

Figure 5.20 Electrodes for detecting fetal electrocardiogram during labor, by means of intracutaneous needles. (a) Suction electrode. (b) Cross-sectional view of suction electrode in place, showing penetration of probe through epidermis. (c) Helical electrode, which is attached to fetal skin by corkscrew-type action.

the deeper layers of the epidermis. On the back of the suction electrode is a reference electrode that contacts the fluid, and the signal seen between these two electrodes is the voltage drop across the resistance of the stratum corneum. Thus, although the amniotic fluid essentially places all the body of the fetus at a common potential, the potentials beneath the stratum corneum can be different, and fetal ECGs having peak amplitudes of the order of 50–700 μV can be reliably recorded.

Another intradermal electrode that is widely applied for detecting fetal ECG during labor is the helical electrode developed by Hon (1972). It consists of a stainless steel needle, shaped approximately like one turn of a helix, mounted on a plastic hub. The back surface of the hub contains an additional stainless steel reference electrode. When labor has proceeded far enough, this electrode can be attached to the fetal presenting part by rotating it so that the needle twists just beneath the surface of the skin as would a corkscrew shallowly penetrating a cork. This electrode remains firmly attached, and due to the shortness of the helical needle, it does not penetrate deep enough into the skin to cause serious damage. It operates under the same basic principle as the suction electrode. See Figure 5.20(c).

Often when radio telemetry is used, we want to implant electrodes within the body and not penetrate the skin with the wires. In this case the radio transmitter must be implanted in the body. As in the other cases in this section, there is a wide variety of electrodes used in this application. Only a few examples are given here.

The simplest electrode for this application is shown in Figure 5.21(a). Insulated multistranded stainless steel wire suitable for implantation has one end stripped so that an eyelet can be formed from the strands of stainless steel. This is best done by individually taking each strand and forming the eyelet either by twisting the wires together one by one at the point at which the insulation stops, or by spot-welding each strand to the wire mass at this point. The eyelet can then be sutured to the point in the body at which electrical contact is to be established.

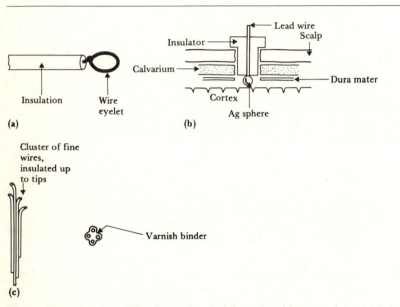

Figure 5.21 Implantable electrodes for detecting biopotentials. (a) Wire-loop electrode. (b) Silver-sphere cortical-surface potential electrode. (c) Multi-element depth electrode.

Figure 5.21(b) shows another example of an implantable electrode for obtaining cortical-surface potentials from the brain. This electrode has been applied by Critchfield and coworkers (1971) for the radio telemetry of subdural EEGs. The electrode consists of a 2-mm-diameter silver sphere located at the tip of the cylindrical Teflon insulator through which the electrode lead wire passes. The calvarium is exposed through an incision in the scalp and a burr hole is drilled. A small slit is made in the exposed dura, and the silver sphere is introduced through this opening so that it rests on the surface of the cerebral cortex. The assembly is then cemented in place onto the calvarium using a dental acrylic material.

Deep cortical potentials can be recorded from multiple points using the technique described by Delgado (1964), as shown in Figure 5.21(c). This kind of electrode consists of a cluster of fine insulated wires held together by a varnish binder. Each wire has been cut transversely to expose an uninsulated cross section that serves as the active electrode surface. By staggering the ends of the wires as shown, we can produce electrodes located at known differences in depth in an array. The other ends of the electrodes can be attached to appropriate implantable electronic devices or to a connector cemented on the skull to allow connection to an external recording apparatus.

5.8 Microelectrodes

In studying the electrophysiology of excitable cells, it is often important to measure potential differences across the cell membrane. To be able to do this, we must have an electrode within the cell. Such electrodes must be small with respect to the cell dimensions to avoid causing serious cellular injury, thereby changing the cell's behavior. In addition to being small, the electrode used for measuring intracellular potential must also be strong, so that it can penetrate the cell membrane and remain mechanically stable.

Electrodes that meet these requirements are known as *microelectrodes*. These have tip sizes ranging from approximately 0.05 to 10 μm. Microelectrodes can be formed from solid-metal needles, from metal contained within or on the surface of a glass needle, or from a glass micropipet having a lumen filled with an electrolytic solution. Examples of each type are given in the following paragraphs. More detailed descriptions can be found in Geddes (1972), Ferris (1974), and Cobbold (1974).

Metal microelectrodes

The metal microelectrode is essentially a fine needle of a strong metal that is insulated with an appropriate insulator up to its tip, as shown in Figure 5.22. A metal needle is prepared in such a way as to produce a very fine tip. This is usually done by electrolytic etching, using a cell in which the metal needle is the anode. The needle is etched as it is slowly withdrawn from the electrolyte solution. Very fine tips can be formed in this way, but a great amount of patience and practice are required to gain the skill to make them. Suitable strong metals for these microelectrodes are stainless steel, platinum-iridium alloy, and tungsten. The compound tungsten carbide is also frequently used because of its great strength.

The etched metal needle is then supported in a larger metallic shaft that can be insulated, and that serves as a sturdy mechanical support for the microelectrode, as well as a means of connecting it to its lead wire. The microelectrode and supporting shaft are usually insulated by a film of some polymeric material or varnish. Only the extreme tip of the electrode remains uninsulated.

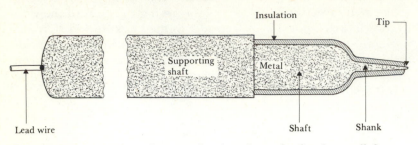

Figure 5.22 Structure of a metal microelectrode for intracellular recordings.

Supported-metal microelectrodes

The properties of two different materials are used to advantage in supported-metal microelectrodes. A strong insulating material that can be drawn to a fine point makes up the basic support, and a metal with good electrical conductivity constitutes the contacting portion of the electrode.

Figure 5.23 shows examples of supported metal microelectrodes. The classical example of this form is a glass tube drawn to a micropipet structure with its lumen filled with an appropriate metal. Often this type of microelectrode, as shown in Figure 5.23(a), is prepared by first filling a glass tube with a metal that has its melting point near the softening point of the glass. The tube can then be heated to the softening point and pulled to form a narrow constriction. When it is broken at the constriction, two micropipets filled with metal are formed. In this type of structure the glass not only provides the mechanical support, but also serves as the insulation. The active tip is the only metallic area exposed in cross section where the pipet was broken away. Metals such as silver-solder alloy and platinum and silver alloys are used. In some cases metals with low melting points, such as indium or Wood's metal, are used.

New supported-metal electrode structures have been developed using techniques employed in the semiconductor microelectronics industry. Figure 5.23(b) shows the cross section of the tip of a deposited-metal-film microelectrode. A solid glass rod or glass tube is drawn to form the micropipet. A metal film is deposited uniformly on this surface to a thickness of the order of tenths of a micrometer. A polymeric insulation is then coated over this, leaving just the tip, with the metal film exposed.

The technology used to produce beam-lead transistors and integrated circuits has been applied by Wise *et al.* (1970) to produce a microelectrode array. The basic structure is shown in Figure 5.23(c). It consists of gold (Au) strips deposited on an Si substrate, the surface of which has been first insulated by growing an SiO_2

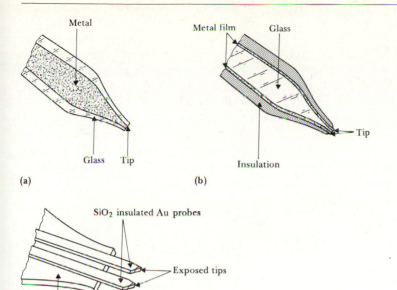

Figure 5.23 Structures of several types of supported metal microelectrodes. (a) Metal-filled glass micropipet. (b) Glass micropipet or probe, coated with metal film. (c) Beam-lead electrode based on semiconductor microelectronic technology. (Based on Figure 7 in K.D. Wise, J.B. Angell, and A. Starr, "An Integrated Circuit Approach to Extracellular Microelectrodes." Reprinted, with permission, from *IEEE Trans. Biomed. Eng.*, vol. BME-17, pp. 238–246, 1970. Copyright © 1970 by The Institute of Electrical and Electronics Engineers.)

film. The Au strips are then further insulated by depositing SiO_2 over their surface. The Si substrate is etched to a thin, narrow structure just large enough to accommodate the Au electrodes in the region of the tip. It is then etched back from the tip several millimeters, so that only the Au strips and the SiO_2 insulation remain. The latter is then etched away from the very tip of the Au strips to expose the contacting surface of the electrodes. Although this technology cannot produce tips as small as can be produced with the glass technology previously described, it is possible to make multielectrode arrays and to maintain the geometry between individual electrodes of the array very closely.

Micropipet electrodes

Glass micropipet microelectrodes are fabricated from glass capillaries. The central region of a piece of capillary tubing, as shown in Figure 5.24(a), is heated with a burner to the softening point. It is then rapidly stretched to produce the constriction shown in Figure 5.24(b). The two halves of the structure are broken apart at the constriction to produce a pipet structure having a tip diameter of the order of 1 μm. This pipet is fabricated into the electrode form shown in Figure 5.24(c). It is filled with an electrolyte solution that is frequently 3M KCl. A cap containing a metal electrode is then sealed to the pipet, as shown. The metal electrode contacts the electrolyte within the pipet. The electrode is frequently a silver wire prepared with an electrolytic AgCl surface. Platinum or stainless steel wires are also occasionally used.

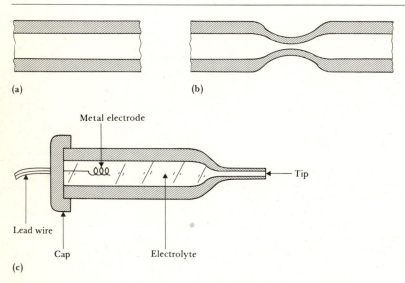

(a)   (b)

Metal electrode

Tip

Lead wire

Cap   Electrolyte

(c)

Figure 5.24 A glass micropipet electrode filled with an electrolytic solution. (a) Section of fine-bore glass capillary. (b) Capillary narrowed through heating and stretching. (c) Final structure of glass-pipet microelectrode.

Electrical properties of microelectrodes

To understand the electrical behavior of microelectrodes, we must derive an electrical equivalent circuit from physical considerations. This circuit differs for metal and micropipet electrodes.

Figure 5.25 shows metal microelectrodes. The microelectrode contributes a series resistance R_s due to the resistance of the metal itself. A major contributor to this resistance is the metal in the shank and tip portion of the microelectrode, since the ratio of its length to its cross-sectional area is much higher in this portion than it is for the shaft. Since the metal is coated with an insulating material over all but its most distal tip, a capacitor is set up between the metal and the extracellular fluid. This is a distributed capacitance

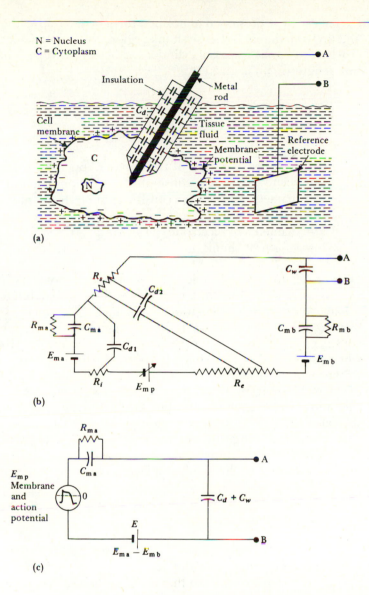

Figure 5.25 Equivalent circuit of metal microelectrode. (a) Electrode with tip placed within a cell, showing origin of distributed capacitance. (b) Equivalent circuit for situation in (a). (c) Simplified equivalent circuit. (From L.A. Geddes, *Electrodes and the Measurement of Bioelectric Events*, Wiley-Interscience, 1972. Used with permission of John Wiley and Sons, New York.)

C_d that can be represented in lumped form by separating the shank and tip from the shaft. In the shank region, we can consider the microelectrode to be a coaxial cylinder capacitor; the capacitance per unit length (F/m) is given by

$$\frac{C_{d1}}{L} = \frac{2\pi\epsilon_r\epsilon_0}{\ln(D/d)} \tag{5.16}$$

where

ϵ_0 = dielectric constant of free space (Appendix A.1)
ϵ_r = relative dielectric constant of insulation material
D = diameter of cylinder consisting of electrode plus insulation
d = diameter of electrode
L = length of shank

Of course, this coaxial-cable approximation is not a very good approximation for the shank region, which is tapered, but it is reasonable for a rough calculation. Since insulation thicknesses are usually of the order of 1 μm in the shank and tip, it is important to consider the structure using the coaxial cylinder analog. However, when we consider the shaft portion of the electrode, if the thickness of the insulation is still approximately 1 μm, the diameter of the metal shaft can be on the order of several millimeters. Here the ratio of diameters would be practically unity, so we can simplify the calculation by unwrapping the circumferential surface of the shaft and considering the system to be a parallel-plate capacitor of area equal to the circumferential surface area and thickness equal to t, the thickness of the insulation layer. The capacitance per unit length (F/m) is given by

$$\frac{C_{d2}}{L} = \frac{\epsilon_r\epsilon_0\pi d}{t} \tag{5.17}$$

It is important to note that this capacitance comes from only that portion of the electrode shaft that is submerged in the extracellular fluid. Often only the shank is submerged, so C_{d2} is zero.

The other significant contributions to the equivalent circuit from the metal microelectrode are the components contributed by the metal-electrolyte interface, R_{ma}, C_{ma}, and E_{ma}. A similar set of components, C_{mb}, R_{mb}, and E_{mb}, are associated with the reference electrode. Due to the much larger surface area of the reference electrode compared with the tip of the microelectrode, the impedance due to these components is much lower. Of course, the half-cell potential due to the reference electrode is unaffected by the surface area. Since the tip of the microelectrode is within a cell, there is a series resistance R_i associated with the electrolyte within the cell membrane and another series resistance R_e due to the extracellular fluid. The cell membrane itself can be modeled simply as a variable potential, E_{mp}, but in more detailed analyses an equivalent circuit of greater complexity is required. Some of the distributed capacitance of the shank, C_{d1}, is between the microelectrode and the extracellular fluid, as shown in the equivalent circuit, whereas the remainder of it is between the microelectrode and the intracellular fluid.

There is also a capacitance associated with the lead wires, C_w. The physical basis for this equivalent circuit is shown in Figure 5.25(a); the actual equivalent circuit is shown in Figure 5.25(b). Often it is acceptable to simplify this equivalent circuit to that shown in Figure 5.25(c), which neglects the impedance of the reference electrode and the series-resistance contribution from the intracellular and extracellular fluid and lumps all the distributed capacitance together. Under circumstances in which the input impedance of the amplifier connected to this electrode is not sufficiently large, we see that this circuit can behave as a high-pass filter and significant waveform distortion can result.

The effective impedance of metal microelectrodes is frequency-dependent, and can be of the order of 10 to 100 MΩ. We can, however, lower this impedance by increasing the effective surface area of the tip of the microelectrode through the application of platinum black, as was done in the case of the hydrogen electrode. Impedance reduction of one or two orders of magnitude can be achieved in this way. At lower frequencies, the impedance can be reduced by applying an Ag-AgCl surface to the electrode tip. Care must be taken in doing this, however, because of the mechanically fragile nature of this film and its tendency to flake off.

The equivalent circuit for the micropipet electrode is somewhat more complicated than that of the metal microelectrode. The physical situation is illustrated in Figure 5.26(a), with the resulting equivalent circuit shown in Figure 5.26(b). The internal electrode in the micropipet gives the metal-electrolyte interface components R_{ma}, C_{ma}, and E_{ma}. In series with this is a resistive element R_t corresponding to the resistance of the electrolyte in the shank and tip region of the microelectrode. Connected to this is the distributed capacitance C_d corresponding to the capacitance across the glass in this region. The distributed capacitance due to the shaft region has been neglected because the glass wall of the electrode is much thicker in this region, and the capacitive contribution is quite small.

There are two potentials associated with the tip of the micropipet microelectrode. The *liquid-junction potential E_j* corresponds to the liquid junction set up between the electrolyte in the micropipet and the intracellular fluid. In addition, there is a potential known as the *tip potential E_t*, which comes from the fact that the thin glass wall surrounding the tip region of the micropipet behaves like a glass membrane and has an associated membrane potential.

The equivalent circuit also includes resistances corresponding

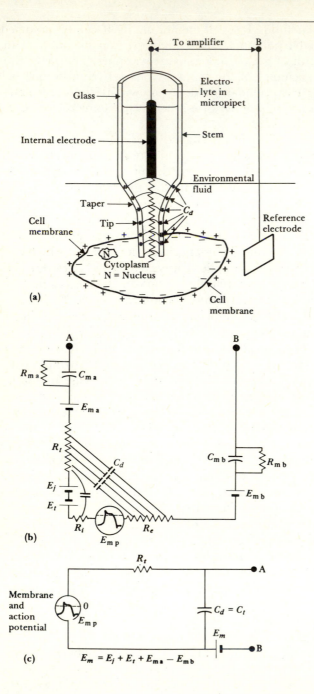

Figure 5.26 Equivalent circuit of glass micropipet microelectrode. (a) Electrode with its tip placed within a cell, showing origin of distributed capacitance. (b) Equivalent circuit for situation in (a). (c) Simplified equivalent circuit. (From L.A. Geddes, *Electrodes and the Measurement of Bioelectric Events,* Wiley-Interscience, 1972. Used with permission of John Wiley and Sons, New York.)

to the intracellular R_i and extracellular R_e fluids. These are coupled to the microelectrode through the distributive capacitance C_d, as is the case for the metal microelectrode. The equivalent circuit for the reference electrode remains unchanged from that in Figure 5.25(b).

Unlike the metal microelectrode, the micropipet's major impedance contribution is resistive. This can be illustrated by approximating the equivalent circuit to give that shown in Figure 5.26(c). Here the overall series resistance of the electrode is lumped as R_t. This resistance generally ranges in value from 1 to 100 MΩ. The total distributed capacitance is lumped together to form C_t, which can be on the order of tens of picofarads. And all the associated dc potentials are lumped together in the source E_m, which is given by

$$E_m = E_j + E_t + E_{ma} - E_{mb} \tag{5.18}$$

Note that the micropipet-type microelectrode behaves as a low-pass filter. The high series resistance and distributed capacitance cause the electrode output to respond slowly to rapid changes in cell-membrane potential. To reduce this problem, positive-feedback, negative-capacitance amplifiers (see Section 6.6) are used to reduce the effective value of C_t.

Example 5.5   A glass micropipet microelectrode has the following dimensions and properties.

Tip diameter	1.5 μm
Tip lumen diameter	1.0 μm
Shank length	3 mm
Resistivity of electrolyte	2.0 Ω · cm
Relative dielectric constant of glass	1.82

The microelectrode is to be used in an ac measurement. Determine a simple approximate ac equivalent circuit for it. What is the maximum frequency for a flat (to within 3 dB) frequency response for this electrode?

Answer   We can use the equivalent circuit of Figure 5.26(c), but it will not be necessary to include dc voltage source E_m, since we are concerned only with the ac equivalent circuit. The series resistance is primarily the resistance of the electrolyte in the shank. This is found by

$$R = \rho \frac{L}{A} \tag{E5.13}$$

where ρ = resistivity of electrolyte
L = length of shank
A = cross-sectional area of tip lumen

Therefore

$$R = 2.0 \ \Omega \cdot cm \times \frac{3 \ mm}{(\pi/4)(1.0 \ \mu m)^2} = 76.4 \ M\Omega \qquad (E5.14)$$

The capacitance can be found from (5.16).

$$C_{d1} = \frac{2\pi\epsilon_r\epsilon_0 L}{\ln (D/d)} = \frac{2\pi \times 1.82 \times 8.8 \times 10^{-12} \ F/m \times 3 \ mm}{\ln (1.5/1.0)}$$

$$C_{d1} = 7.43 \times 10^{-13} \ F \qquad (E5.15)$$

The equivalent circuit thus consists of a 76.4-MΩ resistor in series with the membrane potential of the cell being measured with a 0.743-pF capacitor shunting the output.

The maximum frequency for a flat frequency response is the corner frequency of the low-pass filter formed by the equivalent circuit. This is given by

$$f = \frac{1}{2\pi RC} = \frac{1}{2\pi \times 7.64 \times 10^7 \times 7.43 \times 10^{-13}} = 2.80 \ kHz$$

$$(E5.16)$$

Since some intracellular potentials can have frequency components up to 10 kHz, this electrode may cause some undesirable distortion.

5.9 Electrodes for electrical stimulation of tissue

Electrodes used for the electrical stimulation of tissue follow the same general design as those for the recording of bioelectric potentials. They differ in that currents of the order of milliamperes cross the electrode-electrolyte interface in stimulating electrodes. Examples of specific electrodes used in cardiac pacemakers and cardiac defibrillators are given in Chapter 12. Other types of stimulating electrodes are of the same form as the potential recording electrodes described in this chapter.

In considering stimulating electrodes, we must bear in mind that the net current across the electrode-electrolyte interface is not always zero. If a biphasic stimulating pulse is used, the average current over long periods of time is zero. However, over the stimulus cycle, there are periods of time during which the net current across the electrode is in one direction at one time and in the other direction at a different time. Also the magnitudes of the currents in the two directions may be unequal. In studying the electrical characteristics of the electrode-electrolyte interface under such circumstances, we may well imagine that the equivalent circuit changes as the stimulus progresses. Thus the effective equivalent circuit for the electrode is determined by the stimulus parameters, principally the current and the duration of the stimulus.

Rectangular biphasic or monophasic pulses are frequently used for electrical stimulation. However, other waveshapes, such as decaying exponentials or sine waves, have also been used. Frequently a stimulus that is either constant current or constant voltage during the pulse is used. The response of a typical electrode to this type of stimulus is illustrated in Figure 5.27.

A constant-current stimulus pulse is applied to the stimulating electrodes in Figure 5.27(a), giving the voltage response shown. Note that the resulting voltage pulse is not constant. This is reasonable when we consider that there is a strong reactive component to the electrode-electrolyte interface, or in other words, polarization occurs. The initial rise in voltage corresponding to the leading edge of the current pulse is due to the voltage drop across the resistive components of the electrode-electrolyte interface, but we see that the voltage continues to rise with the constant current. This is due to the establishment of a change in the distribution of charge concentration at the electrode-electrolyte interface; or, in other words, a change in polarization resulting from the unidirectional current. As stated in the description of the simplified electrode-electrolyte equivalent circuit of Figure 5.9, this polarization effect can be represented by a capacitor. Again it is important to remember that the size of this capacitor is determined by several factors, one of which is the current density at the interface, so the equivalent circuit for stimulating electrodes changes with the stimulus.

When the current falls back to its low value, the voltage across the electrodes drops, but not back to its initial value. Instead, after the initial steep fall, there is a slower decay corresponding to the dissipation of the polarization charge at the interface.

Constant-voltage stimulation of the electrodes is shown in Figure 5.27(b). In this case the current corresponding to the rising edge of the voltage pulse is seen to jump in a large step and, as the distribution of the polarization charge becomes established, to fall back to a lower steady-state value. When the voltage pulse falls, the current is seen to change direction and then slowly return to its initial zero value. This is a result of the dissipation of the polarization charge built up at the electrode-electrolyte interface.

The choice of materials for stimulating electrodes must take into consideration chemical reactions occurring at the electrode-electrolyte interface. If a stimulating current causes the material of the electrode to be oxidized, the electrode is consumed, thereby limiting its lifetime and also increasing the concentration of the ions of electrode material in the vicinity of the electrode. This could be toxic to the tissue. When electrodes such as the Ag-AgCl electrode are used, the stimulating current can result in either the formation of additional Cl^- or the reduction of what is already formed, thereby greatly changing the characteristics of the elec-

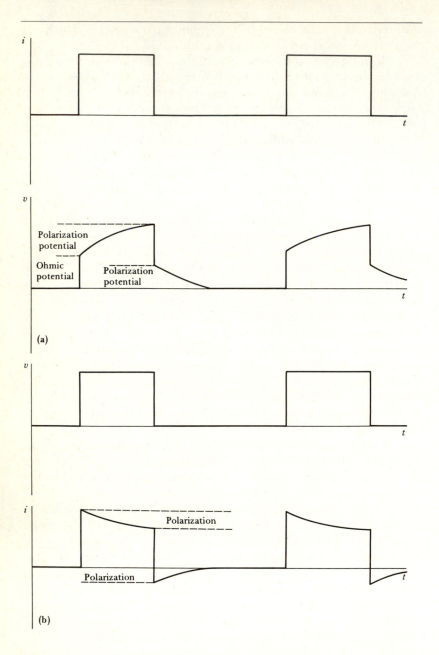

Figure 5.27 Current and voltage waveforms seen with electrodes used for electrical stimulation. (a) Constant-current stimulation. (b) Constant-voltage stimulation.

trode. Thus the best stimulating electrodes are made from noble metals (or at least stainless steel) which undergo only minimal chemical reactions. Of course, the polarization of these electrodes is large, and the waveforms, such as shown in Figure 5.27, are less rectangular than they would be with nonpolarizable electrodes.

5.10 Practical hints in using electrodes

In using metal electrodes for measurement and stimulation, we should understand a few practical points not mentioned elsewhere in this chapter. The first point is the importance of constructing the electrode and any parts of the lead wire that may be exposed to the electrolyte *all of the same material*. Furthermore, a third material such as solder should not be used to connect the electrode to its lead wire unless it is certain that this will not be in contact with the electrolyte. It is far better either to weld the lead wire to the electrode or at least to form a mechanical bond through crimping or peening. Dissimilar metals should not be used in contact because their half-cell potentials are different. And, since they are connected and in contact with the same electrolyte, it is more than likely that an electrochemical reaction will be set up between them that can result in additional polarization and often in corrosion of one of the metals. This factor also tends to make half-cell potentials less stable, thereby contributing to increased electrical noise from the electrode.

When pairs of electrodes are used for measuring differentials, such as in detecting surface potentials on the body or internal potentials within it, it is far better to use the same material for each electrode, since the half-cell potentials are approximately equal. This means that the net dc potential seen at the input to the amplifier connected to the electrodes is relatively small, possibly even zero. This minimizes possible saturation effects in the case of high-gain, direct-coupled amplifiers.

Electrodes placed on the skin's surface have a tendency to come off. Frequently, this is due to a loss of effectiveness of the tack on the tape holding them in place. However, the problem need not arise if the electrodes are well designed. Lead wires to these surface electrodes should be extremely flexible, yet strong. If they are, only tension on the lead wire can apply a force that is likely to remove the electrode. If the lead wire remains loose, it cannot apply any forces to the electrode because of its high flexibility.

The point at which the lead wire enters the electrode is a frequent point of failure. Even though the insulation appears intact, the wire within may be broken as a result of severe repeated flexing at this point. Well-designed electrodes can minimize this problem by providing strain relief at this point, so that there is a gradual transition between the wire and the solid material of the electrode.

Using a tapered region of insulation gradually increasing from the diameter of the wire to one closer to that of the electrode often minimizes this problem and distributes the flexing forces over a greater portion of wire.

Another point to consider is that the insulation of the lead wire and the electrode can also present problems. Electrodes are often in a high-humidity environment or are continually soaked in extracellular fluid, or even in cleaning solution (if they are of the reusable type). The insulation of these electrodes is usually made of a polymeric material, so it can absorb water. Some of these materials can become more conductive when they absorb this water, and, in the case of implantable electrodes, there may be some high resistance contact with the lead wire as well as at the electrode itself. If the lead wire is made of a material different from that of the electrode, the problems just described can result, thereby increasing the observed electrical noise and possibly leading to the weakening of the lead wires due to corrosion. Thus it is important to understand the insulation material used with the electrode, and to make sure that there is a layer of it thick enough to prevent this problem from occurring in the particular application in which the electrode is used.

One final point regarding electrodes for measuring biopotentials: In deriving the equivalent circuit for electrodes such as those shown in Figure 5.9, we stressed that for high-fidelity recordings of the measured biopotential, the input impedance of the amplifier to which the electrodes are connected must be much higher than the source impedance represented by the equivalent circuit. If this condition is not met, not only will the amplitude of the recorded signal be less than it should be, but also significant distortion will be introduced into the waveform of the signal. This is demonstrated by Geddes (1966) for electrodes used to record electrocardiograms. Geddes shows how lowering the input impedance of the amplifier causes the recorded signal to take on a more and more biphasic character, as well as a reduced amplitude.

Problems

5.1 A set of biopotential electrodes made of silver are attached to the chest of a patient to detect the electrocardiogram. When current passes through the anode, it causes silver to be oxidized, producing silver ions in solution. There is a 10-μA leakage current between these electrodes. Determine the number of silver ions per second entering the solution at the electrode-electrolyte interface.

5.2 When electrodes are used to record the electrocardiogram, an electrolyte paste is usually put between them and the surface of the skin. This makes it possible for the metal of the electrode to form metallic ions that move into the electrolyte paste. Often, after prolonged use, this electrolyte paste begins to dry out and change the characteristic of the electrodes. Draw an equivalent circuit for the electrode while the electrolyte paste is fresh. Then discuss and illustrate the way you expect this equivalent circuit to change as the electrolyte paste dries out. In the extreme case when there is no electrolyte paste left, what does the equivalent circuit of the electrode look like? How will this affect the quality of the recorded electrocardiogram?

5.3 A zinc wire and an aluminum wire accidentally come in contact with a part of the body that has been saturated with a physiologic saline solution. Is there a potential difference between these two wires? If your answer is yes, quantitatively state the value of this potential under open-circuit conditions.

5.4 A pair of biopotential electrodes is used to detect the electrocardiogram of an adult male. It has become necessary to determine the equivalent-source impedance of this electrode pair so that a particular experiment can be performed. Describe an experimental procedure that can be used to determine this quantity, using a minimum of test equipment.

5.5 A pair of biopotential electrodes is placed in a saline solution and connected to a stimulator, which passes a direct current through the electrodes. It is noted that the offset potential from each electrode is different. Explain why this happens during the passage of current. Sketch the distribution of ions about each electrode while the current is on.

5.6 Electrodes having a source resistance of 4 kΩ each are used in a bipolar configuration with a differential amplifier having an input impedance of 70 kΩ. What will be the percentage reduction in the amplitude of the biopotential signal?

5.7 A nurse noticed that one electrode of a pair of Ag-AgCl cardiac electrodes used on a chronic cardiac monitor was dirty, and cleaned it by scraping it with steel wool (Brillo) until it was again shiny and bright. The nurse then placed the electrode back on the patient. How did this procedure affect the signal observed from the electrode?

5.8 A metal microelectrode has a tip that can be modeled as being cylindrical. The metal itself is 1 μm in diameter and the tip region is 3 mm long. The metal has a resistivity of 1.2×10^{-5} $\Omega \cdot$ cm and is coated over its circumference with an insulation material that is 0.2 μm thick. The insulation material has a relative dielectric constant of 1.67. Only the base of the cylinder is free of insulation.

   a What is the resistance associated with the tip of this microelectrode?
   b What is the area of the surface of the electrode that contacts the electrolytic solution within the cell? The resistance associated with the electrode-electrolyte interface of

this material is $10^3 \ \Omega/cm^2$. What is the resistance due to this microelectrode's contact with the electrolyte?

c What is the capacitance associated with the tip of the microelectrode when the capacitances at the interface of the electrode-electrolytic solution are neglected?

d Draw an approximate equivalent circuit for the tip portion of this microelectrode.

e At what frequencies do you expect to see distortion when the electrode is connected to an amplifier having a purely resistive input impedance of 10 MΩ? You may assume that the reference electrode has an impedance low enough so that it will not enter into the answer to this question. If the amplifier's input impedance is raised to 100 MΩ, how does this affect the frequency response of the system? Is this difference significant for most intracellular biologic applications?

5.9 A micropipet electrode has a lumenal diameter of 3 μm at its tip. At this point, the glass wall is only 0.5 μm thick and 2 mm long. The resistance of the electrolyte in the tip is 40 MΩ. The glass has a relative dielectric constant of 1.63. Estimate the frequency response of this electrode when it is connected to an infinite-input-impedance amplifier. How can this frequency response be improved?

5.10 A pair of biopotential electrodes are used to monitor a bioelectric signal from the body. The monitoring electronic circuit has a low-input impedance that is of the same order of magnitude as the source impedance in the electrodes.

a Sketch an equivalent circuit for this situation.

b Qualitatively describe what you expect the general characteristics of the frequency response of this system to be. It is not necessary to plot an analytic Bode plot.

5.11 An identical pair of stainless steel electrodes is designed to be used to stimulate skeletal muscles. The stimulus consists of a rectangular constant-voltage pulse applied to the electrodes. The pulse has an amplitude of 5 V with a duration of 10 ms. Draw an equivalent circuit for the load seen by the constant-voltage pulse generator, based on the equivalent circuits of each of the electrodes. Simplify your circuit as much as possible. What is the waveshape of the current at the generator terminals? Remember that a constant-voltage generator has a source impedance of zero. Explain and sketch the resulting current waveform.

5.12 An exotic new animal, recently discovered, has an unusual electrolyte makeup in that its major anion is Br$^-$ rather than Cl$^-$. Scientists want to measure the EEG of this animal, which is less than 25 μV. Electrodes made of Ag-AgCl seem to be noisy. Can you suggest a better electrode system, and explain why it is better?

5.13 Needle-type EMG electrodes are placed directly in a

muscle. Figure P5.1 shows their simplified equivalent circuit, and also the equivalent circuit of the input stage of an amplifier. The value of the capacitor C_2 in the amplifier may be varied to any desired quantity.

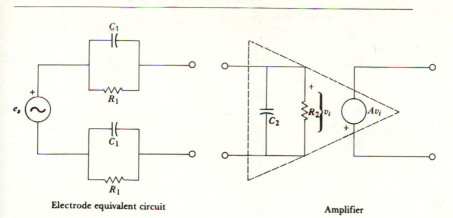

Electrode equivalent circuit   Amplifier

Figure P5.1

a Assuming $C_2 = 0$ and an amplifier gain of A, write an equation showing the output voltage of the amplifier as a function of e_s (the signal) and frequency.

b Determine a value for C_2 which gives electrode-amplifier characteristics that are independent of frequency.

c What is the amplifier's output voltage in part (b) when the signal is e_s?

References

Caldwell, C.W., and J.B. Reswick, "A percutaneous wire electrode for chronic research use." *IEEE Trans. Biomed. Eng.*, 1975, BME-22, 429–432.

Cobbold, R.S.C., *Transducers for biomedical measurements: Principles and applications.* New York: Wiley, 1974.

Critchfield, F.H., C. Xinteras, B. Johnson, and M.R. Neuman, "Surgical and engineering techniques for the supra-cephalic mounting of a multichannel EEG telemeter." *Dig. Int. Conf. Med. Biol. Eng.*, 1971, paper number 22-4.

Delgado, J.M.R., "Electrodes for extracellular recording and stimulation," in W.L. Nastuk (ed.), *Physical techniques in biological research.* New York: Academic, 1964, Vol. 5A.

Ferris, C.D., *Introduction to bioelectrodes.* New York: Plenum, 1974.

Geddes, L.A., *Electrodes and the measurement of bioelectric events.* New York: Wiley, 1972.

Geddes, L.A., and L.E. Baker, "The relationship between input impedance and electrode area in recording the ECG." *Med. Biol. Eng.*, 1966, 4, 439–450.

Geddes, L.A., and L.E. Baker, "Chlorided silver electrodes." *Med. Res. Eng.*, 1967, 6, 33–34.

Geddes, L.A., L.E. Baker, and A.G. Moore, "Optimum electrolytic chloriding of silver electrodes." *Med. Biol. Eng.*, 1969, 7, 49–56.

Geddes, L.A., C.P. DaCosta, and G. Wise, "The impedance of stainless steel electrodes." *Med. Biol. Eng.*, 1971, 9, 511–521.

Hon, E.H., R.H. Paul, and R.W. Hon, "Electronic evaluation of fetal heart rate. XI: Description of a spiral electrode." *Obstet. Gynecol.*, 1972, 40, 362–363.

Janz, G.J., and D.J.G. Ives, "Silver-silver chloride electrodes." *Ann. N.Y. Acad. Sci.*, 1968, 148, 210–221.

Ko, W.H., and J. Hynecek, "Dry electrodes and electrode amplifiers," in H.A. Miller and D.C. Harrison (eds.), *Biomedical electrode technology.* New York: Academic, 1974, pp. 169–181.

Miller, H.A., and D.C. Harrison (eds.), *Biomedical electrode technology.* New York: Academic, 1974.

Neuman, M.R., "Flexible thin film skin electrodes for use with neonates." *Dig. Int. Conf. Med. Biol. Eng.*, 1973, paper no. 35.11.

Richardson, P.C., "The insulated electrode." *Proc. Ann. Conf. Eng. Med. Biol.*, 1967, paper no. 15.7.

Robinson, D.A., "The electrical properties of metal microelectrodes." *Proc. IEEE*, 1968, 56, 1065–1071.

Schwan, H.P., "Determination of biological impedances," in W.L. Nastuk (ed.), *Physical techniques in biological research.* New York: Academic, 1963, pp. 323–407.

Tam, H.W., and J.G. Webster, "Minimizing electrode motion artifact by skin abrasion." *IEEE Trans. Biomed. Eng.*, 1977, BME-24, 134–139.

Webster, J.G., "Interference and motion artifact in biopotentials," *IEEE 1977 Region 6 Conference Record*, 1977: 53–64.

Wise, K.D., J.B. Angell, and A. Starr, "An integrated circuit approach to extracellular microelectrodes." *IEEE Trans. Biomed. Eng.*, 1970, BME-17, 238–246.

Yon, E.T., M.R. Neuman, R.N. Wolfson, and W.H. Ko, "Insulated active electrodes." *IEEE Trans. Ind. Electron. Control Instrum.*, 1970, IECI-17, 195–197.

Chapter six

Biopotential amplifiers

Michael R. Neuman

Amplifiers are an important part of modern instrumentation systems for measuring biopotentials. Such measurements involve voltages that are often at low levels and have high source impedances, or both. Amplifiers are required to increase signal strength while maintaining high fidelity. Amplifiers that have been designed specifically for this type of processing of biopotentials are known as *biopotential amplifiers*. In this chapter we examine some of the basic features of biopotential amplifiers and also look at specialized systems.

6.1 Basic requirements

The essential function of a biopotential amplifier is to take a weak electrical signal of biologic origin and increase its amplitude so that it may be further processed, recorded, or displayed. Usually such amplifiers are in the form of voltage amplifiers, since they are capable of increasing the voltage level of a signal. Nonetheless, voltage amplifiers also serve to increase power levels, so they can be considered power amplifiers as well. In some cases, biopotential amplifiers are used to isolate the load from the source. In this situation, the amplifiers provide only current gain, leaving the voltage levels essentially unchanged.

To be useful biologically, all biopotential amplifiers must meet certain basic requirements. They must have high input impedance, so that they provide minimal loading of the signal being measured. The characteristics of biopotential electrodes can be affected by the electrical load which they see, and when loading is excessive, this can result in distortion of the signal. Loading effects are minimized by making the amplifier input impedance as high as possible, thereby reducing this distortion. Modern biopotential amplifiers have input impedances of at least 2 MΩ, with 10 MΩ being a desirable value for many applications.

The input circuit of a biopotential amplifier must also provide protection to the organism being studied. Any current or potential appearing across the amplifier input terminals is capable of affecting the biologic potential being measured. In clinical systems, electric currents produced by the biopotential amplifier and seen at its input terminals can generate micro- or macroshocks in the patient being studied—a situation that can have grave consequences. To avoid these problems, the amplifier input should have isolation and protection circuitry, so that current through the electrode circuit can be kept at safe levels and any artifact generated by such current can be minimized.

The output circuit of a biopotential amplifier does not present as many critical problems as the input circuit. Its principal function is to drive the amplifier load, usually an indicating or recording device, in such a way as to maintain maximum fidelity and range in this readout. Therefore the output impedance of the amplifier must be low with respect to the load impedance and the amplifier must be capable of supplying the power required by the load.

Biopotential amplifiers must operate in that portion of the frequency spectrum in which the biopotentials that they amplify exist. Because of the low level of such signals, it is important to limit the bandwidth of the amplifier so that it is just great enough to process the signal adequately. In this way, we can obtain optimal signal-to-noise ratios. Biopotential signals usually have amplitudes of the order of a few millivolts or less. Such signals must be amplified to levels compatible with recording and display devices. This means that most biopotential amplifiers must have high gains, of the order of 1000 or greater.

Very often biopotential signals are obtained from bipolar electrodes. These electrodes are often symmetrically located, electrically, with respect to ground. Under such circumstances, the most appropriate biopotential amplifier is a differential one. Since such bipolar electrodes frequently have a common-mode voltage with respect to ground which is much larger than the signal amplitude, and since the symmetry with respect to ground can be distorted, such biopotential differential amplifiers must have high common-mode rejection ratios to minimize artifact due to the common-mode signal.

A final requirement for biopotential amplifiers that are used both in medical applications and in the laboratory is that they make possible a quick calibration. In recording biopotentials, the scientist and clinician need to know not only the waveforms of these signals, but also their amplitudes. To provide this information, the gain of the amplifier must be well calibrated. Frequently biopotential amplifiers have a standard signal source that can be momentarily connected to the input, at the push of a button, to check the calibration.

Biopotential amplifiers have additional requirements that are application-specific and that can be ascertained from an examination of each application. To illustrate some of these, let us first consider the electrocardiogram (ECG), the most frequently used application of biopotential amplifiers.

6.2 The electrocardiograph

To learn more about biopotential amplifiers, we shall examine a typical clinical electrocardiograph. Before we do so, let us review the ECG itself.

The ECG

As we learned in Section 4.6, the beating heart generates an electrical signal that can be used as a diagnostic tool for examining some of the functions of the heart. This electrical activity of the heart can be approximately represented as a vector quantity. Thus we need to know the location at which signals are detected, as well as the time-dependence of the amplitude of the signals. Electrocardiographers have developed a simple model to represent the electrical activity of the heart. In this model, the heart consists of an electric dipole located in the partially conducting medium of the thorax.

Figure 6.1 shows a typical example of this. This particular field and the dipole that produces it represent the electrical activity of the heart at a particular instant of time. At the next instant of time, the dipole can change its magnitude and its orientation, thereby resulting in a change in the electric field. Once we accept this model (it is an oversimplification when we consider the real heart in the real torso), we need not draw a field plot every time we want to discuss the dipole field of the heart. Instead, we can represent it by its dipole moment, a vector extending from the negative charge to the positive charge, and having a magnitude proportional to the amount of charge (either positive or negative) multiplied by the separation of the two charges. In electrocardiography, this dipole moment, known as the *cardiac vector*, is depicted by **M**, as shown in Figure 6.1. As we progress through a cardiac cycle, the magnitude and direction of **M** varies, since the dipole field varies.

The electric potentials generated by the heart appear throughout the body and on its surface. Potential differences are determined by placing electrodes on the surface of the body and measuring the voltage between them, being careful to draw little current (ideally there should be no current at all, since current distorts the electric field that produces the potential differences). If the two electrodes are located on different equal-potential lines of the electric field of the heart, a nonzero potential difference is measured. Different pairs of electrodes at different locations generally yield different results due to the spatial dependence of the electric field of the heart. Thus it is important to have certain standard positions for clinical evaluation of the ECG. The limbs make fine

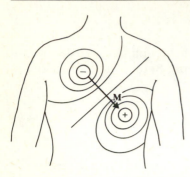

Figure 6.1 Rough sketch of dipole field of heart when R wave is maximum. Dipole consists of the points of equal positive and negative charge separated from one another and denoted by the dipole moment vector **M**.

guideposts for locating the ECG electrodes. We shall look at this in more detail later.

In the simplified dipole model of the heart, it would be convenient if we could predict the voltage, or at least its waveform, in a particular set of electrodes at a particular instant of time when the cardiac vector is known. We can do this if we define a *lead vector* for the pair of electrodes. This vector is a unit vector, defining the direction a constant-magnitude cardiac vector must have to generate maximum voltage in the particular pair of electrodes. A pair of electrodes, or combination of several electrodes through a resistive network that gives an equivalent pair, is referred to as a *lead*.

For a cardiac vector **M**, as shown in Figure 6.2, the voltage induced in a lead represented by the lead vector $\mathbf{a}_1$ is given by the component of **M** in the direction of $\mathbf{a}_1$. In vector algebra, this can be denoted by the dot product

$$v_{a1} = \mathbf{M} \cdot \mathbf{a}_1 \tag{6.1}$$

where v_{a1} is the scalar voltage seen in the lead that has the vector, $\mathbf{a}_1$. Let us consider another lead, represented by the lead vector $\mathbf{a}_2$, as seen in Figure 6.2. In this case, the vector is oriented in space so as to be perpendicular to the cardiac vector **M**. The component of **M** along the direction of $\mathbf{a}_2$ is zero, so that no voltage is seen in this lead as a result of the cardiac vector. If we measured the ECG generated by **M** using one of the two leads shown in Figure 6.2 alone, we could not uniquely describe the cardiac vector. However, by using two leads with different lead vectors, both of which lie in the same plane as the cardiac vector, we can describe **M**.

In clinical electrocardiography, more than one lead must be recorded to fully describe the heart's electrical activity. In practice, several leads are taken in the *frontal* (the plane of your body parallel to the ground when you are lying on your back) and *transverse*

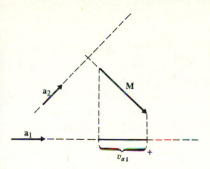

Figure 6.2 Relationships between two lead vectors $\mathbf{a}_1$ and $\mathbf{a}_2$ and cardiac vector $\mathbf{M}$. The component of $\mathbf{M}$ in the direction of $\mathbf{a}_1$ is given by the dot product of these two vectors and denoted on the figure by v_{a1}. Lead vector $\mathbf{a}_2$ is perpendicular to cardiac vector, so there is no voltage component seen in this lead.

(the plane of your body parallel to the ground when you are standing erect) *planes*.

Three basic leads make up the *frontal-plane* ECG. These are derived from the various permutations of pairs of electrodes when one electrode is located on the right arm (RA in Figure 6.3), the left arm (LA), and the left leg (LL). Very often an electrode is also placed on the right leg (RL) and grounded or connected to special circuits, as shown in Figure 6.19. The resulting three leads are lead I, LA to RA; lead II, LL to RA; and lead III, LL to LA. The lead vectors formed can be approximated as an equilateral triangle, known as *Eindhoven's triangle,* in the frontal plane of the body, as shown in Figure 6.3. The components of a particular cardiac vector can be easily determined by placing the vector within the triangle and determining its components along each side. The process can also be reversed, allowing us to determine the cardiac vector when

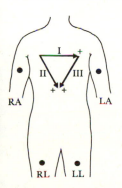

Figure 6.3 Lead vectors for standard limb leads taken from electrodes on right arm (RA), left arm (LA), and left leg (LL) make up the Eindhoven triangle in frontal plane of body.

we know the components along the three lead vectors, or at least two of them. It is this latter problem that usually concerns the electrocardiographer.

Three additional leads in the frontal plane—as well as a group of leads in the transverse plane—are routinely used in taking clinical ECGs. These leads are based on signals obtained from more than one pair of electrodes. They are often referred to as *unipolar leads* because they consist of the potential appearing on one electrode taken with respect to an equivalent reference electrode, which is the average of the signals seen at two or more electrodes.

One such equivalent reference electrode is the *Wilson central terminal,* shown in Figure 6.4. Here the three-limb electrodes just described are connected through equal-valued resistors to a common node. The voltage at this node, which is the Wilson central terminal, is the average of the voltages at each electrode. The signal between LA and the central point is known as VL; that at RA, as VR; and that at the left foot, VF. Note that for each of these leads, one of the resistances R shunts the circuit between the central terminal and the limb electrode. This tends to reduce the amplitude of the signal observed, and we can modify these leads to

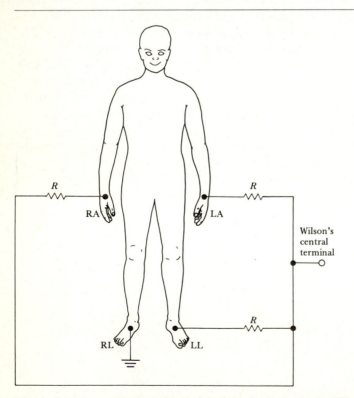

Figure 6.4 Connection of electrodes to the body to obtain Wilson's central terminal.

augmented leads by removing the connection between the limb being measured and the central terminal. This does not affect the direction of the lead vector, but results in a 50% increase in amplitude of the signal.

The augmented leads—known as aVL, aVR, and aVF—are illustrated in Figure 6.5, which also illustrates their lead vectors, along with those of leads I, II, and III. Note that when the negative direction for aVR is considered with the other five, all six vectors are equally spaced, by 30°. It is thus possible for the cardiologist looking at an ECG consisting of these six leads to estimate the position of the cardiac cycle by seeing which of the six leads has the greatest signal amplitude at that point in the cycle.

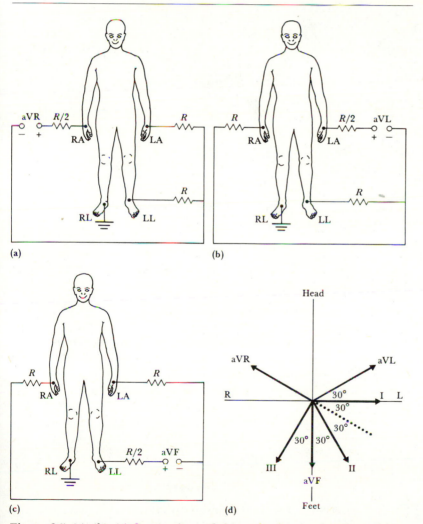

Figure 6.5 (a), (b), (c) Connections of electrodes for the three augmented limb leads. (d) Vector diagram showing standard and augmented lead-vector directions in the frontal plane.

When physicians look at the ECG in the transverse plane, they use *precordial* (chest) leads. They place an electrode at various anatomically defined positions on the chest wall, as shown in Figure 6.6. The potential between this electrode and Wilson's central terminal is the electrocardiogram for that particular lead. Figure 6.6 also shows the lead-vector positions. Physicians can obtain ECGs from the posterior side of the heart by means of an electrode placed in the esophagus. This structure passes directly behind the heart, and the potential between the esophageal electrode and Wilson's central terminal gives a posterior lead.

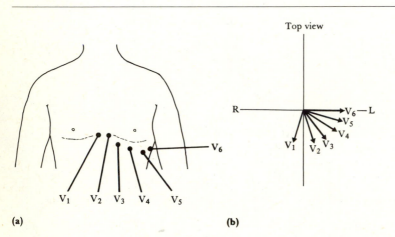

(a)   (b)

Figure 6.6 (a) Positions of precordial leads on chest wall. (b) Directions of precordial lead vectors in transverse plane.

Example 6.1 Show that the voltage in lead aVR is 50% greater than that in lead VR at the same instant of time.

Answer Considering the connections for aVR and VR, we can draw the equivalent circuits of Figure E6.1. v_a, v_b, and v_c are the voltages between each limb and ground. When no current is drawn by the voltage-measurement circuit, the negative terminal for aVR (the modified Wilson's central terminal) will be at a voltage of v'_w with respect to ground, which can be determined by

$$i_1 = \frac{v_b - v_c}{2R}$$

$$v'_w = i_1 R + v_c = \frac{v_b - v_c}{2R} R + v_c = \frac{v_b + v_c}{2} \tag{E6.1}$$

Since no current is drawn, the positive aVR terminal (RA) will be at a voltage v_a with respect to ground. Then aVR will be

$$aVR = v_a - \frac{v_b + v_c}{2} = \frac{2v_a - v_b - v_c}{2} \tag{E6.2}$$

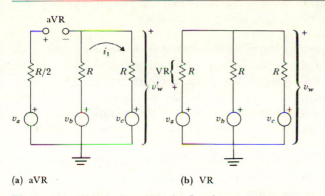

(a) aVR   (b) VR

Figure E6.1 Equivalent circuits for determining aVR and VR.

We can determine VR from Figure E6.1(b). To find the Wilson's central terminal voltage v_w, we can simplify the circuit by taking the Thévenin equivalent circuit of the two right-hand branches. This gives the circuit of Figure E6.2, where v'_w comes from (E6.1). Now v_w is

$$v_w = \frac{v_a - v'_w}{3R/2}\frac{R}{2} + v'_w = \frac{v_a + 2v'_w}{3} \tag{E6.3}$$

$$v_w = \frac{v_a + 2(v_b + v_c)/2}{3} = \frac{v_a + v_b + v_c}{3} \tag{E6.4}$$

Thus

$$VR = v_a - v_w = \frac{2v_a - v_b - v_c}{3} \tag{E6.5}$$

which shows that

$$aVR = \tfrac{3}{2}VR$$

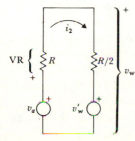

Figure E6.2 Simplified circuit of Fig. E6.1(a).

Specific requirements of the electrocardiograph

The Committee on Electrocardiography of the American Heart Association has made recommendations for the standardization of direct-writing electrocardiographs (Pipberger, 1975). Some of the recommendations are as follows.

1 Linearity and distortion Deviation from linearity should be less than 5% of the peak-to-peak output for signal peak-to-peak output amplitides between 5 and 50 mm on the chart. For peak-to-peak amplitudes less than 5 mm, the deviation from linearity should be no greater than 0.25 mm. This requirement covers signals composed of frequency components between 0.05 and 100 Hz.

2 Input range Specifications should be met for input signals ranging in amplitude up to 10 mV p–p.

3 Input impedance and current The input impedance between an electrode terminal and ground should be no less than 5 MΩ. During the measurement all other electrodes should be grounded. The instrument should not allow currents greater than 1.0 μA to flow through the patient. (Today leakage currents of not greater than 10 μA are considered acceptable.)

4 Central terminal The resistance networks needed to establish the central terminal should not cause any distortion greater than an additional 2% of that already specified for the machine (item 1). Along with the input-impedance requirements, this sets the minimum value of resistances to determine the central terminal at 3.3 MΩ.

5 Gain There should be three fixed gain settings: 5, 10, and 20 mm/mV.

6 Frequency response The instrument's response should be flat to within ± 0.5 dB over the frequency range of from 0.14 to 25 Hz. For signals having a peak-to-peak amplitude of less than or equal to 5 mm on the chart at 25 Hz, the response to a constant-amplitude sinusoidal input up to a frequency of 100 Hz should not be reduced by more than 3 dB.

7 Common-mode-rejection ratio (CMRR) For each position of the lead selector switch, with the recorder gain set at 10 mm/mV and with all input electrode lines connected, a 60-Hz, 120-V rms source with one terminal grounded and the other terminal applied to the junction of the leads through a series capacitance of 22 pF shall cause no more than 20-mm peak-to-peak deflection. This specification must still be met when a resistance of 100 kΩ is placed in series with one or more input lines in any combination.

8 Calibration A 1.0-mV standardizing voltage should be available to check the calibration of the gain.

9 Chart speed The standard chart speed of 25 mm/s is to be used. In addition, the higher speed of 50 mm/s should be available. Speed accuracy should be $\pm 2\%$.

10 Output The output impedance should be less than 100 Ω. Full scale output should be ± 1 V.

11 Event marker A manually controlled marker should be

provided at the edge of the chart to allow the operator to encode recordings.

The above recommendations are voluntary. However, the standard developed for the Food and Drug Administration (Schoenberg *et al.*, 1977a) will likely become a mandatory, Class II performance standard (Section 1.10).

Functional blocks of the electrocardiograph

Figure 6.7 shows a block diagram of a typical electrocardiograph. To understand the overall operation of the system, let us consider each block separately.

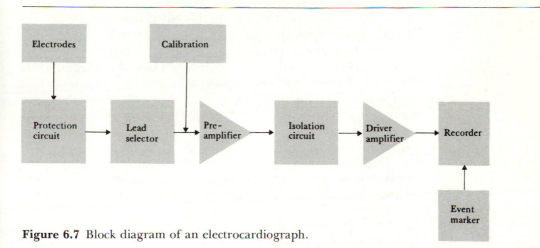

Figure 6.7 Block diagram of an electrocardiograph.

1 Isolation and protection circuit The circuitry of this block protects the patient from dangerous currents that could be generated in the electrocardiograph. It provides some type of isolation between the electrodes, the remainder of the machine, and the power lines. Often this circuit includes protection devices so that high voltages that may appear across the input to the electrocardiograph under certain conditions do not damage it.

2 Lead selector Each electrode connected to the patient is attached to the lead selector of the electrocardiograph. The function of this block is to determine which electrodes are necessary for a particular lead and to connect these to the remainder of the circuit. It is this part of the electrocardiograph in which the connections for the central terminal are made. Generally, the central component of this block is a selector switch that the operator can position for the particular lead desired.

3 Calibration signal A 1-mV calibration signal can be momentarily introduced into the electrocardiograph by the operator's pressing a button.

4 Preamplifier The input preamplifier stage carries out the initial amplification of the ECG. This stage should have very high input impedance and a high common-mode-rejection ratio (CMRR). A typical preamplifier stage used is the differential amplifier consisting of three operational amplifiers, shown in Figure 3.5. A gain-control switch giving the electrocardiograph the three gains described above is often included as a part of either this stage or the driver-amplifier stage.

5 Isolation circuit The circuitry of this block contains a barrier to the passage of 60-Hz current. For example, if the patient came in contact with a 120-V line, this barrier would prevent dangerous currents from flowing from the patient through the amplifier to the ground of the recorder.

6 Driver amplifier Circuitry in this block amplifies the ECG to a level at which it can appropriately deflect the pen of the recorder. Its input should be ac-coupled so that offset voltages amplified by the preamplifier are not seen at its input. These dc voltages, when amplified by this stage, might cause it to saturate. This stage also carries out the bandpass filtering of the electrocardiograph to give the frequency characteristics described previously. Also it often has a zero-offset control that is used to position the pen on the chart paper. This control adjusts the dc level of the output signal.

7 Recorder The recorder is usually an oscillograph-type recorder that meets the specifications of chart speed and frequency response given above. Frequently, heated-stylus recorders are used with thermally sensitive paper to record the ECG. This avoids problems associated with inking systems. When this type of recorder is used, an additional control is provided on the electrocardiograph to adjust the current supplied to the thermostylus which, in turn, determines the intensity of the trace. Recently pressurized-ink systems have been used in recording pens. Ink is provided to the stylus under pressure, thereby avoiding many of the problems of clogged pens that previously made ink-type recorders undesirable. An additional pen is provided on the recorder which contacts the paper only during the time that the event-marker button is depressed.

6.3 Problems frequently encountered

There are many factors that must be taken into consideration in the design and application of the electrocardiograph. Not only must the medical engineer be aware of these factors, but also the individual who operates the electrocardiograph must be aware of them. In the following paragraphs, we shall describe a few of the more common problems encountered, and indicate some of their causes.

Frequency distortion

The electrocardiograph does not always meet the frequency-response standards described above. When this happens, frequency distortion is seen in the ECG. Figure 6.8 illustrates how frequency distortion can change an ECG.

Figure 6.8(a) shows a normal ECG taken with an instrument that has a frequency response wider than the prescribed 0.05 to 100 Hz.

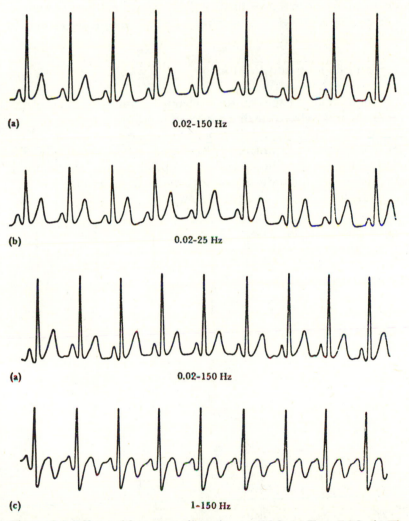

(a)   0.02-150 Hz

(b)   0.02-25 Hz

(a)   0.02-150 Hz

(c)   1-150 Hz

Figure 6.8 Effects of frequency distortion on ECG. (a) True ECG. (b) The same ECG when passed through a circuit that has diminished gain at high frequencies. This pattern is said to have high-frequency distortion. (c) The same ECG as in (a) when passed through an amplifier that has inadequate gain for low frequencies. This type is said to have low-frequency distortion.

Figure 6.8(b) shows the original ECG when recorded with a machine that has a frequency response of from 0.02 to 25 Hz. In this case we have what is known as *high-frequency distortion*, which results in rounding off the sharp corners of the waveforms, as well as in diminishing the amplitude of the QRS complex.

Figure 6.8(c) shows this same ECG when recorded by an instrument that has a frequency response of 1–150 Hz. Note the distortion in the baseline of this ECG. It is no longer horizontal, especially immediately following any event in the tracing. Note, furthermore, that monophasic waves in the ECG appear to be more biphasic in nature in this recording. Such effects may be considered together and referred to as *low-frequency distortion* of the ECG.

Saturation or cutoff distortion

High offset voltages at the electrodes or improperly adjusted amplifiers in the electrocardiograph can produce saturation or cutoff distortion that can greatly modify the appearance of the ECG. Figure 6.9(a) shows a normal ECG. Figure 6.9(b) shows how the waveform is distorted by saturation. In this case, the combination of input-signal amplitude and offset voltage drives a portion of the

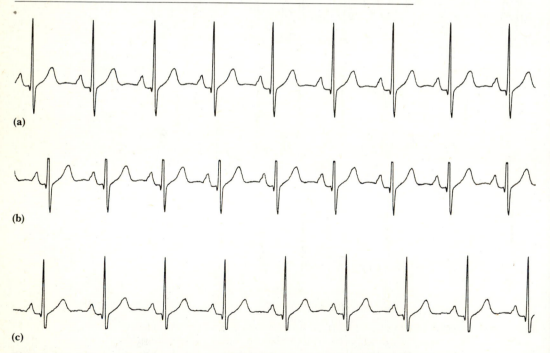

(a)

(b)

(c)

Figure 6.9 Effects of saturation or cutoff distortion on ECG. (a) Undistorted ECG. (b) Clipping of peak of the ECG in (a) due to positive-saturation effects in the amplifier. (c) Clipping of lower voltages in the ECG of (a) due to negative saturation or cutoff effects in amplifier.

amplifier into saturation (Section 3.2). The peaks of the QRS complex are thereby cut off, since the output of the amplifier cannot exceed the saturation voltage.

Figure 6.9(c) shows a similar occurrence in which the lower portions of the ECG are cut off. This can be the result of negative saturation of a portion of the amplifier. Note that in this case the baseline is perfectly flat. Peaks of the P and T waves may still be seen in the recordings, or they may be below the cutoff level, so that only the R wave appears.

Ground loops

Patients having their ECGs taken on either a clinical electrocardiograph or continuously on a cardiac monitor are often connected to other pieces of electrical apparatus. Each electrical device has its own ground connection, either through the power line, or, in some cases, through a heavy ground wire attached to some ground point in the room.

A *ground loop* can exist when the situation of Figure 6.10(a) occurs. Here two machines are connected to the patient. Both the electrocardiograph and machine X have a ground electrode attached to the patient. The electrocardiograph is grounded through the power line at a particular socket, which we denote as ground A. Machine X is also grounded through the power line, but it is plugged into an entirely different outlet across the room, which has a different ground, denoted as ground B. If ground B is at a slightly higher potential than ground A, a current from ground B flows to machine X's electrode on the patient and then through the patient to the ground electrode of the electrocardiograph and along its lead wire to ground point A. In addition to this current presenting a safety problem, it can elevate the patient's body potential to some voltage above the lowest ground (in this case ground A) to which the instrumentation is attached. In the example in Figure 6.10(a), the patient would be at some potential between that of ground B and that of ground A. This produces common-mode voltages on the electrocardiograph which, if it has a poor common-mode-rejection ratio, can increase the amount of artifact seen.

The current path between the two grounds, as shown in Figure 6.10(a), is referred to as a ground loop. It is something that should be avoided in medical-instrumentation systems.

A much more appropriate situation is shown in Figure 6.10(b). Here both machines are grounded at the same point. There are no loops in the ground circuit. Ground potential on the electrocardiograph and on machine X should be the same unless one or the other of these machines, due to faulty operation, is passing a fairly large current through its grounding circuit to the

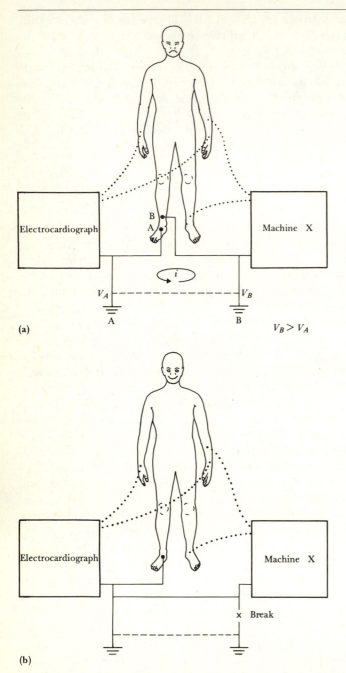

(a)

$V_B > V_A$

(b)

Figure 6.10 (a) Example of a ground loop between an electrocardiograph and another electrical machine connected to the same patient. Each machine is grounded separately and also connected to the patient, so that there is a closed path from ground A on the electrocardiograph to ground B on machine X. Current returns through dashed line representing connection between grounds in the wall, and thereby establishes the loop. (b) Ground loop can be eliminated by connecting both machines to the same ground and having only one connection to the patient.

ground point. In such a case, there could be a voltage drop along the ground conductor that caused the machine to be at a higher potential than the ground point. Even so, the patient is grounded through only one machine, so that no current can flow in the ground circuit through the patient. Normally, both machines have the same ground potential, so no current can flow through the ground connection to the patient, even if the patient is accidentally grounded to more than one machine.

Another problem caused by the ground currents shown in Figure 6.10(a) is related to the fact that, since the ground lead of the electrocardiograph usually runs alongside the signal leads, magnetic fields caused by the current in the grounding circuit can induce small voltages in the signal lead wires. This can produce artifact on the tracing.

By their very nature, ground loops represent closed current paths. Thus they must subtend some geometric area within the loop. If this area is large and in a region of a strong time-varying magnetic field (such as could be produced by other electrical devices connected to the power line, or, for that matter, the power line itself), a current can be induced in the ground loop. This process, which we shall describe in more detail later, can cause a ground current to flow through the patient, as in the case described above, or it can cause common-mode voltages.

Open lead wires

Frequently one of the wires connecting a biopotential electrode to the electrocardiograph can become disconnected from its electrode or broken as a result of excessively rough handling, in which case the electrode is no longer connected to the electrocardiograph. Relatively high potentials can often be induced in the open wire due to electric fields emanating from the power lines or other sources in the vicinity of the machine. This results in a wide, constant-amplitude deflection of the pen on the recorder at the power-line frequency, as well as, of course, signal loss. Such a situation also arises when an electrode is not making good contact with the patient. A circuit for detecting poor electrode contact is described in Section 6.9.

Artifact from large electrical transients

In some situations in which a patient is having an ECG taken, cardiac defibrillation may be required (Section 12.2). In such a case, a high-voltage, high-current electrical pulse is applied to the chest of the patient, so that transient potentials can be observed across the electrodes. These potentials can be several orders of magnitude higher than the normal potentials encountered in the ECG. Other electrical sources can cause similar transients. When this situation occurs, it can cause an abrupt deflection in the ECG, as shown in Figure 6.11. This is due to the saturation of the amplifiers in the electrocardiograph caused by the relatively high-amplitude pulse at its input. This pulse is sufficiently large to cause the buildup of charge on coupling capacitances in the amplifier, resulting in its remaining saturated for a finite period of time following the pulse, and then slowly drifting back to the original baseline with a time constant determined by the low corner frequency of the amplifier. The slowly recovering waveform is shown in Figure 6.11.

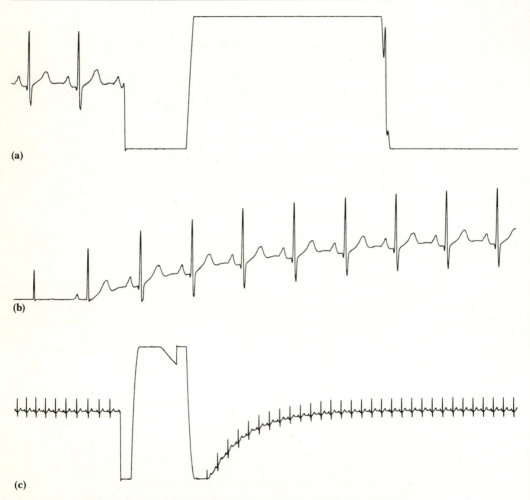

(a)

(b)

(c)

Figure 6.11 Effect of a voltage transient on an ECG recorded on an electrocardiograph in which the transient causes the amplifier to saturate and a finite period of time is required for the charge to bleed off enough to bring the ECG back into the amplifier's active region of operation. (a) Initiation of the transient. (b) Continuation of (a), showing recovery. (c) Similar transient at reduced gain to illustrate first-order recovery of system.

Transients of the type just described can be generated by means other than defibrillation. Serious artifact caused by motion of the electrodes can produce variations in potential greater than ECG potentials. Another source of artifact is the patient's encountering a built-up static electric charge that can be partially discharged through the body.

This problem is greatly alleviated by reducing the source of the artifact. Since we do not have time to disconnect an electrocardiograph when a patient is being defibrillated, we can include electronic protection circuitry, such as described in Section 6.4, in the machine itself. In this way, we can limit the maximum input voltage across the ECG amplifier so as to minimize the saturation and charge buildup effects due to the high-voltage input signals. This results in a more rapid return to normal operation following the transient. Such circuitry is also important in protecting the electrocardiograph from any damage that might be caused by such pulses.

Artifact caused by static electric charge on personnel can be noticeably lessened by reducing the buildup of static charge through the use of conductive clothing, shoes, and flooring, as well as by having personnel touch the bed before the patient. Motion artifact from the electrodes can be decreased by using the techniques described in Chapter 5.

Example 6.2 Figure 6.22 shows a practical ECG amplifier circuit. The final stage is coupled through a 1-μF capacitor. Suppose that a 100-mV transient appears across the input which lasts long enough to charge this capacitor to its peak value. How long will it take the baseline to return to within 1 mV of its original value?

Answer Since the nominal gain of the previous dc-coupled stages is 25, the 100-mV transient will have an amplitude of 2.5 V at the coupling capacitor. Thus it will be charged to that voltage. It must discharge through the 3.3-MΩ resistor, so the input voltage of the follower-with-gain stage is

$$v_i = (2.5 \text{ V}) \exp\left(-\frac{t}{3.3 \text{ M}\Omega \times 1.0 \ \mu\text{F}}\right)$$

$$= (2.5 \text{ V}) \exp\left(-\frac{t}{3.3}\right) \tag{E6.6}$$

A 1-mV baseline offset at the input is equivalent to a 25-mV offset at the input of the follower-with-gain stage. The time it takes the amplifier to recover to this point is

$$0.025 \text{ V} = (2.5 \text{ V}) \exp\left(-\frac{t}{3.3}\right) \tag{E6.7}$$

$$t = -3.3 \times \ln (0.01) = 15.2 \text{ s} \tag{E6.8}$$

Interference from electrical devices

A major source of artifact when one is recording or monitoring the ECG is the electric-power system. Besides providing power to the electrocardiograph itself, power lines are connected to other pieces of equipment and appliances in the typical hospital room or physician's office. There are also power lines in the walls, floor, and ceiling running past the room to other points in the building. These power lines can affect the recording of the ECG and introduce interference at the line frequency in the recorded trace, as illustrated in Figure 6.12(a). Such interference appears on the recordings as a result of two mechanisms, each operating singly, or, in some cases, together.

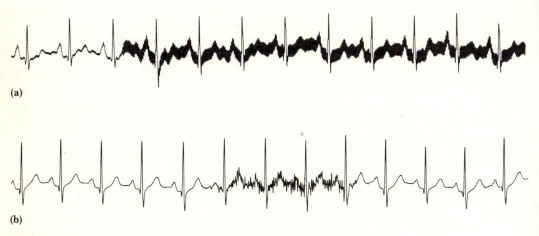

(a)

(b)

Figure 6.12 (a) 60-Hz power-line interference. (b) Electromyographic interference on the ECG. Severe 60-Hz interference is also shown on the bottom tracing in Figure 4.14.

Electric-field coupling between the power lines and the electrocardiograph and/or the patient is a result of the electric fields surrounding main power lines and the power cords connecting different pieces of apparatus to electrical outlets. These fields can be present even when the apparatus is not turned on, since current is not necessary to establish the electric field. These fields couple into the patient, the lead wires, and the electrocardiograph itself. It is almost as though small capacitors joined these entities to the power lines, as shown by the crude model in Figure 6.13.

The current through the capacitance C_3 coupling the ungrounded side of the power line and the electrocardiograph itself flows to ground and does not cause interference. C_1 represents the capacitance between the power line and one of the leads. Current i_{d1} does not flow into the electrocardiograph because of its high input impedance, but rather through the skin-electrode resistances

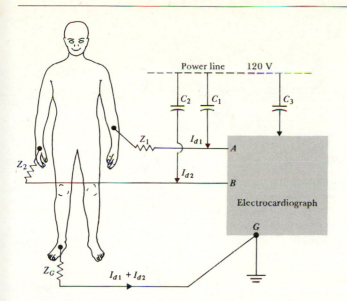

Figure 6.13 A mechanism of electric-field pickup of an electrocardiograph due to the power line. Coupling capacitance between hot side of power line and lead wires causes current to flow through skin-electrode impedances on its way to ground.

Z_1 and Z_G to ground. Similarly, i_{d2} flows through Z_2 and Z_G to ground. Body impedance, which is about 500 Ω, can be neglected when compared with the other impedances shown. The voltage amplified is that appearing between input A and B, $v_A - v_B$.

$$v_A - v_B = i_{d1}Z_1 - i_{d2}Z_2 \tag{6.2}$$

Huhta and Webster (1973) suggest that if the two leads run near each other, $i_{d1} \cong i_{d2}$. In this case,

$$v_A - v_B = i_{d1}(Z_1 - Z_2) \tag{6.3}$$

Values measured for 9-m cables show that $i_d \cong 6$ nA. Skin-electrode impedances may differ by as much as 20 kΩ. Hence

$$v_A - v_B = (6 \text{ nA})(20 \text{ k}\Omega) = 120 \ \mu\text{V} \tag{6.4}$$

which would be an objectionable level of interference. This can be minimized by shielding the leads and grounding each shield at the electrocardiograph. This is, in fact, done in most modern electrocardiographs. Lowering skin-electrode impedances is also helpful.

Figure 6.14 shows that current also flows from the power line into the body. The displacement current i_{db} flows through the

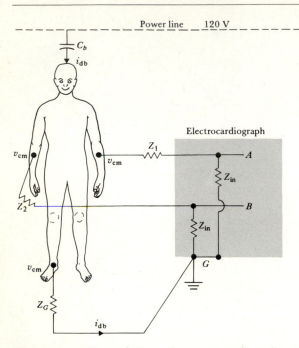

Figure 6.14 Current flows from power line through body and ground impedance, thus creating a common-mode voltage everywhere on the body.

ground impedance Z_G to ground. The resulting voltage drop causes a common mode voltage v_{cm} to appear throughout the body.

$$v_{cm} = i_{db} Z_G \tag{6.5}$$

Substituting typical values yields

$$v_{cm} = (0.2 \ \mu A)(50 \ k\Omega) = 10 \ mV \tag{6.6}$$

In poor electrical environments in which $i_{db} > 1 \ \mu A$, v_{cm} can be greater than 50 mV. For a perfect amplifier, this would cause no problem, because a differential amplifier rejects common-mode voltages (Section 3.4). However, real amplifiers have finite input impedances Z_{in}. Thus v_{cm} is decreased because of the attenuator action of the skin-electrode impedances and Z_{in}. That is,

$$v_A - v_B = v_{cm} \left(\frac{Z_{in}}{Z_{in} + Z_1} - \frac{Z_{in}}{Z_{in} + Z_2} \right) \tag{6.7}$$

Because Z_1 and Z_2 are much less than Z_{in},

$$v_A - v_B = v_{cm} \left(\frac{Z_2 - Z_1}{Z_{in}} \right) \tag{6.8}$$

Substituting typical values yields

$$v_A - v_B = (10 \text{ mV})(20 \text{ k}\Omega/5 \text{ M}\Omega) = 40 \text{ }\mu\text{V} \qquad (6.9)$$

which would be noticeable on an ECG and would be very objectionable on an EEG. This can be minimized by lowering skin-electrode impedance and raising amplifier input impedance.

Thus we see that the difference between the skin-electrode impedances is an important consideration in the design of biopotential amplifiers. Some common-mode voltage is always present, so the input imbalance and Z_{in} are critical factors determining the common-mode rejection, no matter how good the differential amplifier itself is.

The other source of artifact from power lines is magnetic induction. Current in power lines establishes a *magnetic field* in the vicinity of the line. Magnetic fields can also sometimes originate from transformers and ballasts in fluorescent lights. If such magnetic fields pass through the effective single-turn coil produced by the electrocardiograph, lead wires, and the patient, as shown in Figure 6.15, a voltage is induced in this loop. This voltage is proportional to the magnetic-field strength and the area of the effective single-turn coil. It can be reduced by either (1) reducing the magnetic field through shielding, or by (2) keeping the electrocardiograph and leads away from potential magnetic-field regions (both of which are rather difficult to achieve in practice), or (3) by reducing the effective area of the single-turn coil. This last effect can

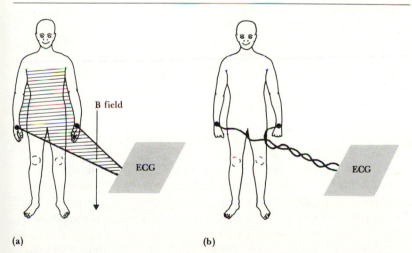

(a)   (b)

Figure 6.15 Magnetic-field pickup by the electrocardiograph. (a) Lead wires for lead I make a closed loop (shaded area) when patient and electrocardiograph are considered in the circuit. The change in magnetic field passing through this area induces a current in the loop. (b) This effect can be minimized by twisting the lead wires together and keeping them close to the body so as to subtend a much smaller area.

be easily achieved by twisting the lead wires together over as much of the distance between the electrocardiograph and the patient as possible.

Other sources of electrical interference

Electrical interference from sources other than the power lines can also affect the electrocardiograph. *Electromagnetic interference* from nearby high-power radio, television, or radar facilities can be picked up and rectified by the electronics in the electrocardiograph, and sometimes even by the electrode-electrolyte interface on the patient. The lead wires and the patient serve as an antenna. Once the signal is detected, the demodulated signal appears as interference on the electrocardiogram.

Electromagnetic interference can also be generated by high-frequency generators in the hospital itself. Electrosurgical and diathermy (Section 12.7) equipment is a frequent offender. Grobstein and Gatzke (1977) show both proper use of electrosurgical equipment and the design of ECG amplifier required to minimize interference. Electromagnetic radiation can be generated from x-ray machines or switches and relays on heavy-duty electrical equipment in the hospital as well. Even arcing in a fluorescent light that is flickering and in need of replacement can produce serious interference.

Electromagnetic interference can usually be minimized by shunting the input terminals to the electrocardiograph amplifier with a small capacitor. The reactance of this capacitor is quite high over the frequency range of the ECG, so it does not appreciably lower the input impedance of the electrocardiograph. However, with today's modern high-input-impedance machines, it is important to make sure that this is really the case. At radio frequencies, its reactance is low enough to cause effective shorting of the electromagnetic interference picked up by the lead wires and keep it from appearing at the amplifier input.

There is also a source of electrical artifact that can have an effect on ECGs located within the body itself. There is always muscle located between the electrodes making up a lead of the electrocardiograph. Any time that this muscle is contracting, it generates its own electromyographic signal that can be picked up by the lead along with the ECG and can result in interference on the ECG, as shown in Figure 6.12(b). When we look only at the ECG and not at the patient, it is sometimes very difficult to determine whether interference of this type is muscle artifact or the result of electromagnetic radiation. However, while the ECG is being taken, we can easily separate the two sources, since the EMG artifact is associated with the patient's muscle contractions.

6.4 Transient protection

The isolation circuits described in Section 13.9 are primarily for the protection of the patient, in that they eliminate the hazard of electric shock resulting from the interaction between the patient, the electrocardiograph, and other electrical devices in the patient's environment. There are also times when the patient can present a risk to the machine. For example, in the operating suite, patients undergoing surgery usually have their ECGs continuously monitored during the procedure. If the surgical procedure involves the use of an electrosurgical unit (Section 12.7), it can introduce onto the patient relatively high voltages that can enter the electrocardiograph or cardiac monitor through the patient's electrodes. If the ground connection to the electrosurgical unit is faulty or if higher-than-normal resistance is present, the patient's voltage with respect to ground can become quite high during coagulation or cutting. These high potentials enter the electrocardiograph or cardiac monitor and can be large enough to cause damage to the electronic circuitry. They can also cause severe transients on the recording, of the type shown in Figure 6.11.

Ideally, cardiac monitors and electrocardiographs should be designed so that they are unaffected by such transients. Unfortunately, this cannot be completely achieved. However, it is possible to reduce the effects of these electrical transients and to protect the equipment from serious damage. Figure 6.16 shows the basic arrangement of such protective circuits. Two-terminal voltage-limiting devices are connected between each patient electrode and electrical ground.

Figure 6.17(a) shows the typical current-voltage characteristic of such a device. At voltages less than V_b, the breakdown voltage, the device allows very little current to flow and ideally appears as an open circuit. Once the voltage across the device attempts to exceed

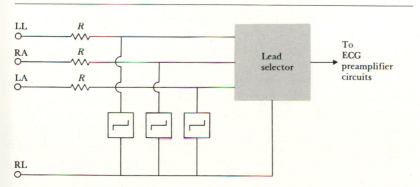

Figure 6.16 A voltage-protection scheme at the input of an electrocardiograph to protect machine from high-voltage transients. Circuit elements connected across limb leads on left-hand side are voltage-limiting devices.

V_b, the characteristics of the device sharply change and current passes through the device to such an extent that the voltage cannot exceed V_b due to the voltage drop across the series resistors R (in Figure 6.16). Under these conditions, the device appears to behave as a short circuit in series with a constant-voltage source of magnitude, V_b.

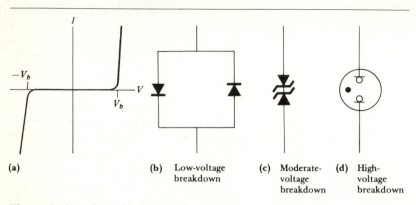

(a)   (b)   Low-voltage   (c)   Moderate-   (d)   High-
                           breakdown   voltage   voltage
                                             breakdown   breakdown

Figure 6.17 Voltage-limiting devices. (a) Current-voltage characteristics of a voltage-limiting device. (b) Parallel silicon-diode voltage-limiting circuit. (c) Back-to-back silicon Zener-diode voltage-limiting circuit. (d) Gas-discharge tube (neon light) voltage-limiting circuit element.

In practice, there are several ways that one can achieve a characteristic approaching this idealized characteristic. Figure 6.17 indicates three of these. *Parallel silicon diodes,* as shown in Figure 6.17(b), give a characteristic with a breakdown voltage of approximately 600 mV. The diodes are connected so that the terminal voltage on one has a polarity that is opposite to that on the other. Thus, when the voltage reaches approximately 600 mV, one of the diodes is forward-biased. And, even though the other is reverse-biased, its bias voltage is limited to the forward voltage drop. When the voltage across the network is reversed, roles of the two diodes are reversed, again limiting the voltage across the network to approximately 600 mV. The transition from the nonconducting to the conducting state, however, is not as sharp as shown in the characteristic curve, and signal distortion can begin to appear from these diodes at voltages of approximately 300 mV. Although the ECG itself does not approach such a voltage, it is possible under extreme conditions to achieve dc-offset potentials of that order of magnitude resulting from faulty electrodes. The main advantage of this circuit is its low breakdown voltage, so that the maximum transients at the amplifier input are only approximately 600 mV peak amplitude.

If the breakdown voltage of this circuit is too small, it can be increased simply by connecting two or more diodes in series instead of using single diodes in each branch. This has the advantage of not only increasing the breakdown voltage by multiplying the initial 600 mV by the number of diodes in series, but also increasing the resistance of the circuit, both in the conducting and nonconducting state.

When we want higher breakdown voltages, we can use the circuit of Figure 6.17(c). This consists of two silicon diodes, usually *zener diodes*, connected back to back. When a voltage is connected across this circuit, one of the diodes is biased in the forward direction and the other in the reverse direction. The breakdown voltage in the forward direction is approximately 600 mV, but that in the reverse direction is much higher. It generally covers the range of 3 to 20 V. Thus this circuit does not conduct until its terminal voltage exceeds the reverse breakdown of the diode by approximately 600 mV. Again, when the polarity of the circuit terminal voltage is reversed, the roles of the two diodes are interchanged. This circuit gives a sharp *V-I* characteristic at voltages ranging from approximately 3 to 20 V.

A device that gives a higher breakdown voltage is the *gas-discharge tube* illustrated in Figure 6.17(d). This device appears as an open circuit until it reaches its breakdown voltage. It then switches to the conducting state and maintains a voltage that is usually several volts less than the breakdown voltage. Breakdown voltages ranging from 50 to 90 V are typical for this device.

Designers of biopotential amplifiers often use miniature neon lamps as voltage limiters. They are very inexpensive and have a symmetrical characteristic, requiring only a single device per electrode pair. Their resistance in the nonconducting state is nearly infinite, so there is no loading effect on the electrodes—a feature that is most desirable when the biopotential amplifier has very high input impedance.

6.5 Common-mode and other interference-reduction circuits

As stated earlier, common-mode voltages can be responsible for much of the interference in biopotential amplifiers. Although having an amplifier with a high common-mode-rejection ratio minimizes the effects of common-mode voltages, a better approach to this problem is to discover the source of the voltage and try to eliminate it. In this section, we shall look at some of the sources of this and other types of interference and discover ways in which they can be minimized.

Electric- and magnetic-field pickup

As we saw in Section 6.3, electrical artifact can be introduced in systems of biopotential measurement through capacitive coupling and magnetic induction. We can minimize these interfering signals by trying to eliminate the sources of the signals by means of shielding techniques. Electrostatic shielding, as illustrated in Figure 6.18, is accomplished by placing a grounded conducting plane between the source of the electric field and the measurement system. The measurement of very low level biopotentials, such as the EEG, has traditionally been carried out in a shielded enclosure of this type to minimize noise. Many hospitals have shielded rooms for their EEG laboratories, with all the walls of the room containing either continuous solid-metal panels or at least grounded copper screening.

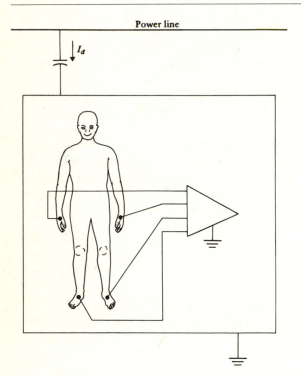

Figure 6.18 Electrostatic shielding to eliminate electric-field interference on an electrocardiograph. The electrostatic shielding is a conductor that surrounds patient and preamplifier of electrocardiograph to minimize electrostatic pickup. Displacement current from capacitive coupling to power lines is returned to ground through the shield rather than through electrocardiograph and patient.

This type of shielding is ineffective for magnetic fields unless the metal panels have a high permeability (such as sheet steel). In other words, the panels must be good magnetic conductors as well as good electrical conductors. Such rooms are available to provide magnetic shielding, but a much less expensive way of achieving a reduction of magnetically induced signals is to reduce the effective surface area between the differential inputs to the biopotential amplifier, in the case of differential signals, and between the inputs and ground, in the case of common-mode signals. Something as simple as a twisted pair of lead wires, as illustrated in Figure 6.15(b), may greatly improve the situation.

Elimination of ground loops

Ground loops, as described in Section 6.3, can generate common-mode voltages through flow of current in the grounding circuit. This can be caused by the existence of slightly different ground potentials in different electrical devices connected to the patient, or by magnetic induction. In either case, the method of eliminating the common-mode voltage is simple: Eliminate all ground loops. All measurement systems, as well as other electrical devices associated with the patient, should be grounded at a common point. Figure 6.10(b) illustrates how the ground-loop example given in Figure 6.10(a) can be modified to eliminate the loop. In setting up a biopotential instrumentation system, the engineer should design grounding circuits so that there is a single unique path between each component and ground, as well as a single unique path between the ground circuit of one component and that of any other component in the system. The grounding circuit should look like a star, with the ground point at its center and rays extending to each component of the system.

Driven-right-leg system

In many modern electrocardiographic systems, the patient is not grounded at all. Instead, the right-leg electrode is connected (as shown in Figure 6.19) to the output of an auxiliary op amp. The common-mode voltage on the body is sensed by the two averaging resistors R_a, inverted, amplified, and fed back to the right leg through R_o. This negative feedback drives the common-mode voltage to a low value. The body's displacement current does not flow to ground, but rather to the op-amp output circuit. This reduces the pickup as far as the ECG amplifier is concerned and effectively grounds the patient. Even lower common-mode voltage can be achieved by connecting R_f to RL instead of to the op amp output.

The circuit is also valuable in terms of electrical safety. If an abnormally high voltage should appear between the patient and ground due to electrical leakage or other means, the auxiliary op amp in Figure 6.19 saturates. This effectively ungrounds the patient, since the amplifier can no longer drive the right leg. Now the resistance R_o is between the patient and ground. It can be several megohms in value, and thus large enough to protect the patient.

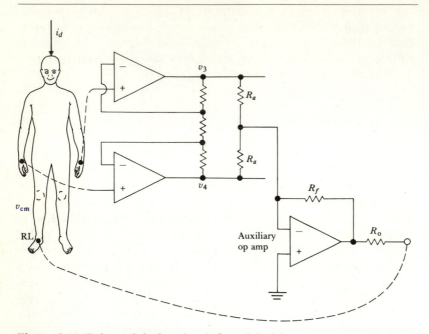

Figure 6.19 Driven-right-leg circuit for minimizing common-mode interference. The circuit derives common-mode voltage from a pair of
averaging resistors connected to v_3 and v_4 in Figure 3.5. The right leg is
not grounded, but is connected to output of auxiliary op amp.

Example 6.3 Determine the common-mode voltage v_{cm} on the
patient in the driven-right-leg circuit of Figure 6.19 when a displacement current i_d flows to the patient from the power lines.
Choose appropriate values for the resistances in the circuit so
that the common-mode voltage is minimal and there is only a
high-resistance path to ground when the auxiliary operational amplifier saturates. What is v_{cm} for this circuit when $i_d = 0.2\ \mu\text{A}$?

Answer The equivalent circuit for the circuit of Figure 6.19 is
shown in Figure E6.3. Note that, since the common-mode gain of
the input stage is 1 (Section 3.4), and since the input stage as shown
has a very high input impedance v_{cm} at the input is isolated from
the output circuit. Summing the currents at the negative input of
the operational amplifier, we get

$$\frac{2v_{cm}}{R_a} + \frac{v_o}{R_f} = 0 \tag{E6.9}$$

This gives

$$v_o = -\frac{2R_f}{R_a}\,v_{cm} \tag{E6.10}$$

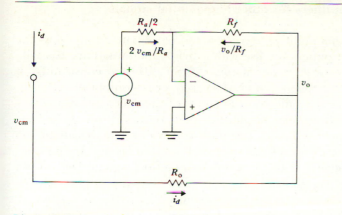

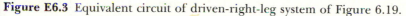

Figure E6.3 Equivalent circuit of driven-right-leg system of Figure 6.19.

but

$$v_{cm} = R_o i_d + v_o \tag{E6.11}$$

Thus, substituting (E6.10) into (E6.11), we find

$$v_{cm} = \frac{R_o i_d}{1 + 2R_f/R_a} \tag{E6.12}$$

The effective resistance between the right leg and ground is the resistance of the output resistor divided by 1, plus the gain of the auxiliary operational-amplifier circuit. When the amplifier saturates, as would occur during a large transient v_{cm}, its output appears as the saturation voltage v_s. The right leg is now connected through this source and R_o to ground. Under these conditions we want to isolate the patient from ground. Thus R_o should be large. Values as high as 5 MΩ are used.

When the amplifier is not saturated, we would like v_{cm} to be as small as possible, or, in other words, to be an effective low-resistance path to ground. This can be achieved by making R_f large and R_a relatively small. R_f can be equal to R_o, but R_a can be much smaller.

A typical value of R_a would be 25 kΩ. The effective resistance between the right leg and ground would now be

$$\frac{5 \text{ M}\Omega}{1 + \dfrac{2 \times 5 \text{ M}\Omega}{25 \text{ k}\Omega}} = 12.5 \text{ k}\Omega$$

For the 0.2-μA displacement current, the common-mode voltage is

$$v_{cm} = 12.5 \text{ k}\Omega \times 0.2 \text{ μA} = 2.5 \text{ mV}$$

6.6 Amplifiers for other biopotential signals

Up to this point we have stressed biopotential amplifiers for the ECG. Amplifiers for use with other biopotentials are basically the same. However, other signals do put different constraints on some aspects of the amplifier. The frequency content of different biopotentials covers different portions of the spectrum. Some biopotentials have higher amplitudes than others. Both these facts place gain and frequency-response constraints on the amplifiers used. Figure 6.20 shows the ranges of amplitudes and frequencies covered by several of the common biopotential signals. Depending on the signal, frequencies range from dc to about 10 kHz. Amplitudes can range from tens of microvolts to approximately 100 mV. The amplifier for a particular biopotential must be designed to handle that potential and provide an appropriate signal at its output.

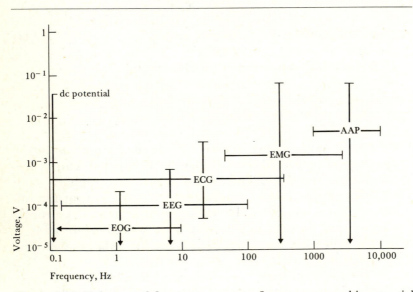

Figure 6.20 Voltage and frequency ranges of some common biopotential signals: dc potentials include intracellular voltages as well as voltages measured from several points on the body. EOG is the electrooculogram, EEG is the electroencephalogram, ECG is the electrocardiogram, EMG is the electromyogram, and AAP is the axon action potential. (From J.M.R. Delgado, "Electrodes for Extracellular Recording and Stimulation," in *Physical Techniques in Biological Research*, edited by W.L. Nastuk, New York: Academic Press, 1964.

The electrodes used to obtain the biopotential place certain constraints on the amplifier input stage. To achieve the most effective signal transfer, the amplifier must be matched to the electrodes. Also the amplifier input circuit must not promote the generation of artifact by the electrode, as could occur with excessive offset current. Let us look at a few requirements placed on different types of biopotential amplifiers by the measurement being made.

EMG amplifier

Figure 6.20 shows that electromyographic signals range in frequency from 25 Hz to several kilohertz. Signal amplitudes range from 100 μV to 90 mV, depending on the type of signal and electrodes used. Thus EMG amplifiers must have a wider frequency response than ECG amplifiers, but they do not have to cover as low a frequency range as the ECGs. This is desirable because motion artifact contains mostly low frequencies that can be more effectively filtered in EMG amplifiers than in ECG amplifiers, without affecting the signal.

If skin-surface electrodes are used to detect the EMG, the levels of signals are generally low, having peak amplitudes of the order of 0.1 to 1 mV. Electrode impedance is relatively low, ranging from about 200 to 5000 Ω, depending on the type of electrode, the electrode-electrolyte interface, and the frequency at which the impedance is determined. Thus the amplifier must have somewhat higher gain than the ECG amplifier for the same output-signal range, and its input characteristics should be almost the same as the ECG amplifier. If intramuscular needle electrodes are used, the EMG signals can be an order of magnitude stronger, thus requiring an order of magnitude less gain. Furthermore, the surface area of the EMG electrode is much less, so its source impedance is higher. Thus a higher amplifier input impedance is desirable for quality signal reproduction.

Amplifiers for use with glass micropipet intracellular electrodes

Intracellular electrodes or microelectrodes that can measure the potential across the cell membrane generally detect potentials of the order of 50 to 100 mV. Their small size and small effective surface-contact area give them a very high source impedance, and their geometry results in a relatively large shunting capacitance. These features place the constraint on the amplifier of requiring an extremely high input impedance. Furthermore, the high shunting capacitance of the electrode itself affects the frequency-response characteristics of the system. Often positive-feedback schemes are used in the biopotential amplifier to provide an effective negative capacitance that can compensate for the high shunt capacitance of the source.

The frequency response of microelectrode amplifiers must be quite wide. Intracellular electrodes are often used to measure the dc potential difference across a cell membrane, so the amplifier must be capable of responding to dc signals. When excitable cell-membrane potentials are to be measured, such as in muscle cells and nerve cells, rise times can contain frequencies of the order of 10 kHz and the amplifiers must be capable of passing these too. The fact that the potentials have relatively high potentials means that the voltage gain of the amplifier does not have to be as high as in previous examples.

A preamplifier circuit that is especially useful with microelectrodes is the negative-input-capacitance amplifier shown in Figure 6.21. The basic circuit consists of a low-gain, very-high-input-

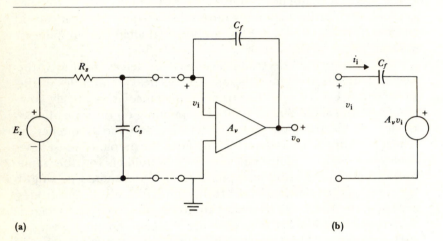

(a)   (b)

Figure 6.21 (a) Basic arrangement for negative-input capacitance amplifier. Basic amplifier is on right-hand side; equivalent source with lumped series resistance R_s and shunt capacitance C_s on the left. (b) Equivalent circuit of basic negative-input capacitance amplifier.

impedance, noninverting amplifier with a capacitor C_f providing positive feedback to the input. If we look at the equivalent circuit for this amplifier, as shown in Figure 6.21(b), we can relate the input voltage and current:

$$v_i = \frac{1}{C_f} \int i_i \, dt + A_v v_i \tag{6.10}$$

where A_v is the amplifier gain, provided the operational amplifier itself draws no current. This can be rearranged to be

$$v_i = \frac{1}{(1 - A_v)C_f} \int i_i \, dt \tag{6.11}$$

Thus the equivalent capacitance at the amplifier input is $(1 - A_v)C_f$. If A_v is greater than unity, this equivalent capacitance is negative. The amplifier is connected to the microelectrode, with its high source resistance R_s. The shunt capacitance from the electrode and cable is C_s. The total circuit capacitance is:

$$C = C_s + (1 - A_v)C_f \qquad (6.12)$$

This is zero when

$$C_s = (A_v - 1)C_f \qquad (6.13)$$

This condition can be met by adjusting either the amplifier gain A_v or the feedback capacitance C_f.

In practical negative-input-capacitance amplifiers, the idealized condition of (6.13) cannot be met, since the gain of any amplifier has some frequency dependence. There are thus frequencies wherein the input capacitance of the amplifiers does not cancel the source capacitance and the circuit does not have an ideal transient response. Since the amplifier employs positive feedback and does not have an ideal frequency response, it is possible for the conditions of oscillation to be met at some frequency, and the amplifier will then become unstable. Thus it is important that the amplifier be carefully adjusted to meet the condition of (6.13) as closely as possible without becoming unstable. Another consequence of the positive feedback is that the amplifier tends to be noisy. This, however, is not a serious problem, since the voltages from microelectrodes are usually relatively high.

EEG amplifiers

Figure 6.20 shows that the EEG requires an amplifier with a frequency response of from 0.1 to 100 Hz. When surface electrodes are used, as in clinical electroencephalography, amplitudes of signals range from 25 to 100 μV. Thus amplifiers with relatively high gain are required. These electrodes are smaller than those used for the ECG, so they have somewhat higher source impedances, and a high input impedance is essential in the EEG amplifier. Because the signal levels are so small, common-mode voltages can have more serious effects. Therefore more stringent efforts must be made to reduce common-mode artifact, as well as to use amplifiers with higher common-mode-rejection ratios and low noise.

6.7 Example of a biopotential preamplifier

As we have seen, biopotential amplifiers can be used for a variety of signals. The gain and frequency response are two important variables that relate the amplifier to the particular signal. An important factor common to all amplifiers is the first stage, or preamplifier. This stage must have low noise, since its output must be amplified through the remaining stages of the amplifier, and any noise is amplified along with the signal. It must also be coupled directly to the electrodes (i.e., no series capacitors) to provide optimal low-frequency response as well as to minimize charging effects on coupling capacitors from input offset current. Of course, every attempt should be made to minimize this current, since, even without coupling capacitors, it can polarize the electrodes, resulting in polarization overpotentials that produce a large dc offset voltage at the amplifier's input. It is for this reason that preamplifiers often have relatively low voltage gains. Since the offset potential is coupled directly to the input, it could saturate high-gain preamplifiers, cutting out the signal altogether. To eliminate the saturating effects of this dc potential, the preamplifier can be capacitor-coupled to the remaining amplifier stages. A final consideration of the preamplifier is that it must have a very high input impedance, since it represents the load on the electrodes.

Often, for safety reasons, the preamplifier either is electrically isolated from the remaining amplifier stages (and hence from the power lines) (Section 13.9), or is located near the signal source to minimize noise pickup on the high-impedance lead wires. In the latter case, we can use for the circuit a battery-powered preamplifier with low power consumption or a power supply that is electrically isolated.

Figure 6.22 shows the circuit of an ECG amplifier. The instrumentation amplifier of Figure 3.5 is used to provide very high input impedance. High common-mode rejection is achieved by adjusting the potentiometer to about 47 kΩ. Electrodes may produce an offset potential of up to 0.2 V. Thus, to prevent saturation, the dc-coupled stages have a gain of only 25. Coupling capacitors are not placed at the input because this would block the op-amp bias current. Adding resistors to supply the bias current would lower the Z_{in}. Coupling capacitors placed after the first op amps would have to be impractically large. Therefore the single 1-μF coupling capacitor plus the 3.3-MΩ resistor form a high-pass filter. The resulting 3.3-s time constant passes all frequencies above 0.05 Hz. The output stage is a follower with gain having a gain of 32 (Section 3.3).

A second 3.3-MΩ resistor is added to balance bias-current source impedances. The 150 kΩ to 0.01 μF low-pass filter attenuates frequencies above 100 Hz. Switch S_1 may be momentarily closed when the output saturates. This is required after defibrillation or lead switching to rapidly charge the 1-μF capacitor to the new value and return the output to the linear region. Switch closure may be automatic, using a circuit that detects when the output is in saturation, or it may be manual. Although the 741 op amp is

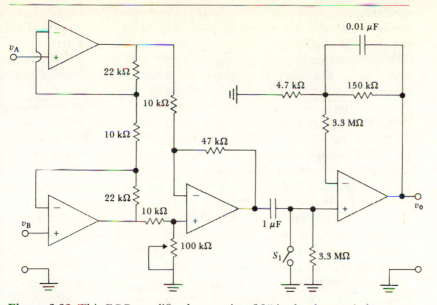

Figure 6.22 This ECG amplifier has a gain of 25 in the dc-coupled stages. The high-pass filter feeds a follower-with-gain stage having a gain of 32. The total gain is 25 × 32 = 800. Using μA 776 op amps, the circuit was found to have a CMRR of 86 dB at 100 Hz and noise level of 40 mV peak to peak at the output. The frequency response was 0.04 to 150 Hz for ±3 dB and was flat over 4 to 40 Hz.

satisfactory in this circuit, an op amp such as the 308, which has lower bias current, may be preferred.

6.8 Other biopotential signal processors

Up to now we have looked at amplifiers as biopotential signal processors. Although the amplifier is always an important constituent of a biopotential signal processor, it can be a part of systems containing additional circuitry that can further process the signal. In this section we shall look at some of the more common processors that are used to handle biopotential signals.

Cardiotachometers

A cardiotachometer is a device for determining heart rate. The signal most frequently used is the ECG. However, circuitry for deriving heart rate from signals such as the arterial pressure waveform or heart sounds has also been developed.

There are two basic kinds of cardiotachometers. The averaging cardiotachometer determines average heart rate by counting the pulse over a known period of time. The beat-to-beat cardiotachometer, on the other hand, determines the reciprocal of the time interval between heartbeats for each beat and presents it as the heart rate for that particular interval. If there is any slight variability in the interval between beats, it shows up as a variation in the instantaneous heart rate determined by this method.

A typical averaging cardiotachometer is shown in block-diagram form in Figure 6.23. Its input consists of an amplified ECG with an amplitude of approximately 1 V p–p. This signal is passed through a bandpass filter that serves two purposes: It removes low-frequency noise and baseline drift, so that the signal can be threshold-detected. It also passes only those frequencies that are associated with the QRS complex, thereby providing optimal reduction of noise. Of course, much of the electrocardiogram is lost because of this filtering, as indicated by the waveforms, but it is still possible to use this device to determine heart rate.

Bandpass filters in adult cardiotachometers typically cover the frequency range from 10 to 50 Hz. The signal is passed through a threshold detector that indicates when the signal amplitude is greater than a fixed level. When this occurs, the threshold detector causes a pulse generator to generate a pulse of fixed duration that is longer than the Q–S interval. This allows only one pulse to be generated per QRS complex. All pulses generated have the same amplitude and width. They are fed to the same low-pass active-filter circuit, as shown in Figure 3.13(a). The circuit determines the average amplitude of the pulse train coming from the pulse generator. The resistor bleeds off charge from the capacitor, so that a fixed average voltage is reached for any particular pulse rate. For this to occur, the time constant of the RC circuit must be at least several beats in duration. (Typically, the values of 5 to 15 s are used.) The higher the heart rate, the more frequent the appearance of pulses from the pulse generator. These cause a larger charge to build up on the capacitor, which in turn increases the output voltage from the circuit. Since the resistor R shunts the output to the virtual ground, the increased heart rate results in increased current through the resistor. This current must come from the capacitor charge, so after several beats an equilibrium voltage is reached. The waveform emanating from this circuit is not pure dc. Each pulse increases the charge on the capacitor, and this charge can then bleed off between pulses to give a sawtooth waveform. However, on some averaging cardiotachometers, we can see the pulsations if we look carefully at the meter.

Cardiotachometers often have *alarm circuits* to indicate when heart rates have exceeded or gone below certain preset levels. Figure 6.23 shows an example of such an alarm circuit. It consists of a comparator circuit connected to the output of the low-pass filter. A variable voltage is available at one of the comparator inputs to set the trigger level for the comparator. When the heart-rate voltage increases above or decreases below the upper or lower point set on the comparator, the circuit turns on an alarm. Cardiotachometers that have an analog-meter indicator sometimes carry out the comparison function by a meter relay. Small electrical or light-beam relay contacts are housed in the meter body, so that when the pointer exceeds a preset high level or falls beneath a preset low level, the contacts are closed and the alarm circuit is energized.

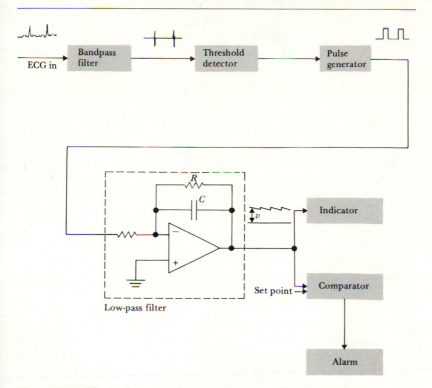

Figure 6.23 Block diagram of an averaging cardiotachometer.

Figure 6.24 shows a beat-to-beat cardiotachometer. As with the averaging cardiotachometer, the ECG initially passes through a bandpass filter, which passes QRS complexes while reducing artifact and most of the P and T waves. The threshold detector triggers the first 10-μs monostable multivibrator, which produces pulse P_1, as shown in the timing diagram of Figure 6.25.

The falling edge of pulse P_1 triggers a second monostable multivibrator that also produces a 10-μs duration pulse P_2. This pulse occurs 10 μs after the initiation of pulse P_1, as shown in the timing diagram. These two pulses control a NOR (not OR) circuit, which has output P_3. This signal is high during the interval when P_1 and P_2 are not occurring. Immediately following the initiation of a QRS complex, pulse P_3 goes low for a total of 20 μs and is then returned to its initial level. The signal controls an AND gate, so that a

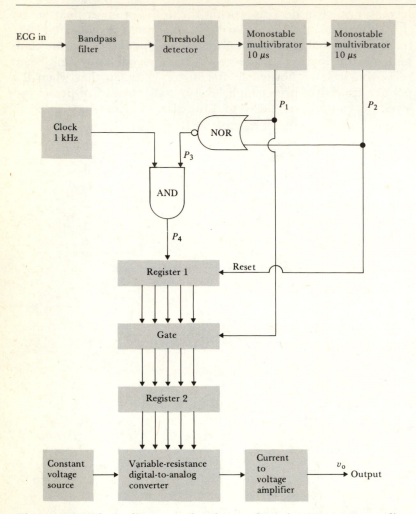

Figure 6.24 Block diagram of a beat-to-beat instantaneous cardiota-chometer.

1-kHz clock signal is allowed to enter a counting register whenever P_3 is high. Since P_3 is high during the interval between QRS complexes, the 1-ms pulses coming from the clock (P_4) accumulate in register 1 during this period. If the register is initially at zero, the number of pulses in the register by the time the next QRS complex arrives equals the number of milliseconds in the interval between this QRS complex and the previous one. Once the gate prohibits additional clock pulses from entering register 1, pulse P_1 enables the signal in this register to be stored in a second register, which serves as a memory. The second register is connected to a digital-to-analog converter of the type that produces a resistance proportional to the digital signal at its input. The resistance is proportional to the time interval between QRS complexes. Resistance is connected across a constant-voltage source, yielding a current given by

$$i = \frac{v}{R} = \frac{k}{T_R} \tag{6.14}$$

where k is a constant and T_R is the interval between QRS complexes. We see that the current in the circuit is proportional to the reciprocal of the beat-to-beat time interval of the original ECG, or in other words, it is proportional to the heart rate. The signal is amplified through a current-to-voltage amplifier, giving the output voltage v_0, as shown in Figure 6.25. Note that this voltage shifts with each heartbeat and that its amplitude is proportional to the duration of the previous beat-to-beat interval.

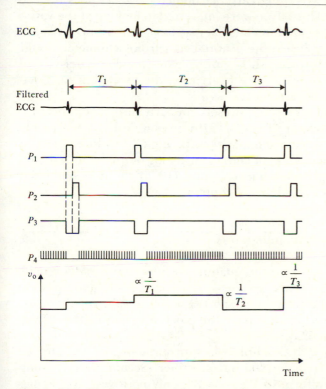

Figure 6.25 Timing diagram for beat-to-beat cardiotachometer in Figure 6.24.

It is important to note that the contents of register 1 must be zero before the gate is opened to let the clock pulses enter that register. It is for this reason that, once the contents of register 1 have been transferred to register 2, pulse P_2 enters the reset terminal of register 1, sets it to zero, and prepares it to count the next beat-to-beat interval.

Alarm circuits may also be used with this type of cardiota-chometer. Often these circuits consist of digital rather than analog comparators, which compare the signal in register 1 to determine whether an interval of longer than a preset value has occurred (which could happen when the heart rate was too low). An additional comparator can monitor the signal in register 2 to determine whether it is less than a preset value, a situation that would occur if the heart rate were too high. In either case, the comparators can then be used to activate appropriate alarms.

In comparing the averaging and beat-to-beat cardiotachom-eters, we see that the latter respond more rapidly to changes in heart rate. Since the interval between QRS complexes usually changes slightly from one beat to the next, the output from the beat-to-beat cardiotachometer varies slightly with each beat. On the other hand, the averaging cardiotachometer usually does not see such variations. Thus, if we were interested in looking at the variability in heart rate (a parameter that may be of importance in monitoring of the fetal heart) the beat-to-beat cardiotachometer would be the only way to proceed. If, on the other hand, we were more concerned with trends in the heart rate, the averaging cardiota-chometer would be adequate.

Ludwig and Ng (1967) present an early design of a beat-to-beat cardiotachometer. Taylor (1975) gives a design for a highly accurate digital cardiotachometer with digital readout. Hartley (1976) presents a method of getting an analog output from a digital rate-determining circuit. Fichtenbaum (1976) shows a simplified design based on a divide-by-N counter.

Electromyogram integrators

It is often of interest to quantify the amount of EMG activity measured by a particular system of electrodes. Such quantification often assumes the form of taking the absolute value of the EMG and integrating it, as shown by the block diagram of the system shown in Figure 6.26.

The raw EMG, amplified appropriately, is fed to an absolute-value circuit or full-wave rectifier (Section 3.6). As indicated in the waveform of Figure 6.27, only positive-going signals (v_2) result following this block. The negative-going portions of the signal have been inverted, making them positive. The signal is then integrated in the operational-amplifier integrator (Section 3.8). The feedback capacitor is charged according to the integral of the incoming waveform. Once the integrator output has exceeded a preset threshold level, a comparator at the output of the integrator fires a monostable multivibrator. The pulse emanating from the multivibrator closes a switch that discharges the integrator's capacitor. The duration of the pulse from the multivibrator must be at least five times greater than the time constant of the capacitor and

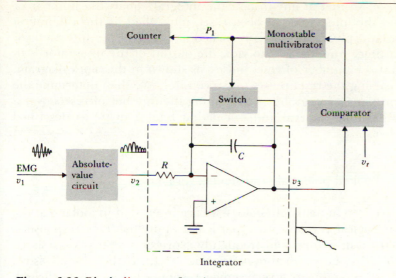

Figure 6.26 Block diagram of an integrator for EMG signals.

closed-switch circuit to ensure nearly complete discharge of the capacitor. The integrator then reinitiates integration of the EMG until the cycle repeats itself.

We can view the output from the integrator in two ways. The actual voltage output from the integrator can be recorded on a conventional strip-chart recorder to give the actual integral at any instant in time. The total integral necessary to reset the integrator is

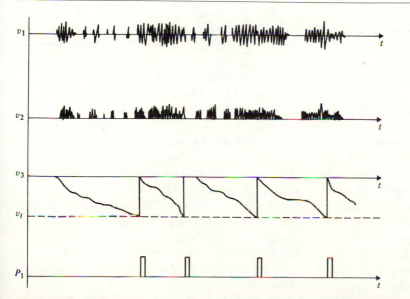

Figure 6.27 The various waveforms for EMG integrator circuit in Figure 6.26.

known, so that at any instant the integral equals the number of times the integrator has been reset, multiplied by this calibration constant, plus whatever is recorded as being in the integrator at that time. Another way to view the output of the integrator is to count the number of reset pulses, as shown in the block diagram, by passing the reset pulses into a counter. We then determine the approximate integral by determining the number of resets over a specific time interval and calculating total activity, as described earlier.

Evoked potentials and signal averagers

Often in neurophysiology we are interested in looking at the neurological response to a particular stimulus. This response is electrical in nature, and frequently represents a very weak signal with a very poor signal-to-noise ratio (SNR). If the stimulus is repeated, the same or a very similar response is repeatedly elicited. This is the basis for biopotential signal processors, which can obtain an enhanced response by means of repeated application of the stimulus.

Figure 6.28 shows the principle. The basic idea is to record the responses. This process is then repeated for the second sample point, the third, and so on. The sum of the individual responses can then be displayed, as shown at the bottom of Figure 6.28, with the stimulus serving as reference point. The number of repeated samples averaged together can be higher than 1000.

The noise on the individual responses is random with respect to the stimulus. This means that if a large enough sample is taken, some positive-going noise pulses at a particular instant after the stimulus partially cancel some negative-going noise spikes at the same instant. Thus the net sum of the noise at any instant following the stimulus increases as $\sqrt{n}$, where n is the number of responses. The evoked response, on the other hand, follows the same time course after each stimulus. Thus there is no cancellation in this signal as the individual responses are summed. Instead, the amplitude of the evoked response increases in direct proportion to n. By repetitive summing, one is thus able to enhance the SNR by the factor $n/\sqrt{n} = \sqrt{n}$.

This technique is frequently used with the EEG. As stated earlier in this chapter, EEGs obtained from surface electrodes are very weak and consequently can have a high noise component. If a repetitive stimulus (such as electric shock, flashing light, or repeating sound) is applied to the test subject, it is often difficult to ascertain the response in a directly recorded EEG. However, if we apply this signal summing or averaging technique, it is possible to obtain the evoked response.

The hardware necessary to carry out signal averaging varies

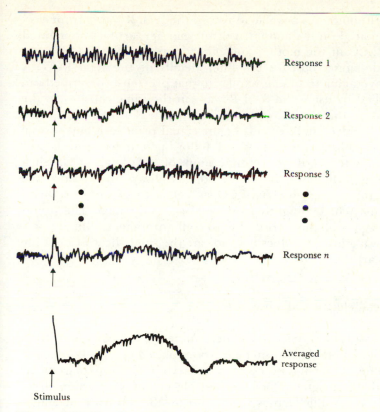

Response 1

Response 2

Response 3

Response n

Averaged response

Stimulus

Figure 6.28 Signal-averaging technique for improvement of SNR in signals that are repetitive or respond to a known stimulus.

from general-purpose digital-computing systems, which have to be specifically programmed for signal averaging, to smaller, less expensive, dedicated computing circuitry, which can carry out only this function. Such systems are referred to as *average-response computers*. The basic scheme involves digitizing the signal and then locating the stimulus. The first sample of the response is stored in a given register, the second sample is stored in the next register, and so on. After the second application of the stimulus, the signal is again digitized and the stimulus is located. The first sample after the stimulus is added to what is already in the first register, and the sum remains in that register. The second sample is added to the contents of the second register and remains there, and so on. The group of registers contains the summed signal and can be read in succession to display that signal on an oscilloscope or chart recorder. The operator of the system can look at the sum after each application of the stimulus to determine how many stimuli are necessary to adequately extract the signal from the noise.

This technique can be used without applying the external stimulus. One example of its use is the recording of the ECG of a fetus. Although it is possible to record the fetal R waves from electrodes placed on the abdomen of the mother, artifacts generated by the ECG of the mother and other biopotentials, as well as by electrode noise, obscure the finer details of the fetal ECG. A signal-averaging technique similar to that previously described can be applied by using the fetal R wave in the same capacity as the stimulus. In this case the computer locates the R wave and averages several hundred milliseconds of the signal prior to it and several hundred milliseconds of the signal following it, in order to recover the complete P-QRS-T configuration of the fetal ECG. Such averaging techniques, however, do not always work, since the various intervals of the fetal ECG, as well as the waveforms themselves, may change slightly from one beat to the next. The sum is an average of all the recorded ECG configurations and might provide a waveform that does not indicate the single-beat ECG of the fetal heart.

Fetal electrocardiography

As we said, physicians can determine the ECG of a fetus from a pair of biopotential-sensing electrodes placed on the abdomen of the mother. Often it is necessary to try several different placements to get the best signal. Once the best placement is determined, we obtain a recording such as that shown in the top trace of Figure 6.29. For comparison, Figure 6.29 also shows a direct ECG of the same fetus and a direct ECG of the same mother. The fetal ECG signal is usually quite weak, generally having an amplitude of around 50 μV or less. This makes it extremely difficult to record the heartbeat of the fetus using electrodes attached to the abdomen of the mother during labor, when the mother is restless and motion artifact as well as EMG interfere. There is also considerable interference from the ECG of the mother.

Note that the QRS complexes of the mother are much stronger than those of the fetus, which makes it difficult to determine the fetal heart rate electronically from recordings of this type. This information can be obtained by hand, however, by measuring the fetal R–R interval on the chart and converting this to heart rate.

Several methods have been devised for improving the quality of fetal ECGs obtained by attaching electrodes to the mother's abdomen. In addition to the signal-averaging technique previously described, physicians have applied various forms of anticoincidence detectors to eliminate the maternal QRS complexes (Offner and Moisand, 1966; and Walden and Birnbaum, 1964). This method, as shown in the block diagram of Figure 6.30, uses at least three electrodes: one on the mother's chest; one at the upper part or fundus of the uterus; and one over the lower part of the uterus.

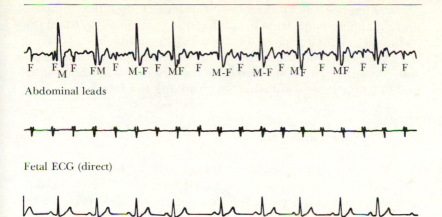

Abdominal leads

Fetal ECG (direct)

Maternal ECG

Figure 6.29 Typical fetal ECG obtained from maternal abdomen. F represents fetal QRS complexes: M represents maternal QRS complexes. Maternal ECG and fetal ECG (recorded directly from fetus) are included for comparison. (From "Monitoring of Intrapartum Phenomena," by J.F. Roux, M.R. Neuman, and R.C. Goodlin, in *C.R.C. Critical Reviews in Bioengineering*, **2**, pp. 119–158, January 1975, © C.R.C. Press. Used by permission of C.R.C. Press, Inc.)

The ECG of the mother is obtained from the top two electrodes and the fetal-plus-maternal signal is obtained from the bottom two. The center electrode is common to both. A threshold detector determines the mother's QRS complexes and uses this information to turn off an analog switch between the electrodes recording the fetal ECG and the recording apparatus. Therefore, whenever a maternal QRS complex is detected, the signal from the abdominal

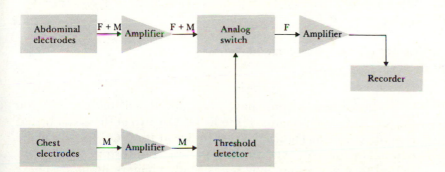

Figure 6.30 Block diagram of a scheme for isolating fetal ECG from abdominal signal that contains both fetal and maternal ECGs. (From "Monitoring of Intrapartum Phenomena," by J.F. Roux, M.R. Neuman, and R.C. Goodlin, in *C.R.C. Critical Reviews in Bioengineering*, **2**, pp. 119–158, January 1975, © C.R.C. Press. Used by permission of C.R.C. Press, Inc.)

leads is temporarily blocked until the end of the QRS complex, thereby eliminating it from the abdominal recording. Note that this technique also eliminates any fetal QRS complexes occurring simultaneously with the maternal ones. Modern systems incorporate computing circuits to recognize the absence of this fetal signal and to compensate for it when determining the fetal heart rate.

The vectorcardiograph

In Section 6.2 we looked at the basis of the ECG and defined the cardiac vector. The ensuing description of the electrocardiograph showed how a particular component of the cardiac vector could be recorded. Such scalar ECGs are the type that are usually taken. However, we can obtain far more information from a *vectorcardiogram* (VCG). A VCG shows a three-dimensional—or at least a two-dimensional—picture of the orientation and magnitude of the cardiac vector throughout the cardiac cycle. It is difficult for practical machines to display the VCG in three dimensions, but it is relatively simple to display it in two dimensions—or, in other words, in a particular plane of the body.

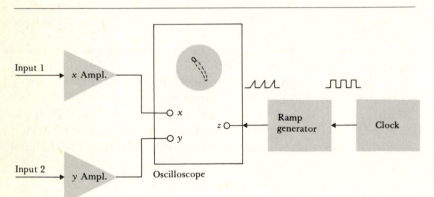

Figure 6.31 Block diagram of a vectorcardiograph for displaying the vector loop in a single plane.

Special lead systems have been developed that can provide the *x*, *y*, and *z* components of the ECG. Any two of these can be fed into the circuit of Figure 6.31, to arrive at the VCG for the plane defined by the axes. The signal from the lead for one axis is connected to input 1 and that for the other enters input 2. These signals, amplified by appropriate identical amplifiers, are fed to the *x* and *y* deflection circuits of a cathode-ray oscilloscope. For each heartbeat, a vector loop representing the locus of the tip of the cardiac vector when its tail is at the origin is then traced on the oscilloscope screen.

This type of display does not give any information on how the ECG signals are changing with respect to time. The scalar ECG is best able to provide this information, but it is of interest to see the time course of the vector loop as well. For this reason, the z (intensity) axis of the oscilloscope is modulated by a ramp generator driven by a precision clock. The ramp signal produced for every clock pulse gives a segment of the vector loop that corresponds to the duration of the ramp. The viewer can tell the direction of the vector loop, as well as its time course, since the ramp causes one end of the segment to be at low intensity while the other is at high intensity. Often triggering circuits are included in the vectorcardiograph, so that only one cardiac cycle is displayed, thereby avoiding overlap.

With the type of vectorcardiograph described in Figure 6.31, the VCG is displayed on the cathode-ray-tube screen. If we wish to get a permanent record of the VCG, we must take a photograph of the pattern. Most vectorcardiographs of this type come equipped with a camera to make it possible for us to obtain permanent records.

Vectorcardiographs have recently been produced that contain a memory that can store the signals from the two axes to make up a vector loop. These memories are read into an oscilloscope at a rapid and repeating rate to give a no-fade display of the vector loop. The memories can also be read at a slow rate into an x-y recorder to give a permanent record.

6.9 Cardiac monitors

There are several clinical situations in which continuous observation of the ECG and heart rate are important to the care of the patient. Continuous observation of the ECG during the administration of anesthesia helps doctors monitor the patient's condition while the patient is on the operating table. Constant monitoring of the ECG and heart rate of the myocardial-infarction patient during the danger period of several days following the initial incident has made possible the early detection of cardiac arrhythmias that could have led to death if they had gone unnoticed when they occurred. Continuous monitoring of the fetal heart rate during labor helps in the early detection of fetal distress.

These and other clinical applications of continuous monitoring of the ECG and heart rate are made possible by *cardiac monitors* and *cardioscopes*. Figure 6.32 shows the basic cardiac monitor in block-diagram form. Its front-end circuitry is similar to that of the electrocardiograph. A pair of electrodes, usually located on the anterior part of the chest, pick up the ECG and are connected by lead wires to the input circuit of the monitor. The input circuit contains patient-isolation circuitry, as described in Section 6.2, and protec-

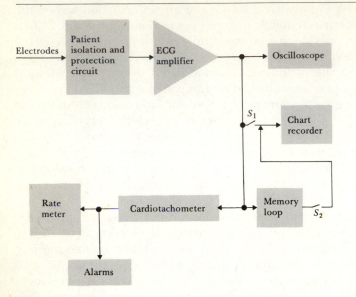

Figure 6.32 Block diagram of a cardiac monitor.

tion circuitry, as described in Section 6.4, to protect the monitor from high-voltage transients that can occur during defibrillation procedures.

The next stage of the monitor is a standard biopotential amplifier designed to amplify the ECG. Although it is best to have the frequency-response characteristics described in Section 6.2, often cardiac monitors have a slightly higher low corner frequency than would be acceptable for a standard electrocardiograph. The reason for this is that much of the motion-artifact signal seen during movement of the patient is at very low frequencies and, by filtering out some of these low frequencies, one can obtain a vast improvement in SNR and recording stability without seriously affecting the information pertaining to cardiac rhythm in the ECG. These low corner frequencies are usually found in the range of from 0.1 to 1 Hz.

The output from the amplifier can take several routes. It is fed directly to a cathode-ray-tube oscilloscope which has a sweep rate that can show the ECG as it would appear on an electrocardiograph. The oscilloscopes in modern cardiac monitors contain memory units, so that the ECG is displayed without flicker or fading due to the low sweep rate.

If the cardiac monitor is required to show only the ECG, the three blocks are all that are necessary. A monitor of this type is called a *cardioscope.* It is this type that is frequently used in the operating room to monitor the patients during surgery.

Often a physician wants to have a permanent record of the

ECG being monitored. For this reason, many cardiac monitors have a small chart recorder built into them that can be switched on (S_1) by the operator to record a particularly interesting ECG as it appears on the oscilloscope screen.

It is frequently desirable to have a record of the events in the ECG that lead up to a serious arrhythmia. This can be done if the amplifier output is fed first to a memory loop, which delays the ECG signal by about 15 s. The output from the memory loop can then be fed to the chart recorder via S_2. Thus, if the operator of the monitor sees an interesting ECG waveform on the oscilloscope, the operator can switch on the chart recorder through the memory loop and obtain a record of the events leading up to that particular pattern.

The ECG from the amplifier is also fed to a cardiotachometer. The output of the cardiotachometer is displayed on a rate meter, so that the operator can immediately tell the patient's heart rate. Alarm circuitry to warn of high and low heart rate is also associated with the cardiotachometer. Frequently, the alarm circuit automatically turns on the chart recorder and connects it to the output of the memory loop so that a recording of what precipitated the alarm is produced. This can be a valuable aid to clinicians in selecting appropriate therapy for the alarm-producing event.

Cardiac monitors may be used with individual patients on a ward by bringing a portable monitor to that patient. Most hospitals also utilize them in an organized system, called a coronary-care unit. In such units, there are often individual monitors at each patient's bedside that consist of a cardioscope and a cardiotachometer with a rate meter and alarms. These individual monitors are connected to a central unit located at the nursing station. The unit contains a cardioscope, which shows the ECGs for all patients being monitored, and a rate meter and slave alarm* unit for each patient. Memory loops and a chart recorder are also located at the central display. The chart recorder can be activated either at the central station or by remote control from the individual monitors at the patient's bedside.

Computers are also being applied to coronary-care units. Special-purpose machines can be made to recognize cardiac arrhythmias and to record the frequency of their occurrence. The machines can also prepare hard-copy charts showing trends in the patient's monitored parameters and keep records of various therapeutic measures taken by the clinical staff. The computer can also be a big help in the coronary-care unit by carrying out many observational and secretarial functions, thereby freeing the clinical staff to care for the patient.

The availability of microcomputers has made it possible to

---

* An alarm placed at the patient's bedside is "master" to a "slave" alarm that is placed at the nurse's station.

combine the monitoring of ambulatory patients with detection of cardiac arrhythmias. Portable tape recorders connected to ECG amplifiers can collect data from ambulatory patients; these data are analyzed later by a computer (Jurgen, 1976).

Figure 6.33 shows the block diagram of a system that carries this monitoring one step further—a microprocessor-based arrhythmia-detection system. The system utilizes an Intel 8080 microprocessor. All components of the system are connected to the 8080 data bus (Section 3.16). The initial approach uses a "bootstrap" method of programming, in which the arrhythmia-detection program is loaded into the system from a larger minicomputer system. The program is then stored in RAM for the portable unit. In a final unit, this program would be stored in a ROM, so that it is not lost when power to the unit is turned off. The patient-interactive devices consist of a four-digit display (liquid crystal to conserve power), a push-button, and a buzzer. The display shows the current heart rate and the push-button causes the instrument to transmit an R–R interval histogram and a sample ECG strip. The device may be connected to a central-processing facility through a telephone *modem* (modulator-demodulator). Power is provided by two lithium batteries. The unit measures $5 \times 13 \times 20$ cm, and weighs 1.3 kg.

The system, which is discussed in more detail by Walters (1976), provides a number of useful functions. For example, the instrument not only gathers ECG information, but also provides

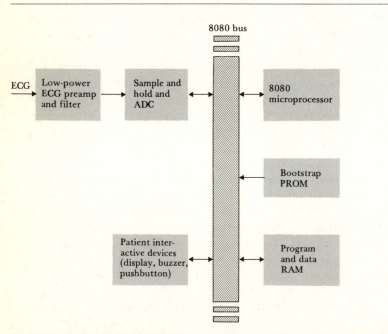

Figure 6.33 Simplified block diagram of a portable microprocessor-based system for real-time arrhythmia analysis.

immediate feedback to the patient regarding suggested actions to take or avoid. The patient may be reminded to take medication, cautioned to change physical activity, and requested to describe behavior or to call a central-processing station to dump processed data. In this manner, clinicians can obtain information more rapidly and monitor patients under more varied conditions than would be possible without the use of the microcomputer.

In situations in which cardiac monitors are used to observe a patient's ECG over a long period of time, artifact and failure of the monitor can occur as a result of a poor electrode–patient interface. The longer the electrodes remain on the patient, the more often this occurs. Frequently in coronary-care units electrodes are routinely changed—sometimes once a shift, sometimes once a day—to ensure against this type of breakdown. Some cardiac monitors also have alarm circuits that indicate when electrodes fall off the patient or the electrode–patient connection degenerates.

Figure 6.34 shows a block diagram of a typical lead fall-off alarm. A 50-kHz high-impedance source is connected across the electrodes. Peak amplitudes of the current can be hundreds of microamperes without any risk to the patient, because the microshock hazard to excitable tissue decreases as the frequency increases above 50 Hz (Figure 13.3). The current passes through the body between the electrodes, and, as long as there is good electrode contact, the voltage drop is relatively small. If the electrode connections become poor, as can happen when the electrolyte paste begins to dry, or if one of the electrodes falls off, the impedance between the electrodes jumps considerably. This causes the voltage produced by the 50-kHz source to rise. The high-frequency signal is separated from the ECG by the filtering scheme, as shown. The ECG passes through a low-pass filter with approximately a 150-Hz corner frequency, and is processed in the usual way. A bandpass

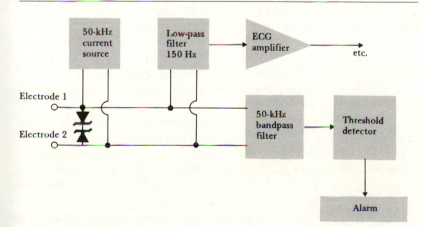

Figure 6.34 Block diagram of a system used with cardiac monitors to detect either increased electrode impedance or electrode fall-off.

filter with a 50-kHz center frequency passes the voltage resulting from the current source to a threshold detector. This detector sets off an alarm when the voltage exceeds a certain threshold, which would correspond to poor electrode contact. When an electrode falls off the patient, the interelectrode impedance should increase to infinity, resulting in the possibility of 50-kHz voltages high enough to cause some damage to the electronic devices. For this reason, a high-voltage protection circuit, such as described in Section 6.4, is frequently connected across the input terminals to the monitor. In the case shown in Figure 6.34, back-to-back zener diodes are shown.

Schoenberg (1977b) provides information on use of cardiac monitors, including specifications, performance, and problems, and also gives 370 references.

6.10 Radiotelemetry

Biopotential and other signals are often processed by radiotelemetry, a technique that provides a wireless link between the patient and the majority of the signal-processing components. By using a miniature radio transmitter attached to the patient to broadcast the information over a limited range, clinicians can monitor a patient or study a research animal while they have full mobility. This technique also provides the best method of isolation of the patient from the recording equipment and the power lines. For a single-channel system of biopotential radiotelemetry, a miniature battery-operated radio transmitter is connected to the electrodes on the patient. This transmitter broadcasts the biopotential over a limited range to a remotely located receiver, which detects the radio signals and recovers the signal for further processing. In this situation there is obviously negligible connection or stray capacitance between the electrode circuit connected to the radio transmitter and the rest of the instrumentation system. The receiving system can even be located in a room separate from the patient's. Hence the patient is completely isolated, and the only risk of electric shock that the patient encounters is due to the battery-powered transmitter itself. Thus, if the transmitter power supply is kept at a low voltage, there is negligible risk to the patient.

There are many types of radiotelemetry systems used in biomedical instrumentation. These are reviewed by MacKay (1970). The basic configuration of the system, however, is pretty much the same for all. Figure 6.35 shows a single-channel radiotelemetry system for the ECG. A preamplifier amplifies the ECG signal to a level at which it can modulate the radiofrequency (RF) carrier generated by an oscillator. Frequency modulation is often applied on single-channel systems, but more recent designs use pulse-duration or pulse-position modulation with pulse-code modulation applied

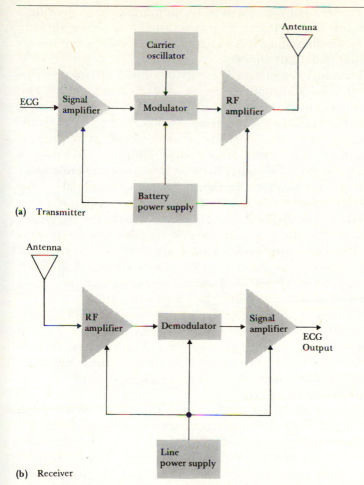

(a) Transmitter

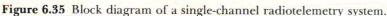

(b) Receiver

Figure 6.35 Block diagram of a single-channel radiotelemetry system.

where ultrahigh reliability is required. The modulated RF signal can be either directly applied to the radiating antenna (which in some cases might merely be a coil around the transmitter package) or amplified through an RF amplifier to provide higher signal levels. The entire transmitter is powered by a small battery pack. It is carried by the patient, usually attached by means of a special harness. Ultraminiature radio transmitters can be attached by surgical tape directly to the patient's skin. In research with experimental animals, experimenters can surgically implant the tiny transmitters within the bodies of the animals so that no external connections or wires are required.

In the receiving system, a pickup antenna receives the modulated RF signal, which is amplified through a tuned RF amplifier. The signal is then demodulated to recover the original information from the carrier. The signal can be further amplified to provide a usable output. The receiver system is usually powered directly from the power line, since it is in a permanent location and not attached to the patient in any way.

Multichannel radiotelemetry systems consist of two or more channels of data transmitted over a single carrier wave. The method of combining the various channels of information into a single signal is known as *multiplexing*. There are two basic methods of multiplexing. *Frequency-division multiplexing* makes use of continuous-wave subcarrier frequencies. Figure 6.36 shows a simple three-channel frequency-division multiplex radiotelemetry system. In the transmitter the signals frequency-modulate three different subcarrier oscillators, respectively, each being at a frequency so that its modulated signal does not overlap the frequency spectrums of the other two modulated signals. The frequency-modulated signals from each channel are then added together through a summing amplifier to give a composite signal in which none of the parts overlap in frequency. This signal then modulates the RF carrier of the transmitter, and is broadcast.

At the receiver for the frequency-division multiplexing system, the RF signal is amplified and detected to give a signal equivalent to the sum of the three modulated subcarriers. Each of these is then separated by a bandpass filter tuned to the frequencies that it contains. The separated signal is then demodulated and sent to the appropriate recording device.

The bandwidth of signal information that can be contained in any one channel depends on the frequency deviation of the subcarrier modulator and the bandwidth of the subcarrier channel itself. Of course, as more subcarrier channels are used, they have to occupy higher and higher frequencies so that they do not overlap. And the RF channel has to have a wider bandwidth to handle the information. Figure 6.36(c) shows how the individual subcarriers and their surrounding sidebands, which contain the modulated information, are positioned in the frequency domain to avoid overlapping.

The second multiplexing scheme that is used in multichannel radiotelemetry is the *time-division method*. Figure 6.37 shows a three-channel time-division multiplexing system. In this case, the three signals are amplified and applied to a commutator circuit. This circuit is an electronic switch that is rapidly scanning the three signals and a fourth "frame reference signal" in succession. For the sake of this description, let us consider the three input signals (v_1, v_2, and v_3) to be constant voltages. The frame reference signal v_4 is already at a constant voltage. An oscillator drives the commutator circuit so that it samples each voltage for a small instant of time, thereby giving a pulse-train sequence for v_1, v_2, and v_3, as shown in Figure 6.37(b). When the commutator reaches the frame reference

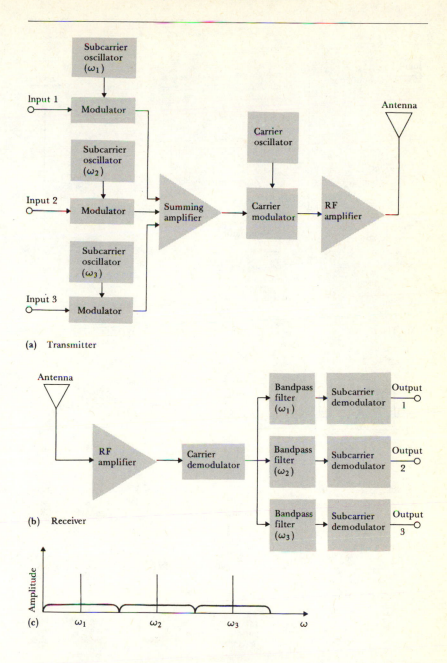

(a)   Transmitter

(b)   Receiver

(c)

Figure 6.36 A three-channel frequency-division multiplexed radiotelemetry system. (a) Transmitter with three subcarrier oscillators. (b) Receiver with bandpass filters. (c) Frequency spectrum of subcarrier channels, showing frequency spread to avoid overlap.

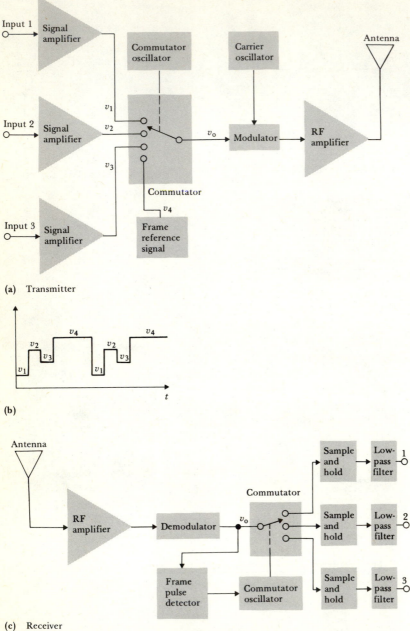

(a) Transmitter

(b)

(c) Receiver

Figure 6.37 Block diagram of a three-channel time-division multiplexed radiotelemetry system. (a) Transmitter. (b) Example of output waveform from commutator in transmitter. (c) Receiver.

signal v_4, it samples this for a longer period of time to give a wider pulse. This is necessary so that it is easy to recognize the frame-reference signal in the receiving system.

The receiver consists of a conventional radio receiver and de-modulator that recovers the signal shown in Figure 6.37(b). This signal must be demultiplexed by another commutator, which is driven by an oscillator in the receiver. The frame-reference pulse is used to achieve this synchronization. The frame-pulse-detector circuit recognizes the longer frame-reference pulse and uses this to tell the commutator oscillator to set the commutator so that the next pulse it receives is v_1, which is then followed by v_2 and finally by v_3. In this way the receiving commutator follows the transmitting commutator. Each separated pulse at the receiver is then applied to a sample-and-hold circuit that holds its amplitude until the next pulse is received. A low-pass filter follows this sample-and-hold circuit and removes the artifact generated by the commutating technique.

The bandwidth of each signal channel of this system is deter-mined by the rate at which it is sampled. Ideally, the rate of sampling must be at least twice that of the highest frequency com-ponent to be transmitted, but in practical circuits the rate of sampling is usually at least five times that of the highest frequency component.

It is important to note that, although radiotelemetry systems provide ideal isolation with no patient ground required, they are not completely immune from problems of electrical noise. Since coupling is achieved by a radiated electromagnetic signal, other electromagnetic signals at similar frequencies can interfere and cause artifacts. In extreme cases, these other signals can even bring about complete loss of signal.

In addition, the relative orientation between transmitting and receiving antennas is important. There can be orientations in which none of the signals radiated from the transmitting antenna are picked up by the receiving antenna. In such cases, there is no transmission of signals. In high-quality radiotelemetry systems, it is therefore important to have a means of indicating when signal interference or signal dropout is occurring, so that steps can be taken to rectify this problem, and so that the clinical staff realizes that the information being received is noise and should be disregarded.

Problems

6.1 Design an electrocardiograph with an input-switching system such that we can record the six frontal-plane leads by means of changing the switch.

6.2 What position of the cardiac vector at the peak of the R wave of an electrocardiogram gives the greatest sum of voltages for leads I, II, and III?

6.3 What position of the cardiac vector during the R wave gives identical signals in leads II and III? What does the ECG seen in lead I look like for this orientation of the vector?

6.4 Discuss the factors entering into the choice of a resistance value for the three resistors used to establish the Wilson central terminal. Describe the advantages and disadvantages of having this resistance either very large or very small.

6.5 Silicon diodes having a forward resistance of 2 Ω are to be used as voltage-limiting devices in the protection circuit of an electrocardiograph. They are connected as shown in Figure 6.17(b). The protection circuit is shown in Figure 6.16. If voltage transients as high as 500 V can appear at the electrocardiograph input during defibrillation, what is the minimum value of R that the designer can choose so that the voltage at the preamplifier input does not exceed 800 mV? Assume that the silicon diodes have a breakdown voltage of 600 mV.

6.6 A physician wishes to obtain two simultaneous ECGs in the frontal plane from leads having lead vectors at right angles. The signal will be used to generate a VCG using the system of Figure 6.31. Describe how you would go about obtaining these two signals and suggest a test to determine whether the leads are truly orthogonal.

6.7 An engineer sees no purpose for $R/2$ in Figure 6.5(a) and replaces it with a wire in order to simplify the circuit. What is the result?

6.8 The central-terminal requirements for an electrocardiograph that meets the recommendations of the Committee on Electrocardiography of the American Heart Association sets the minimum value of the resistances at 3.3 MΩ. Show that this value is a result of the specifications given in Section 6.2.

6.9 Design a technique for automatically calibrating an electrocardiograph at the beginning of each recording. The calibration can consist of a 1-mV standardizing pulse.

6.10 The circuit in Figure 6.10(a) is in a hospital in which there is 0.1-Ω resistance between ground A and ground B. An improperly connected electric lamp with a 150-W bulb is connected in the power circuit in such a way that the neutral connection is open and the current returns through the ground circuit passing from ground B to ground A.

    a What is the maximum potential that can appear between the two ground electrodes on the patient?

    b What is the maximum common-mode voltage at the input of the electrocardiograph as a result of this ground loop?

    c What must be the common-mode rejection ratio of the electrocardiograph amplifier to prevent more than 50 μV of interference from appearing on the ECG?

6.11 Design a biopotential preamplifier that is battery-powered and isolated in such a way that there is less than 0.5-pF coupling capacitance between the input and output terminals. The amplifier should have a nominal gain of 10 and an input impedance greater than 10 MΩ differentially and greater than 10 GΩ with respect to ground. The output impedance should be less than 100 Ω and single-ended.

6.12 A student attempts to measure his own ECG on an oscilloscope having a differential input. For Figure 6.14, $Z_{in} = 1$ MΩ, $Z_1 = 20$ kΩ, $Z_2 = 10$ kΩ, $Z_G = 30$ kΩ, and $i_{db} = 0.5$ μA. Calculate the power-line interference the student observes.

6.13 Design a driven-right-leg circuit and show all resistor values. For 1 μA of 60-Hz current flowing through the body, the common-mode voltage should be reduced to 2 mV. The circuit should supply no more than 5 μA when the amplifier is saturated at ±12 V.

6.14 An ECG lead is oriented such that its electrodes are placed on the body in positions that pick up an electromyogram from the chest muscles as well as the electrocardiogram. Design a circuit that separates these two signals as best as possible and discuss the limitations of such a circuit.

6.15 A cardiac monitor is found to have 1 mV p–p of 60-Hz interference. Describe a procedure that you could use to determine whether this is due to an electric field or a magnetic field pickup.

6.16 Contrast averaging and beat-to-beat cardiotachometers in terms of what would happen to the output signal of each if they were both connected to a patient who suddenly went into cardiac arrest.

6.17 Design a full-wave rectifier circuit that provides a signal corresponding to the absolute value of an electromyogram. The electromyogram coming from the electrodes has a maximum peak amplitude of 1 mV. What are the limitations of such a rectifier?

6.18 In an evoked-response experiment in which the EEG is studied after a patient is given the stimulus of a flashing light, the experimenter finds that the response has approximately the same amplitude as the random noise of the signal. If a signal averager is used, how many samples must be averaged to get an SNR of 10:1? If we want an SNR 100:1, would it be practical to use this technique?

6.19 A single-channel radiotelemetry system is used to continuously monitor a patient's ECG. Occasionally, because of improper orientation of the antenna or the transmitter getting out of range, there is a loss of signal. Design a system to indicate this signal loss at the telemetry receiver.

6.20 The ECG shown in Figure P6.1 is distorted due to an instrumentation problem. Discuss possible causes of this distortion and suggest means of correcting the problem.

6.21 Figure P6.2 shows ECGs from simultaneous leads I and II. Sketch the vector loop for this QRS complex in the frontal plane.

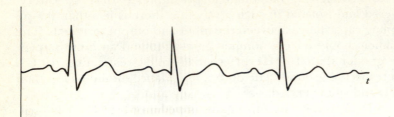

Figure P6.1

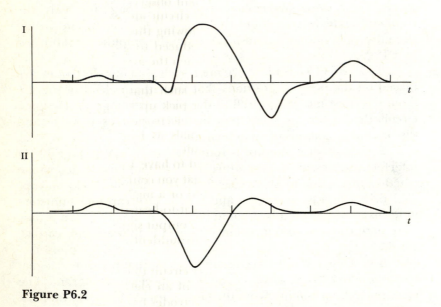

Figure P6.2

References

Cobbold, R.S.C., *Transducers for biomedical measurements: Principles and applications.* New York: Wiley, 1974.

Delgado, J.M.R., "Electrodes for extracellular recording and stimulation." In W.L. Nastuk, *Physical techniques in biological research.* New York: Academic, 1964, pp. 88–139.

Fichtenbaum, M., "Counter inverts period to measure low frequency." *Electron.*, March 4, 1976, 49, 100.

Geddes, L.A., and L.E. Baker, *Principles of applied biomedical instrumentation,* 2nd ed. New York: Wiley, 1975.

Grobstein, S.R., and R.D. Gatzke, "A battery-powered ECG monitor for emergency and operating room environments." *Hewlett-Packard Journal,* September 1977, 29(1), 26–32.

Hartley, R., "Analogue-display rate meter built around digital switching elements." *Med. Biol. Eng.,* 1976, 14, 107–108.

Huhta, J.C., and J.G. Webster, "60-Hz interference in electrocardiography." *IEEE Trans. Biomed. Eng.,* 1973, BME 20, 91–101.

Jurgen, R.K., "Software (and hardware) for the 'medics'." *IEEE Spectrum,* April 1976, 13(4), 40–43.

Ludwig, H., and Y-K Ng, "Heart rate meter with digital timing and linear beat-to-beat readout." *Med. Biol. Eng.,* 1967, 5, 615–621.

Mackay, R.S., *Bio-medical telemetry,* 2nd ed., New York: Wiley, 1970.

Offner, F., and B. Moisand, "A coincidence technique for fetal electrocardiography." *Amer. J. Obstet. Gynecol.,* 1966, 95, 676.

Pipberger, H.V., *et al.,* "Recommendations for standardization of leads and of specifications for instruments in electrocardiography and vectorcardiography." *Circ.,* August 1975, 52(2), 11–31.

Plonsey, R., *Bioelectric phenomena.* New York: McGraw-Hill, 1969.

Plonsey, R., "The biophysical basis for electrocardiography." *Crit. Rev. Bioeng.,* 1971, 1, 1–48.

Roux, J.F., M.R. Neuman, and R. Goodlin, "Monitoring intrapartum phenomena." *Crit. Rev. Bioeng.,* January 1975, 119–158.

Schoenberg, A.A., *et al.,* "Standard for electrocardiographic devices." Utah Biomedical Test Laboratory, FDA MDS-021-0006, UBTL TR 227–003, 20 January 1977a.

Schoenberg, A.A. A study of cardiac monitor safety and efficacy. Utah Biomedical Test Laboratory, UBTL TR 173–008, 19 July 1977b.

Svetz, P., and N. Duane, "The α β γ of bioelectric measurements." *Electron. Des.,* August 2, 1975, 23(16), 68.

Taylor, K., and M. Mandelberg, "Precision digital instrument for calculation of heart rate and R–R interval." *IEEE Trans. Biomed. Eng.,* May 1975, BME 22, 255–257.

Walden, W.D., and S.J. Birnbaum, "Fetal electrocardiography with cancellation of maternal complexes." *Amer. J. Obstet. Gynecol.,* 1964, 94, 596.

Walters, J.B., "A microprocessor based arrhythmia monitor for ambulatory subjects." Biomedical Engineering Center for Clinical Instrumentation Rept N BMEC TR004. Cambridge, MA: MIT, September 1976.

Chapter seven

Blood pressure and sound

Robert A. Peura

Determining an individual's blood pressure is a standard clinical measurement whether taken in a physician's office or in the hospital during a specialized surgical procedure. Blood-pressure values in the various chambers of the heart and in the peripheral vascular system help the physician determine the functional integrity of the cardiovascular system. A number of direct (invasive) and indirect (noninvasive) techniques are being used to measure blood pressure in the human. The accuracy of each should be established as well as its suitability for a particular clinical situation.

Fluctuations in pressure recorded over the frequency range of hearing are called *sounds*. The sources of heart sounds are the vibrations set up by the accelerations and decelerations of blood. A complete clinical work-up of a patient with suspected cardiac problems includes phonocardiography as a valuable adjunct to cardiac catheterization.

7.1 Direct measurements

Blood-pressure transducer systems may be divided into two general categories, according to the location of the transducer element. The most common clinical method for directly measuring pressure is to couple the vascular pressure to an *external* transducer element via a liquid-filled catheter. In the second general category, the liquid coupling is eliminated by incorporating the transducer into the tip of a catheter that is placed in the vascular system. This device is known as an *intravascular pressure transducer*.

A number of different kinds of transducer elements may be used: strain gage; linear-variable differential transformer; variable inductance; variable capacitance; electro-optical; piezoelectric; and semiconductor devices. Cobbold (1974) compares the significant electrical and mechanical properties of commercial pressure transducers. This section describes the principles of operation of an extravascular and an intravascular system. Description of other transducers is similar to the material covered in Chapter 2.

Extravascular transducers

The extravascular transducer system, as shown in Figure 7.1, is made up of a catheter connected to a three-way stopcock, and then to the dome of the pressure transducer. The catheter-transducer system, which is filled with a saline-heparin solution, must be flushed with the solution every few minutes to avoid blood clotting at the tip.

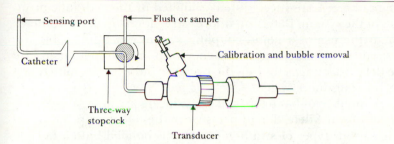

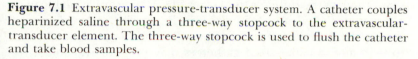

Figure 7.1 Extravascular pressure-transducer system. A catheter couples heparinized saline through a three-way stopcock to the extravascular-transducer element. The three-way stopcock is used to flush the catheter and take blood samples.

The physician inserts the catheter either by means of a *surgical cut-down,* which exposes the artery or vein, or by means of *percutaneous insertion,* which involves the use of a special needle or guide-wire technique. Blood pressure is transmitted via the catheter liquid column to the transducer dome and, finally, to the diaphragm, which is deflected. Figure 7.2 shows that the displacement of the diaphragm is transmitted to a system composed of a moving armature and an unbonded strain gage. The reason these systems are used so frequently is that they have high stability and sensitivity. The strain on one pair of gages, *B* and *C,* is increased, while that on the other pair, *A* and *D,* is decreased. This strain-gage system is connected in a Wheatstone-bridge circuit, as was shown in Figure 2.2, and is inherently temperature stable. Section 2.3 describes the operation of bridge circuits.

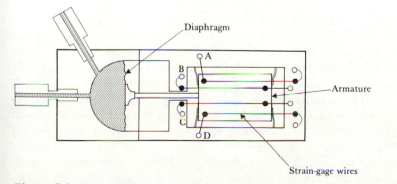

Figure 7.2 Unbonded strain-gage pressure transducer. The diaphragm is directly coupled by an armature to an unbonded strain-gage system. With increasing pressure, the strain on gage pair B and C is increased, while that on gage pair A and D is decreased.

Intravascular transducers

Catheter-tip transducers have the advantage that the hydraulic connection via the catheter, between the source of pressure and the transducer element, is eliminated. The frequency response of the catheter-transducer system is limited by the hydraulic properties of the system. Detection of pressures at the tip of the catheter without the use of a liquid-coupling system can thus enable the physician to obtain a high frequency response and eliminate the time delay encountered when the pressure pulse is transmitted in a catheter-transducer system.

A number of basic types of transducers are being used commercially for the detection of pressure in the catheter tip. These include various types of strain-gage systems bonded onto a flexible diaphragm at the catheter tip. Gages of this type are available in the F 5 catheter (1.67 mm OD) size. In the French scale (F), used to denote the diameter of catheters, each unit is approximately equal to 0.33 mm. Smaller-sized catheters may become available as the technology improves and the problems of temperature and electrical drift, fragility, and nondestructive sterilization are solved more completely. A disadvantage of the catheter-tip pressure transducer is that it is more expensive and may break after only a few uses, thus increasing its cost per use.

The fiber-optic intravascular pressure sensor can be made in sizes comparable to those described above, but at a lower cost. The fiber-optic device measures the displacement of the diaphragm optically by the varying reflection of light from the back of the deflecting diaphragm (Lindstrom, 1970). (Recall that Section 2.14 detailed the principles of transmission of light along a fiber bundle.) These devices are inherently safer electrically, but unfortunately lack a convenient way to measure relative pressure without an additional lumen either connected to a second pressure transducer or vented to the atmosphere.

Other types of transducers

Special-purpose pressure transducers of many types have been developed. Figure 7.3 shows the details of a *passive-pressure endoradiosonde* (Collins, 1970). This device consists of two spiral coils attached to diaphragms on opposite faces of a miniature box. As the pressure surrounding the box changes, the box deforms and effects a change in the relative spacing between the coils. There is then a change in the mutual inductance and stray capacitance between the coils. An RF signal is coupled from an external oscillator into the high-Q resonant circuit of the implanted coil, so the change in resonant frequency can be determined and the pressure measured.

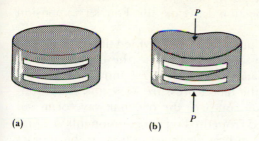

(a)   (b)

Figure 7.3 Passive-pressure endoradiosonde. (a) Two spiral coils are attached to diaphragms on opposite faces of a miniature box. (b) Changes in pressure cause deformations of the box; mutual inductance and stray capacitance between coils is sensed by monitoring the resonant frequency of the circuit.

Miniature pressure transducers have been used for implantation studies in animals (Konigsberg and Russell, 1968). Diameters on the order of 2 to 3 mm are typical for the transducer element consisting of silicon strain gages bonded to a metal diaphragm.

7.2 Harmonic analysis of blood-pressure waveforms

The basic sine-wave components of any complex time-varying periodic waveform can be dissected into an infinite sum of properly weighted sine and cosine functions of the proper frequency which, when added, reproduce the original complex waveform (Section 1.9). It has been shown that researchers can apply techniques of Fourier analysis when they want to characterize the oscillatory components of the circulatory and respiratory systems, because two basic postulates for Fourier analysis—periodicity and linearity—are usually satisfied (Attinger *et al.*, 1970).

Cardiovascular physiologists and some clinicians have been employing Fourier-analysis techniques in the quantification of pressure and flow since this method was established in the 1950s. They have carried out Fourier analysis using bandpass filters. More recent analysts have used computer techniques to obviate the need for special hardware. The advantage of the technique is that it allows for a quantitative representation of a physiologic waveform; thus it is quite easy to compare corresponding harmonic components of pulses.

O'Rourke (1971) points out that the modern physician who turns for assistance in the interpretation of the arterial pulse to a standard medical textbook is likely to be confused, misled, and disappointed. He further indicates that analysis of the frequency components of the pulse in recent years appears to have given more information on arterial properties than any other approach. He proposes that the arterial pulse be represented in terms of its frequency components. (Section 1.9 gave the Fourier expansion for a periodic function.)

The blood-pressure pulse may be divided into its fundamental component (of the same frequency as the blood-pressure wave) and its significant harmonics. Figure 7.4 shows the first six harmonic components of the blood-pressure wave and the resultant sum of these. When we compare the original waveform and the waveform reconstructed from the Fourier components, we find that they agree quite well, indicating that the first six harmonics give a fairly good reproduction. Note that the amplitude of the sixth harmonic is approximately 12% of the fundamental. We can achieve more faithful reproduction of the original waveform by adding higher harmonic components.

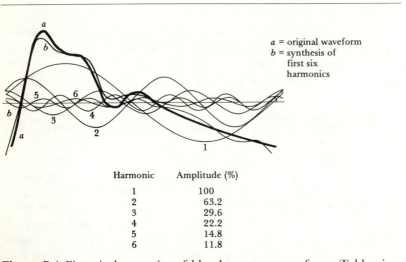

a = original waveform
b = synthesis of
    first six
    harmonics

Harmonic	Amplitude (%)
1	100
2	63.2
3	29.6
4	22.2
5	14.8
6	11.8

Figure 7.4 First six harmonics of blood-pressure waveform. Table gives relative values for amplitudes. (From T.A. Hansen, "Pressure Measurement in the Human Organism," *Acta Physiologica Scandinavica*, 1949, **19,** Suppl. 68, 1–227. Used with permission.)

7.3 Dynamic properties of pressure-measurement systems

An understanding of the dynamic properties of a pressure-measurement system is important if we wish to preserve the dynamic accuracy of the measured pressure. Errors in measurement of dynamic pressure can have serious consequences in the clinical situation. For instance, an underdamped system can lead to an overestimation of pressure gradients across *stenotic* (narrowed) heart valves. The liquid-filled catheter transducer is a hydraulic system that can be represented by either distributed or lumped-parameter models. Distributed-parameter models are described in the literature (Fry, 1960, and Hansen, 1949, 1950, and Hansen and Warberg, 1950), which gives an accurate description of the dynamic behavior of the catheter-transducer system. However, distributed-parameter models are not normally employed, because the single-degree-of-freedom (lumped-parameter) model is easier to work with, and the accuracy of the results obtained by using these models is acceptable for the clinical situation.

Analogous electrical systems

The modeling approach taken here develops a lumped-parameter model for the catheter and transducer separately and shows how, with appropriate approximations, it reduces to the lumped-parameter model for a second-order system. Figure 7.5 shows the physical model of a catheter-transducer system. An increase in pressure at the input of the catheter causes a flow of liquid to the right from the catheter tip, through the catheter, and into the transducer. This liquid shift causes a deflection of the transducer diaphragm, which is sensed by an electromechanical system. The subsequent electrical signal is then amplified.

A liquid catheter has inertial, frictional, and elastic properties represented by inertance, resistance, and compliance, respectively. Similarly, the transducer has these same properties, in addition to the compliance of the diaphragm. Figure 7.5(b) shows an electrical analog of the pressure-measuring system, wherein the analogous elements for hydraulic inertance, resistance, and compliance are electrical inductance, resistance, and capacitance, respectively.

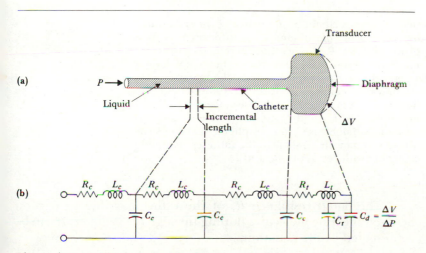

Figure 7.5 (a) Physical model of catheter-transducer system. (b) Analogous electrical system for catheter-transducer system. Each segment of the catheter has its own resistance R_c, inertance L_c and compliance C_c. In addition the transducer has resistance R_t, inertance L_t, and compliance C_t. C_d is the compliance of the diaphragm.

The analogous circuit in Figure 7.5(b) can be simplified to that in Figure 7.6(a). The compliance of the transducer diaphragm is much larger than that of the liquid-filled catheter or transducer cavity, provided that the saline solution is bubble free and the catheter material is relatively noncompliant. The resistance and inertance of the liquid in the transducer can be neglected with respect to that of the liquid in the catheter. Let us now derive equations relating the resistance and inductance to the properties of the system.

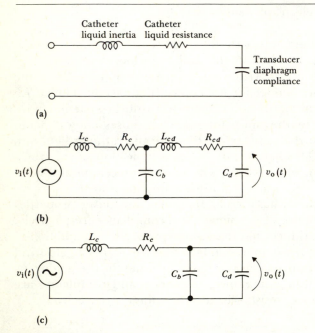

Figure 7.6 (a) Simplified analogous circuit. Compliance of the transducer diaphragm is larger than compliance of catheter or transducer cavity for a bubble-free, noncompliant catheter. Resistance and inertance of the catheter is larger than that of the transducer, since the catheter has longer length and smaller diameter than the transducer. (b) Analogous circuit for catheter-transducer system with a bubble in the catheter. Catheter properties proximal to the bubble are inertance L_c and resistance R_c. Catheter properties distal to the bubble are L_{cd} and R_{cd}. Compliance of the diaphragm is C_d; compliance of the bubble is C_b. (c) Simplified analogous circuit for catheter-transducer system with a bubble in the catheter, assuming that L_{cd} and R_{cd} are negligible with respect to R_c and L_c.

The liquid resistance R_c of the catheter is due to friction between shearing molecules flowing through the catheter. It can be represented by the equation:

$$R_c = \frac{\Delta P}{F} \ (\text{Pa} \cdot \text{s/m}^3) \tag{7.1}$$

or

$$R_c = \frac{\Delta P}{\bar{u}A}$$

where

P = pressure difference across the segment in Pa (pascal = N/m²)
F = flow rate, m³/s
$\bar{u}$ = average velocity, m/s
A = cross-sectional area, m²

Poiseuille's equation enables us to calculate R_c when we are given the values of catheter length L, in meters, radius r, in meters, and liquid viscosity η, in pascal-seconds. The equation applies for laminar or Poiseuille flow:

$$R_c = \frac{8\eta L}{\pi r^4} \tag{7.2}$$

The liquid inertance L_c of the catheter is due primarily to the mass of the liquid. It can be represented by the equation:

$$L_c = \frac{\Delta P}{dF/dt} \; (\text{Pa} \cdot \text{s}^2/\text{m}^3) \tag{7.3}$$

or

$$L_c = \frac{\Delta P}{aA}$$

where a = acceleration, m/s².
This equation reduces further to

$$L_c = \frac{m}{A^2}$$

or

$$L_c = \frac{\rho L}{\pi r^2} \tag{7.4}$$

where

m = mass of liquid, kg, and ρ = density of liquid, kg/m³.
Equations (7.2) and (7.4) show that we can neglect the resistive and inertial components of the transducer with respect to those of the liquid catheter. The reason for this is that the liquid-filled catheter is longer than the cavity of the transducer, and of smaller diameter. Geddes (1970) develops a more refined model of fluid inertance, based on kinetic energy considerations, in which he considers that the effective mass is four-thirds times that of the fluid in the catheter.

The compliance C_d of the transducer diaphragm is given by the equation,

$$C_d = \frac{\Delta V}{\Delta P} = \frac{1}{E_d}$$

where E_d is the volume modulus of elasticity of the transducer diaphragm.

We can find the relationship between the input voltage v_i, analogous to applied pressure, and output voltage v_o, analogous to pressure at the diaphragm, by using Kirchhoff's voltage law. Thus,

$$v_i(t) = \frac{L_c C_d \, d^2 v_o(t)}{dt^2} + \frac{R_c C_d \, dv_o(t)}{dt} + v_o(t) \tag{7.5}$$

Using the general form of a second-order system equation derived in Section 1.9, we can show that the natural undamped frequency ω_n is $1/(L_c C_d)^{1/2}$, and the damping ratio ζ is $(R_c/2)(C_d/L_c)^{1/2}$. For the hydraulic system under study, we can show by substituting (7.2) and (7.4) into the expressions for ω_n and ζ that

$$f_n = \frac{r}{2}\left(\frac{1}{\pi \rho L}\frac{\Delta P}{\Delta V}\right)^{1/2} \tag{7.6}$$

and

$$\zeta = \frac{4\eta}{r^3}\left(\frac{L(\Delta V/\Delta P)}{\pi \rho}\right)^{1/2} \tag{7.7}$$

Here are a number of useful relationships and pertinent constants.

η for water at 20°C = 0.001 Pa · s
η for water at 37°C = 0.0007 Pa · s
η for air at 20°C = 0.000018 Pa · s
ρ for air at 20°C = 1.21 kg/m³
$\Delta V/\Delta P$ for water = 0.53 × 10⁻¹⁵ m⁵/N per milliliter volume
η for blood $\cong 4 \times \eta$ for water

We can study the transient and frequency response of the catheter-transducer system by means of the analogous electrical circuit. In addition, we can study the effects of changes in the hydraulic system by adding appropriate elements to the circuit. For example, an air bubble in the liquid makes the system more compliant. Thus its effect on the system is the same as that caused by connecting an additional capacitor in parallel to that representing the diaphragm compliance. Example 7.1 illustrates how the analogous circuit is used.

Example 7.1 A 5-mm-long air bubble has formed in the rigid-walled catheter connected to a Statham P23Dd transducer. The catheter is 1 m long, 6 French diameter, and filled with water at 20°C. (The isothermal compression of air $\Delta V / \Delta P = 1$ ml per cm H_2O pressure per liter of volume.) Plot the frequency response curve of the system with and without the bubble. (Internal radius of catheter = 0.46 mm; volume modulus of elasticity of the diaphragm = 0.49×10^{15} N/m⁵.)

Answer The analogous circuit for the hydraulic system with and without the bubble is shown in Figure 7.6(b) and (c). We can calculate the values of the natural frequency f_n and damping ratio ζ without the bubble by using (7.6) and (7.7). That is,

$$f_n = \frac{r}{2} \left(\frac{1}{\pi L} \frac{\Delta P}{\rho \Delta V} \right)^{1/2}$$

$$= \frac{0.046 \times 10^{-2}}{2} \left(\frac{1}{\pi (1)} \frac{0.49 \times 10^{15}}{1 \times 10^3} \right)^{1/2} = 91 \text{ Hz}$$

$$\zeta = \frac{4\eta}{r^3} \left(\frac{L}{\pi \rho} \frac{\Delta V}{\Delta P} \right)^{1/2}$$

$$= \frac{4(0.001)}{(0.046 \times 10^{-2})^3} \left(\frac{1}{\pi} \frac{1}{(1 \times 10^3)(0.49 \times 10^{15})} \right)^{1/2} = 0.033$$

The frequency response for the catheter-transducer system is shown in Figure 7.7.

The next step is to calculate the new values of ζ and f_n for the case in which a bubble is present. Since the two capacitors are in parallel, the total capacitance for the circuit is equal to the sum of these two. That is,

$$C_t = C_a + C_b \tag{7.8}$$

or

$$C_t = \frac{\Delta V}{\Delta P_a} + \frac{\Delta V}{\Delta P_b}$$

The value of $\Delta V / \Delta P_a = 1/E_a = 2.04 \times 10^{-15}$ m⁵/N. The volume of the bubble is 3.33×10^{-6} liter, and thus $\Delta V / \Delta P_b = 3.38 \times 10^{-14}$ m⁵/N. Consequently, $C_t = 3.58 \times 10^{-14}$ m⁵/N. We can find the new values for f_n and ζ by referring to (7.6) and (7.7) and assuming that the only parameter that changes is the value of $\Delta V / \Delta P$. Thus

$$f_{n,\text{bubble}} = f_{n,\text{no bubble}} \left(\frac{\Delta P / \Delta V_{\text{total}}}{\Delta P / \Delta V_{\text{no bubble}}} \right)^{1/2}$$

or

$$f_{n,\text{bubble}} = 92 \left(\frac{3.58 \times 10^{+14}}{(1/2.04) \times 10^{+15}} \right)^{1/2} = 22 \text{ Hz}$$

and

$$\zeta_{\text{bubble}} = \zeta_{\text{no bubble}} \left(\frac{\Delta V/\Delta P_{\text{total}}}{\Delta V/\Delta P_{\text{no bubble}}} \right)^{1/2} = 0.137$$

The frequency response for the system with the bubble present is shown in Figure 7.7. Note that the bubble lowers f_n and increases ζ. This lowering of f_n may cause distortion problems with the higher harmonics of the blood-pressure waveform.

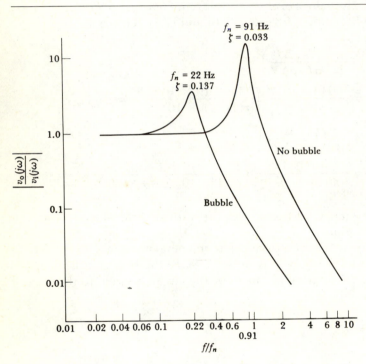

Figure 7.7 Frequency-response curves for catheter-transducer system with and without bubbles. Natural frequency decreases from 91 to 22 Hz and damping ratio increases from 0.033 to 0.137 with the bubble present.

Example 7.2 Water is not a perfect liquid, since it has a finite volume modulus of elasticity. Therefore a theoretical upper limit of high-frequency response exists for a water-filled transducer-catheter system. Find the maximum f_n for a transducer that has a 0.50-ml liquid chamber and that is connected to the pressure source by means of a #20 ($r = 0.29$ mm) 50-mm-long steel needle.

Answer Since a steel needle is used for the catheter, the volume modulus of elasticity of the catheter is assumed to be zero. We do not consider the volume modulus of elasticity of the diaphragm because we want the theoretical upper limit of high-frequency response. Thus $\Delta V/\Delta P$ for this example is that of water = 0.53×10^{-15} m^5/N per milliliter volume. The total volume of the water is equal to the volume of the liquid chamber of the transducer plus the volume of the cylindrical steel needle.

$$V_t = 0.5 + \pi(0.029)^2(5) \text{ ml} = 0.513 \text{ ml}$$

Thus

$$\left(\frac{\Delta V}{\Delta P}\right)_{\text{water}} = (0.53 \times 10^{-15})(0.513) = 0.272 \times 10^{-15} \text{ m}^5/\text{N}$$

Then

$$f_n = \frac{0.029 \times 10^{-2}}{2} \left(\frac{1}{\pi(0.05)(1000)(0.27 \times 10^{-15})}\right)^{1/2}$$

$$= 700 \text{ Hz}$$

7.4 Measurement of system response

The response characteristics of a catheter-transducer system can be determined by two methods. The simplest and most straightforward technique involves measuring the transient step response for the system. A potentially more accurate method—but more complicated because it requires special equipment—involves measuring the frequency response of the system.

Transient step response

The basis of the transient-response method is to apply a sudden step input to the pressure catheter and record the resultant damped oscillations of the system. This is also called the *pop* technique, for reasons that will become evident in the following discussion. The transient response can be found by the method shown in Figure 7.8. For a complete discussion of practical problems involving manometric testing, see Gabe (1972).

The catheter, or needle, is sealed in a tube by a screw adaptor that compresses a rubber washer against the insert. Flushing of the system is accomplished by passing excess liquid out of the three-way stopcock. The test is performed by securing a rubber membrane over the tube by means of an O ring. Surgical-glove material is an excellent choice for the membrane. The technician pressurizes the system by squeezing the sphygmomanometer bulb, punctures the balloon with a burning match or hot soldering iron, and observes the response. The response should be observed on a

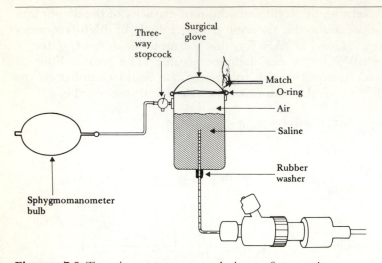

Figure 7.8 Transient-response technique for testing a pressure-transducer–catheter-transducer system.

strip-chart recorder running at a speed that makes it possible to distinguish the individual oscillations. However, if the frequency bandwidth of the recorder is inadequate, the technician can use a recording oscilloscope or oscilloscope photograph.

Figure 7.9 shows an example of the transient response. In this case the response represents a second-order system. The technician can measure the amplitude ratio of successive positive peaks and determine the logarithmic decrement Λ. Equation (1.33) yields the damping ratio ζ. The observer can measure T, the time between successive positive peaks, and determine the undamped natural frequency from $\omega_n = 2\pi/T(1 - \zeta^2)^{1/2}$.

Note that this method is reliable for the simple second-order

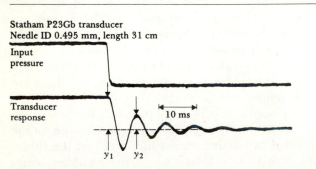

Figure 7.9 Pressure-transducer transient response. Negative-step input pressure is recorded on top channel; bottom channel is transducer response for a Statham P23Gb transducer connected to a 31-cm needle (0.495 mm ID). (From I.T. Gabe, "Pressure Measurement in Experimental Physiology," in D.H. Bergel, ed., *Cardiovascular Fluid Dynamics*, vol. I, New York: Academic Press, 1972.)

model proposed for the catheter-transducer system. For higher-order systems, we can fortunately still use this method to determine the parameters of the second-order system. Figure 7.10 shows a response for a catheter-transducer system wherein an 83-Hz signal is riding on the lower basic 15-Hz frequency. This higher resonant frequency should not affect the system, because it is higher than the significant harmonics of the blood pressure for humans, provided that there are not any artifacts (such as catheter whip) present at this higher resonant frequency.

Statham P23Gb transducer. No 7 cardiac catheter 125 cm long, I.D. 0·0177cm

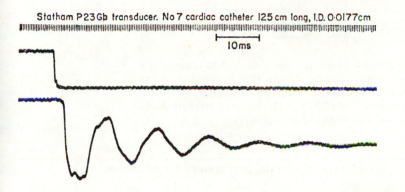

10ms

Figure 7.10 Pressure-transducer transient response for a higher-order system. (From I.T. Gabe, "Pressure Measurement in Experimental Physiology," in D.H. Bergel, ed., *Cardiovascular Fluid Dynamics*, vol. I, New York: Academic Press, 1972.)

Sinusoidal frequency response

As mentioned previously, the sinusoidal frequency-response method is more complex because it requires more specialized equipment. Figure 7.11 shows a schematic diagram of a sinusoidal pressure-generator test system. A pump produces sinusoidal pressures that are normally monitored at the pressure source by a pressure transducer with known characteristics. This is used because the amplitudes of the source-pressure waveforms are not normally constant for all frequencies. The source pressure is coupled to the catheter transducer under test by means of bubble-free saline. The air is removed by boiling the liquid. Inexpensive sinusoidal pressure-generator systems built from commercially available units appear in the literature (King, 1972; Stegall, 1967).

We can find an accurate model for the catheter-transducer system by determining the amplitude and phase of the output as a function of frequency without the constraint of the second-order system model required in the transient-response case. In some cases resonance at more than one frequency may be present.

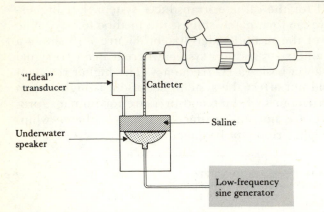

"Ideal" transducer

Catheter

Saline

Underwater speaker

Low-frequency sine generator

Figure 7.11 A sinusoidal pressure-generator test system. A low-frequency sine generator drives underwater-speaker system that is coupled to the catheter of the pressure transducer under test. An "ideal" pressure transducer, with a frequency response from 0 to 100 Hz, is connected directly to the test chamber housing and monitors input pressure.

7.5 Effects of system parameters on response

We have shown in our discussion of the model of the catheter-transducer system that the values of the damping ratio ζ and natural frequency ω_n are functions of the various system parameters. This section reports on experimental verification of these theoretical derivations (Shapiro and Krovetz, 1970). By use of step transient-response and sinusoidal pressure-generation techniques similar to those described above, these investigators determined the effects on the performance of the catheter-transducer system of deaerating water and of using various catheter materials and connectors. They found that even minute air bubbles, which increase the compliance of the catheter manometer system, drastically decreased the damped natural frequency $\omega_d = 2\pi/T$. For a PE-190 catheter of lengths 10 to 100 cm, the damped natural frequency decreased by approximately 50 to 60% for an unboiled-water case compared to a boiled-water case. Length of the catheter was shown to be inversely related to the damped natural frequency for Teflon and polyethylene catheters for the diameters (0.58 to 2.69 mm) tested. The theoretical linear relationship between the damped natural frequency and $1/(\text{catheter length})^{1/2}$ seemed to hold within experimental errors. They found a linear relationship between the inner diameter of the catheter and the damped natural frequency for both polyethylene and Teflon catheters, as predicted by the model equations.

In comparing the effect of catheter material on frequency response, they found that since Teflon is slightly stiffer than polyethylene, it has a slightly higher frequency response at any given length. As expected, the increased compliance of Silastic tubing caused a marked decrease in frequency response. The authors concluded that Silastic is a poor material for determining parameters other than mean pressure.

They examined the effect of connectors on the system response by inserting—in series with the catheter—various connecting needles that added little to the overall length of the system. They found that the damped natural frequency was linearly related to the needle bore for needles of the same length. The connector serves as a simple series hydraulic damper that decreases the frequency response. They suggested that the fewest possible number of connectors be used, and that all connectors be tight-fitting and have a water seal.

In further tests, they found that coils and bends in the catheter cause changes in the resonant frequency. However, the magnitude of these changes was insignificant when compared with changes caused by factors affecting compliance.

7.6 Bandwidth requirements for measuring blood pressure

When we know the representative harmonic components of the blood-pressure waveform—or, for that matter, any periodic waveform—we can specify the bandwidth requirements for the instrumentation system. As with all biomedical measurements, bandwidth requirements are a function of the investigation.

For example, if the mean blood pressure is the only parameter of interest, it is of little value to try to achieve a wide bandwidth system. It is generally accepted that harmonics of the blood-pressure waveform higher than the tenth may be ignored. As an example, the bandwidth requirements for a heart rate of 120 beats/min (or 2 Hz) would be 20 Hz.

For a perfect reproduction of the original waveform, there should be no distortion in the amplitude or phase characteristics. The waveshape can be preserved, however, even if the phase characteristics are not ideal. This is the case if the relative amplitudes of the frequency components are preserved but their phases are displaced in proportion to their frequency. Then the synthesized waveform gives the original waveshape, except that it is delayed in time, depending on the phase shift.

Measurements of the derivative of the pressure signal increase the bandwidth requirements, because the differentiation of a sinusoidal harmonic increases the amplitude of that component by a factor proportional to its frequency. Figure 7.12 shows a record of left-ventricular pressure and its derivative measured by an implanted semiconductor device with an amplitude response flat to 105 Hz (Gabe, 1972). As with the original blood-pressure waveform, the bandwidth requirements for the derivative of the

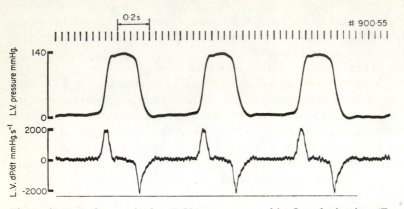

Figure 7.12 Left-ventricular (L.V.) pressure and its first derivative. (From I.T. Gabe, "Pressure Measurement in Experimental Physiology," in D.H. Bergel, ed., *Cardiovascular Fluid Dynamics*, vol. I, New York: Academic Press, 1972.)

blood pressure can be estimated by a Fourier analysis of the derivative signal. The amplitude-versus-frequency characteristics of any catheter-manometer system used for the measurement of ventricular pressures that are subsequently differentiated must remain flat to within 5%, up to the twentieth harmonic (Gersh *et al.*, 1971).

7.7 Typical pressure-waveform distortion

Accurate measurements of blood pressure are important in both clinical and physiological research. This section gives examples of typical types of distortion of blood-pressure waveform due to an inadequate frequency response of the catheter-transducer system. There may be serious consequences when an underdamped system leads to an overestimation of the pressure gradients across a stenotic (narrowed) heart valve.

Figure 7.13 shows examples of distortion of pressure waveform. The actual blood-pressure waveform [Figure 7.13(a)] was recorded with a high-quality pressure transducer with a bandwidth from dc to 100 Hz. Note that in the underdamped case, the amplitude of the higher-frequency components of the pressure wave are amplified, whereas for the overdamped case these higher-frequency components are attenuated. The actual peak pressure [Figure 7.13(a)] is approximately 130 mm Hg (17.3 kPa). The underdamped response [Figure 7.13(b)] has a peak pressure of about 165 mm Hg (22 kPa), which may lead to a serious clinical error if this peak pressure is used to assess the severity of aortic-valve stenosis. The minimum pressure is also in error, − 15 mm Hg (− 2 kPa) compared with the actual value of 5 mm Hg (0.7 kPa). There is also a time delay of approximately 30 ms in the underdamped case.

The overdamped case [Figure 7.13(c)] shows a significant time delay of approximately 150 ms and an attenuated amplitude,

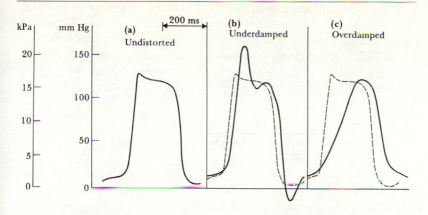

Figure 7.13 Pressure-waveform distortion. (a) Recording of an undistorted left-ventricular pressure waveform using a pressure transducer with bandwidth dc to 100 Hz. (b) Underdamped response, where peak value is increased. A time delay is also evident in this recording. (c) Overdamped response that shows a significant time delay and an attenuated amplitude response.

120 mm Hg (16 kPa) compared with the actual value of 130 mm Hg (17.3 kPa). This type of response can occur in the presence of a large air bubble or a blood clot at the tip of the catheter.

An underdamped catheter-transducer system may be transformed to an overdamped system by pinching the catheter. This procedure reduces the damping ratio ζ, with little effect on the natural frequency. (See Problem 7.6.)

Another example of distortion in blood-pressure measurements in known as *catheter whip*. Figure 7.14 shows these low-

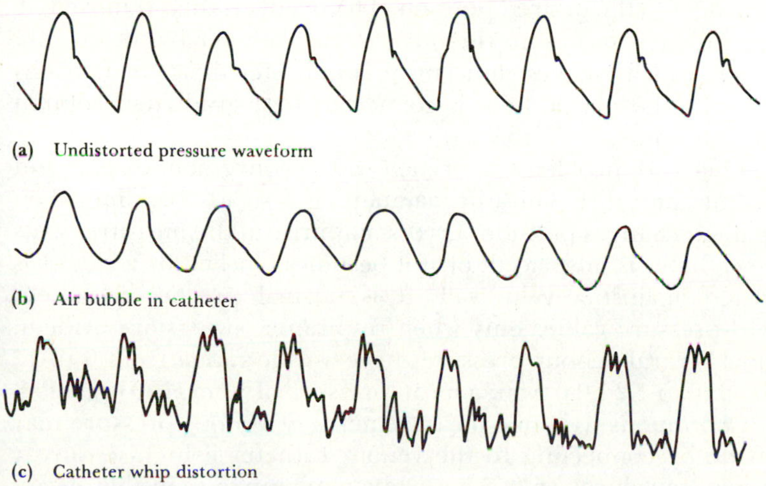

(a) Undistorted pressure waveform

(b) Air bubble in catheter

(c) Catheter whip distortion

Figure 7.14 Distortion during recording of arterial pressure. Bottom trace is response when pressure catheter is bent and whipped by accelerating blood in regions of high pulsatile flow.

frequency oscillations that appear in the blood-pressure recording. This may occur when an aortic ventricular catheter, in a region of high pulsatile flow, is bent and whipped about by the accelerating blood. This type of distortion may be minimized by the use of stiff catheters or by careful placement of catheters in regions of low flow velocity.

7.8 Systems for measuring venous pressure

Measurements of venous pressure are an important aid to the physician for determining the function of the capillary bed and the right heart. The pressure in the small veins is lower than the capillary pressure and reflects the value of the capillary pressure. The intrathoracic venous pressure determines the diastolic filling pressure of the right ventricle (Rushmer, 1970). The central venous pressure is measured in a central vein or in the right atrium. It fluctuates above and below atmospheric pressure as the subject breathes, while the extrathoracic venous pressure is 2 to 5 cm H_2O (0.2 to 0.5 kPa) above atmospheric. The reference level for venous pressure is at the right atrium.

Central venous pressure is an important indicator of myocardial performance. It is normally monitored on surgical and medical patients to assess proper therapy in cases of heart dysfunction, shock, hypo- or hypervolemic states, or circulatory failure. It is used as a guide to determine the amount of liquid a patient should receive.

Physicians usually measure steady-state or mean venous pressure by making a percutaneous venous puncture with a large-bore needle, inserting a catheter through the needle into the vein, and advancing it to the desired position. The needle is then removed. A plastic tube is attached to the intravenous catheter by means of a stopcock, which enables clinicians to administer drugs or fluids as necessary. The plastic tube is connected to a graduated column filled with saline.

There are problems associated with inconvenient display and recording, and difficulties in maintaining a steady baseline when the patient changes position. Errors may arise in the measurements if the catheter is misplaced, or if it becomes blocked by a clot or is impacted against a vein wall. It is normal practice to accept venous-pressure values only when respiratory swings are evident. Normal central venous pressures have a wide range from 0 to 12 cm H_2O (0 to 1.2 kPa), with a mean pressure of 5 cm H_2O (0.5 kPa).

Continuous dynamic measurements of venous pressure may be made by connecting to the venous catheter a high-sensitivity pressure transducer with a lower dynamic range than that necessary for arterial measurements.

7.9 Heart sounds

The auscultation of the heart provides valuable information to the clinician concerning the functional integrity of the heart. More information becomes available when clinicians compare the temporal relationships between the heart sounds and the mechanical and electrical events of the cardiac cycle. This latter approach is known as *phonocardiography.*

There is a wide diversity of opinion concerning the theories that attempt to explain the origin of heart sounds and murmurs. More than 40 different mechanisms have been proposed to explain the first heart sound. A basic definition shows the difference between heart sounds and murmurs (Rushmer, 1970). *Heart sounds* are vibrations or sounds due to the acceleration or deceleration of blood, whereas *murmurs* are considered vibrations or sounds due to blood turbulence.

Mechanism and origin

Figure 7.15 shows the correlation of the four heart sounds with the electrical and mechanical events of the cardiac cycle. The first heart sound is associated with the movement of blood during ventricular systole (Rushmer, 1970). As the ventricles contract, blood shifts toward the atria, closing the atrioventricular valves with a consequential oscillation of blood. The first heart sound further originates from oscillations of blood between the distending root of the aorta and ventricle and vibrations due to blood turbulence at the aortic and pulmonary valves. Splitting of the first heart sound is defined as an asynchronous closure of the tricuspid and the mitral valves. The second heart sound is a low-frequency vibration associated with the deceleration and reversal of flow in the aorta and pulmonary artery and the closure of the semilunar valves. This second heart sound is coincident with the completion of the T wave of the ECG.

The third heart sound is attributed to the sudden termination of the rapid-filling phase of the ventricles from the atria and the associated vibration of the ventricular muscle walls, which are relaxed. This low-amplitude, low-frequency vibration is audible in children and in some adults.

The fourth or atrial heart sound—which is not audible, but which may be recorded by the phonocardiogram—occurs when the atria contract and propel blood into the ventricles.

The sources of most murmurs, developed by turbulence in rapidly moving blood, are known. Murmurs are common in children during the early systolic phase; they are normally heard in nearly all adults after exercise. Abnormal murmurs may be caused

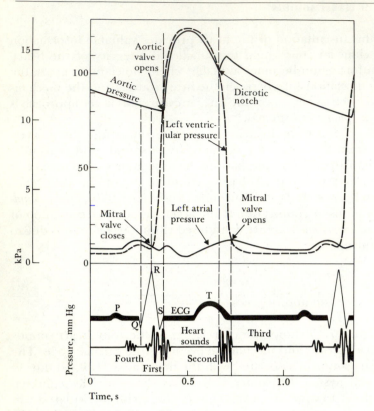

Figure 7.15 Correlation of four heart sounds with electrical and mechanical events of cardiac cycle.

by stenoses and insufficiencies (leaks) at the aortic, pulmonary, and mitral valves. They are detected by noting the time of their occurrence in the cardiac cycle and their location at the time of measurement.

Auscultation techniques

Heart sounds travel through the body from the heart and major blood vessels to the body surface. Because of the acoustical properties of the transmission path, sound waves are attenuated and not reflected. The largest attenuation of the wavelike motion occurs in the most compressible tissues, such as the lungs and fat layers.

There are optimal recording sites for the various heart sounds, sites at which the intensity of sound is the highest because the sound is being transmitted through solid tissues or through a

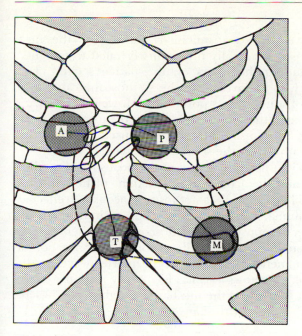

Figure 7.16 Auscultatory areas on the chest. A, aortic; P, pulmonary; T, tricuspid and M, mitral areas. (From A.C. Burton, *Physiology and Biophysics of the Circulation*, 2nd ed. Copyright © 1972 by Year Book Medical Publishers, Inc., Chicago. Used by permission.)

minimal thickness of inflated lung. There are four basic chest locations at which the intensity of sound from the four valves is maximized (Figure 7.16).

Heart sounds and murmurs have extremely small amplitudes, with frequencies from 0.1 to 2000 Hz. Two difficulties may occur because of this frequency range. At the low end of the spectrum (below about 20 Hz), the amplitude of heart sounds is below the threshold of audibility. The high-frequency end is normally quite perceptible to the human ear, since this is the region of maximum sensitivity. However, if a phonocardiogram is desired, the recording device must be carefully selected for high frequency-response characteristics. That is, a standard pen strip-chart recorder would be inadequate, whereas a light-beam or ink-jet recorder would be adequate.

Since heart sounds and murmurs are of low amplitude, extraneous noises must be minimized in the vicinity of the patient. It is standard procedure to record the phonocardiogram for non-bedridden patients in a specially designed acoustically quiet room. Artifacts from movements of the patient appear as baseline wandering.

Stethoscopes

Stethoscopes are used to transmit heart sounds from the chest wall to the human ear. Originally physicians listened to patients' heart sounds by putting their ears on the patient's chest. For reasons of propriety and convenience the stethoscope came into use. An advantage of using it is its portability. However, the variability in interpretation of the sounds stems from the user's auditory acuity and training. Moreover, the technique used to apply the stethoscope can greatly affect the sounds perceived.

Ertel *et al.* (1966a) have investigated the acoustics of stethoscope transmission and the acoustical interactions of human ears with stethoscopes. They found that stethoscope acoustics reflected the acoustics of the human ear when worn: Younger individuals revealed slightly better responses to a stethoscope than their elders. The mechanical stethoscope amplifies sound because of a standing-wave phenomenon, which occurs at quarter wavelengths of the sound. Figure 7.17 shows a typical frequency-response curve for a stethoscope; it shows that the mechanical stethoscope has an uneven frequency response, with many resonance peaks.

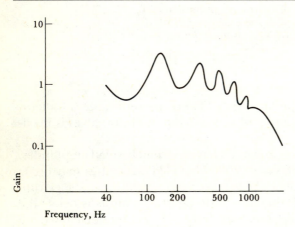

Frequency, Hz

Figure 7.17 Typical frequency-response curve for a stethoscope, found by applying a known audiofrequency signal to the bell of a stethoscope by means of a headphone-coupler arrangement. Audio output of stethoscope earpiece was monitored by means of a coupler microphone system. (From P.Y. Ertel, M. Lawrence, R.K. Brown, and A.M. Stern, *Stethoscope Acoustics* I, "The Doctor and his Stethoscope." Circulation 34, 1966; by permission of American Heart Association.)

In a follow-up study of the transmission and filtration patterns of stethoscope acoustics, Ertel *et al.* (1966b) tested four groups of basic bell-type stethoscopes. They found attenuation at high frequencies with both shallow bells and single-tubing-design stethoscopes, whereas deep trumpet-shaped bells with double-tubing design may provide amplification at higher frequencies. They emphasized that the critical area of the performance of a stethoscope—i.e., the clinically significant sounds near the listener's threshold of hearing—may be totally lost if the stethoscope attenuates them as little as 3 dB. A physician may miss sounds with one instrument that can be heard with another.

When the stethoscope chest piece is firmly applied, low frequencies are attenuated more than high frequencies. The stethoscope housing is in the shape of a bell. It makes contact with the skin, which serves as the diaphragm at the bell rim. The diaphragm becomes taut with pressure, thereby causing an attenuation of low frequencies.

Loose-fitting earpieces cause additional problems, because the leak that develops reduces the coupling between the chest wall and the ear, with consequent decrease in the listener's perception of heart sounds and murmurs. A further difficulty in using a stethoscope is that it is very hard to give a verbal description of the sounds. Such descriptions are known to be notoriously inadequate (Rushmer, 1970).

Many types of electronic stethoscopes have been proposed by engineers. These devices have selectable frequency-response characteristics ranging from the "ideal" flat-response case and selected bandpasses to typical mechanical-stethoscope responses. Physicians, however, have not generally accepted these electronic stethoscopes, mainly because they are unfamiliar with the sounds heard with them. Their size, portability, convenience, and resemblance to the mechanical stethoscope are other important considerations.

7.10 Phonocardiography

A phonocardiogram is a recording of the heart sounds and murmurs. It is valuable in that it not only eliminates the subjective interpretation of these sounds, but also makes possible an evaluation of the heart sounds and murmurs with respect to the electrical and mechanical events in the cardiac cycle. In the clinical evaluation of a patient, a number of other heart-related variables are recorded simultaneously with the phonocardiogram. These include the ECG, carotid arterial pulse, jugular venous pulse, and apex cardiogram. (See Figure 7.18.) The indirect carotid, jugular, and apex-cardiogram pulses are recorded by using a microphone system with a low frequency response (less than 0.2 to 0.5 Hz).

Technicians measure the *indirect carotid pulse* by applying the sensor directly over the point of carotid pulsations in the midneck region. They either hold it in position manually or secure it by a low-pressure inflatable cuff. Artifacts may appear due to movements of the patient's muscles under the cuff or air leaks in the mechanical coupling between the sensor and the sensing crystal ele-

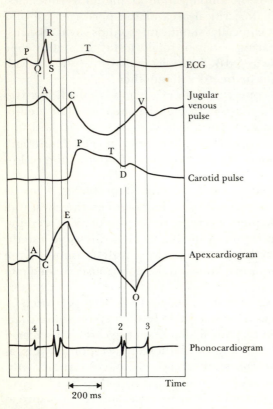

ECG

Jugular
venous
pulse

Carotid pulse

Apexcardiogram

Phonocardiogram

Time

200 ms

Figure 7.18 Correlation of various sounds, and electrical and pulsatile events associated with heart dynamics. The A wave of jugular pulse is due to right-atrial contraction; C wave results mainly from onset of contraction of right ventricle (tricuspid-valve closure); V wave is caused by atrial filling while the tricuspid valve is closed. Carotid pulse rises steeply with aortic pressure to its peak; the percussion wave P occurs approximately at maximum ejection. A second wave (the tidal wave T) follows late in systole; its shape is a function of peripheral vascular tone. The dicrotic notch D indicates closure of aortic valve. The A wave of the apexcardiogram is caused by left atrial contraction. The C wave occurs at beginning of isovolumetric contraction. The E point occurs at beginning of ejection of left ventricle. Mitral valve opens at point O. (From M.E. Tavel, *Clinical Phonocardiography and External Pulse Recording*. Copyright © 1972 by Year Book Medical Publishers, Inc., Chicago. Used by permission.)

ment. The waveshape for the carotid pulse is essentially the same as the waveshape for the aortic pulse, except that an appreciable time delay exists between these two. Closure of the aortic valve is reflected in the carotid pulse as the dicrotic notch.

The *indirect jugular venous pulse* is measured using a cup-shaped sensor placed over the internal jugular vein near its inferior bulb and held in place manually. The jugular venous pulse reflects the mechanical events in the right atrium.

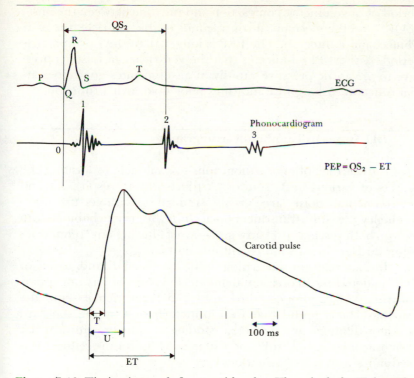

Figure 7.19 Timing intervals for carotid pulse. These include: T time, the time it takes to reach one-half maximum value; U time, the time it takes to reach maximum value; and ET, the ejection time, or time from pulse onset to dicrotic notch. The pre-ejection period, PEP, is measured from the Q wave of the ECG to the onset of carotid upstroke (corrected for time delay). The carotid pulse is corrected for time delay by shifting the carotid pulse such that the dicrotic notch is synchronous with S_2. Also $PEP = QS_2 - ET$.

The *apexcardiogram* reflects the mechanical pulsations of the heart muscle transmitted to the body surface. A single pickup device is subject to movement artifacts of the *precordium* (the chest wall in front of the heart). A differential-pressure system can be used to eliminate this artifact. It has value in that it serves as a timing reference for the phonocardiogram; also, in pathological situations, its shape assumes certain characteristic patterns.

The cardiologist evaluates the results of a phonocardiograph on the basis of changes in waveshape and in a number of timing parameters. Figure 7.19 shows the timing intervals for the carotid pulse. The period of isovolumetric contraction is indirectly measured from the Q wave of the ECG to the onset of the carotid upstroke, after it has been corrected for time delay. This parameter is called the *pre-ejection period*, PEP. The PEP is best calculated by subtracting the ejection time from the time period from the Q wave to the second heart sound (Tavel, 1972). The PEP is the sum of the period of isovolumetric contraction and the time between the onset of QRS and the mechanical contractions of the ventricle (the electromechanical interval). The PEP is longer than the isovolumetric period. A short PEP indicates that the ventricle can raise its pressure to the aortic pressure rapidly; it also indicates good myocardial function. A long PEP indicates poor myocardial function.

7.11 Intracardiac phonocardiography

Intracardiac phonocardiographs are valuable in locating the sources of various heart sounds. Artifacts due to respiratory and environmental noise are greatly reduced. Catheter-tip high-frequency pressure transducers placed in the heart chambers can pick up both vascular pressure and—after filtering out frequencies below 20 Hz—heart sounds and murmurs.

Intracardiac phonocardiography has been found to be of value in detecting an occasional undetected abnormality not apparent from surface phonocardiography. Small ventricular-septal defects have been found that were undetermined by the standard indicator-dilution or hydrogen studies. However, intracardiac phonocardiography is still not a standard clinical procedure; it is used more in research situations.

7.12 Heart-sound instrumentation systems

Microphones

Heart-sound microphones operate on the basis of either the piezoelectric effect (the *crystal* microphone) or Faraday's principle (the *dynamic* microphone). Figure 7.20 shows that the piezoelectric microphone is more sensitive than the dynamic microphone at low frequencies. The crystal microphone can be used for essentially all phonocardiographic measurements. The dynamic microphone, on the other hand, has a higher output voltage than the crystal. But it cannot be used for pulse-wave recordings because of its inadequate low-frequency response.

There are two basic categories of heart-sound and pulse-wave microphones: contact and air-coupled. The *contact* microphone is applied directly to the skin, whereas the air-coupled system has an air-filled tube between a cup on the skin and the transducer. The *air-coupled* crystal microphone is generally used to measure carotid pulse and jugular venous pulse, and to make apexcardiograms. A system time constant of 2 s is specified for acceptable pulse recording. When an air-coupled microphone is used, all air leaks

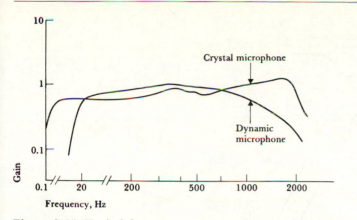

Figure 7.20 Typical frequency response for crystal and dynamic micro-phones.

must be eliminated in order to maintain the desired frequency response.

Filtering

The microphone sensing element may be coupled to the patient's skin surface either through a bell-shaped cone that uses the principle of air conduction between the skin and transducer or through a diaphragm that conducts the sound to the sensing element. *Mechanical* filtering of heart sounds and murmurs is possible by a careful selection of the size of the diaphragm and microphone bell. The larger the diameter of the diaphragm, the lower the maximum frequency response of the system. As the pressure is increased on a microphone bell, the skin becomes more taut and the microphone system becomes more sensitive to higher frequencies and less sensitive to lower frequencies. *Electronic* filtering can be used to selectively record or listen to desired frequency bands.

Signal conditioning

In order to reproduce the heart sounds, the total system must have a frequency response of 25 to 2000 Hz for heart sounds and murmurs and 0.1 to 100 Hz for pulse waves. The recording device must be capable of reproducing signals over this frequency range. It is possible to compensate for an inadequate frequency response in the recording device by pre-emphasizing these heart-sound frequencies in the amplifier. Figure 7.21 shows how an optical galvanometer with a bandwidth of 500 Hz can be compensated by inserting a frequency-compensation network in the amplifier.

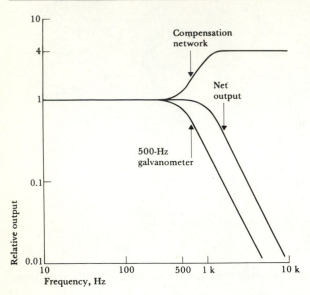

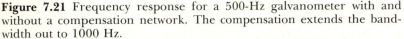

Figure 7.21 Frequency response for a 500-Hz galvanometer with and without a compensation network. The compensation extends the bandwidth out to 1000 Hz.

Example 7.3 Figure 7.21 shows the frequency response for a compensated-galvanometer system used to record heart sounds. Design an appropriate compensation network that will increase the bandwidth from 500 to 1000 Hz when connected in series with the galvanometer.

Answer We can extend the second-order response of the galvanometer from 500 to 1000 Hz by connecting a system in series with the galvanometer with the "opposite" frequency characteristics. Assume that the high-frequency response of the galvanometer is critically damped ($\zeta = 1$). One solution to this problem would be to insert two equivalent first-order systems in series with the individual frequency response shown in Figure 7.22(a). The frequency response of the one-section compensator is somewhat like that of the high-pass filter that we saw in Figure 3.11, except that it requires a response at dc. We achieve this by placing a resistor in parallel with the input capacitor of Figure 3.13(b), as shown in Figure 7.22.

The low-frequency corner frequency f_{c1} is given by $1/2\pi R_1 C = 500$ Hz. If we choose $R_1 = 10$ kΩ, then $C = 0.032$ μF. The high-frequency corner frequency f_{c2} is given by $(R_1 + R_2)/R_1 R_2 2\pi C = 1$ kHz. Then $R_2 = 10$ kΩ. At low frequencies the capacitor has a very high impedance and the gain should be 1.0. Hence we choose $R_3 = 20$ kΩ. The two sections are placed in series to form the total compensation.

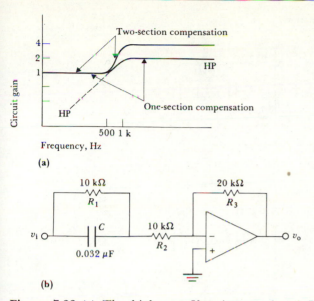

Figure 7.22 (a) The high-pass filter is reproduced from Figure 3.11. (b) One-section compensation is accomplished by placing a resistance across the input capacitor of Figure 3.13(b). Place two circuits in series to achieve the two-section compensation shown in (a).

If high-frequency noise is a problem, then an alternative design with a sharper high-frequency attenuation can be employed.

High-frequency heart sounds may be displayed on a low-frequency-response direct-writing pen recorder as follows. The heart sounds are envelope-detected and the signal is then modulated by an 80-Hz carrier. The amplitude and the temporal relationships of heart sounds to pulse waves and murmurs are accurately reproduced. However, in order to analyze the frequency content, the technician must obtain the signal prior to envelope detection.

Hot-wire anemometer

A new phonocardiographic transducer utilizing the hot-wire anemometer principle has been introduced (Laughlin and Mahoney, 1972). Movement of the skin is amplified pneumatically by sealing a plastic cup to the skin and mounting a thermistor and a wire sensing element in the center of a small exit port plugged into a hole in the cup (Figure 7.23). The system employs a pair of fine heated wires to detect heart sounds (50 to 1000 Hz) and a pair of heated thermistors to detect pulses (0.2 to 15 Hz). The thermistors

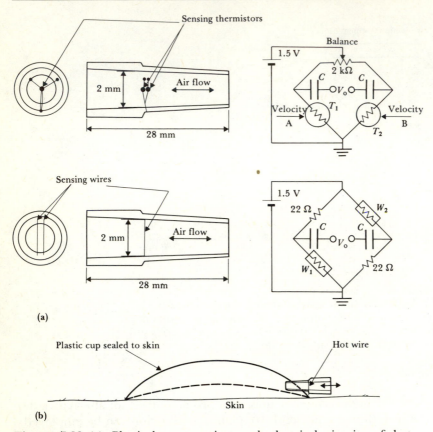

(a)

(b)

Figure 7.23 (a) Physical construction and electrical circuits of hot-thermistor sensors (T_1, T_2) and hot-wire sensors (W_1, W_2). (b) Skin cup and sensor elements. Dashed line indicates how skin moves to push air through sensor lumen. (From D.E. Laughlin and R.P. Mahoney, "New Phonocardiographic Transducers Utilizing the Hot-Wire Anemometer Principle," *Med. Biol. Eng.*, 1972, **10**, 43–55. Used with permission.)

respond to cardiac pulses because they are heated; but because of their relatively high thermal inertia they do not respond to heart sounds. Two thermistors are placed in a longitudinal position in an airstream and are connected in two arms of a Wheatstone bridge that produces a biphasic unbalancing of the bridge as the direction of airflow reverses. The airflow is caused by the inward and outward movements of the skin. The thermistor closest to the flow cools more than the more distant one, thus causing a bridge unbalance. When the flow is reversed, an unbalance of opposite polarity appears at the bridge terminals. Heart sounds are detected by two wires, also connected as arms of another Wheatstone bridge. Both wires are cooled by the moving air, and detect the small fluctuations in sound that are superimposed on the large pulse wave. An increased air velocity cools the wires, thus decreasing their resistance and unbalancing the bridge.

Figure 7.23(a) shows the physical construction and electrical circuits of the hot-wire and hot-thermistor sensors. The skin cup and sensor elements are shown in Figure 7.23(b). This compact, low-impedance transducer has a high SNR and is insensitive to ambient sounds. The quality of superficial pulse recordings has proved to be equal to comparable devices. Reliable recordings of low-frequency heart sounds have been demonstrated.

Signal analysis

The spectral phonocardiogram has been used successfully in a recording that displays frequency, time, and an intensity-modulated gray scale that indicates amplitude (Kingsley and Segal, 1974). This method allows for an analysis of the instantaneous sound energy during 5-ms intervals throughout the heartbeat. Gupta *et al.* (1975) have reported a spectral-analysis technique of arterial sounds for studying arterial disease.

7.13 Cardiac catheterization

The cardiac-catheterization procedure is a combination of several techniques that are used to assess hemodynamic function and cardiovascular structure. Cardiac catheterization is performed in virtually all patients in whom heart surgery is contemplated. This procedure yields information that may be crucial in defining the timing, risks, and anticipated benefit for a given patient (Grossman, 1974). Catheterization procedures are performed in specialized laboratories equipped with x-ray equipment for visualizing heart structures and the position of various pressure catheters. In addition, measurements are made of cardiac output, blood and respiratory gases, blood-oxygen saturation, and metabolic products. The injection of radiopaque dyes into the ventricles or aorta makes it possible for the clinician to assess ventricular or aortic function. In a similar fashion, injection of radiopaque dyes into the coronary arteries makes possible a clinical evaluation of coronary-artery disease. In the following paragraphs, we shall discuss a number of specific procedures carried out in a catheter laboratory.

Clinicians can measure pressures in all four chambers of the heart and in the great vessels by positioning catheters during fluoroscopy in such a way that they can recognize the characteristic pressure waveforms. They measure pressures across the four valves to determine their pressure gradients.

An example of a patient with aortic stenosis helps to illustrate the procedure. Figure 7.24(a) shows the pressures of the stenotic patient before the operation: Note the pressures in the left ventricle and the aorta, and the systolic pressure gradient. Figure 7.24(b) shows the stenotic patient after the operation: Note the marked decrease in the pressure gradient brought about by the insertion of a ball-valve aortic prosthesis. These pressures may be measured by using a two-lumen catheter positioned so that the valve is located between the two catheter openings. The clinician can find the various time indices describing the injection and filling periods of the heart directly from the recordings of blood pressure in the heart.

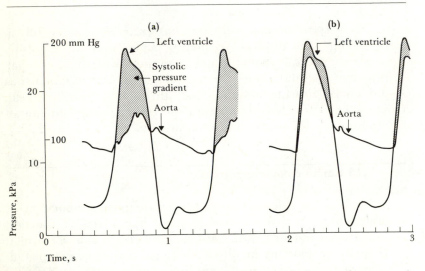

Figure 7.24 (a) Systolic pressure gradient (left ventricular-aortic pressure) across a stenotic aortic valve. (b) Marked decrease in systolic pressure gradient with insertion of an aortic ball valve.

Clinicians can also use balloon-tipped, flow-directed catheters without fluoroscopy (Ganz and Swan, 1974). An inflated balloon at the catheter tip is carried by the bloodstream from the intrathoracic veins through the right atrium, ventricle, pulmonary artery, and into a small pulmonary artery—where it is wedged, blocking the local flow. The wedge pressure in this pulmonary artery reflects the mean pressure in the left atrium because a column of stagnant blood on the right side of the heart joins the free-flowing blood beyond the capillary bed.

Blood samples may be drawn from within the various heart chambers and vessels where the catheter tip is positioned. These blood samples are important in determining the presence of shunts between the heart chambers or great vessels. For example, a shunt from the left to the right heart is indicated by a higher-than-normal

O_2 content in the blood in the right heart in the vicinity of the shunt. The O_2 content is normally determined by an oximeter (recall Section 2.15). Cardiac blood samples are also used to assess metabolic end products such as lactate, pyruvate, CO_2, and other substances (injected), such as radioactive materials and colored dyes.

The measurement of cardiac output is very important to those who want to assess the pumping function of the heart. Cardiac output can be determined by a number of methods, including the Fick method, dye dilution, thermodilution, or impedance cardiography (see Chapter 8).

Angiographic visualization is an essential tool used to evaluate cardiac structure. Radiopaque dye is injected rapidly into a cardiac chamber or blood vessel and the hemodynamics are viewed and recorded on x-ray film, cinemovie film, or videotape. (Section 11.6 will discuss the principles of radiography and fluoroscopy.) Specially designed catheters and power injectors are used in order that a bolus of contrast material can be delivered rapidly into the appropriate vessel or heart chamber. Standard angiographic techniques are employed, where indicated, in the evaluation of the left and right ventricles (*ventriculography*), the coronary arteries (*coronary arteriography*), the pulmonary artery (*pulmonary angiography*), and the aorta (*aortography*). During heart catheterization, ectopic beats and/or cardiac fibrillation frequently occur. These are usually caused by a mechanical stimulus from the catheter or from a jet of contrast material. For this reason, clinicians must have a functional defibrillator (Section 12.2) readily available in the catheterization laboratory.

Areas of a valve orifice can be calculated from basic fluid-mechanics equations (Herman *et al.*, 1974). Physicians can assess valvular stenosis by measuring the pressure gradient across and the flow through the valve of interest.

Bernoulli's equation for frictionless flow is (Burton, 1972):

$$P_t = P + \rho g h + \frac{\rho u^2}{2} \tag{7.12}$$

where

P_t = fluid total pressure
P = local fluid static pressure
ρ = fluid density
g = acceleration of gravity (Appendix A.1)
h = height above reference level
u = fluid velocity

We first assume frictionless flow for the model shown in Figure 7.25, and equate total pressures at locations 1 and 2. We

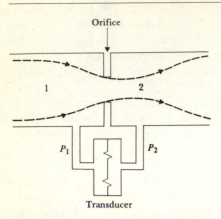

Figure 7.25 Model for deriving equation for heart-valve orifice area: P_1 and P_2 are upstream and downstream static pressures. Velocity u is calculated for minimum flow area A at location 2.

assume that the difference in heights is negligible and that the velocity at location 1 is negligible compared with u, the velocity at location 2. Then (7.12) reduces to

$$P_1 - P_2 = \frac{\rho u^2}{2} \tag{7.13}$$

from which

$$u = \left[\frac{2(P_1 - P_2)}{\rho} \right]^{1/2}$$

At location 2, the flow $F = Au$, where A is the area; hence

$$A = \frac{F}{u} = F \left[\frac{\rho}{2(P_1 - P_2)} \right]^{1/2} \tag{7.14}$$

In practice, there are losses due to friction and the minimum flow area is smaller than the orifice area. Hence (7.14) becomes

$$A = \frac{F}{c_d} \left[\frac{\rho}{2(P_1 - P_2)} \right]^{1/2} \tag{7.15}$$

where c_d is a discharge coefficient. It has been empirically found that for semilunar values, septal defects, and patent ductus, $c_d = 0.85$, whereas for mitral valves, $c_d = 0.6$ (Yellin *et al.*, 1975).

Example 7.4 Calculate the approximate area of the aortic valve for the patient with the aortic and left-ventricular pressures shown in Figure 7.24(a). The patient's cardiac output was measured by thermodilution as 6400 ml/min and the heart rate as 78 beats/min. Blood density is 1060 kg/m³.

Answer From Figure 7.24(a), the ejection period is 0.31 s and the average pressure drop is 7.33 kPa. During the ejection period, the flow (in SI units) is

$$F = (6.4 \times 10^{-3} \text{ m}^3/\text{min})(1/78 \text{ min/beat})(1/0.31 \text{ beat/s})$$
$$= 264 \times 10^{-6} \text{ m}^3/\text{s}$$

From (7.15) we have

$$A = \frac{264 \times 10^{-6}}{0.85} \left[\frac{1060}{2(7330)} \right]^{1/2}$$
$$= 83 \times 10^{-6} \text{ m}^2 = 83 \text{ mm}^2$$

7.14 Effects of potential and kinetic energy on pressure measurements

In certain situations, the effects of potential- and kinetic-energy terms in the measurement of blood pressure may yield inaccurate results.

Bernoulli's equation (7.12) shows that the total pressure of a fluid remains constant in the absence of dissipative effects. The static pressure P of the fluid is the desired pressure; it is measured in a blood vessel when the potential- and kinetic-energy terms are zero.

We first examine the effect of the potential-energy term on the static pressure of the fluid. When measurements of blood pressure are taken with the patient in a supine (on-the-back) position and with the transducer placed in a position so that it is at heart level, no corrections need be made for the potential-energy term. However, when the patient is sitting or standing, the long columns of blood in the arterial and venous pressure systems contribute a hydrostatic pressure, $\rho g h$.

For a patient in the erect position, the arterial and venous pressure both increase to approximately 85 mm Hg (11.3 kPa) at the ankle. When the arm is held above the head, the pressure in the wrist becomes about 40 mm Hg (5.3 kPa). The transducer diaphragm should be placed at the same level as the pressure source. If this is not possible, the difference in height must be accounted for. For each 1.31-cm increase in height of the source, 1.0 mm Hg (133 Pa) must be added to the transducer reading.

The kinetic-energy term $\rho u^2/2$ becomes important when the velocity of blood flow is high. When a blood-pressure catheter is inserted into a blood vessel or into the heart, two types of pressures may be determined—side (static) or end (total) pressures. "Side pressure" implies that the end of the catheter has openings at right angles to the flow. In this case the pressure reading is accurate because the kinetic-energy term is minimal. However, if the catheter pressure port is in line with the flow stream, then the kinetic energy of the fluid at that point is transformed into pressure. If the catheter pressure port faces *up*stream, the recorded pressure is the side pressure plus the additional kinetic-energy term $\rho u^2/2$. On the other hand, if the catheter pressure port faces *down*stream, the value is approximately $\rho u^2/2$ less than the side pressure. If the catheter is not positioned correctly, artifacts may develop in the pressure reading.

Table 7.1 shows the relative importance of the kinetic-energy term in different parts of the circulation (Burton, 1972). As Table 7.1 shows, there are situations in the aorta, venae cavae, and pulmonary artery in which the kinetic-energy term is a substantial part of the total pressure. For the laminar-flow case, this error decreases as the catheter pressure port is moved from the center of the vessel to the vessel wall, where the average velocity of flow is less. The kinetic-energy term could also become important in a disease situation in which an artery becomes narrowed.

Vessel	Vel (cm/s)	KE (mm Hg)	Systolic (mm Hg)	(kPa)	% KE of total
Aorta (systolic)					
At rest	100	4	120	(16)	3
Cardiac output at 3 × rest	300	36	180	(24)	17
Brachial artery					
At rest	30	0.35	110	(14.7)	0.3
Cardiac output at 3 × rest	90	4	120	(16)	3
Venae cavae					
At rest	30	0.35	2	(0.3)	12
Cardiac output at 3 × rest	90	3.2	3	(0.4)	52
Pulmonary artery					
At rest	90	3	20	(2.7)	13
Cardiac output at 3 × rest	270	27	25	(3.3)	52

Table 7.1 Relative importance of the kinetic-energy term in different parts of the circulation (From A. C. Burton, *Physiology and Biophysics of the Circulation*. Copyright 1972 by Year Book Medical Publishers, Inc., Chicago. Used by permission.)

7.15 Indirect measurements of blood pressure

Indirect measurement of blood pressure is an attempt to measure intraarterial pressures noninvasively. The most standard manual techniques employ either the palpation or audible detection of the pulse distal to an occlusive cuff. Figure 7.26 shows a typical system for indirect measurement of blood pressure. It employs a sphygmomanometer consisting of an inflatable cuff for occlusion of the blood vessel, a rubber bulb for inflation of the cuff, and either a mercury or aneroid manometer for detection of pressure.

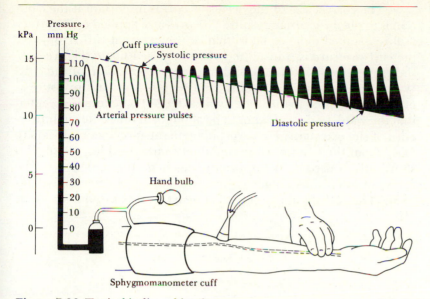

Figure 7.26 Typical indirect blood-pressure measurement system. Sphygmomanometer cuff is inflated by a hand bulb to pressures above the systolic level. Pressure is then slowly released and blood flow under the cuff is monitored by a microphone or stethoscope placed over a downstream artery. The first Korotkoff sound detected indicates systolic pressure, while the transition from muffling to silence brackets diastolic pressure. (From R.F. Rushmer, *Cardiovascular Dynamics*, 3rd ed., 1970. Philadelphia: W.B. Saunders Co. Used with permission.)

Blood pressure is measured in the following way. The occlusive cuff is inflated until the pressure is above systolic pressure, and then is slowly bled off (2–3 mm Hg/s) (0.3–0.4 kPa/s). When the systolic peaks are higher than the occlusive pressure, the blood spurts under the cuff and causes a palpable pulse in the wrist (*Riva-Rocci method*). Audible sounds (*Korotkoff sounds*) generated by the flow of blood and vibrations of the vessel under the cuff may be heard through a stethoscope. At the first detection of the pulse, the manometer pressure indicates the systolic pressure. As the pressure in the cuff is decreased, the audible Korotkoff sounds pass through five phases (Geddes, 1970). The period of transition from muffling (phase IV) to silence (phase V) brackets the diastolic pressure.

It is generally accepted that the palpation method of detecting blood pressure requires a sensitive tactile sense. Claims that this method can be used to consistently measure diastolic pressures have not held up in extensive testing.

In employing the palpation and auscultatory techniques, you should take several measurements, since normal respiration and vasomotor waves modulate the normal blood-pressure levels. These techniques also suffer from the disadvantage of failing to give accurate pressures for infants and hypotensive patients.

The correct size of the occlusive cuff is important if the clinician is to obtain accurate results. The pressure applied to the artery wall is assumed to be equal to that of the external cuff. However, the cuff pressure is transmitted via interposed tissue. Figure 7.27 shows the effects of proper and improper application of the cuff. With a cuff of sufficient width and length, the cuff pressure is evenly transmitted to the underlying artery. It is generally accepted that the width of the cuff should be about 0.40 times the circumference of the extremity. However, no general agreement appears to exist about the length of the pneumatic cuff (Geddes, 1970). If a short cuff is used, it is important that it be positioned over the artery of interest. A longer cuff reduces the problem of misalignment. The cuff should be placed at heart level to avoid hydrostatic effects.

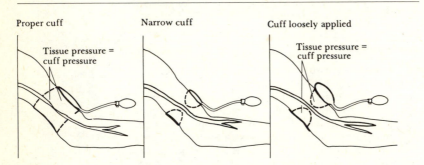

Proper cuff

Tissue pressure =
cuff pressure

Narrow cuff

Cuff loosely applied

Tissue pressure =
cuff pressure

Figure 7.27 Effects of proper and improper application of cuff. A properly designed system transmits pressure applied to cuff directly to tissue surrounding the vessel. A narrow cuff or a loosely applied one does not faithfully transmit cuff pressure to the interposed tissue and thus to the artery. (From R.F. Rushmer, *Cardiovascular Dynamics,* 3rd ed., 1970. Philadelphia: W.B. Saunders Co. Used with permission.)

The auscultatory technique is simple and uses a minimum of equipment. However, it cannot be used in a noisy environment, whereas the palpation technique can. The hearing acuity of the user must be good for low frequencies from 20 to 300 Hz, the bandwidth required for these measurements. Bellville and Weaver (1969) have determined the energy distribution of the Korotkoff sounds for normals and for patients in shock. When there is a fall in blood pressure, the sound spectrum shifts to lower frequencies. The failure of the auscultation technique for hypotensive patients may be due to low sensitivity of the human ear to these low-frequency vibrations (Geddes, 1970).

There is a common misconception that a normal human blood pressure is 120/80, meaning that the systolic value is 120 mm Hg (16 kPa) and that the diastolic value is 80 mm Hg (10.7 kPa). This is not the case. A careful study (by Master *et al.,* 1952) showed that the age and sex of an individual determine the "normal value" of blood pressure. Figure 7.28 shows the range of normal values of systolic and diastolic pressures as a function of sex and age.

A number of techniques have been proposed to automatically measure the systolic and diastolic blood pressure indirectly in humans (Cobbold, 1974). The basic technique involves an automatic sphygmomanometer that inflates and deflates an occlusive cuff at a predetermined rate. A sensitive detector is used to measure the distal pulse. A number of kinds of detectors have been employed, including ultrasonic, piezoelectric, photoelectric, electroacoustic, thermometric, electrocardiographic, rheographic, or tissue impedance (Greatorex, 1971). Two of the commonly used automatic techniques are described in the following paragraphs.

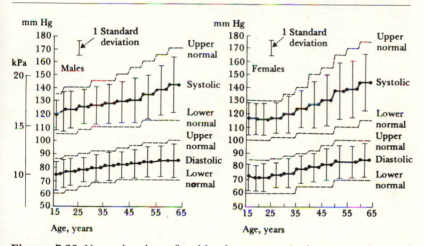

Figure 7.28 Normal values for blood pressure in human males and females, according to age, showing mean systolic and diastolic pressures and plus-and-minus-one standard-deviation range. Limit of normality is given as ±40% of the observations on either side of the mean. [From L.A. Geddes, *The Direct and Indirect Measurement of Blood Pressure.* Copyright © 1970 by Year Book Medical Publishers, Inc., Chicago. Used by permission. (Plotted from data in A.M. Master *et al.*, *Normal Blood Pressure and Hypertension.* Philadelphia: Lea & Febiger, 1952; with permission.)]

The first technique is an automated auscultatory device wherein a *microphone* replaces the stethoscope. The cycle of events that takes place begins with a rapid inflation (20 to 30 mm Hg/s) (2.7 to 4 kPa/s) of the occlusive cuff to a preset pressure about 30 mm Hg higher than the suspected systolic level. The flow of blood beneath the cuff is stopped due to collapse of the vessel. Cuff pressure is then slowly reduced (2 to 3 mm Hg/s) (0.3 to 0.4 kPa/s). The first Korotkoff sound is detected by the microphone, at which time the level of the cuff pressure is stored. The muffling and silent period of the Korotkoff sounds is detected and the value of the diastolic pressure is also stored. After a few minutes, the instrument displays the systolic and diastolic pressures and recycles the

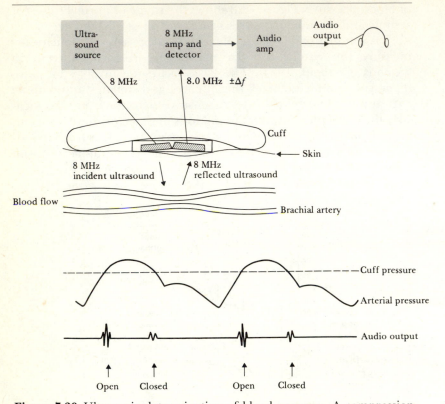

Figure 7.29 Ultrasonic determination of blood pressure. A compression cuff is placed over the transmitting (8 MHz) and receiving (8 MHz $\pm$ Δf) crystals. The opening and closing of the blood vessel is detected as the applied cuff pressure is varied. (From H.F. Stegall, M.B. Kardon, and W.T. Kemmerer, "Indirect Measurement of Arterial Blood Pressure by Doppler Ultrasonic Sphygmomanometry," *J. Appl. Physiol.*, 1968, **25**, 793–798. Used with permission.)

operation. Design considerations for various types of automatic indirect methods of measurement of blood pressure can be found in the literature (Greatorex, 1971).

The *ultrasonic* determination of blood pressure employs a transcutaneous Doppler transducer that detects the motion of the blood-vessel walls in various states of occlusion. Figure 7.29 shows the placement of the compression cuff over two small transmitting and receiving ultrasound crystals (8 MHz) on the arm (Stegall *et al.*, 1968). The Doppler ultrasonic transmitted signal is focused on the vessel wall and the blood. The reflected signal (shifted in frequency) is detected by the receiving crystal and decoded (Section 8.4). The difference in frequency, in the range of 40 to 500 Hz, between the transmitted and received signals is proportional to the velocity of the wall motion and the blood velocity. As the cuff pressure is increased above diastolic but below systolic, the vessel opens and closes with each heartbeat, since the pressure in the artery oscillates above and below the applied external pressure in the cuff. The opening and closing of the vessel is detected by the ultrasonic system.

As the applied pressure is further increased, the time between the opening and closing decreases until they coincide. This point is the *systolic pressure*. Conversely, when the pressure in the cuff is reduced, the time between opening and closing increases until the closing signal from one pulse coincides with the opening signal from the next. This point is the *diastolic pressure* when the vessel is open for the complete pulse.

The advantages of the ultrasonic technique are that it may be used with infants and hypotensive individuals and in high-noise environments. A disadvantage is that movements of the subject's body cause changes in the ultrasonic path between the transducer and the blood vessel. Complete reconstruction of the arterial-pulse waveform is also possible by using the ultrasonic method. A timing pulse from the ECG signal is used as a reference. The clinician uses the pressure in the cuff when the artery opens versus the time from the ECG R wave to plot the rising portion of the arterial pulse. Conversely, the clinician uses the cuff pressure when the artery closes versus the time from the ECG R wave to plot the falling portion of the arterial pulse.

7.16 Tonometry

The basic principle of tonometry is that, when a pressurized vessel is partly collapsed by an external object, the circumferential stresses in the vessel wall are removed and the internal and external pressures are equal. This approach has been used quite successfully to measure intraocular pressure and, with limited success, to determine intraluminal arterial pressure.

Pressman and Newgard (1963) developed an arterial tonometer that uses a flat plate to compress the surface of the skin directly over an artery. Figure 7.30 shows this arterial tonometer. An arterial rider, cylindrical in shape and smaller than the arterial width, senses the radial stress of the artery by means of a force transducer, since the circumferential stresses in the arterial wall are removed by the plate.

An improved arterial tonometer, based on the previous technique, has been developed. It employs electronic feedback to correct for variations in mean blood pressure by changing the force with which the plate presses against the skin (Bahr and Petzke, 1973). It can be used over a greater mean variation in pressure and its use of a solid-state pressure transducer makes it fairly insensitive to motion artifacts. Calibration of absolute pressure is accomplished by means of a mercury manometer. Further testing is necessary for hypo- and normotensive subjects.

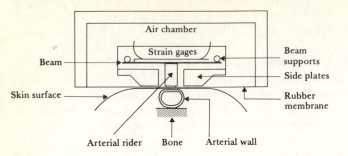

Figure 7.30 An arterial tonometer. Transducer is held in a fixed position against skin surface. Underlying artery must be over a bone. Effects of skin tension in the vertical direction are set to zero by side plates that flatten the skin. Perpendicular force components are due to arterial pulsations and not to skin-motion artifact. The arterial-rider strain-gage-transducer system detects these arterial pulsations. Pressure is found by dividing the force by the contact area of the arterial rider. (From G.L. Pressman and P.M. Newgard, "A Transducer for the Continuous External Measurement of Arterial Blood Pressure," *IEEE Trans. Biomed. Electronics,* 1963, **10,** 73–81. Reprinted with permission of IEEE Transactions on Biomedical Engineering, 1963, New York.)

This force-balance technique can be used to measure intra-ocular pressure. Based on the Imbert-Fick law, the technique enables the clinician to find intraocular pressure by dividing the ap-planation force by the area of applanation. Goldmann (1957) developed an *applanation tonometer,* which is the currently accepted clinical standard. With this technique, the investigator measures the force required to flatten a specific optically determined area. Mackay and Marg (1960) developed a transducer probe that is ap-plied to the corneal surface; the cornea is flattened as the probe is advanced. The intraocular pressure is detected by a force trans-ducer in the center of an annular ring, which unloads the bending forces of the cornea from the transducer.

Forbes *et al.* (1974) developed an applanation tonometer that measures introocular pressure without touching the eye. An air pulse of linearly increasing force deforms and flattens the central area of the cornea, and does so within a few milliseconds. The in-strument consists of three major components: The first is a pneu-matic system that delivers an air pulse whose force increases lin-early with time. The air pulse causes a progressive reduction of the convexity of the cornea, and finally a return to its original shape as the air pulse decays.

The second component, the system that monitors the applan-ation, determines the occurrence of applanation with microsecond resolution by continuously monitoring the status of the curvature of the cornea. Figure 7.31(a) and (b) shows the systems of optical

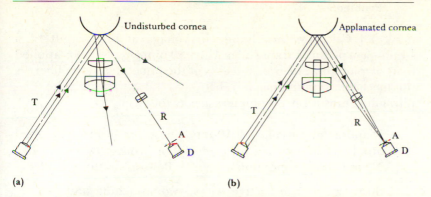

(a)   (b)

Figure 7.31 Monitoring system for noncontact applanation tonometer. (From M. Forbes, G. Pico, Jr., and B. Grolman, "A Noncontact Applanation Tonometer, Description and Clinical Evaluation," *J. Arch. Ophthalmology*, 1975, **91**, 134–140. Copyright © 1975, American Medical Association. Used with permission.)

transmission and detection and the light rays reflected from an undisturbed and an applanated cornea, respectively.

Two obliquely oriented tubes are used to detect applanation. Transmitter tube T directs a collimated beam of light at the corneal vertex, while a telecentric receiver R observes the same area. The light reflected from the cornea passes through the aperture A and is sensed by the detector D. In the case of the undisturbed cornea, little or no light is received by the detector. As the cornea's convexity is progressively reduced to the flattened condition, the amount of light detected is increased. When the cornea is applanated, it acts like a plano mirror with a consequential maximum detected signal. When the cornea becomes concave, a sharp reduction in light detection occurs. The current source for the pneumatic solenoid is immediately shut off when applanation is detected in order to minimize further air-pulse force impinging on the cornea. A direct linear relationship has been found between the intraocular pressure and the time interval to applanation.

The third component of the system is the optical-electronic alignment system. This system is intended to facilitate visual alignment of the noncontacting tonometer and the cornea. An overriding system of verification of automatic alignment disallows measurement unless the specified spatial criteria are satisfied.

A small digital computer is used to control the three segments of the noncontacting tonometer, process the acquired information, and display the intraocular pressure in millimeters of mercury (pascals). The procedure can be safely used on a routine clinical basis without the use of topical anesthesia, and it can be accomplished within a few milliseconds before intervention by a blink reflex.

Problems

7.1 Calculate the change in voltage at the output of a strain-gage pressure transducer when 30 mm Hg (4 kPa) is applied to its diaphragm. The transducer is of the unbonded type. There is no mechanical multiplication between the wires and the diaphragm. Transducer parameters are as follows.

> Diaphragm: Circular: 0.10-mm phosphor bronze; clamped at edges: radius = 12 mm; phosphor bronze: $E_Y = 1 \times 10^{11}$ N/m² (Young's modulus); ($1/m$ = Poisson's ratio = 0.33)

> Strain gage: Four active wires, two stretching and two relaxing; gage factor = 2 (fractional change in resistance/fractional change in length); R_0 of each leg = 150 Ω; effective length of each leg = 80 mm

> Circuit: Unloaded bridge; excitation voltage = 10 V.

Hint: Maximum deflection of the diaphragm at the center, y_c, is equal to

$$y_c = \frac{3(m^2 - 1)r^4 P}{16\, m^2\, E_Y t^3}$$

where

> P = pressure difference normal to diaphragm
> t = thickness = 0.1 mm.

7.2 Compare the transient-step and sinusoidal-frequency methods for determining the response characteristics of a catheter-transducer system.

7.3 Find (a) the damping ratio, (b) the undamped frequency, and (c) the frequency-response curve of the pressure transducer whose transient response to a step change in pressure is shown in Figure P7.1.

7.4 Find the frequency-response curve of the transducer in Problem 7.3, given that its chamber is filled with whole blood at body temperature (37°C). Original data in Problem 7.3 were obtained with water at 20°C.

7.5 What happens to the frequency response of a P23Dd transducer, 6 F, 1-m, water-filled catheter system (at 20°C) when a tiny pinhole leak occurs at the junction of the catheter and transducer? The leak allows a 0.40 ml/min flow for a pressure head of 100 mm Hg (13.3 kPa). Plot frequency-response curves for the system with and without leak. (An intentional leak is often desirable to permit constant flushing of the catheter and thus inhibit formation of clots).

7.6 A low-pass filter is added to the catheter of a

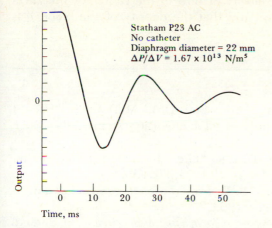

Statham P23 AC
No catheter
Diaphragm diameter = 22 mm
$\Delta P/\Delta V = 1.67 \times 10^{13}$ N/m^5

Figure P7.1 Transient response to a step pressure change. (Used by courtesy of Measurement Systems Division of Gould, Inc.)

pressure-transducer-catheter system by pinching the catheter. The system consists of a Statham P23Dd transducer and a 1-m, 6 F, polyethylene catheter. The pinch effectively reduces the diameter of the catheter to 25% of its original diameter.

    a How long must the pinch be for the system's damping factor to be equal to 0.7?

    b Sketch the frequency response for the system with and without the pinch.

    c Sketch the time response for the system with and without the pinch when excited by a 100-mm-Hg step input.

    d Discuss how faithfully the two systems will reproduce the blood-pressure waveform for humans, dogs, and shrews with heart-rate variations of 1 to 3.3 beats/s, 1.5 to 5 beats/s, and 12 to 22 beats/s, respectively.

    7.7 A heart murmur has a frequency of 300 Hz. Give the block diagram and sketch waveforms for the special instrumentation that enables us to show the occurrence of this murmur on a 0–80-Hz pen recorder.

    7.8 Name the two basic causes of abnormal heart murmurs. For each type, give an example and sketch when it occurs relative to systole and diastole.

    7.9 In block-diagram form show the elements required for an automatic indirect system for measuring blood pressure.

    7.10 A patient who has been vomiting for several days is dehydrated. Liquid is infused through a venous catheter at the rate of 250 ml/h. Sketch the resulting central venous pressure versus time and explain any large change in the slope of the curve. How does the jugular venous pulse change during this procedure?

    7.11 Determine whether the kinetic-energy term is significant for measurements of pressure in the human descending aorta.

Assume that the peak velocity of flow in the center of the aorta is approximately 1.5 m/s and that the density of the blood ρ is 1060 kg/m³.

References

Attinger, E.O., A. Anne, and D.A. McDonald, "Use of Fourier series for the analysis of biological systems." *Biophys. J.* 1970, 6, 291–304.

Bahr, D.E., and J. Petzke, "The automatic arterial tonometer," *Proc. Conf. Eng. Med. Biol.*, 1973, 26, 259.

Bellville, J.W., and C.S. Weaver, *Techniques in clinical physiology.* New York: MacMillan, 1969.

Burton, A.C., *Physiology and biophysics of the circulation*, 2nd ed. Chicago: Year Book, 1972.

Cobbold, R.S.C., *Transducers for biomedical measurements: Principles and applications.* New York: Wiley, 1974.

Collins, C.C., "Biomedical transensors: A review." *J. Biomed. Syst.*, 1970, 1, 23–39.

Ertel, P.Y., M. Lawrence, R.K. Brown, and A.M. Stern, "Stethoscope acoustics I. The doctor and his stethoscope." *Circ.*, 1966a, 34, 889–898.

Ertel, P.Y., M. Lawrence, R.K. Brown, and A.M. Stern, "Stethoscope acoustics II. Transmission and filtration patterns." *Circ.*, 1966b, 34, 899–908.

Fleming, D.G., W.H. Ko, and M.R. Neuman (eds.), *Indwelling and implantable pressure transducers.* Cleveland: CRC Press, 1977.

Forbes, M., G. Pico, Jr., and B. Grolman, "A noncontact applanation tonometer, description and clinical evaluation." *J. Arch. Ophthal.*, 1974, 91, 134–140.

Fry, D.L., "Physiologic recording by modern instruments with particular reference to pressure recording." *Physiol. Rev.*, 1960, 40, 753–788.

Gabe, I.T., "Pressure measurement in experimental physiology," in D.H. Bergel (ed.), *Cardiovascular fluid dynamics.* New York: Academic, 1972, Vol. I.

Ganz, W., and H.J.C. Swan, "Balloon-tipped flow-directed catheters," in W. Grossman (ed.), *Cardiac catheterization and angiography.* Philadelphia: Lea & Febiger, 1974.

Geddes, L.A., *The direct and indirect measurement of blood pressure.* Chicago: Year Book, 1970.

Gersh, B.J., C.E.W. Hahn, and C.P. Roberts, "Physical criteria for measurement of left ventricular pressure and its first derivative." *Cardiovasc. Res.*, 1971, 5, 32–40.

Goldmann, H., "Applanation tonometry," in F.W. Newell (ed.), *Glaucoma: Transactions of the second conference, December 1956, Princeton, N.J.* Madison, NJ, Madison Printing, 1957, pp. 167–220.

Greatorex, C.A., "Indirect methods of blood-pressure measurement," in B.W. Watson (ed.), *IEE Medical Electronics Monographs 1–6,* London: Peter Peregrinus, 1971.

Grossman, W., *Cardiac catheterization and angiography.* Philadelphia: Lea & Febiger, 1974.

Gupta, R., J.W. Miller, A.P. Yoganathan, B.M. Kim, F.E. Udwadia, and W.H. Corcoran, "Spectral analysis of arterial sounds: A noninvasive method of studying arterial disease." *Med. Biol. Eng.,* 1975, 13, 700–705.

Hansen, A.T., "Pressure measurement in the human organism." *Acta Physiol. Scand.* 1949, 19(Suppl. 68), 1–227.

Hansen, A.T., and E. Warberg, "A theory for elastic liquid-containing membrane manometers: General part." *Acta Physiol. Scand.,* 1950, 19, 306–332.

Hansen, A.T., "The theory for elastic liquid-containing membrane manometers: Special part." *Acta Physiol. Scand.,* 1950, 19, 333–343.

Herman, M.V., P.F. Cohn, and R. Gorlin, "Resistance to blood flow by stenotic valves: Calculation of orifice area," in W. Grossman (ed.), *Cardiac catheterization and angiography.* Philadelphia: Lea & Febiger, 1974.

King, G., "An experiment station for teaching cardiovascular manometry." *Med. Res. Eng.,* 1972, 11, 26–28.

Kingsley, B., and B.L. Segal, "Cardiovascular vibratory phenomena," in C. Ray (ed.), *Medical engineering.* Chicago: Year Book, 1974.

Konigsberg, E., and R.H. Russell, "A battery-operated miniature pressure transducer amplifier system," in R.D. Allison (ed.), *Biomedical sciences instrumentation,* New York: Plenum, 1968, Vol. IV.

Laughlin, D.E., R.P. Mahoney, "New phonocardiographic transducers utilizing the hot-wire anemometer principle." *Med. Biol. Eng.,* 1972, 10, 43–55.

Lindstrom, L.H., "Miniaturized pressure transducer intended for intravascular use." *IEEE Trans. Biomed. Electron.,* 1970, BME-17, 207–219.

Mackay, R.S., and E. Marg, "Fast automatic ocular pressure measurement based on an exact theory." *IRE Trans. Med. Electron.,* 1960, ME-7, 61–67.

Master, A.M., C.I. Garfield, and M.B. Walters, *Normal blood pressure and hypertension.* Philadelphia: Lea & Febiger, 1952.

O'Rourke, P.L., "The arterial pulse in health and disease." *Amer. Heart J.,* 1971, 82, 687–702.

Pressman, G.L., and P.M. Newgard, "A transducer for the continuous external measurement of arterial blood pressure," *IEEE Trans. Biomed. Electron.,* 1963, 10, 73–81.

Rushmer, R.F., *Cardiovascular dynamics,* 3rd ed. Philadelphia: Saunders, 1970.

Shapiro, G.G., and L.J. Krovetz, "Damped and undamped frequency responses of underdamped catheter manometer systems," *Amer. Heart J.*, 1970, 80, 226–236.

Stegall, H.F., "A simple inexpensive sinusoidal pressure generator," *J. Appl. Physiol.*, 1967, 22, 591–592.

Stegall, H.F., M.B. Kardon, and W.T. Kemmerer, "Indirect measurement of arterial blood pressure by Doppler ultrasonic sphygmomanometry." *J. Appl. Physiol.*, 1968, 25, 793–798.

Tavel, M.E., *Clinical phonocardiography and external pulse recording,* 2nd ed. Chicago: Year Book, 1972.

Yellin, E.L., R.W.M. Frater, and C.S. Peskin, "The application of the Gorlin equation to the stenotic mitral valve." In A.C. Bell and R.M. Nerem (eds.), *1975 Advances in Bioengineering,* Am. Soc. Mech. Engr., New York, 1975.

Chapter eight

Measurement of flow and volume of blood

John G. Webster

One of the primary measurements the physician would like to acquire from a patient is that of the concentration of O_2 and other nutrients in the cells. Such quantities are normally so difficult to measure that the doctor is forced to accept the second-class measurements of blood flow and changes in blood volume, which usually correlate with concentration of nutrients. If blood *flow* is difficult to measure, the physician may settle for the third-class measurement of blood *pressure*, which usually correlates adequately with blood flow. If blood pressure cannot be measured, the physician may fall back on the fourth-class measurement of the ECG, which usually correlates adequately with blood pressure.

Note that the measurement of blood flow—the main subject of this chapter—is the one that most closely reflects the primary measurement of concentration of O_2 in the cells. However, measurement of blood flow is usually more difficult to make and more invasive than that of blood pressure or of the ECG.

Commonly used flowmeters, such as the orifice or turbine flowmeters, are unsuitable for measuring blood flow because they require cutting the vessel and can cause formation of clots. The specialized techniques described in this chapter have therefore been developed.

8.1 Indicator-dilution method that uses continuous infusion

The indicator-dilution methods described in this chapter do not measure instantaneous pulsatile flow, but flow averaged over a number of heartbeats.

Concentration

When a given quantity m_0 of an indicator is added to a volume V, the resulting concentration C of the indicator is given by $C = m_0/V$. When an additional quantity m of indicator is then added, the incremental increase in concentration is $\Delta C = m/V$.

When the fluid volume in the measured space is continuously removed and replaced, as in a flowing stream, then, in order to maintain a fixed change in concentration, the clinician must continuously add a fixed quantity of indicator per unit time. That is, $\Delta C = (dm/dt)/(dV/dt)$. From this equation, we can calculate flow (Bassingthwaighte, 1974):

$$F = \frac{dV}{dt} = \frac{dm/dt}{\Delta C} \tag{8.1}$$

Example 8.1 Derive (8.1), using principles of mass transport.

Answer The rate at which indicator enters the vessel is equal to the indicator's input concentration C_i times the flow F. The rate at which indicator is injected into the vessel is equal to the quantity per unit time, dm/dt. The rate at which indicator leaves the vessel is equal to the indicator's output concentration C_o times F. For steady state, $C_iF + dm/dt = C_oF$ or $F = (dm/dt)/(C_o - C_i)$.

Fick technique

We can use (8.1) to measure *cardiac output* (blood flow from the heart) as follows.

$$F = \frac{dm/dt}{C_a - C_v} \tag{8.2}$$

where

$$F = \text{blood flow, liters/min}$$
$$dm/dt = \text{consumption of } O_2, \text{ liters/min}$$
$$C_a = \text{arterial concentration of } O_2, \text{ liters/liter}$$
$$C_v = \text{venous concentration of } O_2, \text{ liters/liter}$$

Figure 8.1 shows the measurements required. The blood returning to the heart from the upper half of the body has a different concentration of O_2 from that of the blood returning from the lower half, because the amount of O_2 extracted by the brain is different from that extracted by the kidneys, muscles, and so forth. Therefore we cannot accurately measure C_v in the right atrium. We must measure it in the pulmonary artery after it has been mixed by the pumping action of the right ventricle. The physician may float the catheter into place by the method of temporarily inflating a small balloon surrounding the tip. This is done through a second lumen in the catheter.

As the blood flows through the lung capillaries, the subject adds the indicator (the O_2) by breathing in pure O_2 from a spirometer (see Figure 9.6). The exhaled CO_2 is absorbed in a soda-

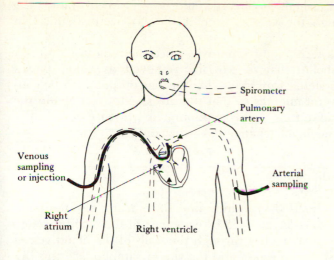

Spirometer

Pulmonary artery

Venous sampling or injection

Arterial sampling

Right atrium

Right ventricle

Figure 8.1 Several methods of measuring cardiac output. In the Fick method, the indicator is O_2; consumption is measured by a spirometer. The arterial-venous concentration difference is measured by drawing samples through catheters placed in an artery and in the pulmonary artery. In the dye-dilution method, dye is injected into the pulmonary artery and samples taken from an artery. In the thermodilution method, cold saline is injected into the right atrium and temperature is measured in the pulmonary artery.

lime canister, so the consumption of O_2 is indicated directly by the net gas-flow rate.

The clinician can measure the concentration of the oxygenated blood C_a in any artery, since blood from the lung capillaries is well mixed by the left ventricle and there is no consumption of O_2 in the arteries. Usually an arm or leg artery is used.

Example 8.2 Calculate the cardiac output, given the following data: spirometer O_2 consumption, 250 ml/min; arterial O_2 content, 0.20 ml/ml; venous O_2 content, 0.15 ml/ml.

Answer From (8.2),

$$F = \frac{dm/dt}{C_a - C_v}$$

$$= \frac{0.25 \text{ liter/min}}{(0.20 \text{ liter/liter}) - (0.15 \text{ liter/liter})} \qquad (8.3)$$

$$= 5 \text{ liters/min}$$

The units for the concentrations of O_2 represent the volume of O_2 that can be extracted from a volume of blood. This concentration is very high for blood because large quantities of oxygen can be bound to hemoglobin. It would be very low if water were flowing through the vessels, even if the Po_2 were identical in both cases.

The Fick technique is nontoxic, since the indicator (O_2) is a normal metabolite that is partially removed as blood passes through the systemic capillaries. The cardiac output must be constant over several minutes so that the investigator can obtain the slope of the curve for O_2 consumption. The presence of the catheter causes a negligible change in cardiac output.

Thermodilution

Heat may be used as an indicator, since heat is also nontoxic, and—like oxygen—is removed by each pass of the blood through the body. Heat may be lost through the walls of the blood vessels between the site of injection and the site of sampling, so this distance should be as short as possible. To ensure adequate mixing, however, this distance should be as long as possible. The indicator in this case should not pass through the lungs, since heat loss there is excessive. So the best compromise is to inject the heat into the right atrium, and—after the heat has been mixed with normal blood in the right ventricle—to sample the resulting mixture in the pulmonary artery. For continuous injection it is not practical to inject heated or cooled saline, since the continuous injection of liquid would overexpand the volume of the circulating blood. In an early device (no longer used), the heat was added by an electric heater and the change in temperature was sensed by a thermistor or thermocouple. The flow, in cubic meters per second, is given by

$$F = \frac{q}{\rho_b c_b \, \Delta T}$$ (8.4)

where

q = rate of heat added, W
ρ_b = density of the blood, kg/m^3
c_b = specific heat of the blood, J/(kg · K)
ΔT = temperature change, K

By remembering that temperature is the concentration of heat per unit volume, we see that (8.4) is directly analogous to (8.1).

8.2 Indicator-dilution method that uses rapid injection

Equation

The continuous-infusion method has been largely replaced by the rapid-injection method, which is more convenient. A bolus of indicator is rapidly injected into the vessel and the variation in downstream concentration of the indicator versus time is measured until the bolus has passed. The solid line in Figure 8.2 shows the fluctuations in concentration of the indicator that occur after the injection. The dotted-line extension of the exponential decay shows the curve that would result if there were no recirculation. For this case we can calculate the flow as follows.

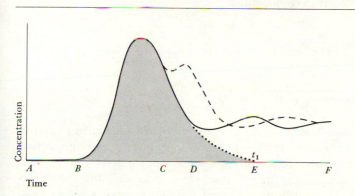

Figure 8.2 Rapid-injection indicator-dilution curve. After the bolus is injected at time A, there is a transportation delay before the concentration begins rising at time B. After the peak is passed, the curve enters an exponential decay region between C and D, which would continue decaying along the dotted curve to t_1 if there were no recirculation. However, recirculation causes a second peak at E before the indicator becomes thoroughly mixed in the blood at F. The dashed curve indicates the rapid recirculation that occurs when there is a hole between the left and right sides of the heart.

An increment of blood of volume dV passes the sampling site in time dt. The quantity of indicator dm contained in dV is the concentration $C(t)$ times the incremental volume. Hence $dm = C(t)dV$. Dividing by dt, we obtain $dm/dt = C(t)dV/dt$. But $dV/dt = F_i$, the instantaneous flow; therefore $dm = F_iC(t)dt$. Integrating over time through t_1, when the bolus has passed the downstream sampling point, we obtain

$$m = \int_0^{t_1} F_iC(t) \, dt \qquad (8.5)$$

where t_1 is the time at which all effects of the first pass of the bolus have died out (point E in Figure 8.2). Minor variations in the instantaneous flow F_i produced by the heartbeat are smoothed out by the mixing of the bolus and the blood within the heart chambers and the lungs. Thus we may obtain the average flow F from

$$F = \frac{m}{\int_0^{t_1} C(t) \, dt} \qquad (8.6)$$

The integrated quantity in (8.6) is equal to the shaded area in Figure 8.2 and may be obtained by counting squares or using a planimeter. Small special-purpose computers that extrapolate the dotted line in real time and compute the flow are also available (Cromwell, 1973).

If the initial concentration of indicator is not zero—as may be the case if there is residual indicator left over from previous injections—then (8.6) becomes

$$F = \frac{m}{\int_0^{t_1}[\Delta C(t)]\ dt} \tag{8.7}$$

Dye dilution

The most common method of clinically measuring cardiac output is to use a colored dye, *indocyanine green* (cardiogreen). It meets the necessary requirements for an indicator in that it is (1) inert, (2) harmless, (3) measurable, (4) economical, and (5) always intravascular. In addition, its optical absorption peak is 805 nm, the wavelength at which the optical absorption coefficient of blood is independent of oxygenation. The dye is available as a liquid that is diluted in isotonic saline and injected directly through a catheter, usually into the pulmonary artery. About 50% of the dye is excreted by the kidneys in the first 10 min, so repeat determinations are possible.

The plot of the curve for concentration versus time is obtained from a constant-flow pump, which draws blood from a catheter placed in the femoral or brachial artery. Blood is drawn through a colorimeter cuvette (Figure 2.20), which continuously measures the concentration of dye, using the principle of absorption photometry (Section 10.1). The 805-nm channel of a two-channel blood oximeter can be used for measuring dye-dilution curves. The clinician calibrates the colorimeter by mixing known amounts of dye and blood and drawing them through the cuvette.

The shape of the curve can provide additional diagnostic information. The dashed curve in Figure 8.2 shows the result when a left-right shunt (a hole between the left and right sides of the heart) is present. Blood recirculates faster than normal, resulting in an earlier recirculation peak. When a right-left shunt is present, the delay in transport is abnormally short, since some dye reaches the sampling site without passing through the lung vessels.

Thermodilution

A method that is finding increasing clinical use in measuring cardiac output is that of injecting a bolus of cold saline as an indicator. A special four-lumen catheter (Forrester *et al.*, 1972) is floated through the brachial vein into place in the pulmonary artery. A syringe forces a gas through one lumen; the gas inflates a small doughnut-shaped balloon at the tip. The force of the flowing blood carries the tip into the pulmonary artery. The cooled saline indicator is injected through the second lumen into the right atrium. The indicator is mixed with blood in the right ventricle. The resulting drop in temperature of the blood is detected by a thermistor located near the catheter tip in the pulmonary artery. The third lumen carries the thermistor wires. The fourth lumen, which is not used for the measurement of thermodilution, can be used for withdrawing blood samples. The catheter can be left in place for about 24 h, during which time many determinations of cardiac output can be made, something that would not be possible if dye were being used as the indicator. Also it is not necessary to puncture an artery.

In the same way that (8.4) is analogous to (8.1), we can derive the following equation, which is analogous to (8.7):

$$F = \frac{Q}{\rho_b c_b \int_0^{t_1} \Delta T_b(t)\ dt} \quad (\text{m}^3/\text{s}) \tag{8.8}$$

where

Q = heat content of injectate, J $(= V_i\ \Delta T_i \rho_i c_i)$
ρ_b = density of blood, kg/m^3
c_b = specific heat of blood, J/(kg · K)

When an investigator uses the thermodilution method, there are a number of problems that cause errors. (1) There may be inadequate mixing between the injection site and the sampling site. (2) There may be an exchange of heat between the blood and the walls of the heart chamber. (3) There is heat exchange through the catheter walls before, during, and after injection. However, the instrument can be calibrated by simultaneously performing dye-dilution determinations and applying a correction factor that corrects for several of the errors (Almasi, 1976).

8.3 Electromagnetic flowmeters

The electromagnetic flowmeter measures instantaneous pulsatile flow of blood and thus has a greater capability than indicator-dilution methods, which measure only average flow. It operates with any conductive liquid, such as saline or blood.

Principle

The electric generator in a car generates electricity by induction. Copper wires move through a magnetic field, cutting the lines of magnetic flux and inducing an emf in the wire. This same principle is used in the most commonly used blood flowmeter, shown in Figure 8.3. Instead of copper wires, the flowmeter depends on the movement of blood, which has a conductance similar to that of saline. The formula for the induced emf is given by Faraday's law of induction:

$$e = \int_0^{L_1} \mathbf{u} \times \mathbf{B} \cdot d\mathbf{L},$$

where

$\mathbf{B}$ = magnetic flux density, T, or Wb/m²
$\mathbf{L}$ = length between electrodes, m
$\mathbf{u}$ = instantaneous velocity of blood, m/s

For a uniform magnetic field B and a uniform velocity profile u, the induced emf is

$$e = BLu \tag{8.9}$$

where these three components are orthogonal.

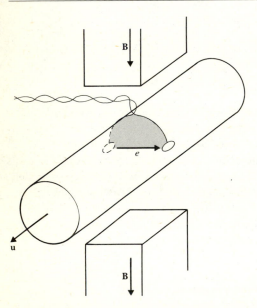

Figure 8.3 Electromagnetic flowmeter. When blood flows in the vessel with velocity **u** and passes through the magnetic field **B**, the induced emf e is measured at the electrodes shown. When an ac magnetic field is used, any flux lines cutting the shaded loop induce an undesired transformer voltage.

Let us now consider real flowmeters, several of which have a number of divergences from this ideal case. If the vessel's cross section were square and the electrodes extended the full length of two opposite sides, the flowmeter would measure the correct average flow for any flow profile. However, the electrodes are small, so velocities near them contribute more to the signal than do velocities farther away.

Figure 8.4 shows the weighting function that characterizes this effect for circular geometry. It shows that the problem is less when the electrodes are located outside the vessel wall. The instrument measures correctly for a uniform flow profile. For axisymmetric nonuniform flow profiles, such as the parabolic flow profile resulting from laminar flow, the instrument measurement is correct if u is replaced by $\bar{u}$, the average flow velocity. Because we usually know the cross-sectional area A of the lumen of the vessel, we can multiply A by $\bar{u}$ to obtain F, the volumetric flow. However, in many locations of blood vessels in the body, as around the curve of the aorta and near its branches, the velocity profile is asymmetric, so errors result.

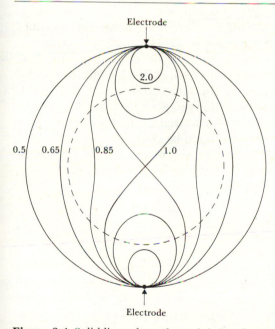

Figure 8.4 Solid lines show the weighting function that represents relative velocity contributions (indicated by numbers) to the total induced voltage for electrodes at top and bottom of circular cross section. If the vessel wall extends from the outside circle to the dashed line, the range of the weighting function is reduced. (Adapted from J.A. Shercliff, *The Theory of Electromagnetic Flow Measurement*, © 1962, Cambridge University Press.)

Other factors can also cause error. (1) Regions of high velocity generate higher incremental emf's than regions of low velocity, so circulating currents flow in the transverse plane. These currents cause varying drops in resistance within the conductive blood and surrounding tissues. (2) The ratio of the conductivity of the wall of the blood vessel to that of the blood varies with the *hematocrit* (percentage of cell volume to blood volume), so the shunting effects of the wall cause a variable error. (3) Fluid outside the wall of the vessel has a greater conductivity than the wall, and hence it shunts the flow signal. (4) The magnetic-flux density is not uniform in the transverse plane; this accentuates the problem of circulating current. (5) The magnetic-flux density is not uniform along the axis, which thus causes circulating currents to flow in the axial direction. To minimize these errors, most workers recommend calibration for animal work by using blood from the animal—and, where possible, the animal's own vessels also. Blood or saline is usually collected in a graduated cylinder and timed with a stopwatch.

Dc flowmeter

The flowmeter shown in Figure 8.3 can use a dc magnetic field, so the output voltage continuously indicates the flow. Although a few early dc flowmeters were built, none were satisfactory, for the following three reasons. (1) The voltage across the electrode's metal-to-solution interface is in series with the flow signal. Even when the flowmeter has nonpolarizable electrodes, the random drift of this voltage is of the same order as the flow signal, and there is no way to separate the two. (2) The ECG has a waveform and frequency content similar to that of the flow signal; near the heart the ECG's waveform is much larger than that of the flow signal, and therefore causes interference. (3) In the frequency range of interest, 0 to 30 Hz, $1/f$ noise in the amplifier is large, which results in a poor SNR.

Ac flowmeter

The clinician can eliminate the problems of the dc flowmeter by operating the system with an ac magnet current of about 400 Hz. Lower frequencies require bulky transducers, whereas higher frequencies cause problems due to stray capacitance. The operation of this carrier system results in the ac flow voltage shown in Figure 8.5. When the flow reverses direction, the voltage changes phase by 180°, so the phase-sensitive demodulator (described in Section 3.15) is required to yield directional output.

Although ac operation is superior to dc operation, the new problem of *transformer voltage* arises. If the shaded loop shown in Figure 8.3 is not exactly parallel to the B field, some ac magnetic flux intersects the loop and induces a transformer voltage proportional to dB/dt in the output voltage. Even when the electrodes and wires are carefully positioned, the transformer voltage is usually many times larger than the flow voltage, as indicated in Figure 8.5.

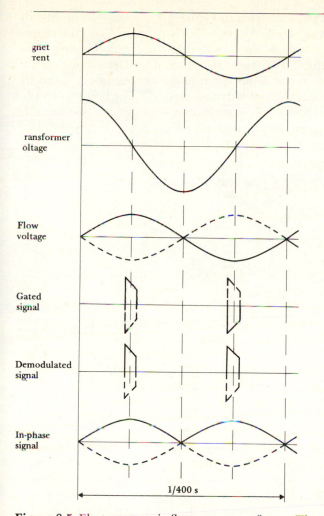

gnet
rent

ransformer
oltage

Flow
voltage

Gated
signal

Demodulated
signal

In-phase
signal

1/400 s

Figure 8.5 Electromagnetic flowmeter waveforms. The transformer voltage is 90° out of phase with the magnet current. Other waveforms are
shown solid for forward flow and dashed for reverse flow. The gated
signal from the gated-sine-wave flowmeter includes less area than the in-
phase signal from the quadrature-suppression flowmeter.

The amplifier voltage is the sum of the transformer voltage and the
flow voltage.

There are several solutions to this problem. (1) It may be
eliminated at the source by use of a *phantom electrode.* One of the
electrodes is separated into two electrodes in the axial direction.
Two wires are led some distance from the electrodes and a potentiometer is placed between them. The signal from the potentiometer
wiper yields a signal corresponding to a "phantom" electrode,
which can be moved in the axial direction. The shaded loop in Figure 8.3 can thus be tilted forward or backward, or placed exactly

parallel to the *B* field. (2) Note in Figure 8.5 that we may sample the composite signal when the transformer voltage is zero. At this time the flow voltage is at its maximum and the resulting *gated signal* measures only the flow voltage. However, if undesired phase shifts cause the gating to be done even a few degrees away from the proper time, large errors and drifts result. (3) The best method for reducing the effects of transformer voltage is to use the *quadrature-suppression* circuit shown in Figure 8.6 (Wyatt, 1971).

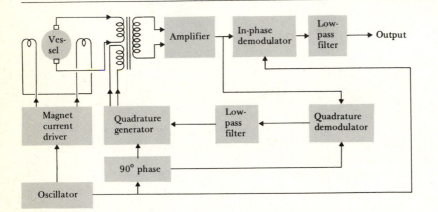

Figure 8.6 The quadrature-suppression flowmeter detects the amplifier quadrature voltage. The quadrature generator feeds back a voltage to buck out the probe-generated transformer voltage.

The magnitude of the voltage in the transformer at the amplifier output is detected by the quadrature demodulator, which has a full-wave-rectified output. This is low-pass-filtered to yield a dc voltage, which is then modulated by the quadrature generator to produce a signal proportional to the transformer voltage. The signal is fed to a bucking coil on the input transformer, thus bucking out the transformer voltage at the input. With enough gain in this negative-feedback loop, the transformer voltage at the amplifier output is reduced by a factor of 50. This low transformer voltage prevents overloading of the in-phase demodulator, which extracts the desired in-phase flow signal shown in Figure 8.5. By choosing low-noise FETs for the amplifier input stage, the proper turns ratio on the step-up transformer (Section 3.13), and full-wave demodulators, we can obtain an excellent SNR.

Some flowmeters, unlike the sine-wave flowmeters described previously, use *square-wave excitation*. In this case, the transformer voltage appears as a very large spike, which overloads the amplifier for a short time. After the amplifier recovers, the circuit samples the square-wave flow voltage and processes it to obtain the flow signal. To prevent overload of the amplifier, *trapezoidal excitation* has also been used.

Probe design

A variety of probes to measure blood flow has been used (Cobbold, 1974). The electrodes for these probes are usually made of platinum. Best results are obtained when the electrodes are platinized (electrolytically coated with platinum) to provide low impedance, and are recessed in a cavity to minimize the flow of circulating currents through the metal. When the electrodes must be exposed, bright platinum is used, since the platinized coating wears off anyway. Bright platinum electrodes have a higher impedance and higher noise level than platinized ones.

Some probes do not use a magnetic core, but they have lower sensitivity. A common *perivascular probe* is shown in Figure 8.7, in which a toroidal laminated Permalloy core is wound with two oppositely wound coils. The resulting magnetic field has low leakage flux. To prevent capacitive coupling between the coils of the magnet and the electrodes, there is an electrostatic shield placed between them. The probe is insulated with a potting material having a very high resistivity and impermeability to salt water (since blood is similar to saline).

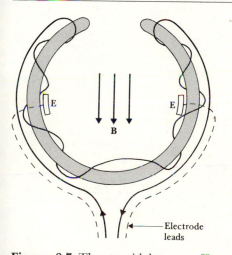

Figure 8.7 The toroidal-type cuff probe has two oppositely wound windings on each half of the core. The magnetic flux thus leaves the top of both sides, flows down in the center of the cuff, enters the base of the toroid, and flows up through both sides.

The open slot on one side of the probe makes it possible to slip it over a blood vessel without cutting the vessel. A plastic key may be inserted into the slot so that the probe encircles the vessel. The probe must fit snugly during diastole so that the electrodes make good contact. This requires some constriction of an artery during systole, when the diameter of the artery is about 7%

greater. So that there can be this snug fit on a variety of sizes of arteries, probes are made in 1-mm increments in the range of 1 to 24 mm. To be able to measure any size of artery requires a considerable expenditure for probes: Costs of individual probes typically range from $200 to $300 each. The probes do not operate satisfactorily on veins, because the electrodes do not make good contact when the vein collapses. Special flow-through probes are used outside the body for measuring the output of cardiac-bypass pumps.

The *catheter-tip probe* (Mills and Shillingford, 1967) shown in Figure 8.8 can be used to measure the velocity of aortic blood in humans. It is similar to the cuff-type probe, but turned inside out. The curved magnetic-field lines external to the probe are perpendicular to the curved electric-field lines, as required by Faraday's law. The weighting function is proportional to $1/r^4$, so the sensitivity varies greatly with the distance of the moving blood from the probe. The probe is inserted into the femoral artery and advanced to the root of the aorta. There is no easy way of finding out whether the probe is centered in the aorta or resting against the wall of the aorta. Hence the flow can only be estimated to within about 20%. Nevertheless, it is valuable in estimating the percent regurgitation through a leaky aortic valve, since it correctly indicates reversal of flow.

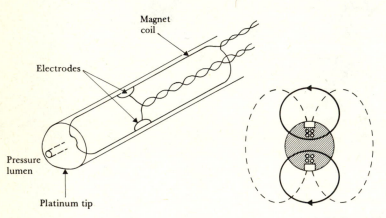

Figure 8.8 Catheter-tip probe coil generates magnetic-field lines (shown solid with arrows) that are perpendicular to the electric-field lines (shown dashed), shown emanating from electrodes at top and bottom. (From C.J. Mills and J.P. Shillingford, *Cardiovascular Research*, 1967, *1*, 263–273.)

Pulsatile arterial blood flow in the limbs can be noninvasively measured by electromagnetic techniques (Doll *et al.*, 1975). A permanent magnet applies a vertical dc magnetic field to a limb. Horizontally placed electrodes detect the aggregate signal from all arteries in the limb. An ECG provides a synchronization signal which makes it possible for the clinician to average waveforms of 64 cycles and thus to minimize random noise. Artifacts that are synchronous with the heart, such as the ECG, are minimized by subtraction techniques. The bandwidth of 0.1 to 50 Hz does not yield the steady-flow component. The height of the pulsatile component is an index of pulsatile flow. The shape of the pulsatile component is an index of the elasticity of the peripheral arterial tree.

8.4 Ultrasonic flowmeters

The ultrasonic flowmeter, like the electromagnetic flowmeter, can measure instantaneous flow of blood. The ultrasound can be beamed through the skin, thus making transcutaneous flowmeters practical. Advanced types of ultrasonic flowmeters can also measure flow profiles. These advantages are making the ultrasonic flowmeter the subject of intensive development. Let us examine some aspects of this development.

Transducers

For the transducer to be used in an ultrasonic flowmeter, we select a piezoelectric material (Section 2.6) that converts power from electric to acoustic form (Wells, 1971). Lead zirconate titanate is a crystal that has the highest conversion efficiency. It may be molded into any shape by melting. As it is cooled through the Curie temperature, it is placed in a strong electric field to polarize the material. It is usually formed into disks, coated on opposite faces with metal electrodes, which are driven by an electronic oscillator. The resulting electric field in the crystal causes mechanical constriction. The pistonlike movements generate longitudinal plane waves, which propagate into the tissue. For maximum efficiency, the crystal is one-half wavelength thick. Any cavities between the crystal and the tissue must be filled with a fluid or watery gel in order to prevent the high reflective losses associated with liquid-gas interfaces.

Since the transducer has a finite diameter, it will produce diffraction patterns, just as an aperture does in optics. Figure 8.9 shows the outline of the beam patterns for several transducer diameters and frequencies. In the *near field*, the beam is mostly contained within a cylindrical outline and there is little spreading. The intensity is not uniform, however: There are multiple maximums and minimums within this region, caused by interference. The near field extends a distance d_{nf} given by

$$d_{nf} = \frac{D^2}{4\lambda}$$

(8.10)

where

D = transducer diameter and λ = wavelength.

In the *far field*, the beam diverges, with the intensity inversely proportional to the square of the distance from the transducer. The angle of beam divergence ϕ, shown in Figure 8.9, is given by

$$\sin \phi = \frac{1.2\lambda}{D} \tag{8.11}$$

Figure 8.9 indicates that we should avoid the far field because of its lower spatial resolution. To achieve near-field operation, we must use higher frequencies and larger transducers.

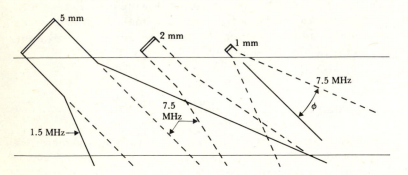

Figure 8.9 Near and far fields for various transducer diameters and frequencies. Beams are drawn to scale, passing through a 10-mm-diameter vessel. Transducer diameters are 5, 2, and 1 mm. Solid lines are for 1.5 MHz; dashed lines, for 7.5 MHz.

To select the operating frequency, we must consider several factors. For a beam of constant cross section, the power decays exponentially because of absorption of heat in the tissue. Since the absorption coefficient is approximately proportional to frequency, this suggests a low operating frequency. However, most ultrasonic flowmeters depend on the power scattered back from moving red-blood cells. The back-scattered power is proportional to f^4, which suggests a high operating frequency. The usual compromise dictates a frequency between 2 and 10 MHz.

Transit-time flowmeter

Figure 8.10(a) shows the transducer arrangement used in the transit-time ultrasonic flowmeter (Cobbold, 1974). The effective velocity of sound in the vessel is equal to the velocity of sound, c, plus a component due to $\hat{u}$, the velocity of flow of blood averaged

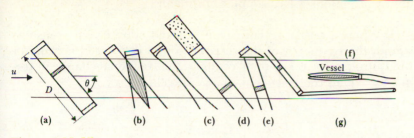

Figure 8.10 Ultrasonic transducer configurations. (a) Transit-time probe requires two transducers facing each other along a path length D inclined from the vessel axis by angle θ. The hatched region represents a single acoustic pulse traveling between the two transducers. (b) In transcutaneous probe, both transducers are placed on the same side of the vessel, so the probe can be placed on the skin. Beam intersection is shown hatched. (c) Any transducer may contain a plastic lens that focuses and narrows the beam. (d) For pulsed operation, the transducer is loaded by backing it with a mixture of tungsten powder in epoxy. This increases losses and lowers Q. Shaded region is shown for a single time of range gating. (e) A shaped piece of Lucite on the front loads the transducer, also refracts the beam. (f) A transducer placed on the end of a catheter beams ultrasound down the vessel. (g) For pulsed operation, the transducer is placed at an angle.

along the path of the ultrasound. For laminar flow, $\hat{u} = 1.33\bar{u}$; and for turbulent flow, $\hat{u} = 1.07\bar{u}$, where $\bar{u}$ is the velocity of the flow of blood averaged over the cross-sectional area. $\hat{u}$ differs from $\bar{u}$ because the ultrasonic path is along a single line rather than averaged over the cross-sectional area. The transit time in the downstream $(+)$ and upstream $(-)$ directions is

$$t = \frac{\text{distance}}{\text{conduction velocity}} = \frac{D}{c \pm \hat{u} \cos \theta} \tag{8.12}$$

The difference between upstream and downstream transit times is

$$\Delta t = \frac{2\, D\hat{u} \cos \theta}{(c^2 + \hat{u}^2 \cos^2 \theta)} \cong \frac{2\, D\hat{u} \cos \theta}{c^2} \tag{8.13}$$

and thus the average velocity $\hat{u}$ is proportional to Δt. A short acoustic pulse is transmitted alternately in the upstream and downstream directions. Unfortunately, the resulting Δt is in the nanosecond range, and complex electronics are required to achieve adequate stability. Like the electromagnetic flowmeter, the transit-time flowmeter and similar flowmeters using a phase-shift principle can operate with either saline or blood as a fluid, since they do not require particulate matter for scattering. However, they do require invasive surgery to expose the vessel.

Continuous-wave Doppler flowmeter

When a target recedes from a fixed source that transmits sound, the frequency of the received sound is lowered because of the Doppler effect. For small changes, the fractional change in frequency equals the fractional change in velocity:

$$\frac{f_d}{f_0} = \frac{u}{c} \tag{8.14}$$

where

f_d = Doppler frequency shift
f_0 = source frequency
u = target velocity
c = velocity of sound.

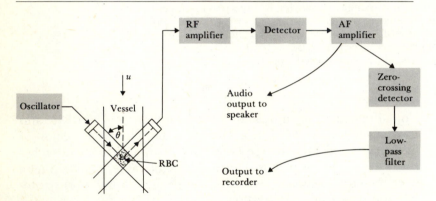

Figure 8.11 Doppler ultrasonic blood flowmeter. In the simplest instrument, ultrasound is beamed through the vessel walls, back-scattered by the red blood cells, and received by a piezoelectric crystal.

The flowmeter shown in Figure 8.11 requires particulate matter such as blood cells to form reflecting targets. The frequency is lowered twice. One shift occurs between the transmitting source and the moving cell that receives the signal. The other shift occurs between the transmitting cell and the receiving transducer.

$$\frac{f_d}{f_0} = \frac{2u}{c + u} \cong \frac{2u}{c} \tag{8.15}$$

The approximation is valid, since $c \cong 1500$ m/s and $u \cong 1.5$ m/s. Since the velocities do not all act along the same straight line, we add an angle factor

$$f_d = \frac{2 f_0 u \cos \theta}{c} \tag{8.16}$$

where θ is the angle between the beam of sound and the axis of the blood vessel, as shown in Figure 8.11. If the flow is not axial, or the transducers do not lie at the same angle, such as in Figure 8.10(b), we must include additional trigonometric factors.

Figure 8.11 shows the block diagram of a simple continuous-wave flowmeter. The oscillator must have a low output impedance to drive the low-impedance crystal. Although at most frequencies the crystal transducer has a high impedance, it is operated at mechanical resonance, where the impedance drops to about 100 Ω (Welkowitz and Deutsch, 1976). The ultrasonic waves are transmitted to the moving cells, which reflect the Doppler-shifted waves to the receiving transducer. The receiving transducer is identical to the transmitting transducer. The amplifier RF (radio frequency) signal plus carrier signal is detected to produce an AF (audio frequency) signal at a frequency given by (8.16).

Listening to the audio output using a speaker, we get much useful qualitative information. A simple *frequency-to-voltage converter* provides a quantitative output to a recorder. The *zero-crossing detector* emits a fixed-area pulse each time the audio signal crosses the zero axis. These pulses are low-pass-filtered to produce an output proportional to the velocity of the blood cells.

Although the electromagnetic blood flowmeter is capable of measuring both forward and reverse flow, the simple ultrasonic-type flowmeter full-wave rectifies the output, and the sense of direction of flow is lost. This results because—for either an increase or a decrease in the Doppler-shifted frequency—the beat frequency is the same. Examination of the field intersections shown in Figure 8.11 implies that the only received frequency is the Doppler-shifted one. However, the received carrier signal is very much larger than the desired Doppler-shifted signal. Some of the RF carrier is coupled to the receiver by the electric field from the transmitter. Because of side lobes in the transducer apertures, some of the carrier signal travels a direct acoustic path to the receiver. Other power at the carrier frequency reaches the receiver after one or more reflections from fixed interfaces. The resulting received signal is composed of a large-amplitude signal at the carrier frequency plus the very low (approximately 0.1%) amplitude Doppler-shifted signal.

The Doppler-shifted signal is not at a single frequency, as implied by (8.16), for several reasons. (1) Velocity profiles are rarely blunt, with all cells moving at the same velocity; rather, cells move at different velocities, producing different shifts of the Doppler frequency. (2) A given cell remains within the beam-intersection volume for a short time. Thus the signal received from one cell is a pure frequency multiplied by some time-gate function, yielding a band of frequencies. (3) Acoustic energy traveling within the main beam, but at angles to the beam axis, plus energy in the side lobes, causes different Doppler-frequency shifts due to an effective change in θ. (4) Tumbling of cells and local velocities caused by turbulence cause different Doppler-frequency shifts. All these factors combine to produce a band of frequencies. The resulting spectrum is similar to band-limited random noise, and from this we must extract flow information.

We would like to have high gain in the RF amplifier in order to boost the low-amplitude Doppler-frequency components. But the carrier is large, so the gain cannot be too high, or saturation will occur. The RF bandwidth need not be wide, since the frequency deviation is only about 0.001 of the carrier frequency. However, RF-amplifier bandwidths are sometimes much wider than required, to permit tuning to different transducers.

The detector can be a simple square-law device such as a diode. The output spectrum contains the desired difference (beat) frequencies, which lie in the audio range, plus other undesired frequencies.

Example 8.3 Calculate the maximum audio frequency of a Doppler-ultrasonic blood flowmeter having a carrier frequency of 7 MHz, a transducer angle of 45°, a blood velocity of 150 cm/s, and an acoustic velocity of 1500 m/s.

Answer Substitute these data into (8.16):

$$f_a = \frac{2(7 \times 10^6 \text{ Hz})(1.5 \text{ m/s}) \cos (45°)}{1500 \text{ m/s}} \cong 10 \text{ kHz} \qquad (8.17)$$

The dc component must be removed with a high-pass filter in the AF amplifier. Figure 8.12(a) shows that we require a corner frequency of about 100 Hz in order to reject large Doppler signals due to motion of vessel walls. Unfortunately, this high-pass filter also keeps us from measuring slow cell velocities (less than 1.5 cm/s), such as occur near the vessel wall. A low-pass filter removes high frequencies and also noise. The corner frequency is at about 15 kHz, which includes all frequencies that could result from cell motion, plus an allowance for spectral spreading.

In the simplest instruments, the AF output drives a power amplifier and speaker or earphones. Since the output is a band of frequencies, it has a whooshing sound, which for steady flows sounds like random noise. Venous flow sounds like a low-frequency rumble, and may be modulated when the subject breathes. Arterial flow, being pulsatile, rises to a high pitch once each beat, and may be followed by one or more smaller easily heard waves caused by the underdamped flow characteristics of arteries. Thus this simple instrument can be used to trace and qualitatively evaluate blood vessels within 1 cm of the skin in locations in the legs, arm, and neck. We may also plot the spectrum of the AF signal versus time to obtain a more quantitative indication of velocities in the vessel.

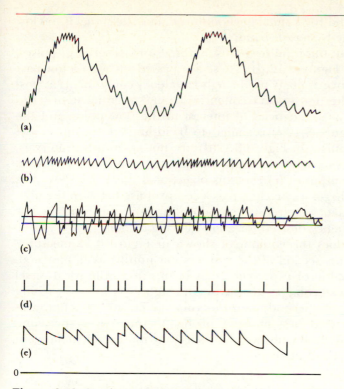

Figure 8.12 Continuous-wave Doppler signal-processing waveforms. (a) Detector output. Large low-frequency waves are caused by vessel-wall motions. Small ripple is the desired signal from the cells. (b) By high-pass filtering in the AF amplifier, wall-motion signals are rejected. (c) Zero-crossing detector has an adjustable hysteresis band, indicated by the horizontal lines. (d) Zero-crossing detector output is a series of equal-area pulses. (e) A low-pass filter yields an output related to cell velocity.

The function of the *zero-crossing detector* is to convert the AF input frequency to a proportional analog output signal. It does this by emitting a constant-area pulse for each crossing of the zero axis. The detector contains a comparator (a Schmitt trigger), so we must determine the amount of hysteresis for the comparator. If the input were a single sine wave, the *signal-to-hysteresis ratio* (SHR) could be varied over wide limits and the output would indicate the correct value. But the input is band-limited random noise. If the SHR is low, many zero crossings are missed. As the SHR increases, the two horizontal lines in Figure 8.12(c) get closer together, and the indicated frequency of the output increases. A SHR of 7 is a good choice, because the output does not vary significantly with changes in SHR. Automatic gain control can be used to maintain this ratio. Very high SHRs are not desirable, since noise may trigger the comparator. Note that the signal in Figure 8.12(c) increases and decreases with time because of the beating of the signal components at the various frequencies. Thus the short-term SHR fluctuates; and for a small portion of the time the signal is too low to exceed the hysteresis band.

The output of the zero-crossing detector is a series of pulses, as shown in Figure 8.12(d). These are passed through a low-pass filter to remove as many of the high-frequency components as possible. The filter must pass frequencies from 0 to 25 Hz in order to reproduce the frequencies of interest in the flow pulse. But the signal in Figure 8.12(c) is similar to band-limited random noise. Hence the pulses in Figure 8.12(d) are not at uniform intervals, even for a fixed flow velocity, but are more like a Poisson process. Hence the output at (e) contains objectional noise. The low-pass filter must therefore be chosen as a compromise between the high corner frequency desired to reproduce the flow pulse and the low corner frequency desired for good filtering of noise.

What does the equipment shown in Figure 8.11 measure? First, the cross section of the vessel is not uniformly illuminated. The intersection of two rectangular beams in a cylindrical vessel has a complex geometry that favors the higher frequencies arising from the center. Second, the zero-crossing detector does not measure the desired first moment of $W(f)$—the power spectrum, which would uniformly weight each contributing element—but rather the second moment,

$$\text{Average zero crossing rate} \cong \left[\frac{\int (f - f_0)^2 W(f)\, df}{\int W(f)\, df}\right]^{1/2} \tag{8.18}$$

where f_0 is the carrier frequency and $(f - f_0)$ equals the Doppler frequency f_d.

This expression also favors the higher frequencies. We thus have two factors that bias the output in favor of the higher frequencies. This is of no consequence for fixed velocity profiles, since the bias is accounted for during calibration. But velocity profiles in the body vary widely with location, obstructions, and time of cardiac cycle. The only case in which we can use the zero-crossing detector with confidence is the case in which $W(f)$ is narrow. This occurs for the intersection of narrow beams [Figure 8.10(c)], for blunt flow profiles, and for range-gated operation.

A major defect of the detector used in simple flowmeters is that it cannot detect the direction of flow. The recorded output looks as it would if the true velocity had been full-wave-rectified. Compared with the electromagnetic flowmeter, this is a real disadvantage, since reverse flow occurs frequently in the body. A first thought might be to translate the Doppler-shifted frequencies not to the region about dc, but to the region about 20 kHz. Forward flow might thus be 30 kHz and reverse flow 10 kHz. The difficulty with this approach is that the high-amplitude carrier signal is translated to 20 kHz. The Doppler signals are so small that considerable effort is required to build any reasonable frequency-to-voltage converter that is not dominated by the 20-kHz signal.

A better approach is to borrow a technique from radar technology, which is used to determine not only the speed an aircraft is flying, but also its direction. This is the quadrature-phase detector.

Figure 8.13(a) shows the analog portion of the *quadrature-phase detector* (McLeod, 1967). A phase-shift network splits the carrier into two components that are in quadrature, which means that they are 90° apart. These reference cosine and sine waves must be several times larger than the RF-amplifier output, as shown in Figure 8.14(a). The reference waves and the RF-amplifier output are linearly summed to produce the RF envelope shown in Figure 8.14(b). We assume temporarily that the RF-amplifier output contains no carrier.

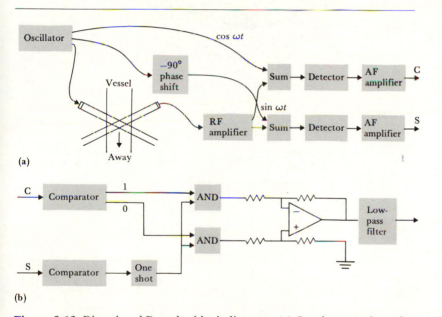

Figure 8.13 Directional Doppler block diagram. (a) Quadrature-phase detector. Sine and cosine signals at the carrier frequency are summed with the RF output before detection. The output C from the cosine channel then leads or lags the output S from the sine channel if the flow is away from or toward the transducer. (b) Logic circuits route one-shot pulses through top or bottom AND gate if the flow is away from or toward the transducer, respectively. Differential amplifier provides bidirectional output pulses that are then filtered.

If the flow of blood is in the same direction as the ultrasonic beam, we consider it as moving away from the transducer, as shown in Figure 8.13(a). For this direction, the Doppler-shift frequency is lower than that of the carrier. The phase of the Doppler wave lags behind that of the reference carrier, and the Doppler vector [see Figure 8.14(a)] rotates clockwise. In Figure 8.14(b), for time 1, the carrier and the Doppler add, producing a larger sum in the cosine channel. The sine channel is unchanged. For time 2, the carrier and the Doppler add, producing a larger sum in the sine channel. Similar reasoning produces the rest of the wave for times 3 and 4. Note that the sine channel lags behind the cosine channel.

If the flow of blood is toward the transducer, the Doppler frequency is higher than the carrier frequency, and the Doppler vector rotates counterclockwise. This produces the dashed waves shown in Figure 8.14(b), and the phase relation between the cosine and sine channels is reversed. Thus, by examining the sign of the phase, we measure direction of flow. The detector produces AF waves that have the same shape as the RF envelope.

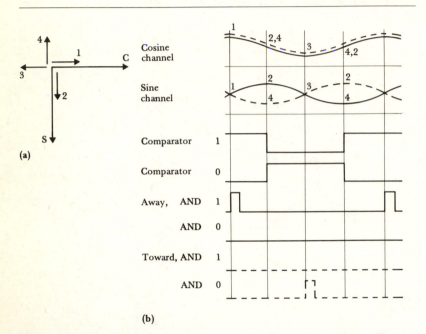

(a)

(b)

Figure 8.14 Directional Doppler signal waveforms. (a) Vector diagram. Sine wave at carrier frequency lags cosine wave by 90°. If flow is away from transducer, Doppler frequency is lower than the carrier. Short vector represents Doppler signal and rotates clockwise, as shown by numbers 1, 2, 3, and 4. (b) Timing diagram. Top two waves represent single-peak envelope of the carrier plus Doppler before detection. Comparator outputs respond to the cosine channel audio signal after detection. One-shot pulses are derived from sine channel and are gated through correct AND gate by comparator outputs. Dashed lines indicate flow toward the transducer.

Figure 8.13(b) shows the logic that detects the sign of the phase. The cosine channel drives a comparator, whose digital output, shown in Figure 8.14(b), is used for gating and does not change with direction of flow of blood. The sine channel triggers a one-shot whose width must be short. Depending on direction of flow, this one-shot triggers either at the beginning or halfway through the period, as shown in Figure 8.14(b). The AND gates then gate it into the top or bottom input of the differential amplifier, thus producing a bidirectional output.

The preceding discussion is correct for a sinusoidal RF signal. Our RF signal is like band-limited random noise. Hence there is some time shifting of the relations shown in Figure 8.14(b). Also, a large fixed component at the carrier frequency is present, which displaces the Doppler vectors away from the position shown. As long as the reference cosine and sine waves are more than twice the amplitude of the total RF output, time shifting of the gating relations is not excessive. These time shifts are not problems in practice, since a short one-shot pulse can shift almost ± 90° before passing out of the correct comparator gate.

It is possible to add another one-shot and several logic blocks to obtain pulse outputs on both positive and negative zero crossings. This doubles the frequency of the pulse train and reduces the fluctuations in the output to 0.707 of their former value.

Pulsed Doppler

Continuous-wave flowmeters provide little information about flow profile. Therefore, several instruments have been built (Cobbold, 1974) that operate in a radarlike mode. The transmitter is excited with a brief burst of signal. The transmitted wave travels in a single packet, and the transmitter can also be used as a receiver, since reflections are received at a later time. The delay between transmission and reception is a direct indication of distance, so we can obtain a complete plot of reflections across the blood vessel. By examining the Doppler shift at various delays, we may obtain a velocity profile across the vessel.

To achieve good range resolution, the transmitted-pulse duration should ideally be very short. To achieve a good SNR and good velocity discrimination, it should be long. The usual compromise is an 8-MHz pulse of 1-μs duration, which produces a traveling packet 1.5 mm long, as shown in Figure 8.10(d). The intensity of this packet is convolved with the local velocity profile to produce the received signal. Thus the velocity profile of the blood vessel is smeared to a larger-than-actual value. Because of this problem, and also because the wave packet arrives at an angle to normal, the location of the vessel walls is indistinct. It is possible, however, to mathematically "deconvolve" the instrument output to obtain a less-smeared representation of the velocity profile.

There are two constraints on pulse repetition rate f_r. First, to avoid *range ambiguities*, we must analyze the return from one pulse before sending out the next. Thus

$$f_r < \frac{c}{2R_m} \tag{8.19}$$

where R_m is the maximum useful range. Second, we must satisfy the *sampling theorem*, which requires that

$$f_r > 2f_d \qquad (8.20)$$

Combining (8.19) and (8.20) with (8.16) yields

$$u_m(\cos \theta)R_{max} < \frac{c^2}{8f_0} \qquad (8.21)$$

which shows that the product of the range and the maximum velocity along the transducer axis are limited. In practice, measurements are constrained even more than indicated by (8.21), because of (1) spectral spreading, which produces some frequencies higher than those expected, and (2) imperfect cutoff characteristics of the low-pass filters used to prevent *aliasing* (generation of fictitious frequencies by the sampling process).

Since we cannot easily start and stop an oscillator in 1 μs, the first stage of the oscillator operates continuously. The transmitter and the receiver both use a common piezoelectric transducer, so a *gate* is required to turn off the signal from the transmitter during reception. A one-stage gate is not sufficient to isolate the large transmitter signals from the very small received signals. Therefore two gates in series are used to turn off the transmitter.

The optimal transmitted signal is a pulse-modulated sine-wave carrier. Although it is easy to generate this burst electrically, it is difficult to transduce this electric burst to a similar acoustic burst. The crystal transducer has a high Q (narrow bandwidth) and therefore rings at its resonant frequency long after the electric signal stops. Therefore the transducer is modified to achieve a lower Q (wider bandwidth) by adding mass to the back [Figure 8.10(d)] or to the front [Figure 8.10(e)]. The Q is not lowered to a desirable value of about 2 to 5, because this would greatly decrease both the efficiency of the transmission and the sensitivity of the reception. The Q is generally 5 to 15, so some ringing still exists.

When we generate a short sine-wave burst, we no longer have a single frequency. Rather, the pulse train of the repetition rate is multiplied by the carrier in time, producing carrier sidebands in the frequency domain. This spectrum excites the transducer, producing a field that is more complex than that for continuous-wave excitation. This causes spectral spreading of the received signal.

Figure 8.15(a) shows a typical received signal. The transmitted signal is large and overloads the RF amplifier for a brief period of time. After the amplifier recovers, there is a large reflection from the relatively stationary near wall of the vessel. Then a small signal is reflected from the moving cells as the pulse passes through the blood vessel. A reflection from the far wall of the vessel completes the observed features. The signal is attenuated

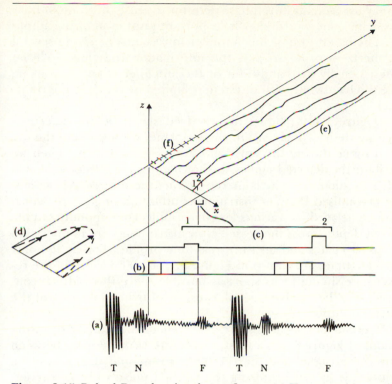

Figure 8.15 Pulsed Doppler signal waveforms. (a) Two repetitions of the received signal. T shows the large transmitted pulse. N is the large reflection from the near wall. F is the reflection from the far wall. (b) The discrete gating times must be correctly positioned between walls. (c) Detected output amplitude of a single gate varies with time 1, time 2, etc. (d) For the parabolic flow profile shown, velocity is higher in center of vessel. (e) Thus audio frequency is higher in the center. x = distance across vessel, y = time axis, z = AF signal amplitude. (f) Tick marks show that successive repetition times must be frequent enough to sample the highest audio frequency present.

throughout this time and becomes negligible before the next sampling time. We want to avoid reflections from within the transducer and from bones behind the vessel.

In the RF amplifier, some type of *switching network* is required to protect the amplifier from overload during transmission and to prevent any voltage from the oscillator from entering the sensitive amplifier during reception. One arrangement uses diodes that conduct for the large signals that are transmitted and do not conduct for the small signals that are received. Amplifiers may use deliberate hard limiting (saturation) to achieve quieting (reduce noise), but the nonlinearities convert the single Doppler sidebands to double sidebands. This prevents us from being able to sense the direction of flow of blood because a sideband corresponding to both directions of the flow is then created. If we use a linear amplifier, we may use a quadrature-phase detector to sense direction of flow. Automatic gain control may help prevent saturation of the amplifier. The bandwidth of the amplifier must be increased to several megahertz in order to pass the information contained in brief pulses. Usually the bandwidth of the amplifier is not a problem, since the bandwidth of the system is limited by the Q of the transducer.

Figure 8.15(a) shows the received signal before detection. Since we desire AF signals in the y-z plane, we must gate the detected signal during the times shown in Figure 8.15(b). Then we distribute the detected signals, as shown in Figure 8.15(c), so that at each x location, we may later reconstruct the desired AF signals. The first pulsed Doppler instruments utilized a single gate, which could be delayed for various lengths of time, corresponding to the desired depth across the vessel. Now instruments are in operation that use 16 gates and measure real-time profiles. For clarity, only four gate times are shown in Figure 8.15(b). The width of the receiver gate should be as short as possible, since this width is convolved with the received signal, causing a further smearing of the spatial resolution.

Certain modifications are required in the signal-processing sections of Figure 8.13(a). First, we require *phase coherence* between the received signal and the reference cosine and sine waves. We achieve this by synchronizing the emitted pulse with the carrier, either with a ripple counter to generate the pulse-repetition frequency or with simple synchronization circuits. The detector outputs are sequentially gated into 16 identical channels. Each contains filters to remove the pulse-repetition frequency and to convert the pulse trains to the desired AF signals. Each channel contains circuits identical to those in Figure 8.13(b). Zero-crossing detectors operate well here, since each channel has a relatively narrow band signal.

The output of the instrument described so far is 16 parallel outputs of curves showing velocity versus time. These can be examined individually or summed with suitable weighting factors to produce a single measurement of average flow of blood. We may also construct a *velocity profile* by rapidly scanning across the 16 channels. The profile is continuously measured in real time and exhibits both forward and reverse flow during the cardiac cycle. Since the entire shape bounces up and down 1 to 3 times per second, it is difficult to observe the detailed profile.

One technique used is to examine single profiles on a storage oscilloscope. Further information is obtained by using the ECG to synchronize the output. By slightly increasing the delay of each profile, we can produce a slow-motion stroboscopic effect. If a tape recorder is available, the moving profile signal may be recorded at high speed and played back at low speed. Péronneau (1977) provides a very complete study of the theory, accuracy, and results of the pulsed Doppler flowmeter, with 218 references.

Random-signal Doppler flowmeter

Figure 8.16 diagrams the random-signal Doppler flowmeter (Bendick and Newhouse, 1974). Waves from a continuous random-noise source are transmitted into the flow stream of blood. The back-scattered waves are received and amplified and the resulting signal is correlated with a delayed version of the original random-noise source. The time delay τ is varied to sample the signal reflected from cells at different distances across the blood vessel in the same manner as the pulsed-Doppler flowmeter.

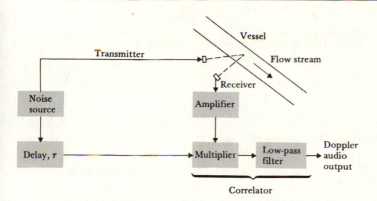

Figure 8.16 Block diagram of a random-signal Doppler flowmeter. When acoustic path delay shown by dashed lines is equal to τ, the correlator yields a large output.

There are two advantages to the random-signal Doppler flowmeter. First, this system suffers neither the ambiguity of range indicated by (8.19) nor the limit of velocity-range product indicated by (8.21), because, for random noise, every signal is different from every other signal. The *correlator* produces a large output only when a section of received random noise lines up with the corresponding section of transmitted random noise. For noncorresponding sections of random noise, the output of the correlator approaches zero. Second, since the random noise operates continuously, the ratio of peak to average transmitted power can be made much smaller in the random-noise system. Thus average power and the resulting received signal can be increased without risking breakdown of the transducer or damage to the cells.

Transmitting noise continuously adds an additional problem. If a single transducer is used to both transmit and receive, reverberation-type echos (*clutter*) from targets outside the desired range add in an uncorrelated manner to the desired signal, thereby worsening the system's SNR. This problem can be overcome by transmitting bursts of noise that are short enough to intercept only one target at a time.

A better means of avoiding clutter is to arrange for separate transmitting and receiving transducer patterns to intercept only in the region of the desired range, as shown in Figure 8.16. Random-signal systems of measuring fluid flow are ideal for long-range use in environments such as the sea, where there are few targets other than the one under observation. However, when used in the body, these systems are plagued by reflections from targets at ambiguous ranges, which worsen the effective SNR. In the case of pulsed-Doppler systems, reflections from stationary or near-stationary targets at ambiguous ranges cause fewer problems because their echoes are transformed into zero or very low-frequency Doppler outputs that can easily be filtered out.

8.5 Thermal-convection velocity sensors

Principle

The thermodilution methods described in Sections 8.1 and 8.2 depend on the mixing of the heat indicator into the entire flow stream. In contrast, thermal velocity sensors depend on convective cooling of a heated sensor and are therefore sensitive only to local velocity.

Figure 8.17(a) shows a simple probe. The thermistor R_u is heated to a temperature difference ΔT above blood temperature by the power W dissipated by current passing through R_u. Experimental observations (Grahn *et al.*, 1969) show that these quantities are related to the blood velocity u by

$$\frac{W}{\Delta T} = a + b \log u \tag{8.22}$$

where a and b are constants. Thus the method is nonlinear, with a large sensitivity at low velocities and a small sensitivity at high velocities.

Probes

Catheter-tip probes are designed with two types of sensors (Cobbold, 1974). The first type uses the thermistors shown in Figure 8.17 and provides a high sensitivity and reasonable resistance values. Since the thermistor shown in Figure 8.17(a) is cooled equally for both directions of velocity, the output of the instrument is a full-wave-rectified replica of the true velocity. To overcome this limitation, the probe shown in Figure 8.17(b) has two additional thermistors located a few tenths of a millimeter downstream and upstream from R_u. Depending on direction of velocity, one or the other is heated by the heat carried through the blood from the thermistor R_u. These two additional thermistors are placed in a bridge that is balanced for zero velocity. A comparator detects the bridge unbalance and switches the output from positive to negative. The probe shown in Figure 8.17(c) uses two velocity sensors arranged so that one is exposed to the fluid velocity while the other is shielded from the fluid velocity.

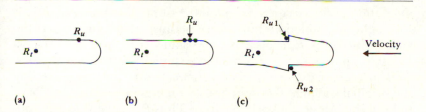

(a)   (b)   (c)

Figure 8.17 Thermal velocity probes. (a) Velocity-sensitive thermistor R_u is exposed to velocity stream. Temperature-compensating thermistor R_t is placed within the probe. (b) Thermistors placed down- and upstream from R_u are heated or not heated by R_u, thus indicating velocity direction. (c) Thermistors exposed to and shielded from flow can also indicate velocity direction.

The second type of sensor uses a glass bead with a thin strip of platinum deposited on its surface. The platinum may be painted on and then fired in a furnace, or it may be *sputtered* (deposited by electrical discharge in a vacuum). A disadvantage of platinum-film sensors is their low resistance (a few ohms) and low sensitivity.

A real question arises about what is actually being measured. When a catheter is inserted into a blood vessel, the sensor may be centered and measuring maximum velocity, or it may be against the wall of the vessel and measuring a low velocity. One way of ensuring that the sensor is not against the wall is to rotate the catheter, searching for the maximum output. Catheters are also sensitive to radial velocity of blood, as well as radial vibrations of the catheter (catheter whip). Thus, in addition to any errors due to measuring velocity, there are errors in trying to estimate flow due to lack of knowledge about location of the sensor. Either type of probe (if made sufficiently small) may be placed at the end of a hypodermic needle and inserted perpendicular to the vessel for measuring velocity profiles.

Circuit

A *constant-current* sensor circuit cannot be used for two reasons. First, the time constant of the sensor embedded in the probe is a few tenths of a second—much too long to achieve the desired frequency response of 0 to 25 Hz. Second, to achieve a reasonable sensitivity at high velocities, the sensor current must be so high that when the flow stops, lack of convection cooling increases the sensor temperature more than 5°C above the blood temperature and fibrin coats the sensor.

The *constant-temperature* sensor circuit shown in Figure 8.18 overcomes both these problems. The circuit is initially unbalanced by adjusting R_1. The unbalance is amplified by the high-gain op amp and its output is fed back to power the resistance bridge. Operation of the circuit is as follows. Assume that thermistor R_u is 5°C higher than blood temperature because of self-heating. If the velocity increases, R_u cools and its resistance increases. A more positive voltage enters the + op-amp terminal, so that v_b increases. This increases bridge power and R_u heats up, thus counteracting the original cooling. The system uses high-gain negative feedback to keep the bridge always in balance. Thus R_u remains nearly constant and therefore its temperature remains nearly constant. The high-gain negative feedback divides the sensor time constant by a factor equal to the loop gain, so frequency response is greatly improved. In effect, if the sensor becomes slightly cooled, the op amp can provide a large quantity of power to rapidly heat it back to the desired temperature.

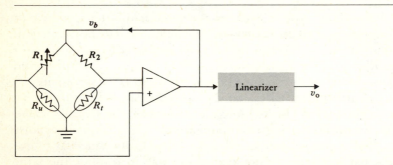

Figure 8.18 Thermal velocity meter circuit. A velocity increase cools R_u, the velocity-measuring thermistor. This increases voltage to the bottom op amp input, which increases bridge voltage v_b and heats R_u. R_t provides temperature compensation.

The circuit operates satisfactorily with only one sensor, R_u, provided that the blood temperature is constant. Should the blood temperature vary, a temperature-compensating thermistor R_t is added to keep the bridge in balance. So that its rise in temperature is very small, R_t must have a much lower resistance-temperature coefficient than R_u, to ensure that R_t is a sensor of temperature and not of velocity. The thermal resistance of R_t can be lowered by making it large in size, using a heat sink, or placing it within the probe so that the effective cooling area is much larger. Another solution is to increase the resistance values for R_2 and R_t, so that their power dissipation is much lower.

A linearizer is required to solve (8.22). We may square v_b to obtain W, then use an antilog converter to obtain v_o. For the directional probe shown in Figure 8.17(b), a unity-gain inverter and switch may be used to yield the direction of flow.

Calibration may be accomplished by using a sinusoidal-flow pump or a cylindrical pan of liquid rotating on a turntable.

The main use of thermal-velocity sensors is to measure the velocity of blood and to compile velocity profiles in studies of animals, although such sensors have also been regularly used to measure velocity and acceleration of blood at the aortic root in human patients undergoing diagnostic catheterization (Roberts, 1972). The same principle has also been applied to the measurement of the flow of air in lungs, by using a heated platinum wire installed in a breathing tube (Cromwell *et al.*, 1973).

8.6 Chamber Plethysmography

Plethysmographs measure changes in volume. The only accurate way to noninvasively measure changes in volume of blood in the extremities is by using a chamber plethysmograph. By timing these volume changes, we can measure flow by computing $F = dV/dt$. A cuff is used to prevent venous blood from leaving the limb—hence the name *venous-occlusion plethysmography*.

Equipment

Figure 8.19 shows the equipment used in a venous-occlusion plethysmograph. The chamber has a rigid cylindrical outer container, and is placed around the leg. As the volume of the leg increases, the leg squeezes some type of bladder and decreases its volume. If the bladder is filled with water, the change in volume may

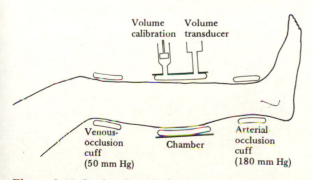

Figure 8.19 In chamber plethysmography, the venous-occlusion cuff is inflated to 50 mm Hg (6.7 kPa), stopping venous return. Arterial flow causes an increase in volume of leg segment, which is measured by the chamber. The text explains the purpose of the arterial-occlusion cuff.

be measured by observing the water rising in a calibrated tube. For recording purposes, some air may be introduced above the water and the change in air pressure measured. Water-filled plethysmographs are temperature-controlled to prevent thermal drifts. Because of their hydrostatic pressure, they may constrict the vessels in the limb and cause undesirable physiological changes.

Air may be used in the bladder and the resulting changes in pressure measured directly. Some systems do not use a bladder. They attempt to seal the ends of a rigid chamber to the limb; but then leaks may be a problem. One device uses a pneumotachometer to measure the flow of air in and out of the chamber. This flow is then integrated to yield changes in volume. This equipment is designed to accommodate a variety of limb sizes, so the chambers and bladders are made in a family of sizes. Alternatively, a single chamber may be used for several sizes of limb. Devices that are capable of doing this are made with iris diaphragms that form the ends of the chamber and close down on the limb.

Method

Figure 8.20 shows the sequence of operations that yield a measurement of flow. A calibration may be marked on the record by injecting into the chamber a known volume of fluid, using the volume-calibration syringe. The venous-occlusion cuff is then applied to a limb and pressurized to 50 mm Hg (6.7 kPa), which prevents venous blood from leaving the limb. Arterial flow is not hindered by this cuff pressure, and the increase in volume of blood in the limb per unit time is equal to the arterial inflow. If the chamber completely encloses the limb distal to the cuff, the arterial flow into the limb is measured. If the chamber encloses only a segment of a limb, as shown in Figure 8.19, an arterial-occlusion cuff distal to the chamber must be inflated to 180 mm Hg (24 kPa) so that the changes in chamber volume measure only arterial flow entering the segment of the limb.

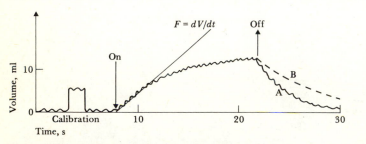

Figure 8.20 After venous-occlusion cuff pressure is turned on, the initial volume-versus-time slope is caused by arterial inflow. After cuff is released, segment volume rapidly returns to normal (A). If a venous thrombosis blocks the vein, return to normal is slower (B).

A few seconds after the cuffs are occluded, the venous pressure exceeds 50 mm Hg (6.7 kPa), venous return commences, and the volume of blood in the limb segment plateaus. When the clinician releases the pressure of the venous-occlusion cuff, the volume of blood in the limb segment rapidly returns to normal (Figure 8.20, curve A). If a venous thrombosis (vein clot) partially blocks the return of venous blood, the volume of blood in the veins returns to normal more slowly (Figure 8.20, curve B). This technique is a useful noninvasive test for venous thrombosis.

Example 8.4 A given chamber plethysmograph has a gas volume of 200 ml. Calculate the slow change in tissue volume that produces a 120-Pa change in chamber pressure.

Answer Slow changes are isothermal (take place at constant temperature), because the heat generated by compression of gas in the chamber has sufficient time to conduct to the chamber wall. Hence, in the chamber,

$$PV = nRT = k \quad \text{a constant}$$

$$P = k(V)^{-1}$$

$$\frac{dP}{dV} = -k(V)^{-2} = -V^{-1}[k(V)^{-1}] = \frac{-P}{V}$$

$$dV = \frac{-dPV}{P} = \frac{-(120)(200)}{101,325} = -0.24 \text{ ml}$$

where P is atmospheric pressure (Appendix A.3). Change in volume of tissue is $+0.24$ ml.

Other plethysmographs

Since chamber plethysmographs are expensive, awkward to use, and complex, clinicians usually use simpler plethysmographs: capacitance plethysmographs, impedance plethysmographs, and elastic-resistance strain-gage plethysmographs.

The *capacitance plethysmograph* (Cromwell, 1973) measures electric capacitance between the skin and a rigid cylindrical outer electrode. The two "plates" of the capacitor are separated by very compliant foam sponges. An increase in volume of blood in a limb segment results in a decrease in separation of the plates and an increase in capacitance, which is measured by an ac bridge. Since the resulting capacitance forms part of a high-impedance circuit, a second rigid screen surrounds the active plate to increase electrical stability.

420 MEASUREMENT OF FLOW AND VOLUME OF BLOOD

Impedance plethysmographs, described in Section 8.7, measure the tissue impedance of the limb segment by use of encircling electrodes.

Elastic-resistance strain-gage plethysmographs (Section 2.2) measure the change in resistance ΔR of a conducting liquid in an extendable rubber tube. The volume of the liquid, which is typically mercury or saline, remains constant, so that, as the length L increases, the area A decreases and

$$R = \frac{\rho L}{A} = \frac{\rho L}{V/L} = kL^2 \tag{8.23}$$

where ρ is the resistivity and k is a constant.

Although this relation is nonlinear, if the excursions are small, the system is close to linear. If a mercury strain gage is used, its resistance is about 1 Ω. This is so low that it is difficult to use in a normal bridge. A solution is to use a transformer to step up the effective impedance of the gage and make measurements in an ac bridge. The mercury strain gage can encircle the limb and detect arterial pulsations, but it is not known how the resulting waveforms correlate with changes in limb volume.

8.7 Electrical-impedance plethysmography

It is simple to attach electrodes to a segment of tissue and measure the resulting impedance of the tissue. As the volume of the tissue changes due to pulsations of blood (as happens in a limb) or the resistivity changes due to increased air in the tissue (as happens in the lung), the impedance of the tissue changes.

Electrical-impedance plethysmography has been used to measure a wide variety of variables, but in many cases the accuracy of the method is poor or unknown.

Principle

Nyboer (1970) developed the equations used in impedance plethysmography in the early 1950s. However, we shall follow Swanson's (1976) derivation, which is conceptually and mathematically simpler. Figure 8.21 shows Swanson's model of a cylindrical limb. The derivation requires three assumptions. (1) The expansion of the arteries is uniform. This is probably valid in healthy vessels, but may not be valid in diseased ones. (2) ρ_b, the resistivity of blood, does not change. In fact, ρ_b decreases with velocity because of alignment of the cells with flow streamlines and movement of cells toward the axis. Also ρ_b is real for dc, but has a small reactive component at higher frequencies. (3) Lines of current are par-

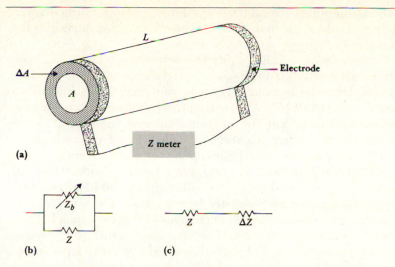

Figure 8.21 (a) A model for impedance plethysmography. A cylindrical limb has length L and cross-sectional area A. With each pressure pulse, A increases by the shaded area ΔA. (b) This causes impedance of the blood, Z_b, to be added in parallel to Z. (c) Usually ΔZ is measured instead of Z_b.

allel to the arteries. This is probably valid for most limb segments, but not for the knee.

The shunting impedance of the blood, Z_b, is due to the additional blood volume ΔV that causes the increase in cross-sectional area ΔA:

$$Z_b = \frac{\rho_b L}{\Delta A} \qquad (8.24)$$

$$\Delta V = L\,\Delta A = \frac{\rho_b L^2}{Z_b} \qquad (8.25)$$

But we must replace the Z_b of Figure 8.21(b) in terms of the normally measured $\Delta Z = [(Z_b \parallel Z) - Z]$ of Figure 8.21(c). Now

$$\Delta Z = \frac{Z Z_b}{Z + Z_b} - Z = \frac{-Z^2}{Z + Z_b} \qquad (8.26)$$

and as $Z \ll Z_b$,

$$\frac{1}{Z_b} \simeq \frac{-\Delta Z}{Z^2} \qquad (8.27)$$

Substituting (8.27) in (8.25) yields

$$\Delta V = \frac{-\rho_b L^2 \Delta Z}{Z^2} \qquad (8.28)$$

If the assumptions are valid, (8.28) shows that we can calculate ΔV from ρ_b (Geddes and Baker, 1975) and from other quantities that are easily measured.

While (8.28) is valid at any frequency, there are several considerations that suggest the use of a frequency of about 100 kHz. (1) It is desirable to use a current greater than 1 mA in order to achieve adequate SNR. At low frequencies this current causes an unpleasant shock. But the current required for perception increases with frequency (Section 13.2). Therefore frequencies above 20 kHz are used to avoid perception of the current. (2) The skin-electrode impedance decreases by a factor of about 100 as the frequency is increased from low values up to 100 kHz. High frequencies are therefore used to decrease both the skin-electrode impedance and the undesirable changes in this impedance due to motion of the patient. (3) If a frequency much higher than 100 kHz is used, the low impedances of the stray capacitances make design of the instrument difficult.

Two or four electrodes

For reasons of economy and ease in application, some impedance plethysmographs use two electrodes, as shown in Figure 8.22. The current i flows through the same electrodes used to measure the voltage v. This causes several problems. (1) The current density

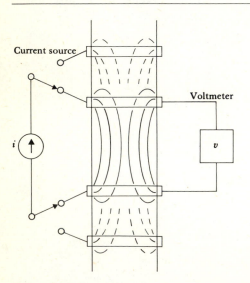

Figure 8.22 In two-electrode impedance plethysmography, switches are in the position shown, resulting in a high current density (solid lines) under voltage-sensing electrodes. In four-electrode impedance plethysmography, switches are thrown to the other position, resulting in a more uniform current density (dashed lines) under voltage-sensing electrodes.

is higher near the electrodes than elsewhere in the tissue. This causes the measured impedance, $Z = v/i$, to weight impedance of the tissue more heavily near the electrodes than elsewhere in the tissue. (2) Pulsations of blood in the tissue cause artifactual changes in the skin-electrode impedance, as well as changes in the desired tissue impedance. Since the skin-electrode impedance is in series with the desired tissue impedance, it is impossible to separate the two and determine the actual change in impedance of the tissue. (3) The current density is not uniform in the region of interest, so (8.28) cannot be used.

To solve these problems, clinicians use the four-electrode impedance plethysmograph shown in Figure 8.22. The current flows through the two outer electrodes, so the current density is more uniform in the region sensed by the two inner voltage electrodes. Variations in skin-electrode impedance cause only a second-order error.

Constant current source

Figure 8.23 shows the circuit of a four-electrode impedance plethysmograph. Ideally the current source i causes a constant current to flow through Z, regardless of changes in ΔZ or other impedances. In practice, however, there is a shunting impedance Z_i due to stray and cable capacitance. At 100 kHz, 15 pF of stray capacitance results in an impedance of about 100 kΩ. Thus changes in Z_1, ΔZ, and Z_4 cause the constant current to divide between Z and Z_i in a changing manner. In practice, this is not a problem, since changes in Z_1, ΔZ, and Z_4 are small and careful design can keep Z_i

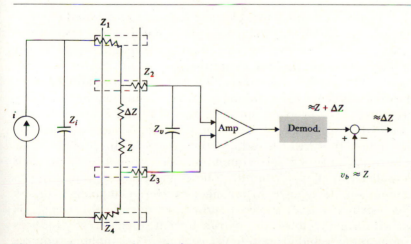

Figure 8.23 In four-electrode impedance plethysmograph, current is injected through two outer electrodes and voltage sensed between two inner electrodes. Amplification and demodulation yield $Z + \Delta Z$. Normally a bucking voltage v_b is applied to produce the desired ΔZ.

large enough. Also, Z and Z_i are close to 90° out of phase, which reduces the effects of the problem. Frequently the constant current is supplied through a low-capacity transformer to prevent ground-loop problems.

Example 8.5 For Figure 8.23, assume that $Z_1 + \Delta Z + Z + Z_4 = Z_t = 200 \ \Omega$ (resistive). How large an error is caused if $Z_i = -j2000 \ \Omega$ (capacitive)?

Answer The error is given by the fractional reduction in the magnitude of the voltage across Z_t:

$$\text{Fractional error} = \frac{(Z_t - |Z_t \| Z_i|)}{Z_t}$$

$$= \frac{\left[200 - \left| \frac{(200)(-j2000)}{200 - j2000} \right| \right]}{200}$$

$$= \frac{\left[200 - \frac{400{,}000}{(200^2 + 2000^2)^{1/2}} \right]}{200}$$

$$= \frac{200 - 199}{200} = 0.005$$

Both Z and ΔZ are proportionally reduced by this amount, which is negligible in physiological applications.

Voltage-sensing amplifier

Figure 8.23 shows that electrodes Z_2 and Z_3 are used to sense the voltage. Ideally the voltage amplifier has an input impedance sufficiently high so that no current flows through Z_2 and Z_3. In practice, however, there is a shunting impedance Z_v due to stray, cable, and amplifier capacitance. Thus changes in Z_2 and Z_3 cause the desired voltage to be attenuated in a changing manner. In practice, this is not a problem, since changes in Z_2 and Z_3 are small and careful design can keep Z_v large enough. Also Z_2 and Z_3 are 90° out of phase with Z_v, which reduces the effects of the problem. Not shown in Figure 8.23 are common-mode impedances from each amplifier input to ground. These impedances can convert common-mode voltages to erroneous differential voltages unless the instrument is carefully designed. Frequently the voltage is sensed through a low-capacity transformer, which greatly reduces common-mode and ground-loop problems. The amplifier requires only modest gain, since a typical voltage sensed is $v = iZ = (0.004)(40) = 0.16$ V.

Demodulation

The output of the amplifier is a large 100-kHz signal, amplitude-modulated a small amount by $i \Delta Z$. This $i \Delta Z$ may be demodulated by any AM detector, such as a diode followed by a low-pass filter. The phase-sensitive detector described in Section 3.15 is a superior demodulator because it is insensitive to the noise and 60-Hz interference that are detected by simpler demodulators.

Methods of balance

The demodulator produces an output $Z + \Delta Z$. Frequently ΔZ contains the useful information, but it may be only 1/1000th of Z. One approach is to use a high-pass filter to pass frequencies above 0.05 Hz and extract ΔZ. This is satisfactory for measuring pulsatile arterial changes, but not venous or respiratory changes. To build a dc-responding instrument, we subtract a bucking voltage v_b from the demodulated signal to yield ΔZ, as shown in Figure 8.23. We may derive v_b from an adjustable dc source, but then slight changes in i produce artifactual changes in ΔZ. A better technique is to derive v_b from a rectified signal from the master oscillator that generates i. Then the system behaves like a Wheatstone bridge: A change in excitation voltage does not unbalance the bridge.

But there still is a problem. When the electrodes are first applied or when the patient moves, Z changes by an amount much larger than ΔZ. The operator must manually adjust v_b to keep ΔZ small, which is necessary if the operator is to be able to adequately amplify and display ΔZ. To eliminate the bother of manual adjustment, an *automatic-reset system* has been developed. Whenever ΔZ saturates its amplifier, a sample-and-hold circuit makes $v_b = Z + \Delta Z$, which momentarily resets ΔZ to zero. The sudden vertical-reset trace is easily distinguished from the slower-changing physiological data.

Guard electrode

Many attempts have been made to measure changes in lung volume by using impedance plethysmography. The optimal placement of electrodes is below the patient's armpits on the sides of the thorax (Geddes and Baker, 1975). However, in this location, most of the current flows through the low-resistance thorax wall and very little through the high-resistance lung tissue. In fact, in experiments on dogs, the lungs can be deflated so that they carry no current, and a normal "respiratory" signal is obtained if the thorax walls are inflated and deflated by the normal amount.

It is possible to force current through the high-resistance tissue of the lungs by using a guard electrode (Cooley and Longini, 1968). Figure 8.24(a) shows that, for small electrodes, some current flows outside the region of the electrode because of fringing. Figure 8.24(b) shows that this effect can be reduced by using large-area electrodes. Figure 8.24(c) shows that we can eliminate fringing for a central electrode by surrounding it with an annular guard electrode. Figure 8.24(d) shows that by supplying the guard-electrode current from a unity-gain follower amplifier, we can measure the current i through the central electrode separately. Application of the guard electrode to the thorax makes it possible to measure resistivity of lung tissue, since the currents through the thorax wall are supplied by the guard electrode. The impedance measured by the central electrode is several times higher than that measured without the guard, because the current density is increased in the region in which the impedance is measured. A two-electrode technique is used.

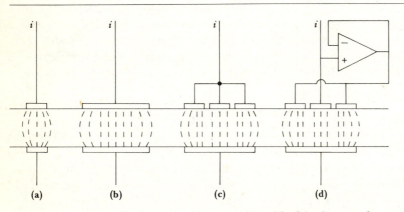

Figure 8.24 (a) Small electrodes have considerable fringing, so they emphasize impedance changes in high-current-density region near electrodes. (b) Large electrodes produce a more uniform current density. (c) Splitting the electrode into a center electrode plus an annular guard electrode does not change current distribution. (d) Driving the guard with a unity-gain follower causes current i to flow only through central region.

Applications

Electrical-impedance plethysmography is used to measure a wide variety of changes in the volume of tissue (Geddes and Baker, 1975). Electrodes placed on both legs provide an indication of whether pulsations of volume are normal or not. If the pulsatile waveform in one leg is much smaller than that in the other, this indicates an obstruction in the first leg. If pulsatile waveforms are reduced in both legs, this indicates an obstruction in their common supply. A clinically useful noninvasive method for detecting venous thrombosis in the leg is that of venous-occlusion plethysmography. When impedance plethysmography measures the changes in volume shown in Figure 8.20, this replaces the cumbersome chamber shown in Figure 8.19.

Electrodes on each side of the thorax provide an excellent indication of rate of ventilation, but a less-accurate indication of volume of ventilation. Electrodes around the neck and around the waist cause current to flow through the major vessels connected to the heart. The resulting changes in impedance provide a rough estimate of beat-by-beat changes in cardiac output (Kubicek *et al.*, 1970). Although Nyboer (1970) and others claim that flow of blood in the limbs can be measured, Swanson (1976) shows their techniques to be poor predictors of flow.

The advantages of electrical-impedance plethysmography are that it is noninvasive and relatively simple to use. The disadvantages are that it is not sufficiently accurate for many of the attempted applications, and even the cause of the changes in impedance is not clear in some cases.

8.8 Photoplethysmography

Light may be transmitted through a capillary bed. As arterial pulsations fill the capillary bed, the changes in volume of the vessels modify the absorption, reflection, and scattering of the light. Although the method is simple and indicates the timing of events such as heart rate, it provides a poor measure of changes in volume, and is very sensitive to motion artifact.

Light sources

Figure 8.25 shows two photoplethysmographic methods, in which sources generate light that is transmitted through the tissue (Geddes and Baker, 1975). A miniature tungsten lamp may be used as the light source, but the heat generated causes vasodilation, which alters the system being measured. This may be considered desirable because a larger pulse is produced. A less bulky unit may be formed using a GaAs LED (Lee *et al.*, 1975), which produces a narrow-band source with a peak spectral emission at a wavelength of 940 nm [Figure 2.21(a)].

Photosensors

Photoconductive cells have been used as sensors, but they are bulky and present a problem, in that prior exposure to light

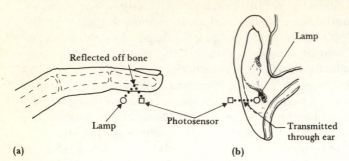

(a)   (b)

Figure 8.25 (a) Light transmitted into finger pad is reflected off bone and detected by photosensor. (b) Light transmitted through aural pinna is detected by photosensor.

changes the sensitivity of the cell. In addition, a filter is required to restrict the sensitivity of the sensor to the near-infrared region. This is required to prevent changes in blood O_2 content that are prominent in the visible-light region from causing changes in sensitivity. A less-bulky unit may be formed using an Si phototransistor. A filter that passes only infrared light is helpful for all types of sensors to prevent 120-Hz signals from fluorescent lights from being detected. This does not prevent dc light from tungsten lights or daylight from causing baseline shifts, so lightproof enclosures are usually provided for these devices.

Circuits

The output from the sensor represents a large value of transmittance, modulated by very small changes due to pulsations of blood. To eliminate the large baseline value, frequencies above 0.05 Hz are passed through a high-pass filter. The resulting signal is greatly amplified to yield a sufficiently large waveform. Any movement of the photoplethysmograph relative to the tissue causes a change in the baseline transmittance that is many times larger than the pulsation signal. These large artifacts due to motion saturate the amplifier; thus it is a good thing to have a means of quickly restoring the output trace.

Example 8.6 Design the complete circuit for a solid-state photoplethysmograph.

Answer A typical LED requires a forward current of 15 mA. Using a 15-V supply would require a series resistor of $R_L = v/i = 15/0.015 = 1 k\Omega$. A typical phototransistor passes a maximum of 150 μA. To avoid saturation, choose a series resistor $R_p = v/i =$

15/0.00015 = 100 kΩ. The largest convenient paper capacitor is 2 μF. The output resistor $R_o = 1/2\pi f_o C = 1/2\pi(0.05)(2 \times 10^{-6}) = 1.6$ MΩ. Figure 8.26 shows the circuit.

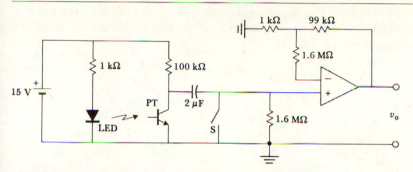
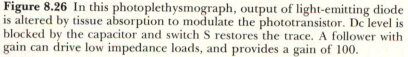

Figure 8.26 In this photoplethysmograph, output of light-emitting diode is altered by tissue absorption to modulate the phototransistor. Dc level is blocked by the capacitor and switch S restores the trace. A follower with gain can drive low impedance loads, and provides a gain of 100.

Applications

For a patient who remains quiet, the photoplethysmograph can measure heart rate. It has an advantage in that it responds to pumping action of the heart and not to the ECG. When properly shielded, it is unaffected by the use of electrocautery, which usually disables the ECG. However, when the patient is in a state of shock, vasoconstriction causes peripheral flow to be greatly reduced, and the resulting small output may make the device unusable. To prevent this problem, the device has been used to transmit light through the nasal septum (Groveman *et al.*, 1966). This monitors terminal branches of the internal carotid artery, and yields an output that correlates with cerebral blood flow.

Problems

8.1 *Clearance* is defined as the minimal volume of blood entering an organ per unit time required to supply the amount of indicator removed from the blood per unit time during the blood's passage through the organ. Derive a formula for renal clearance, given the arterial concentration of the indicator PAH, all of which is excreted by the kidneys into the urine. Give units.

8.2 In Figure 8.2, the final concentration at time F is higher than the initial concentration at time A. Write a formula that yields the circulating blood volume from the information obtained during an indicator dilution test. Give units.

8.3 In the decaying exponential portion of Figure 8.2, the concentrations at times C and D are given. Calculate the shaded area under the dotted curve between times C and E. Give units.

8.4 A physician is using the rapid-injection thermodilution method of finding a patient's cardiac output. Calculate the cardiac output (in milliliters per second and in liters per minute) from the following data.

$$V_i = 10 \text{ ml}, \Delta T_i = -30 \text{ K}$$

$$\rho_i = 1005 \text{ kg/m}^3, c_i = 4170 \text{ J/(kg} \cdot \text{K)}$$

$$\rho_b = 1060 \text{ kg/m}^3, c_b = 3640 \text{ J/(kg} \cdot \text{K)}$$

$$\int_0^{t_1} \Delta T_b \, dt = -5.0 \text{ s} \cdot \text{K}$$

8.5 The maximum average velocity of blood in a dog, 1 m/s, occurs in the dog's aorta, which is 0.015 m in diameter. The magnetic flux density in an electromagnetic blood flowmeter is 0.03 T. What is the voltage at the electrodes?

8.6 In order to determine the frequency response of an electromagnetic flowmeter, the clinician can transiently short-circuit the magnet current by using a microswitch. For steady flow, sketch the resulting output of the flowmeter. Describe the mathematical steps you could implement on a computer in order to convert the resulting transient wave to the flowmeter's frequency response.

8.7 On a common time scale, sketch the waveforms for the magnet current, flow signal, and transformer voltage for the following electromagnetic flowmeters: (1) gated sine wave, (2) square wave, (3) trapezoidal. Indicate the best time for sampling each flow signal.

8.8 For the Doppler ultrasonic flowmeter shown in Figure 8.10(b), suppose that the two transducers are inclined at angles θ and ϕ to the axis. Derive a formula for f_d, the Doppler frequency shift.

8.9 Use information from Section 3.5 to design a comparator with a SHR of 7, as required for the Doppler zero-crossing detector (Section 8.4).

8.10 Suppose that $W(f)$, the Doppler power spectrum, is 1.0 from 5 to 10 kHz and 0 elsewhere. Calculate the average zero-crossing rate.

8.11 For Figure 8.13, show how to add another one-shot and several logic blocks to obtain pulse outputs on both positive and negative zero crossings.

8.12 For a pulsed Doppler flowmeter using an 8-MHz oscillator and a 1-μs pulse, sketch on a common time scale the waveforms for (1) the electrical excitation of the transducer, (2) the acoustical output of the transducer and (3) the signal received from an arterial wall 1 mm thick.

8.13 A pulsed Doppler flowmeter has $f_r = 15$ kHz, $f_0 = 8$ MHz, and $\theta = 45°$. Calculate R_m and u_m.

8.14 Expand Figures 8.18 and 8.17(b) to show a complete block diagram of a directionally sensitive thermal velocity meter and probe.

8.15 The chamber plethysmograph in Figure 8.19 has a volume of 200 ml. Calculate the rapid change in tissue volume that produces a 120-Pa change in chamber pressure. Assume an adiabatic process: $P(V)^{1.4}$ = constant.

8.16 Calculate the arterial inflow for the test shown in Figure 8.20.

8.17 For Figure 8.23, assume $Z + \Delta Z = Z_2 = Z_3 = 100 \, \Omega$ and $Z_v = -j2000 \, \Omega$ (capacitive). How large is the error caused by a 5-Ω change in Z_2? Is an error of this magnitude important?

8.18 For Figure 8.23, show the functional blocks that must be added to provide an automatic-reset system.

8.19 The guard electrode shown in Figure 8.24 is a two-electrode system. If a four-electrode system is possible, show the arrangement of electrodes and connections.

8.20 Sketch the way the field lines would change if the guard-driving amplifier in Figure 8.24(d) had a gain greater than 1.

8.21 Design a circuit that uses the same two electrodes (plus one ground electrode) to monitor respiration by impedance and the conventional ECG, with no cross interference.

References

Almasi, J.J., "A computerized thermal dilution system," In *Computers in cardiology. 1976 conference proceedings.* Long Beach, CA: IEEE Computer Society, 1976.

Baker, D.W., "Pulsed ultrasonic Doppler blood-flow sensing." *IEEE Trans. Sonics Ultrason.*, 1970, SU-17, 170–185.

Bassingthwaighte, J.B., "The measurement of blood flows and volumes by indicator dilution," in C.D. Ray (ed.), *Medical engineering.* Chicago: Year Book, 1974, pp. 246–260.

Bellville, J.W., and C.S. Weaver, *Techniques in clinical physiology.* New York: Macmillan, 1969.

Bendick, P.J., and V.L. Newhouse, "Ultrasonic random-signal flow measurement system." *J. Acoust. Soc. Amer.*, 1974, 56, 860–865.

Bergel, D.H., and U. Gessner, "The electromagnetic flowmeter," in R.F. Rushmer (ed.), *Methods in medical research,* Chicago: Year Book, 1966, Vol. XI.

Calvert, M.H., B.R. Pullan, and D.E. Bone, "A simple method for measuring the frequency response of an electromagnetic flowmeter." *Med. Biol. Eng.*, 1975, 13, 592–594.

Cobbold, R.S.C., *Transducers for biomedical measurements: Principles and applications.* New York: Wiley, 1974.

Cooley, W.L., and R.L. Longini, "A new design for an impedance pneumograph." *J. Appl. Physiol.*, 1968, 25, 429–432.

Cromwell, L., F.J. Weibell, E.A. Pfeiffer, and L.B.Usselman, *Biomedical instrumentation and measurements*. Englewood Cliffs, NJ: Prentice-Hall, 1973.

Doll, H.G., H.J. Broner, and G.G. Nahas, "Non-invasive electromagnetic flowgraphy of peripheral arteries." *Dig. Int. Conf. Biomed. Transducers,* Paris, November 3–7, 1975, paper C3.6.

Forrester, J.S., Ganz, W., Dramond, G., McHugh, T., and Chonette, D.W., "Thermodilution cardiac output determination with a single flow-directed catheter." *Amer. Heart J.,* 1972, 83, 306–311.

Geddes, L.A., and Baker, L.E., *Principles of applied biomedical instrumentation,* 2nd ed. New York: Wiley, 1975.

Grahn, A.R., M.H. Paul, and H.U. Wessel, "A new direction-sensitive probe for catheter-tip thermal velocity measurements." *J. Appl. Physiol.*, 1969, 27, 407–412.

Groveman, J., D.D. Cohen, and J.B. Dillon, "Rhinoplethysmography: Pulse monitoring at the nasal septum." *Anesth. Analg.,* 1966, 45, 63.

Kubicek, W.G., A.H.L. From, R.P. Patterson, D.A. Witsoe, A. Castenda, R.G. Lilleki, and R. Ersek, "Impedance cardiography as a noninvasive means to monitor cardiac function." *J. Assoc. Adv. Med. Instrum.*, 1970, 4, 79–84.

Lee, A.L., A.J. Tahmoush, and J.R. Jennings, "An LED-transistor photoplethysmograph." *IEEE Trans. Biomed. Eng.,* 1975, BME-22, 243–250.

McCutcheon, E.P., *Chronically implanted cardiovascular instrumentation.* New York: Academic, 1973.

McLeod, F.D., "A directional Doppler flowmeter." *Dig. Int. Conf. Med. Biol. Eng.* Stockholm, 1967, 213.

Mills, C.J., and J.P. Shillingford, "A catheter tip electromagnetic velocity probe and its evaluation." *Cardiovasc. Res.,* 1967, 1, 263–273.

Nyboer, J., *Electrical impedance plethysmography,* 2nd ed. Springfield, IL: C.C. Thomas, 1970.

Péronneau, P., "Analyse de l'écoulement sanguin dans les gros vaisseaux par méthode ultrasonore." Docteur de Sciences Thèse à l'Université de Paris-Sud, 1977.

Reneman, R.S., *Cardiovascular applications of ultrasound.* New York: American Elsevier, 1974.

Roberts, V.C., *Blood flow measurements.* Baltimore: Williams & Wilkins, 1972.

Roberts, V.C., "The measurement of flow in intact blood vessels." *Crit. Rev. Bioeng.,* 1973, 1, 419–452.

Shercliff, J.A., *The theory of electromagnetic flow measurement.* Cambridge: Cambridge University Press, 1962.

Swanson, D.K. "Measurement errors and origin of electrical

impedance changes in the limbs." Ph.D. dissertation, Department of Electrical and Computer Engineering, University of Wisconsin, Madison, Wisconsin, 1976.

Wells, P.N.T., "Clinical applications of ultrasonics," in B.W. Watson (ed.), *IEE Medical Electronics Monographs 1–6*. London: Peregrinus, 1971.

Welkowitz, W., and S. Deutsch, *Biomedical instruments: Theory and design*. New York: Academic, 1976.

Wyatt, D.G., "Electromagnetic blood-flow measurements," in B.W. Watson (ed.), *IEE Medical Electronics Monographs 1–6*. London: Peregrinus, 1971.

Chapter nine

Measurements of the respiratory system

Frank P. Primiano, Jr.

This chapter deals with the processes in the lungs that are involved in the exchange of gases between the blood and the atmosphere. Measurement of variables associated with these processes enables the physician to perform two clinically relevant tasks: assess the functional status of the respiratory system (lungs, airways, and chest wall) and intervene in its function.

The objective assessment of respiratory function is clinically performed on two time scales. One is relatively long, involving discrete observations at intervals on the order of days to years. The observations made at these intervals are usually in the form of *pulmonary function tests* (PFT). These are combinations of specified experimental conditions, sets of measurements, and computational procedures used to evaluate parameters of respiratory function. Tests of pulmonary function are used: (1) to screen the general population for disease; (2) to serve as part of periodic physical examinations, especially of individuals with chronic pulmonary conditions; (3) to evaluate acute changes during episodes of disease; and (4) to follow up after treatment.

The second time scale on which respiratory function is assessed is very short, with observations made either continuously or at intervals on the order of minutes to hours. This activity comes under the heading of *patient monitoring,* and is performed in a hospital setting, usually in an intensive-care unit (ICU). It is warranted in crisis situations such as might result from accidental trauma, drug overdose, major surgery, or disease. (See Section 12.5.)

Therapeutic modification of respiratory function can be achieved through surgery, the use of drugs, or physical intervention with respiratory-assist devices. Except for extreme, acute circumstances—such as cardiac surgery, in which the lungs are completely by-passed and blood is arterialized in an extracorporeal oxygenator (Section 12.3)—these approaches attempt to control arterial blood gases by manipulating concentrations and distribution of pulmonary gas and distribution of the flow of pulmonary blood. The same variables used to evaluate lung function can be monitored to provide objective feedback information for this external control of the system.

Since there are a myriad of instruments that have been used to measure variables associated with respiration, some selection process must be invoked if we are to put bounds on a chapter such as this. Consequently, we shall discuss clinically applicable devices that yield accurate, quantitative measures suitable for the computation of parameters routinely evaluated by pulmonary function tests. This eliminates from discussion those devices which have primary applications as patient-monitoring or physical-diagnosis tools. Examples are radiographs (x-ray films), fluoroscopes, magnetometers, variable-resistance extension gages that go around the chest, and transthoracic electrical impedance devices, each used to estimate or detect lung-volume change; nasal thermistors to detect airflow; and force plates to detect body movements associated with breathing.

The literature in respiratory physiology suffers from having a very poor system of notation. This system has evolved, to some extent, from an effort to accommodate the clinically oriented audience. The symbols used in this chapter are a compromise between those that are frequently found in the respiratory literature (Comroe, 1962; Cotes, 1975) and those that are found in the physical sciences literature.

In the respiratory literature, V represents geometrical volume of a container, such as the lungs, and $\dot{V}$ represents the rate of change of the container's volume. However, because the gas in the lungs can be compressed, $\dot{V}$ is not necessarily equal to the volume flow rate of gas entering the lungs through the nose and mouth, although, in many circumstances, $\dot{V}$ is well approximated by this flow. Nevertheless, to emphasize the distinction between rate of change of volume of a container and the rate of flow of a fluid (gas or liquid) into it, we use the symbol Q for flow rate, as is commonly done in physics and fluid mechanics. We could not use F, as is done in the rest of this book, because F is routinely used in respiratory physiology to denote molar fraction (fractional concentration) of a gas species in a mixture. Finally, we follow the standard of having the first modifier after the quantity symbol in small capitals or lower-case letters.

9.1 Modeling the respiratory system

The decision as to which of the many respiratory variables are to be measured is based on the type of behavior under study as well as on a concept of how the system functions. Ideas about how the respiratory system functions are usually formalized in abstract (i.e., verbal or mathematical) models. Not only are the variables that are to be measured specified by models of the respiratory system, but such models also define characteristic parameters of respiratory function and are the basis for the design of experiments to evaluate these parameters. In addition, they motivate control strategies and devices that are used to produce effective respiratory assistance. The definitions and discussions of lung physiology are based on models of the lungs. Therefore, before we attempt measurements, we should understand the essential features of the respiratory system and some approaches to modeling that we can use not only for the respiratory system but also for some of the devices used to test it.

Because it is the respiratory function of living individuals that is to be evaluated, measurements must be minimally invasive, cause minimal discomfort, and be acceptable for use in a clinical environment. This greatly limits the number and types of measurements that can be made and leads to the use of lumped-parameter models. For the sake of discussion, it is convenient to divide respiratory function into two categories: (1) gas transport in the lungs (including extrapulmonary airways and pulmonary capillaries) and (2) mechanics of the lungs and chest wall. The models describing gas transport deal primarily with changes in concentrations of gas species and volume flow of gas, whereas the models dealing with mechanics primarily relate pressure, lung volume, and volume flow of gas. Bear in mind that these two categories are highly interrelated, and tests from one complement those from the other.

Gas transport

Models of gas transport, both in the gas phase and across the alveolar-capillary membrane into the blood, are developed from mass balances for the pulmonary system depicted as a set of compartments. What can be considered as a basic gas-transport unit of the lungs is shown in Figure 9.1(a). It consists of a variable-volume alveolar compartment, with its contents well mixed by diffusion; a well-mixed, flow-through blood compartment that exchanges gases with the alveolar compartment by diffusion; and a constant-volume dead space. Gas moves by convection through the dead space, which acts only as a time-delay conduit between its outer opening and its associated alveolar volume. A *pair* of normal lungs during quiet breathing may be represented satisfactorily by the system in Figure 9.1(a). Descriptions of either normal lungs undergoing maximal volume changes or diseased lungs experiencing abnormal gas transport may require more complicated systems, made of combinations of such units, either in parallel or series or both.

A dynamic mass balance can be written for any chemical species X or set of species of the breathed gas mixture. If the production of X by chemical reaction in a system were negligible, a

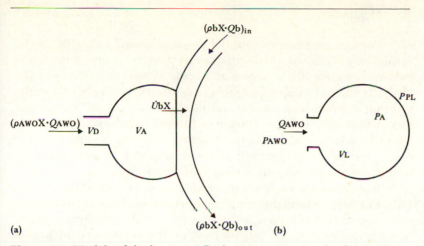

Figure 9.1 Models of the lungs. (a) Basic gas-transport unit of the pulmonary system. $(\rho x \cdot Q)$ is the molar flow of X through the airway opening AWO and the pulmonary capillary blood network, b. $\dot{U}bX$ is the net rate of molar uptake, i.e., the net rate of diffusion of X into the blood. V_D and V_A are the dead-space volume and alveolar volume, respectively. (b) A basic mechanical unit of the pulmonary system. P_A, P_{PL}, and P_{AWO} are the pressures inside the lung, i.e., alveolar compartment, on the pleural surface of the lungs, and at the airway opening, respectively. V_L is the volume of the gas space within the lungs, including the airways; Q_{AWO} is the volume flow of gas into the lungs measured at the airway opening.

species mass balance could be written as

$$
\begin{array}{c}
\text{Rate of mass} \\
\text{accumulation} \\
\text{of X in the} \\
\text{system}
\end{array}
=
\sum_{i=1}^{n}
\begin{array}{c}
\text{Rate of mass} \\
\text{convection} \\
\text{of X through} \\
\text{port } i
\end{array}
-
\begin{array}{c}
\text{Net rate of} \\
\text{diffusion out} \\
\text{of the system}
\end{array}
\qquad (9.1)
$$

This can also be written as a molar balance, since the number of moles N is the ratio of the mass of X to its molecular weight (in mass units). Define $\rho_{AWO}X$ as the mole density (moles per unit volume) of species X and Q_{AWO} as its volume flow (volume per unit time), each measured at the airway opening. Then a molar balance for X in the gas phase in the model of the lungs in Figure 9.1(a) would be

$$
\frac{d(N_L X)}{dt} = (\rho_{AWO} X \cdot Q_{AWO}) - \dot{U}bX \qquad (9.2)
$$

in which $\dot{U}bX$ is the net molar rate of uptake of X by the blood. The number of moles of X in the lungs, $N_L X$, is the sum of the moles in the dead-space volume, $N_D X$, and the alveolar compartment, $N_A X$.

Mechanics

We can conveniently model the mechanical behavior of the respiratory system as a combination of pneumatic and mechanical elements. Figure 9.1(b) shows an idealized mechanical unit of the lungs. It consists of a deformable pressure vessel made of a material that exhibits both elastic and plastic behavior and a nonrigid airway that has a variable resistance to convective flow. The system contains a saturated mixture of ideal gases that exhibits inertia during acceleration through the airway and that undergoes an isothermal process during changes of state.

Even though each of the millions of alveoli and terminal airways could potentially act as a separate mechanical unit, it has been found that the mechanics of a pair of normal lungs during quiet breathing can be represented by the single unit of Figure 9.1(b). However, at high rates of breathing, normal and abnormal pulmonary systems may require models containing combinations of such units. Note that only in rare instances, such as when there is only a single gas space in each model, do compartments of the gas-transport units [Figure 9.1(a)] correspond one-to-one to mechanical units [Figure 9.1(b)] in the same lungs.

An additional deformable pressure vessel representing the chest wall surrounding the lungs has been added to the system in Figure 9.2(a). The chest wall includes all extrapulmonary structures, such as respiratory muscles and abdominal contents, which can undergo motions as a result of breathing. The gap between the lung unit and the chest wall represents the liquid-filled interpleural space.

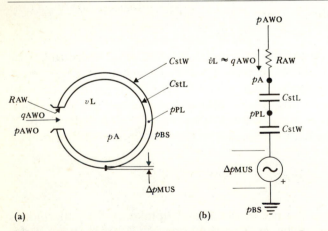

Figure 9.2 Models of normal ventilatory mechanics for small-amplitude, low-frequency (normal lungs, resting) breathing. (a) Mechanical unit enclosed by chest wall. (b) Equivalent circuit for model in Figure 9.2(a).

The mechanics of the respiratory system are described by the relationships between pressure differences across the various subsystems and the changes in volume and flow of gas through them. The subsystems are defined between points in the system at which representative pressures can be computed or measured. Consequently, the difference in pressure across the entire system can be expressed as the algebraic sum of pressure differences across subsystems. Mass balances can be used to follow the path of gas flow through the subsystems, and geometrical constraints determine the distribution of volume changes.

Model of normal respiratory mechanics during quiet breathing

When the flows, changes of volume, or their respective time derivatives are large, the equations describing the mechanical behavior of the respiratory system are highly nonlinear. However, for small flows and changes of volume such as those that occur during resting breathing, linear approximations adequately describe the respiratory system. These linear approximations define the familiar properties such as compliance, resistance, and inertance that are to be evaluated by pulmonary function tests.

The following conventions will be applied throughout this chapter to facilitate writing linearized equations. Lower-case letters for variables will indicate finite perturbations about an operating point or reference level:

$$y = Y - \hat{Y}$$

where $\hat{Y}$ indicates some fixed reference value for Y. All linearized equations, therefore, are written in lower-case variables. A delta Δ will indicate differences between two spatial points,

$$\Delta Y = Yi - Yj$$

where i and j indicate different positions, for example, AWO and PL. Therefore, the change in the pressure difference across the lungs (transpulmonary pressure) would be

$$(P_{AWO} - P_{PL}) - (\hat{P}_{AWO} - \hat{P}_{PL}) = \Delta P_L - \Delta \hat{P}_L = \Delta p_L$$

If the alveoli exhibit predominantly elastic behavior, the following set of linear equations can be used as a simple model of the mechanics of the respiratory system for normal tidal breathing in the atmosphere [Figure 9.2(a)]:

$$p\text{AWO} - p\text{A} = R\text{AW } q\text{AWO} \tag{9.3a}$$

$$p\text{A} - p\text{PL} = \frac{1}{C\text{stL}} v\text{L} \tag{9.3b}$$

$$\Delta p\text{MUS} + (p\text{PL} - p\text{BS}) = \frac{1}{C\text{stw}} v\text{L} \tag{9.3c}$$

in which lower-case letters are used to designate changes in the following variables with respect to an operating point.

P_{AWO} Hydrostatic pressure at the airway opening

P_{A} Representative pressure within the lungs (alveolar pressure)

P_{PL} Representation of the average force per unit area acting on the pleural surfaces (interpleural pressure)

ΔP_{MUS} Representation of the average force per unit area on the chest wall, which would cause the same movements produced by the active contraction of the respiratory muscles during breathing (muscle pressure difference)

P_{BS} Hydrostatic pressure acting on the body surface, except at the airway opening

Q_{AWO} Volume flow of gas at the airway opening

V_{L} Volume of the gas space in the system, assumed to be entirely within the lungs and airways

Three mechanical properties are included in (9.3): airway resistance, R_{AW}, pulmonary static compliance, C_{stL}, and chest-wall static compliance, C_{stw}. We can evaluate these parameters by applying the general definitions of flow resistance through a conduit and compliance of a deformable structure:

$$R \equiv \frac{\partial(\Delta P)}{\partial Q} \tag{9.4}$$

and

$$C\text{st} \equiv \frac{\partial V}{\partial(\Delta P)} \tag{9.5}$$

in which ΔP is the pressure difference across the system under study. Therefore,

$$R_{\text{AW}} = \frac{\partial(P_{\text{AWO}} - P_{\text{A}})}{\partial Q_{\text{AWO}}} \tag{9.6}$$

The partial derivatives in (9.4) through (9.6) are used to indicate that all other variables must be constant when these parameters are evaluated. In particular, Cst can be evaluated only when the system is at static equilibrium, i.e., when all flows and rates of change of volume and pressure in the system are zero. In this situation, $P_{AWO} - P_A = 0$, and $(P_A - P_{PL})$ can be measured as $(P_{AWO} - P_{PL})$. Thus, pulmonary static compliance can be evaluated as

$$C_{stL} \equiv \frac{V_L(t_2) - V_L(t_1)}{\Delta P_L(t_2) - \Delta P_L(t_1)} \qquad (9.7)$$

in which

$$\Delta P_L = (P_{AWO} - P_{PL}) \qquad (9.8)$$

the transpulmonary pressure difference; and t_2 and t_1 are two instants in time at which the system is completely motionless.

It is impossible to measure the muscle pressure difference, ΔP_{MUS}, directly. Consequently, chest-wall static compliance can be evaluated only when $\Delta P_{MUS} = 0$. This occurs by definition when the respiratory muscles are completely relaxed. Defining the difference in pressure across the chest wall as

$$\Delta P_W \equiv P_{PL} - P_{BS} \qquad (9.9)$$

we obtain chest-wall static compliance from

$$C_{stw} \equiv \frac{V_L(t_4) - V_L(t_3)}{\Delta P_W(t_4) - \Delta P_W(t_3)} \qquad (9.10)$$

in which t_4 and t_3 are two instants at which the system is static *and* the respiratory muscles are completely relaxed.

As the lungs change volume and lose or gain gas through the airway opening, the gas inside is compressed or expanded. For fast changes in volume, this produces an inequality between the rate of volume change $\dot{V}_L$ and the volume flow of gas at the mouth, Q_{AWO}. However, for normal, tidal breathing, this effect can be neglected and Q_{AWO} can be taken as a good approximation to $\dot{V}_L$. Therefore (9.3a) and (9.3b) can be combined and rewritten as

$$p_{AWO} - p_{PL} = \frac{1}{C_{stL}} v_L + R_{AW}\dot{v}_L \qquad (9.11)$$

Equations (9.3c) and (9.11), which describe Figure 9.2(a), can also be represented by the analogous equivalent circuit in Figure 9.2(b).

Measurable variables in the respiratory system

Even though a number of variables are included in the simple models of gas transport and mechanics shown in Figures 9.1 and

9.2, only a very limited subset can be measured directly. These include: volume flow of gas through the mouth and nose (and equivalently a measure of its integral, the equivalent volume of gas breathed); pressure near the mouth and nose and body surface; partial pressures or concentrations of various gases in gas mixtures passing the airway opening and in discrete samples of blood; and temperature (including body-core temperature). The values of all other variables in the preceding equations cannot be measured directly, but must be inferred from measurements of other variables. A notable example is change in lung volume, which is routinely obtained from gas flow or volume.

9.2 Measurement of pressure

Two noteworthy characteristics of respiratory pressure measurements are the manner in which pressure is measured and the fact that most of the measurements involve pressure differences. All the pressures included in the respiratory models given in Section 9.1 are described in the respiratory literature as lateral pressure or side pressure, i.e., the pressure measured at the wall of a vessel with the plane of the measurement port parallel to the direction of any flow that might exist. This defines the static or hydrostatic pressure of the fluid dynamicist. The total, or stagnation, pressure and the dynamic pressure at a point are never used in these models. Confusion can arise, however, because of the way in which the terms static and dynamic are used with respect to pressure in the respiratory literature. It is standard practice to express the difference in hydrostatic pressure between two points as the sum of two time-varying components, the static component and the dynamic component. For example, the transpulmonary pressure difference can be written as

$$\Delta P_L = (\Delta P_L)\text{st} + (\Delta P_L)\text{dyn} \tag{9.12}$$

The static component is defined as a function of only the volume change in the system. The dynamic component, which is the hydrostatic pressure difference minus its static component, is related only to flows, rates of change of volume, and their derivatives. The static component of a pressure difference, therefore, can be measured as the hydrostatic pressure difference when all flows, rates of volume change, and their derivatives are zero, i.e., when the system is static.

Pressure transducers

We can conveniently perform dynamic measurements of respiratory pressures using an electronic strain-gage pressure transducer with a tube or catheter as a probe. Section 7.2 described the characteristics of such systems for the circulatory system in which the catheter and transducer are filled with liquid. The same type of analysis can be used for gas-filled systems, with the exception that the acoustic compliance of the gas may be of the same order of magnitude—or even higher than—the compliance of the transducer diaphragm. Therefore, an appropriate shunt capacitor must be included in the equivalent circuit for the device [Figure 7.6(a)].

An additional point must be considered, however, when a pressure difference is measured. Such measurements are usually accomplished with differential pressure transducers that have two chambers separated by a diaphragm connected to strain-sensitive elements. Gas is introduced into each chamber through a catheter. Therefore, the circuit of Figure 7.6(a) represents the mechanical or pneumatic transfer function for only one side of a differential pressure gage. Note that the time-varying pressure that exists in the chamber on each side of the diaphragm is influenced by the transfer characteristics of the respective mechanical-pneumatic circuits between the pressure source and the strain-sensing diaphragm. Thus it is extremely important that the frequency response of the transmission lines on both sides of the transducer be matched over the frequency range of interest. This becomes critical when high-frequency changes in pressure are to be measured with transducers manufactured with chambers that have unequal volumes on either side of the diaphragm.

Intraesophageal pressure

Computing pulmonary mechanical properties—for instance, pulmonary static compliance, from (9.7)—requires a measure of the spatially averaged pressure acting on the pleural surfaces. Direct measurements of the pressure on the visceral pleural surface made by puncturing the thoracic wall and introducing a catheter into the interpleural space are not clinically applicable. Such measurements have shown, however, that a gravity-related pressure gradient exists in the thin liquid film in the interpleural space surrounding the lungs. This nonuniform pressure, which is lowest in the uppermost part of the chest, makes the point at which a representative pressure can be measured uncertain. Fortunately, the determination of mechanical properties from linearized equations such as (9.3) involve only changes in pressure about an operating point. This relaxes the requirement on the measurement of the absolute pressure.

A significant advance in clinical testing of pulmonary function was the development of a method of estimating changes in the average pressure on the visceral pleural surface from measurements of changes in the pressure in a bolus of gas introduced into the esophagus. The most commonly used technique involves passing an air-filled catheter with a small latex balloon on its end through the nose into the esophagus (Milic-Emili *et al.*, 1964; Macklem, 1974).

The esophagus, which is normally a flaccid, collapsed tube, is subjected to the pressure in the interpleural space acting through the parietal pleura and the weight of other thoracic structures, primarily the heart. The pressure in the air trapped in a small balloon situated within the thoracic esophagus depends on the compression, or expansion, caused by these sources. Although the mean esophageal pressure does not equal the mean pressure on the pleural surface measured directly by catheter in the interpleural space, under certain conditions the changes in the pressure in the esophageal balloon reflect the changes in pressure on the pleural surface. The mechanical properties of the balloon and esophagus have minimal effect on the changes in pressure in the balloon if the amount of air in the balloon is small enough so that the balloon remains unstressed and the esophageal wall does not undergo motions large enough to influence the transmission of pressure into the balloon. The balloon should be so located that variations in pressure changes due to motions of other organs competing for space in the thoracic cavity are minimized.

The largest noise signal comes from the heartbeat, which usually has a fundamental frequency (on the order of 1 Hz) much higher than that of resting breathing. A region below the upper third of the thoracic esophagus gives low cardiac interference and provides pressure variations that correspond well in magnitude and phase with directly measured representative changes in pleural pressure. The correspondence decreases as lung volume approaches the minimum achievable volume, i.e., residual volume. The frequency response of an esophageal balloon pressure-measurement system depends on the mechanical properties and dimensions of the pressure transducer, catheter, and the gas within the system. The use of helium instead of air can extend the usable frequency range of these systems (Fry *et al.*, 1952).

9.3 Measurement of gas-flow rate

When the lungs change volume during breathing, a mass of gas is transferred through the airway opening by convective flow. Measurement of variables associated with the movement of this gas is of major importance in studies of the respiratory system. The volume-flow rate and the time integral of volume-flow rate are used to estimate rate of change of lung volume and changes of lung volume, respectively. Even though the devices to be described in the following are calibrated and used to measure volume-flow rate or to estimate its integral, the primary physical process involved is mass flow. Volume-flow rate equals the mass-flow rate divided by the density of the gas at the measurement site. The instruments used to measure volume-flow rate are referred to as *volume flow-meters*. The volume occupied by a given mass (number of moles) of gas under known conditions of temperature and pressure is usually determined by using a spirometer (Section 9.4).

Even though breathing movements are cyclic by nature and involve alternating (bidirectional) gas flow, some tests of pulmonary function, such as those involving the single-breath washout, the forced expiratory vital-capacity maneuver, and the maximum breathing capacity require the measurement of flow in only one direction. In addition, the precision and accuracy demanded of flow measurements vary greatly, depending on the settings in which they are performed, from physiology and clinical function laboratories to mass screening centers to intensive care units. Consequently, there are a variety of instruments that can perform measurements useful in particular applications.

Requirements for respiratory gas-flow measurements

Measurement of the motion of material passing through a system requires that the transducer be placed at a position traversed by a known fraction of the material. In respiratory experiments, especially those involving measurement of breathed gas, the usual practice is to have the entire flow stream pass through or into the instrument. This produces several potential problems. Any pressure imposed at the airway during measurements at the airway opening—for example, by a forced oscillation test or with assisted ventilation involving positive end expiratory pressure (PEEP) or continuous positive airway pressure (CPAP)—must be withstood by the instrument without damage, distortion, or leakage. Also, the device should not obstruct breathing or produce a change in pressure during flow which might affect respiratory performance.

As with any instrument, the gas-flow-measuring instrument must have a stable baseline (reference output) and sensitivity so that measurements are accurate. However, changes in composition and temperature of gas can affect the calibration factors of various flowmeters. These changes occur between inspired and expired gas and during an expiration. Furthermore, particles of dust and dirt inhaled from the atmosphere and aerosolized organic particles from the respiratory system can deposit on sensitive parts of the transducers and contaminate them. This not only affects calibration, but can also transmit disease. Therefore, the instrument must be either sterilizable or disposable.

One of the major contaminants in the expired gas in transducers is water vapor. Unless the instrument is heated to body temperature or above, it acts as a condenser for the water in the saturated expirate. This liquid can foul delicate transducers and change the effective cross-sectional area through which the gas must pass.

The measurement procedure must not alter inspired air by adding excessive heat or toxic substances. Such techniques as laser anemometry (which requires reflecting particles in the stream) or ion anemometry (which produces ozone) are not suitable for measurements at the airway opening. If the instrument is to monitor breathing continuously for a number of breaths, then the dead space of the instrument becomes important. Carbon dioxide must be flushed out and O_2 replenished if the conduit tubing in the system is of such a volume that the patient will experience excessive rebreathing of expired gas.

Commonly used respiratory volume flowmeters fall into one of four categories: rotating vane, ultrasonic, thermal convection, and differential pressure.

Rotating-vane flowmeters

This type of device has a small turbine in the flow path. The rotation of the turbine can be related to the volume flow of gas. Mechanical linkages have been used to display parameters of the flow (e.g., peak flow and integral over an expiration) on indicator dials on the instrument. Interruption of a light beam by the turbine has also been sensed and converted to voltages proportional to flow and/or its integral to be recorded photographically or displayed continuously. In devices such as this, the mass of the moving parts and the friction between them combine to prevent high-frequency motions of the turbine in response to accelerating flows. This precludes their use in the measurement of alternating bidirectional flows and makes them primarily suitable for clinical screening.

Ultrasonic flowmeters

Section 8.4 described the operation and application of ultrasonic devices in the measurement of blood flow. For respiratory measurements, investigators measure the effect of the flowing gas on the transit time of the ultrasonic signal. The transmitter-receiver crystal pair is mounted either externally and obliquely to the axis of the tube through which the gas flows or, more recently, internally and coaxially with the flow (Blumenfeld et al., 1975). The transit time between the transmitter and receiver depends not only on the velocity of the gas between them, but also on the composition and temperature of the gas.

In another approach, a rod is placed in the flow stream to produce a pattern of vortices. An ultrasonic transmitter and receiver are mounted diametrically opposite each other in the walls of the tube. The intensity of the ultrasonic signals passing perpendicular to the flow is modulated by the vortices. The modulating frequency is detected and calibrated as a measure of volume-flow rate. Ultrasonic flowmeters are presently suitable only for clinical monitoring, but they may be developed further into accurate, linear, bidirectional flowmeters.

Thermal-convection flowmeters

Thermal-convection flowmeters employ sensing elements such as metal wires, metal films, and thermistors whose resistance changes with temperature. When operated in the self-heated mode, in which sufficient current is passed through them to maintain an average temperature above that of the surrounding fluid, these elements lose heat at a rate that depends on the local mass flow, temperature, specific heat, kinematic viscosity, and thermal conductivity of the fluid. If a feedback circuit is used to operate the primary sensing element at a constant temperature, then a second unheated element can be included in the circuit to compensate for heat loss due to local, ambient temperature changes. (The thermal response time of the unheated elements can be affected by condensation of water vapor from humid gas mixtures.) Section 8.5 described the details and operation of such devices and circuits.

For situations in which gas properties are sufficiently constant, the output voltage from these circuits is a nonlinear function of mass-flow rate only. Special analog circuits implementing piecewise-linear or polynomial approximations of this function have been developed to provide a linear mass-flow–voltage relationship.

Flowmeters using a single, temperature-compensated, heated wire (hot-wire anemometer) with a linearizing circuit provide unidirectional flow measurements that are satisfactory for testing of pulmonary function. If an investigator wants to use a single hot wire to obtain volume-flow rate continuously, several conditions must be fulfilled. For a gas of constant density, volume-flow rate through a cross section is proportional to the average mass flow (averaged over the cross section). The mass-flow sensing wire is very small (on the order of 5 μm diameter and 1 to 2 mm in length) to satisfy heat-transfer and frequency-response requirements. Consequently, mass flow is measured only locally in a correspondingly small region of the flow stream. The duct in which the sensor is located must be designed so that the position at which the measurement is made yields a value representative of the average mass flow through the entire cross section of the duct at every instant of time. At the low Mach numbers involved in respiratory flows, this requires that the velocity profile be well defined at all flows of interest. The variations in cross-sectional area up- and downstream from the sensor can be optimized for this condition.

Although a single hot-wire sensor provides an output of the same polarity independent of the direction of flow, limiting its use to unidirectional flow, multiple sensors located at separate points along the flow path can be used with the appropriate circuitry to provide directional sensitivity, as described in Section 8.5. However, respiratory measurements involve a changing mixture of gases in the flow stream that affects the heat transfer from the heated wire. The significant variations in composition that occur between inspiration and expiration could invalidate the use of a single calibration factor. During the multibreath N_2 washout test (Section 9.4) the N_2–O_2 ratio in the lung changes from approximately 4 to 1 on the first breath to nearly zero at the end of the test. Fortunately, the differences in thermal properties and densities of N_2 and O_2 offset each other sufficiently well that a linearized, temperature-compensated hot-wire anemometer can be used with a constant calibration factor for volume-flow measurements during the successive expirations of a multibreath N_2 washout. In general, however, the instrument should be calibrated for the particular gas mixture to which it is exposed.

The hot-wire anemometer has a number of features that are advantageous in respiratory applications. It has a good frequency response (the sensor itself can respond to frequencies into the kilohertz range). And, since the sensing element in the flow stream is extremely small, the only back pressure produced is that caused by the flow through the duct. In unidirectional applications rebreathing does not occur, so dead space is irrelevant. Accurate readings can be made at low as well as high flow rates if the system includes an appropriate linearizing circuit. Special circuits can be provided to overheat the sensor to burn off contaminants as necessary. The main disadvantage is the limitation to unidirectional flow. The relatively high cost of overcoming this with a paired hot-wire system may not be justified.

Differential pressure flowmeters (pneumotachometers)

Convective flow occurs as a result of a difference in pressure between two points. From the relationship between pressure difference and volume-flow rate through a system, measurement of the difference in pressure yields an estimate of flow. Flowmeters based on this idea have incorporated several mechanisms to establish the relation between pressure drop and flow, including the venturi, orifice, and flow resistances of various types. The last group, which produces approximately linear pressure-flow relationships, has found the most frequent use in respiratory laboratories and is usually what is referred to when the term *pneumota-*

chometer is used. (In general, pneumotachometer is synonymous with gas volume flowmeter.) Flow-resistance pneumotachometers are easy to use and sensitive to alternating flows. They also have sufficient accuracy, sensitivity, linearity, and frequency response for most clinical applications. In addition, they use the same differential pressure gages and amplifiers required for other respiratory measurements. The following discussion primarily concerns these instruments.

Even though other flow-resistance elements have been incorporated in pneumotachometers (Fry *et al.*, 1957), those most commonly used consist of either a fine mesh screen [Figure 9.3(a)] placed perpendicular to flow (Silverman and Whittenberger, 1950; Lilly, 1950) or a tightly packed bundle of capillary tubes or channels [Figure 9.3(b)] with their axes parallel to flow (Fleisch, 1925). These physical devices exhibit, for a wide range of unsteady flows, a nearly linear pressure-drop–flow relationship, with pressure drop approximately in phase with flow.

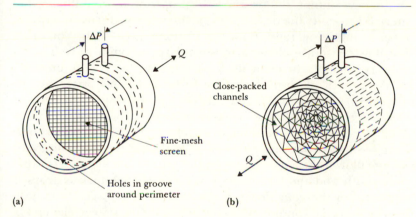

Figure 9.3 Pneumotachometer flow-resistance elements. (a) Screen. (b) Capillary tubes or channels.

In practice, the element is mounted in a conduit of circular cross section. The pressure drop is measured across the resistance element at the wall of the conduit (within the boundary layer of the flow). In the screen-type pneumotachometer, the pressure tap on each side of the screen is either a single hole through the conduit wall or multiple holes from a circumferential channel within the wall, which is connected to a common external tap. The pressure drop in the capillary-bundle pneumotachometer is measured either between two points on one tube in the outermost layer of the bundle or between two single holes in the wall of the conduit on each end of the capillary bundle.

Because the pressure drop is measured at a single radial distance from the center of the conduit, we assume that this pressure drop is representative of the pressure drop governing the total flow through the entire conduit cross section. These flowmeters rely on the flow-resistive element to establish a consistent—though not uniform—velocity profile on each side of the element in the neighborhood of the pressure measurement. This, however, cannot be achieved independent of the ductwork in which the pneumotachometer is placed (Finucane *et al.*, 1972). Therefore, the placement of the pressure ports and the configuration of the tubing that leads from the subject to the pneumotachometer and from the pneumotachometer to the remainder of the system are critical in determining the pressure-drop–flow relationship. This is especially important when alternating and/or high-frequency flow patterns are involved.

A number of tradeoffs exist in the design and use of these devices. A large axial separation between pressure ports may yield a ΔP-Q relationship that is more linear for steady flow than that for small port separation. But during unsteady flow with high-frequency content, the pressure drop may be more influenced by inertial forces. If the device is to avoid excessive formation of vortexes at high flow rates, the cross-sectional area of the conduit at the flow resistance element must be large enough to reduce the velocity through the element. This area may be several times that of the mouth of the subject from which the gas originates, requiring an adapter or diffuser between the mouthpiece and the resistance element. If flow separation and turbulence are to be avoided as the cross-sectional area changes, the adapter should have a shallow internal angle [Figure 9.4(a)] not exceeding 15°. The shallower the angle, however, the greater the distance between the mouth and the flow-resistance element. Symmetric drops in pressure for the same flow rate in either direction require that the geometry of the conduit on both sides of the resistance element be matched. The volume within the adapters and conduit represents a dead space for cyclic breathing. The designer, when designing the device, must balance the effects of decreased angle of the diffuser against the tolerable volume of dead space.

Some experimenters (e.g., Hyatt *et al.*, 1970) have used a bias flow to clear this dead space. Air is drawn through the pneumotachometer from a side hole [Figure 9.4(b)] through a long tube connected to a vacuum pump. This causes a constant bias pressure drop across the pneumotachometer if the bias flow created is constant during the breathing of the patient. This approach can work well when the high-frequency components of the flow pattern are of interest (as in forced-oscillation experiments). But for low frequencies, such as those of tidal breathing, a regulating device may be required to prevent variation of the bias flow as the patient breathes.

The usable frequency range for capillary pneumotachometers is typically smaller than that for the screen type. Depending

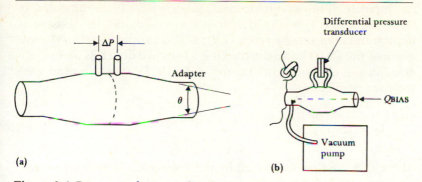

Figure 9.4 Pneumotachometer for measurements at the mouth. (a) Diameter adapter that acts as a diffuser. (b) An application in which a constant flow is used to clear the dead space.

on its design, the screen-type pneumotachometer can exhibit a constant-amplitude ratio of pressure difference to flow, and zero phase shift up to as high as 70 Hz (Peslin *et al.*, 1972b).

In air, the amplitude ratio of the Fleisch (capillary bundle) pneumotachometer is nearly constant at its steady-flow value up to approximately 10 Hz, increasing by 5% at 20 Hz. The phase angle between ΔP and Q increases linearly with frequency to approximately 8.5° at 10 Hz, which corresponds to an approximate 2-ms time delay between flow and pressure difference. These values change with the kinematic viscosity of the gas (Finucane *et al.*, 1972). Peslin *et al.* (1972b) modeled the Fleisch pneumotachometer for frequencies up to 70 Hz by an equation of the form

$$\Delta P = RQ + L\dot{Q} \tag{9.13}$$

L is the inertance (related to mass) of the gas in one capillary tube defined by (7.4) and R is the flow resistance for each capillary tube defined by (7.2). Equation (9.13) can be used as a computational algorithm to compensate the Fleisch pneumotachometer for precise measurements of a gas of constant composition at constant temperature.

An appropriately designed screen pneumotachometer may not require such compensation. But it may instead be subject to equipment-generated, high-frequency noise in clinical applications. An additional point should be stressed: The frequency response of a pneumotachometer is no better than that of its associated differential pressure measurement system. It is essential that the pneumatic (acoustic) impedances, including those of the tubes and connectors between the gage and the pneumotachometer, on each side of the differential pressure gage be balanced.

Equation (7.2) indicates that the resistance of the Fleisch pneumotachometer is proportional to the viscosity of the flowing gas mixture. The screen pneumotachometer can be modeled in terms of a low flow through a porous medium. Its resistance, though not computable from (7.2), is also proportional to the viscosity of the gas. The viscosity of a gas mixture depends on its composition and temperature (Turney *et al.*, 1973). When inertance effects are negligible,

$$Q = \frac{\Delta P}{R(T,[Fx])} \tag{9.14}$$

where Q is the flow measured by the pneumotachometer for a gas mixture with species molar fractions $[Fx] = [N_1/N, N_2/N, \ldots, N_x/N]$ at absolute temperature T. Pneumotachometers are routinely calibrated for steady flow only, and a single calibration factor is used during experiments. But instantaneous values of T and $[Fx]$ are not constant during a single expiration and their mean values change from expiration to inspiration. In particular, changes in viscosity of 10 to 15% occur from the beginning to the end of an experiment in which N_2 is washed out of the lungs by pure O_2. A continuous correction in calibration should be made when accurate results are desired.

The prevention of water-vapor condensation in a pneumotachometer is of particular importance. The capillary tubes and screen pores are easily blocked by liquid water, which decreases the effective cross-sectional area of the flow element and causes a change in resistance. Also, as water condenses, the composition of the gas mixture changes. To circumvent these problems, a common practice is to heat the pneumotachometer element, especially when more than a few consecutive breaths are to be studied. The Fleish pneumotachometer is usually provided with an electrical resistance heater; the screen of the screen pneumotachometer can be heated by passing a current through it. In addition, heating tape is routinely wrapped around any conduit that carries expired gas.

9.4 Lung volume

The most commonly used indexes of the mechanical status of the ventilatory system are the absolute volume and changes of volume of the gas space in the lungs achieved during various breathing maneuvers. Observe Figure 9.5 and assume that a subject's airway opening and body surface are exposed to atmospheric pressure. Then the largest volume to which the subject's lungs can be voluntarily expanded is defined as the *total lung capacity*, TLC. The smallest volume to which the subject can slowly deflate his or her lungs is the *residual volume,* RV. And the volume of the lungs at the end of a quiet expiration when the respiratory muscles are re-

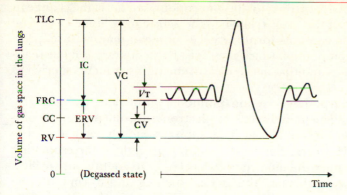

Figure 9.5 Volume ranges of the intact ventilatory system (with no external loads applied). TLC, FRC, and RV are measured as absolute volumes. VC, IC, ERV, and V_T are volume changes. Closing volume (CV) and closing capacity (CC) are obtained from a single-breath washout experiment.

laxed is the *functional residual capacity*, FRC. The difference between TLC and RV is the *vital capacity*, VC, which defines the maximum change in volume the lungs can undergo during voluntary maneuvers. The vital capacity can be divided into the *inspiratory capacity* (IC = TLC − FRC) and the *expiratory reserve volume* (ERV = FRC − RV). The peak-to-peak volume change during a quiet breath is the *tidal volume*, V_T.

Changes in lung volume: Spirometry

The measurement of changes in lung volume has been approached in two ways. One is to measure the changes in the volume of the gas space within the body during breathing by using plethysmographic techniques (discussed in Section 9.5). The second approach involves measurements made in the gas passing through the airway opening. The latter measurements can provide accurate, continuous estimates of changes in lung volume only when compression of the gas in the lungs is sufficiently small. The flow rate of moles of gas at the airway opening can be expressed as

$$\dot{N}_{AWO} = \rho_{AWO} Q_{AWO} = \rho_L \dot{V}_L \qquad (9.15)$$

if we neglect the net rate of diffusion into the pulmonary capillary blood. This equation can be rearranged and, if the densities are essentially constant, it can be integrated from some initial time t_0, as follows:

$$\frac{\rho_{AWO}}{\rho_L} \int_{t_0}^{t} Q_{AWO}\, dt \cong \int_{t_0}^{t} \dot{V}_L\, dt = V_L(t) - V_L(t_0) \equiv v_L \qquad (9.16)$$

in which v_L is, according to the convention used here, the change in the volume of the lungs relative to the reference volume $V(t_0)$. The density ratio accounts for differences in mean temperature, pressure, and composition which may exist between the gas mixture inside the lungs and that in the measurement instrument external to the body.

For purposes of testing pulmonary function, (9.16) is frequently implemented directly by electronically integrating the output of a flowmeter placed at a subject's mouth (with the nose blocked). However, the most common procedure for estimating v_L—in use since the nineteenth century—is to continuously collect the gas passing through the airway opening and to compute the volume it occupied within the lungs. This represents a physical integration of the flow at the mouth; it is performed by a device called a *spirometer*. The widespread and historical use of this device has given rise to the term *spirometry* in reference to the measurement of changes in lung volume for testing of pulmonary function, regardless of whether a spirometer, flowmeter plus integrator, or plethysmograph is used.

A spirometer is basically an expandable compartment consisting of a movable, statically counterbalanced, rigid chamber or bell, a stationary base, and a dynamic seal between them (Figure 9.6). The seal is often water, but dry seals of various types have been used. Changes in internal volume of the spirometer, V_S, are proportional to the displacement of the bell. This motion is traditionally recorded on a rotating drum (Kymograph) through direct mechanical linkage, but any displacement transducer can be used. A simple approach is to attach a single-turn, precision linear potentiometer to the shaft of the counterweight pulley and use it as a voltage divider. The electrical output can then be processed or displayed.

The mouth of the subject (with nose blocked) is connected to the mouthpiece of the spirometer (Figure 9.6). As gas moves into and out of the spirometer, the pressure P_S of the gas in the spirometer changes, causing the bell to move. Analysis of the dynamic mechanics of a spirometer indicates that these variations in pressure are reduced by minimizing: (1) the mass of the bell and counterweight and the moment of inertia of the pulley; (2) the gas space in the spirometer and tubing; (3) the surface area of the liquid seal exposed to P_S; (4) the viscous and frictional losses by appropriate choice of lubricants and type of dynamic seal; (5) the flow resistances of any inlet and outlet tubing and valves. During resting breathing, the pressure changes in the gas within the spirometer can be considered negligible. Therefore only the temperature, average ambient pressure, and change in volume are needed to estimate the amount of gas exchanged with the spirometer. To use the spirometer for estimates of change in lung volume during breathing patterns of higher frequency (>1 Hz) requires, in addi-

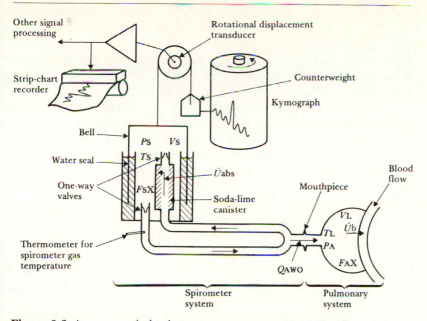

Figure 9.6 A water-sealed spirometer set up to measure slow lung-volume changes. The soda-lime and one-way-valve arrangement prevent buildup of CO_2 during rebreathing.

tion to the variables just mentioned, a knowledge of the acoustic compliance of the gas in the spirometer (see Problem 9.2) and continuous measurement of the change of the spirometer pressure relative to ambient pressure.

The system—i.e., lungs plus spirometer—can be modeled as two gas compartments connected together, such that the number of moles of gas lost by the lungs through the airway opening is equal and opposite to that gained by the spirometer. For rebreathing experiments, most spirometer systems have a chemical absorber (soda lime) to prevent buildup of CO_2. When compression of gas in the lungs and in the spirometer is neglected, mass balances on the system yield

$$\rho_L \dot{V}_L + \dot{U}_b = -\rho_S \dot{V}_S - \dot{U}_{abs} \tag{9.17}$$

The net rates of uptake from the system by the pulmonary capillary blood, $\dot{U}_b$, and the absorber, $\dot{U}_{abs}$, can be assumed constant during steady breathing. Therefore, when (9.17) is integrated with respect to time, the combined effect of these uptakes is a change in volume essentially proportional to time. This can be approximated as a linear baseline drift easily separable from the breathing pattern. Consequently, rearrangement and integration of (9.17) yields

$$v_L \cong -\frac{\rho_S}{\rho_L}(v_S - \text{drift}) = -\frac{\rho_S}{\rho_L}v_S' \qquad\qquad (9.18)$$

from which it can be seen that the change in lung volume is approximately proportional to the volume change of the spirometer corrected for drift v_S'.

The constant of proportionality can be expressed in terms of the measurable quantities, pressure and temperature, by applying an equation of state to the system. With the exception of water vapor in a saturated mixture, all gases encountered during routine respiratory experiments obey the ideal-gas law during changes of state:

$$P = \frac{N}{V}\mathbf{R}T = \rho\mathbf{R}T \qquad\qquad (9.19)$$

where

$\mathbf{R}$ = universal gas constant
T = absolute temperature
ρ = mole density, which, for a well-mixed compartment, equals the ratio of moles of gas N in the compartment to the compartment volume V

This relation holds for an entire gas mixture or for an individual gas species X in the mixture. For the latter, the partial pressure P_X, number of moles N_X, and density $\rho_X = N_X/V$ are substituted into (9.19).

A difficulty in directly substituting (9.19) into (9.18) arises from the presence of water vapor in the system. The gas in the lungs is saturated with water vapor at body-core temperature. The gas in the spirometer is also saturated, even in those with dry seals, after only a few exhalations from the warmer lungs into the cooler spirometer. Water vapor in a saturated mixture does not follow (9.19) during changes of state. Instead, its partial pressure is primarily a function of temperature alone.

Processes in the lungs are approximately isothermal; the change in temperature in the spirometer during most pulmonary function tests is assumed small. Therefore we can compute the partial pressure of the ideal dry gases—i.e., the total gas mixture excluding water vapor—as the mean total pressure (taken to be atmospheric pressure, P_{atm}, for both the spirometer and the lungs) minus the partial pressure of water vapor saturated at the appropriate temperature. Equation (9.18) can then be evaluated as

$$v_L \cong -\left[\frac{(P_{atm} - P_S\text{H}_2\text{O})}{(P_{atm} - P_A\text{H}_2\text{O})}\frac{T_L}{T_S}\right]v_S' \qquad\qquad (9.20)$$

in which $P_A\text{H}_2\text{O}$ is the saturated partial pressure of water vapor in the lung (47 mm Hg (6.27 kPa) at $T_L = 37°C$).

Absolute volume of the lung

Because of the complex geometry and inaccessibility of the lungs, we cannot compute their volume accurately either from direct spatial measurements or from two- or three-dimensional images provided by single or multiple x-ray films. Three procedures have been developed, however, that can give accurate estimates of the volume of gas in normal lungs. Two are based on static mass balances and involve the washout or dilution of a test gas in the lungs. The test gas must have low solubility in the lung tissue. That is, movement of the gas from the alveoli by diffusion into the parenchyma (tissue) and blood must be much less than that occurring by convection through the airways during the experiment. The third procedure is a total body plethysmographic technique employing dynamic mass balances and gas compression in the lungs (see Section 9.5). These estimates of lung volume provide a static baseline value of absolute lung volume that can be added to a continuous measure of the change of lung volume to provide a continuous estimate of absolute lung volume.

The computational formulas for the test-gas procedures described below are routinely derived in the literature in terms of a volume fraction of the test gas in a mixture. The volume fraction of a gas X is an alternative expression of, and is numerically equal to, its molar fraction F_X. When the ideal-gas law [(9.19)] is applied to X alone and to the total mixture containing X, we can express F_X in terms of the partial pressure of X:

$$F_X = \frac{N_X}{N} = \left(\frac{P_X V}{\mathbf{R} T}\right)\left(\frac{\mathbf{R} T}{PV}\right) = \frac{P_X}{P} \tag{9.21}$$

This follows from Dalton's law of partial pressures, for which all gases in a mixture are visualized as having the same temperature and occupying the same volume. On the other hand, the concept of volume fraction lends itself to the use of the spirometer to measure the volume occupied by a mass of gas at a given pressure and temperature. Assume that N_X moles of X at temperature T occupy a volume V_X when subjected to a pressure P. These N_X moles of X are then added to an X-free gas mixture so that the total moles of mixture is N. Applying the ideal-gas law to X before addition to the mixture and to the mixture after the addition of X, we can evaluate F_X for the final mixture as

$$F_X = \frac{N_X}{N} = \left(\frac{PV_X}{\mathbf{R} T}\right)\left(\frac{\mathbf{R} T}{PV}\right) = \frac{V_X}{V} \tag{9.22}$$

Thus the molar fraction F_X can be thought of as either a partial-pressure fraction (9.21) or as an equivalent-volume fraction (9.22), in which the volumes are those that would be occupied by the components of the gas or the gas mixture if each exhibited the *same* temperature and total pressure. However, in some experiments the temperature and/or total pressure changes from one measurement to another. Remember that in the mass balances describing such experiments, Fx represents molar fraction and must be evaluated as such to account for the observed changes in temperature and pressure. Instruments capable of measuring molar fractions and concentrations of gases in a mixture are described in Section 9.7.

Nitrogen-washout estimate of lung volume

Figure 9.7 is a diagram of an apparatus that can be used during a multibreath N_2 washout. The subject inhales only an N_2-free gas mixture (for this example, O_2) because of the one-way valves, but exhales N_2, O_2, CO_2, and water vapor. This experiment is routinely performed to measure FRC, so that the subject is switched into the apparatus at the end of a quiet expiration following normal breathing of atmospheric air. He is allowed to breathe the N_2-free mixture in a relaxed manner around FRC with relatively constant tidal volumes for a fixed period of time (7 to 10 min) or until the N_2 molar fraction in the expirate is sufficiently near zero ($<2\%$).

A static mass (molar) balance on the N_2 in the lungs from before to after the washout yields an estimate of the lung volume at which the first inspiration of O_2 began. Assume that during the experiment, negligible amounts of N_2 diffuse into the alveolar gas from lung tissue and pulmonary capillary blood. Therefore, the change in the number of moles of N_2 in the lungs as a result of the washout is just that which is lost during each expiration (and gained by the spirometer). Assuming that measurements of N_2 fraction are made on a wet-gas basis and that the spirometer contained no N_2 at the start of the experiment, we find that a static mass balance yields

$$F_AN_2(t_1)\frac{V_L(t_1)}{T_L} - F_AN_2(t_2)\frac{V_L(t_2)}{T_L} = F_SN_2(t_2)\frac{V_S(t_2)}{T_S}$$

If the lung volume at the beginning of the washout, t_1, is the same as that at the finish, t_2, then the equation can be rearranged:

$$V_L = \frac{T_L}{T_S}\left[\frac{F_SN_2(t_2)V_S(t_2)}{F_AN_2(t_1) - F_AN_2(t_2)}\right] \qquad (9.23)$$

When this volume is that of the end of a quiet expiration, V_L is the FRC.

All variables on the right-hand side of (9.23) are measurable. The numerator in the brackets in (9.23) represents the equivalent

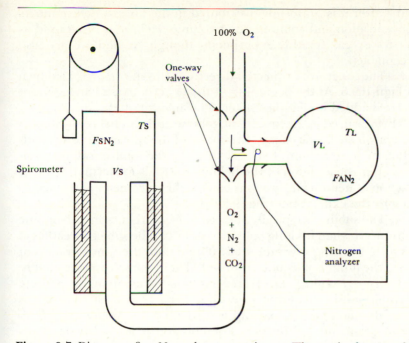

100% O_2

One-way valves

Ts

FsN_2

Spirometer

Vs

VL

TL

FAN_2

O_2
+
N_2
+
CO_2

Nitrogen analyzer

Figure 9.7 Diagram of an N_2 washout experiment. The expired gas can be collected in a spirometer, as shown here, or in a rubberized-canvas or plastic Douglas bag. N_2 content is then determined off-line. An alternative is to measure expiratory flow and nitrogen concentration continuously to determine the volume flow of expired nitrogen, which can be integrated to yield an estimate of the volume of nitrogen expired.

expired N_2 volume for the conditions in the measuring device (the spirometer in Figure 9.7). However, if the nitrogen molar fractions in (9.23) were to be measured on a dry-gas basis rather than on a wet basis as assumed here, the right-hand side would have to be multiplied by the dry-gas partial-pressure ratio ($Patm - PsH_2O$)/($Patm - PAH_2O$).

A washout experiment of this type gives an estimate of the volume of the gas space in the lungs that freely communicates with the airway opening. This is the entire alveolar volume in normal young, adult lungs. In diseased lungs, in which airways are totally or partially obstructed, by mucus, edema, or tumors, for instance, this estimate of the gas volume in the lungs at FRC can be low.

Helium-dilution estimate of lung volume

The procedure described in the previous paragraph involves the removal from the lungs of gas normally resident there in known concentration. An alternative approach is to add a measured amount of a nontoxic, insoluble *tracer* gas to the inspirate, and—after it is uniformly distributed in the lungs—determine its concentration and compute lung volume. Helium is often used as the tracer gas for this experiment, though Ar and Ne are also acceptable.

The lungs are connected directly to the spirometer, as shown in Figure 9.6. At the beginning of the experiment, a fixed amount of He is added to the spirometer. The amount of He added is routinely measured as an equivalent volume at the initial conditions in the spirometer. The change in volume of the spirometer due to addition of pure helium, $VsHe$, divided by the total spirometer volume after the addition of the helium, $Vs(t_1)$, is $FsHe(t_1)$, the molar fraction of helium on a wet-gas basis in the spirometer at the beginning of the experiment [see (9.22)].

The subject is typically allowed to begin rebreathing from the spirometer when his lung volume is at FRC. The subject breathes at his or her resting rate and tidal volume until the concentration of He in the lungs is in equilibrium with that in the spirometer, that is, $FAHe(t_2) = FsHe(t_2)$. The tracer-gas molar fraction in the expirate is continuously measured by withdrawing a small stream of gas from the mouthpiece, passing it through a He analyzer, and returning it to the spirometer. Equilibration is judged to have occurred when the change in the He fraction from one breath to the next is arbitrarily small. As equilibration approaches, the mean spirometer volume is maintained at its original volume $Vs(t_1)$ by the addition of O_2 if required. The experiment is terminated at the end of a quiet expiration (FRC).

The He is redistributed between spirometer and lungs during rebreathing, but the total amount remains essentially constant because no appreciable quantities are lost by diffusion into the tissues. The average total number of moles of dry gas in the system is kept constant by chemically removing the CO_2 added from the blood in the soda-lime canister and replenishing the O_2 taken up. Therefore the system can be considered closed with respect to the test gas only, and a static mass (molar) balance for He may be written as

$$FsHe(t_1) \frac{Vs(t_1)}{Ts(t_1)} = FsHe(t_2) \frac{Vs(t_2)}{Ts(t_2)} + FAHe(t_2) \frac{VL(t_2)}{TL}$$

for molar fractions measured on a wet basis. This can be rearranged and evaluated when the He fractions in the lungs and spirometer are equal:

$$VL = \frac{Vs(t_1)}{FsHe(t_2)} \left[\frac{TL}{Ts(t_1)} FsHe(t_1) - \frac{TL}{Ts(t_2)} FsHe(t_2) \right] \qquad (9.24)$$

VL is an estimate of FRC for the experiment performed as described above. Equation (9.24) is frequently rewritten in terms of the equivalent volume of He originally added to the system, $VsHe$:

$$V_L = \frac{T_L}{T_{S(t_1)}} \left(\frac{V_sHe}{F_sHe(t_2)} \right) - \frac{T_L}{T_{S(t_2)}} \left(\frac{V_sHe}{F_sHe(t_1)} \right) \tag{9.25}$$

If the molar fractions are measured on a dry basis, the temperature ratios in (9.24) and (9.25) must be multiplied by their corresponding dry-gas partial-pressure ratios, that is, $[P_{atm} - P_sH_2O(t_1)]/(P_{atm} - P_AH_2O)$ and $[P_{atm} - P_sH_2O(t_2)]/(P_{atm} - P_AH_2O)$, respectively.

The volume computed from (9.24) and (9.25) is a measure of the volume of gas space in the lungs for which the final He molar fraction in the spirometer $F_sHe(t_2)$ is a representative value. If some parts of the lung do not communicate freely with the airway opening, as in obstructive lung disease, then these equations can provide a low estimate of the FRC.

9.5 Alveolar pressure and lung volume by total-body plethysmograph

The term *plethysmography* refers, in general, to the measurement of the volume or change in volume of a portion of the body. In respiratory applications, plethysmography has been approached in two ways: by measuring the electrical impedance of the thoracic cavity (Section 8.7) and by measuring variables associated with the gas within a total-body plethysmograph. *Transthoracic impedance* is related to the gas space within the body; it is useful as a patient-monitoring tool. However, it does not routinely provide measures of change in lung volume sufficiently accurate for testing of pulmonary function. In contrast, the *total-body plethysmograph* (TBP), which is a rigid, constant-volume box in which the subject is completely enclosed, can be used clinically to evaluate not only the absolute volume and volume changes of the lungs, but also a continuous estimate of alveolar pressure, from which airway resistance R_{AW} may be computed.

There are three types or configurations of TBP: pressure, volume displacement, and flow displacement. These names correspond to the primary plethysmographic variable that is measured and used to compute other variables associated with the lungs. Even though these names provide a means of identifying a particular configuration, they are misleading because a number of measurable plethysmographic variables change in all these systems in response to changes in respiratory variables (Primiano and Greber, 1975).

The pressure plethysmograph is a box that acts as though it were closed or gastight at the frequencies at which pressure changes are measured. The volume-displacement plethysmograph and the flow-displacement plethysmograph are referred to as being open, since each has an opening through which gas is intended to enter and leave. A spirometer or a volume flowmeter such as a pneumotachometer is placed at the opening, and pressure changes within these plethysmographs can be kept small by allowing movement of gas between the box and these measuring devices. Consequently, open boxes are suitable for measurements in which large changes in volume occur. For small-volume-amplitude maneuvers, such as panting, any of the boxes can be employed.

General equation for breathing within a total-body plethysmograph

Absolute volume of the lungs and alveolar pressure changes can be inferred from measurements in a TBP in which the subject can breathe within the box. The following analysis is restricted to the *pressure plethysmograph* (Figure 9.8); this is probably the most commonly used configuration. For simplicity, assume that the subject has a normal pulmonary system. Then, a single mechanical unit can be used to model the lungs; the representative alveolar pressure is well defined as the pressure within the alveolar compartment. Figure 9.8 depicts such a lung. The airway exhibits a flow resistance so that, during breathing, P_A does not equal the pressure at the airway opening P_{AWO}. The gas space within the box outside the subject can be considered a single well-mixed compartment containing an unsaturated gas mixture with its own variables, P_B, V_B, N_B, and T_B.

The volume of the plethysmograph V_P is occupied by the tissues of the body, V_{TIS}, the gas space in the lungs, V_L, and the gas space in the box around the subject, V_B:

$$V_P = V_{TIS} + V_L + V_B \tag{9.26}$$

The tissues of the body, composed of liquids and solids, can be considered incompressible when compared with the gas in the lungs. During breathing movements, the tissues change shape, not volume. Also, since the volume of the plethysmograph is a constant (except during calibration procedures), changes in V_P are zero. Consequently, the change in volume of the gas in the lungs is equal and opposite to the change in volume of the gas space in the box:

$$dV_L = -dV_B \tag{9.27}$$

These equal and opposite changes in volume produce changes in pressure within the lungs and within the gas space in the box as a result of thermodynamic processes. For the lungs and the box, each modeled as a well-mixed compartment, the volume, pressure, and number of moles of the ideal gases undergoing these processes can be related by a barotropic relation of the form

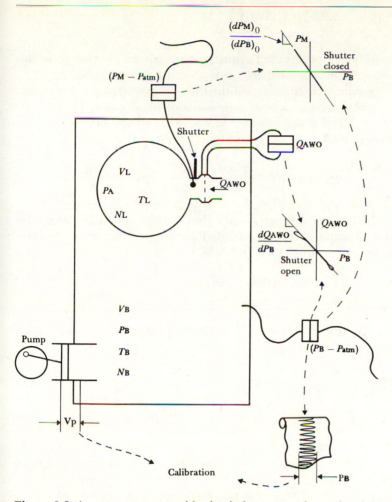

Figure 9.8 A pressure-type total-body plethysmograph, used to determine lung volume with the shutter closed and changes in alveolar pressure with the shutter open. Airway resistance can also be computed if volume flow of gas is measured at the airway opening. Since atmospheric pressure is constant, changes in the pressures of interest can be obtained from measurement made relative to atmospheric pressure.

$$P \left(\frac{V}{N} \right)^{\alpha} = K \tag{9.28a}$$

in which α and K are constants. For an isothermal process, such as occurs in the lungs, $\alpha = 1$; for an adiabatic process, $\alpha = 1.4$ (for a diatomic gas such as air). For any other process, α will be between these two limits. In the box, α approaches the adiabatic limit during rapid breathing movements.

The total derivative of (9.28a) relates the changes in V, P, and N:

$$dV = -\frac{V}{\alpha P} \, dP + \frac{1}{\rho} \, dN \qquad (9.28b)$$

The coefficient of dP is the acoustic compliance C_g of the gas in the container. This is a measure of its absolute compressibility.

Assume that the gas within the plethysmograph is unsaturated and therefore acts as a mixture of ideal gases. Then, evaluating (9.28b) for the mixture in the box and the dry gas only in the lungs and substituting into (9.27) yields

$$-\frac{V_L}{P_A DRY} \, dP_A DRY + \frac{dN_L DRY}{\rho_L DRY} = \frac{V_B}{\alpha_B P_B} \, dP_B - \frac{dN_B}{\rho_B} \qquad (9.29a)$$

The box is sealed, and we assume that the net uptake of gas by the pulmonary capillary blood is negligible. We perform separate mass balances on the lungs and box, which yield

$$dN_L DRY = \rho_{AWO} DRY \, Q_{AWO} \, dt$$
$$dN_B = -\rho_{AWO} \, Q_{AWO} \, dt$$

These can be substituted into (9.29a) to produce, after rearrangement,

$$\frac{V_L}{P_A DRY} \, dP_A DRY$$
$$= -\left[\frac{V_B}{\alpha_B P_B} \, dP_B + \left(\frac{\rho_{AWO}}{\rho_B} - \frac{\rho_{AWO} DRY}{\rho_L DRY} \right) Q_{AWO} \, dt \right] \qquad (9.29b)$$

The ideal-gas law (9.19) can be used to express the densities in (9.29b) in terms of temperatures and pressures. The *mean* (hydrostatic) pressures of the total gas mixtures at the airway opening, within the lungs, and within the box are all equal to atmospheric pressure: $P_{AWO} = P_A = P_B = P_{atm}$. Since the partial pressure of water vapor in the saturated mixture within the lungs is primarily a function of temperature, and since the processes within the lungs are essentially isothermal, then the changes in the total alveolar pressure are simply the changes in partial pressure of the dry gases within the lungs: $dP_A = dP_A DRY$. Consequently (9.29b) can be rewritten as

$$\frac{V_L}{(P_{atm} - P_A H_2O)} \, dP_A = -\left[\frac{V_B}{\alpha_B P_B} \, dP_B \right.$$
$$\left. + \left(\frac{T_B}{T_{AWO}} - \frac{(P_{atm} - P_{AWO} H_2O)}{(P_{atm} - P_A H_2O)} \frac{T_L}{T_{AWO}} \right) Q_{AWO} \, dt \right] \qquad (9.30)$$

Equation (9.30) represents the governing equation for the total-body plethysmograph in which a subject breathes within the box. It may be used in separate experiments—one with the airway occluded, the other with it open—to compute either an estimate of absolute volume of the lungs or a continuous estimate of alveolar pressure, respectively.

Volume of gas within the thoracic cavity

If a subject were to attempt breathing movements within the TBP with his or her airway opening blocked, no gas would flow at that location and $Q_{AWO} = 0$. Then (9.30) could be rewritten as

$$\frac{(dP_A)_0}{(dP_B)_0} = - \frac{(Patm - P_AH_2O)}{V_L} \frac{V_B}{\alpha_B P_B} \tag{9.31}$$

in which the subscript 0 designates zero flow at the airway opening. Equation (9.31) contains V_L, which represents the volume of the gas space within the thoracic cavity at the instant when the airway was blocked. We can compute this volume of thoracic gas, designated V_{TG}, from (9.31) if we know $(V_B/\alpha_B P_B)$, the acoustic compliance of the gas in the box, and if we know the changes in alveolar pressure and pressure in the box during the blocked breathing movements. A two-step clinical procedure can be performed to evaluate these terms. One step involves a calibrating pump and the other requires the subject to attempt to pant.

During airway occlusion, the lungs and the box can each be considered a closed system. Then $dN_B = 0$ and (9.28b) evaluated for the box indicates that $(V_B/\alpha_B P_B)$ can be computed as the ratio of a known change in volume in the gas space in the box to the change in box pressure it causes. The known change in volume is produced by a motor-driven, valveless piston pump mounted in the side of the box (Figure 9.8), which changes the volume V_P of the plethysmograph itself. If the subject stops breathing and blocks his or her nose and mouth while the piston oscillates, the change in volume of the gas space in the box will be only the volume displacement of the pump, $\mathbf{V}_P$. The *amplitude* of the resulting box pressure change, $\mathbf{P}_B$, can be measured. If the frequency of the pump is approximately that of the breathing movements of the subject during the remainder of the experiment, then α_B will have essentially the same value in the two situations and the ratio $\mathbf{V}_P/\mathbf{P}_B$ will yield the acoustic compliance of the gas in the box around the person.

When the airway opening is blocked, for example by a shutter (Figure 9.8), we assume that only compression and expansion of gas occurs within the lungs and that no internal flows take place. Then the pressure at every point in the pulmonary gas space is in equilibrium; and a measurement at any accessible point in communication with the lungs, for instance the mouth, reflects the changes in pressure occurring at every point in the pulmonary system. Therefore, changes in mouth pressure P_M behind the closed shutter during the subject's efforts to breathe are assumed equal to changes in pressure in the alveolar region resulting from the same maneuver, that is, $dP_M = dP_A$ when only compression and expansion of the gas occur.

For these conditions, (9.31) can be rearranged to yield V_{TG} as an estimate of the absolute volume of the lungs:

$$V_{TG} = -(P_{atm} - P_A H_2 O) \frac{V_p}{P_B} \frac{(dP_B)_0}{(dP_M)_0} \tag{9.32}$$

In practice, we evaluate the ratio of change in box pressure to change in mouth pressure by displaying P_M versus P_B simultaneously on the two axes of an oscilloscope (Figure 9.8). Then $(dP_B)_0/(dP_M)_0$ represents the inverse of the average slope of the resulting curve, which for rapid panting movements against a closed shutter should be a straight line that retraces itself.

If the airway is occluded at the end of a quiet expiration, V_{TG} can be used as an estimate of FRC. However, V_{TG} is a measure of the total gas space within the body that is compressed and expanded during the closed-airway panting maneuver (DuBois et al., 1956a). Normally this reflects the gas space contained entirely within the nose, mouth, large airways, and thoracic cavity (plus any volume between the shutter and airway opening), since abdominal gas usually represents a negligible fraction of the gas space within the body. However, this approach cannot distinguish between gas within the lungs and any nondissolved gas within the pleural space (pneumothorax). In a subject with no pneumothorax, V_{TG} is an estimate of the total volume of all gas spaces in the pulmonary system, including those that may not communicate freely with the airway opening. Consequently, for normal subjects, V_{TG} measured at the end of expiration corresponds closely to the FRC estimated by the gas-washout and dilution procedures described in Section 9.4. However, in subjects with obstructive lung disease, V_{TG} is a more accurate estimate of FRC than the lower values calculated from the dilution tests.

Changes in alveolar pressure

For the computation of a continuous estimate of changes in alveolar pressure during flow of gas through the airways, DuBois et al. (1965b) proposed making measurements during a voluntarily produced, high-frequency, low-amplitude pant. Several benefits result from such a maneuver. However, it has two primary advantages related to (9.30). It improves the validity of the assumption that the effects of an exchange of gas between the alveoli and pulmonary capillaries are negligible and it reduces the size of the term involving Q_{AWO}. Since the net uptake by the capillaries can be considered to occur at a nearly constant rate with only slight variation with breathing frequency, its major (low-frequency) component is easily separable from the changes in P_B caused by respiratory movements. At panting frequencies the effects of nonzero net uptake, if seen at all, can be assumed to appear primarily as a baseline drift.

If low volume amplitudes are produced even at high voluntary frequencies, Q_{AWO} will not be large. The coefficient of Q_{AWO} in (9.30) is the difference between two ratios, both of which are near unity. As the conditions at the airway opening approach either those of the gas space in the box or those in the lungs, the difference between these ratios departs from zero. The extent of this departure can limit the application of the procedure of breathing into the box for the estimation of alveolar pressure to small-volume-amplitude maneuvers unless the subject, during the measurements, breathes a gas mixture whose density is very close to that of alveolar gas. During panting, the term involving Q_{AWO} in (9.30) is routinely neglected.

High-frequency maneuvers also decrease the effects of leaks in the box. The combination of a small leak that has a high resistance to flow and the acoustic compliance of the gas in the large gas space in the box (about 10^3 liters) acts as a high-pass filter to differences in pressure and a low-pass filter to the flow between the inside and outside of the plethysmograph. Thus, the higher the frequency of the changes in pressure in the box, the less degradation of the breathing-related signal due to leaks to the atmosphere. Note, however, that the high-pass-filter effects of small, controlled leaks in the box, or of leaky ballast chambers on the reference side of plethysmograph pressure transducers, are sometimes intentionally employed to eliminate slow drift in box-pressure readings. This can be related to increases in temperature of the gas in the box—increases produced by the subject—or to changes in atmospheric pressure such as those caused by the movement of elevators or the closing and opening of doors.

With these considerations in mind, we can simplify (9.30) to yield

$$dP_A \cong - \left(\frac{P_{atm} - P_A H_2O}{V_L} \right) \left(\frac{V_B}{\alpha_B P_B} \right) dP_B \qquad (9.33)$$

This states that for high-frequency, low-amplitude breathing, the change of alveolar pressure will be approximately proportional to changes of pressure in the box, given that the coefficient of dP_B is constant. The dry partial pressure in the lungs, the pressure in the box, and the volume of the gas space in the box change very little

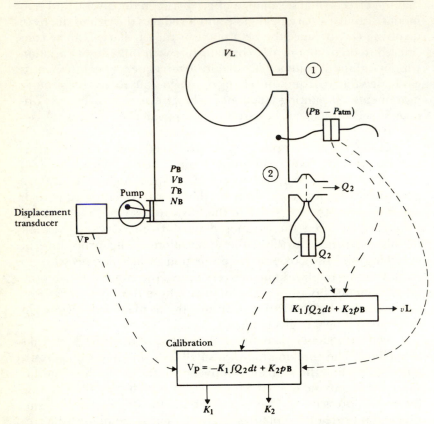

Figure 9.9 A flow-displacement total-body plethysmograph used to continuously measure the volume changes of the lungs. Calculation of v_L and the calibration coefficients K_1 and K_2 are most easily performed by analog computation circuits.

for an individual as a result of breathing movements. However, α_B depends on the frequency of the maneuver, asymptotically approaching the adiabatic limit as frequency increases. Also the volume of the lung can change manyfold from RV to TLC, so that a low-volume-amplitude maneuver is mandatory for V_L to be nearly constant.

Note from the discussion of (9.31) that the coefficient of dP_B in (9.33) can be evaluated from simultaneous measurements of mouth pressure and box pressure during an occluded-airway panting maneuver.

Changes in lung volume by total-body plethysmograph

Figure 9.9 shows a TBP configuration that can be used to provide a continuous measure of the change in the volume of the gas

space within the body. Depicted is a flow-displacement plethysmograph with the subject breathing through a hole (port 1) in the wall
of the box. The gas in the box around the subject can leave the box
only through port 2. It passes through a flowmeter, that is,
$dN_B = -\rho_2 Q_2$. Evaluation of (9.28b) for the gas in the box and im-
position of the plethysmographic constraint (9.27) yields, upon
integration,

$$v_L = \frac{T_B}{T_2} \int_{t_0}^{t} Q_2 \, dt + \frac{V_B}{\alpha_B P_B} p_B \qquad (9.34)$$

in which T_2 is the temperature of the gas at port 2 and $P_B = P_{atm}$
at t_0. This equation describes the pressure-corrected, flow-
displacement plethysmograph (Clément et al., 1969). The system
can be calibrated by simultaneously measuring flow at port 2 and
pressure in the box while the volume of the box is changed by a
known amount by using a valveless piston pump whose cylinder
empties directly into the box (Figure 9.9). During the calibration,
port 1 is closed; the subject remains motionless as the pump is
cycled.

A pressure plethysmograph is not routinely used for this type
of experiment because the large change in pressure that can
accompany large changes in lung volume can be uncomfortable to
the subject (Leith and Mead, 1974). The displacement plethysmographs are sometimes cooled to stabilize their temperature and to
make the subject more comfortable.

9.6 Some tests of respiratory mechanics

Pulmonary function tests can be divided into two groups:
gas-transport tests, concerned with the movement of gas molecules
between the atmosphere and blood (see Section 9.8) and mechanics
tests that deal primarily with the relationships among lung volume,
gas flow, and pressure differences. One of the ultimate objectives
of mechanics tests is to determine whether the defect(s) that produce abnormal pressure-volume-flow relationships can be identified as being intrinsic to the airways (lumen and/or walls), to the
lung parenchyma surrounding and supporting the airways, or to
extrapulmonary structures.

A distinction is often made, in pulmonary medicine, between
obstructive and restrictive disease processes. This distinction is not,
in general, equivalent to asking whether the defect is in the airways
or not; it is based more on the functional impairment caused by a
disease. *Obstruction* has a dynamic mechanics connotation, being associated with an abnormal rate of change of volume or gas flows in

the lungs during breathing movements. *Restriction,* on the other hand, connotes abnormal static mechanics. It is used to refer not only to the lungs but also to extrapulmonary structures (chest wall, muscles, abdominal contents). This condition is indicated if the volume attained by the ventilatory system is inappropriate for the difference in pressure applied or if the differences in pressure that the respiratory muscles are capable of producing are abnormally low. Even though restriction and obstruction may not be completely separable in a given disease state, the presence of either or both can ideally be determined by making measurements on the respiratory system under two sets of conditions: static, when all flows and rates of change of all variables are zero; and dynamic, when these are nonzero.

Static mechanics

When flows and rates of change of flow and volume are zero, the transpulmonary pressure difference, $\Delta P_L = P_{AWO} - P_{PL}$, as indicated by (9.3a) and (9.3b), reduces to a function of volume alone. Therefore the static mechanical characteristics of the lungs can be obtained by simultaneously measuring the lung volume and the transpulmonary pressure difference at various lung volumes while no motions exist in the system. The pulmonary system exhibits a static or plastic hysteresis when cycled through a set of static lung volumes. Consequently, to define the $\Delta P\text{-}V$ relation for the lungs, we must standardize or note the initial volume and direction of change to subsequent volumes. In practice, the expiratory portion of the statically determined $\Delta P\text{-}V$ curve is routinely used to characterize the lungs.

The subject is instructed to inspire to TLC and then to exhale to successively smaller volumes, holding each volume while the pressure in an esophageal balloon is measured relative to pressure at the airway opening. This pressure difference is used as an estimate of transpulmonary pressure (Section 9.2). The lung volume corresponding to each measurement is obtained by spirometer in terms of a change from a reference volume, for example, FRC, determined independently either by gas washout (Section 9.4) or plethysmograph (Section 9.5).

Figure 9.10 shows a facsimile of statically determined expiratory $\Delta P\text{-}V$ curves for a normal subject, for a subject that has restricted, or stiff, lungs (from diseases such as pulmonary fibrosis or pneumonia, for example) and for a subject with very distensible lungs (from pulmonary emphysema, for example). The curves extend from TLC to RV for the corresponding individual and are seen to be nonlinear. Such relations are not routinely described for the entire vital capacity. Instead, for small changes in volume, on

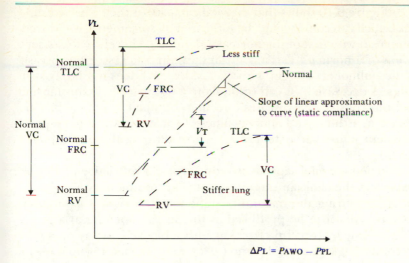

Figure 9.10 Idealized statically determined expiratory pressure-volume relations for the lung. The positions and slopes for lungs with different elastic properties are shown relative to scales of absolute volume and pressure difference.

the order of a tidal volume, straight-line approximations about a volume operating point are used. The slope of the linear approximation to the statically determined ΔP-V curve is the static compliance, as defined by (9.7).

Assuming that the compliance of each of the curves in Figure 9.10 is computed at the respective FRCs, we find, as would be expected, that the stiffer lung has a lower compliance and the less-stiff lung has a higher compliance than normal. Therefore, we can identify a restricted, or stiff, lung by computing lung compliance at a standardized lung volume. However, even though an increased compliance can be associated in certain cases with obstructive pulmonary diseases, such as emphysema, lungs affected by other obstructive diseases, such as those involving partial blockage of the lumen of large airways, frequently exhibit a normal compliance. Consequently, even when compliance is normal, the dynamic behavior of the system must also be studied to rule out obstruction.

Although pulmonary compliance is a desirable parameter to obtain when the physician suspects restrictive lung disease, it is not routinely measured because the esophageal balloon is very unpleasant for the subject. Instead, the observation, made very early in the history of the study of ventilatory mechanics, that TLC, RV, and the difference between them, VC, are reproducible and easily attained, is the basis of a simple test to rule out restrictive disease in the absence of measurements of changes in esophageal pressure.

Figure 9.10 shows that the vital capacity of the restricted subject, which can conveniently be estimated by spirometry, is reduced compared with that of the normal individual. Therefore the observation of a normal VC is a contraindication of a restrictive disease in the pulmonary system. However, a low VC does not imply stiff lungs. A decreased VC can result from a number of circumstances, including obstructive diseases affecting the small airways (e.g., emphysema, asthma) and abnormalities of the chest wall and respiratory neuromuscular system (e.g., as a result of scoliosis and poliomyelitis).

When the vital capacity is reduced and a restrictive process is suspected, the clinician can investigate extrapulmonary abnormality by measuring the maximum static inspiratory and expiratory pressures that can be produced at the airway opening at a given lung volume by forceful efforts against a blocked airway opening. By combining (9.3a), (9.3b), and (9.3c), we note that, for no flows in the system,

$$p\text{AWO} - p\text{BS} = \left[\frac{1}{C\text{stL}} + \frac{1}{C\text{stw}}\right] v\text{L} - \Delta p\text{MUS} \qquad (9.35)$$

where the pressure on the body surface is usually taken to be atmospheric. If a patient is instructed to try to exhale or inhale maximally against a closed nose and mouthpiece while the pressure changes in the mouth are measured, these changes in pressure reflect the forces produced by the respiratory muscles in excess of the forces produced by the stretched elastic components of the lungs and chest wall. If the respiratory muscles, the nerve cells controlling them, and the kinematics of the chest wall are not impaired, then $p\text{AWO} - p\text{BS}$ should approximate that attained by a normal person at the corresponding point in his or her vital capacity (usually FRC) at which the test is performed.

We can infer an obstructive process from a reduced vital capacity if we also know some measure of absolute lung volume such as TLC or RV. In most cases of obstructive disease, the TLC is approximately normal or increased and the vital capacity tends to be reduced (Figure 9.10) as the residual volume increases, due to the obstructor's inability to empty his or her lungs efficiently. However, some obstructive processes, such as those in the larger airways or the initial phases of small airways disease, may not lead to a reduced vital capacity. Consequently, the dynamic behavior of the system should also be studied.

Dynamic mechanics

Equations (9.3a) and (9.3b) indicate that, during resting breathing, changes in transpulmonary pressure can be expressed as a function of the changes in lung volume and gas volume flow rate if the alveoli were purely elastic structures. However, the alveoli are not purely elastic, in that they are able to exhibit a viscoelastic type of behavior. Inclusion of this into (9.3a) and (9.3b) yields

$$(p_{AWO} - p_{PL}) = \frac{1}{C_{stL}} v_L + R_{LT} \dot{v}_L + R_{AW} q_{AWO} \tag{9.36}$$

in which R_{LT} is the resistance of the lung tissue and R_{AW} is the airway resistance defined by (9.6). R_{AW} represents a direct measure of obstruction in the airways. Because of the viscoelastic behavior of the alveolar tissue, the computation of R_{AW} from (9.36) is not convenient. Instead, we compute R_{AW} directly from (9.6). The pressure and flow at the airway opening required by (9.6) are easily measured. However, estimating changes in a representative alveolar pressure while there is flow in the airways requires the total-body plethysmograph, as discussed in Section 9.5.

As an example of a TBP procedure for estimating R_{AW}, consider a subject situated inside a pressure plethysmograph (Figure 9.8). The individual (with nose blocked) breathes within the box through a mouthpiece and flowmeter with an associated shutter that can be closed to block flow at the mouth. While the shutter is open, the pressure at the airway opening (external to the mouthpiece and flowmeter) is the pressure within the plethysmograph. That portion of the pressure drop between the alveoli and box that results from the mouthpiece assembly is taken into account by expressing the total alveolar-to-box resistance [given by (9.6) for this arrangement] as the sum of R_{AW} and the mouthpiece assembly resistance R_{MP}. For a panting maneuver, (9.33) indicates that changes in the representative alveolar pressure are proportional to changes in P_B. Consequently (9.6) can be rewritten

$$R_{AW} + R_{MP} = \left[1 + \frac{(P_{atm} - P_A H_2O) V_B}{V_L \, \alpha_B \, P_B} \right] \frac{\partial P_B}{\partial Q_{AWO}} \tag{9.37}$$

The fraction within the brackets in (9.37) is much greater than unity, since the volume of the gas space in the box V_B is much larger ($> 100:1$) than the volume within the lungs V_L [($P_{atm} - P_A H_2O)/\alpha_B P_B$ being of order 1]. Consequently, as shown by (9.31), a closed-shutter panting maneuver, in which mouth pressure (behind the shutter) and box pressure are measured simultaneously, can be used to evaluate the square-bracketed term in (9.37). We can obtain an approximation to the partial derivative of box pressure P_B with respect to gas flow rate at the airway opening Q_{AWO} by displaying these two variables, measured simultaneously with the shutter open, on orthogonal axes of an oscilloscope (Figure 9.8). For very small changes in volume (a condition of the panting maneuver) and the accelerations associated with panting, normal lungs exhibit a relatively straight P_B-Q_{AWO} relation with very slight looping. Box pressure changes are then essentially a function of flow in the airways alone. Thus $\partial P_B / \partial Q_{AWO}$ can be evaluated as the inverse of the slope of the oscilloscope figure dP_B / dQ_{AWO}, and R_{AW} can be computed as

$$R_{AW} = \frac{(dP_M)_0}{(dP_B)_0} \frac{dP_B}{dQ_{AWO}} - R_{MP} \tag{9.38}$$

for which R_{MP} can be evaluated independently.

In some instances, however, the P_B-Q_{AWO} plot produced on the oscilloscope screen is highly nonlinear and can display exaggerated looping (dynamic hysteresis). Because of this, it is difficult to determine a representative slope for the plot. A convention has therefore been adopted for the evaluation of R_{AW}. The representative slope is that corresponding to a straight line drawn between the points on the plot at which flow is $+0.5$ liter/s and -0.5 liter/s in the region corresponding to the end of inspiration and the beginning of expiration. This straddles the point $Q_{AWO} = 0$; it is usually fairly straight and involves small changes in volume. The representative slope and the parameter R_{AW} computed from it are the only pieces of information from this procedure routinely used for the clinical evaluation of airway mechanics.

At least three phenomena associated with the respiratory system can cause exaggerated looping and/or nonlinearity of the P_B-Q_{AWO} relationship in this experiment. (1) Equation (9.33) may not be a good approximation to (9.30) for the conditions of the experiment. (2) The pulmonary system being tested may not act as a single mechanical unit. Hence the concept of a single representative alveolar pressure in phase with flow may be inappropriate. (3) The mechanical properties of the lungs and airways may be so abnormal that even during a panting maneuver, significant changes in dimension (primarily in diameter) of the airways occur, so that the P_B-Q_{AWO} relationship becomes quite bizarre (nonlinear). The latter two situations can be evaluated by additional independent pulmonary function tests.

It has been shown that the aggregate resistance of the smaller airways that play a major role in the final distribution of gas to the alveoli is small in comparison with that of the larger, upper airways (Macklem and Mead, 1967). Consequently, R_{AW} easily reflects obstruction in the larger airways. However, only when the smaller airways are so affected by pulmonary disease that their aggregate resistance is drastically increased do they significantly affect R_{AW}. Thus the parameter R_{AW} is not a sensitive indicator of the initial phases of diseases of the small airways.

Two other parameters that yield information about obstruction in the larger airways are the *peak expiratory flow* (PEF) and the *maximum breathing capacity*, (MBC). The PEF is the highest instantaneous flow at the airway opening that a subject can produce during a maximally forced expiration from TLC. The MBC is the average expiratory flow produced by a subject who is instructed to continually inhale and exhale as deeply and rapidly as possible. Usually this maneuver is performed for only 12 to 15 s to prevent a large reduction in arterial P_{CO_2}. The gas expired during this time period is collected and its volume is measured by spirometer. Using (9.20), the clinician converts this volume to the volume that the gas would occupy at the temperature and pressure existing within the lungs, and routinely expresses the result on a per-minute basis. As with R_{AW}, the PEF and MBC reflect small airway obstruction only when it is major. However, unlike R_{AW}, these parameters can also be affected by neuromuscular impairment.

Small-volume-amplitude, high-frequency behavior of the ventilatory system

Even though ventilatory mechanics are frequently represented in terms of a single resistance and a single compliance (viscoelastic system), this description is not complete. When rates of breathing in excess of those produced at rest are imposed on the system, a more detailed model is required. In addition, as frequency is increased above the frequencies voluntarily produced, the forces required to accelerate the gas in the airways increase and become measurable.

We can demonstrate this by means of a forced-oscillation system such as is shown in Figure 9.11 (Hyatt, 1970). Gas can leave by two ports. Port 1 is normally used to transmit flow or changes in pressure to the lung. The other port is either closed or connected to a long (8.5-m), large-diameter (3-cm) tube that acts predominantly as a pneumatic inertance element (analog of inductance). Combined with the acoustic compliance of the gas in the chamber ($V \cong 30$ liters), this inertance produces a low-pass filter. Changes in pressure at frequencies on the order of the fundamental of the resting breathing pattern cause gas to flow from the system at port 2. Therefore, at low frequencies, $Q_1 \simeq Q_2$; at higher frequencies, $Q_2 \simeq 0$. As the subject breathes through the device at port 1, small-amplitude variations in pressure can be superimposed upon the subject's breathing pattern. These changes in pressure can be of almost any frequency and amplitude within the operating range of the speaker.

Forcing functions can therefore run the gamut from pure sine waves to white noise. A flowmeter and pressure tap situated in the tube leading to the subject's mouth make it possible for the clinician to determine the driving-point characteristics of the respiratory system in the form of a P_{AWO}-Q_{AWO} relation if P_{AWO} is measured relative to the pressure at the body surface. (This does not

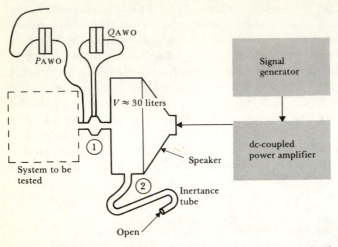

Figure 9.11 Speaker-driven forced-oscillation system. Such a system can be used to obtain the driving-point impedance of the total respiratory system during spontaneous breathing and to measure the acoustic impedance and/or frequency responses of laboratory apparatus.

follow the notation used in the rest of this chapter, inasmuch as the driving pressure should be written $P_{AWO} - P_{BS} = \Delta P_{TR}$, the transrespiratory pressure difference. However, P_{AWO} alone is used to stress the point that the pressure at the AWO is being manipulated, as distinct from other experiments in which P_{BS} is manipulated and P_{AWO} is exposed to atmosphere. The latter yields transfer characteristics.)

If the imposed changes in pressure and resulting flows are sufficiently small (peak-to-peak $P_{AWO} < 3$ cm H_2O (300 Pa) and $Q_{AWO} < 1$ liter/s) so that the P_{AWO}-Q_{AWO} relationship is approximately linear, then the frequency spectrum of the response can be obtained either by varying P_{AWO} sinusoidally at various discrete frequencies (Peslin *et al.*, 1972a) or by employing a waveshape with a desired frequency content and using the Fourier transform to analyze the response (Michaelson *et al.*, 1975). An appropriate characterization of the respiratory system as a whole under these circumstances is the total respiratory acoustical impedance $Z_{TR}(\omega)$. This is a complex number analogous to electrical impedance, with P_{AWO} as the analog of voltage and Q_{AWO} as the analog of current:

$$Z_{TR}(\omega) = \frac{\mathbf{P}_{AWO}(\omega)}{\mathbf{Q}_{AWO}(\omega)} \underline{/\phi(\omega)} \tag{9.39}$$

in which $\mathbf{P}_{AWO}(\omega)$ and $\mathbf{Q}_{AWO}(\omega)$ are the amplitudes of the spectral components of pressure and flow, respectively, at radian frequency ω; and $\phi(\omega)$ is the phase angle between them.

Use of the acoustical impedance makes it possible to represent the respiratory system and its components in terms of an equivalent circuit (either pneumatic, mechanical, or electrical). Figure 9.2(b) is such a representation.

When the frequency of the imposed pressure P_{AWO} is increased, we can find a frequency ω_n, the *natural frequency* (often referred to as "resonant frequency" in pulmonary literature), for which P_{AWO} is in phase with Q_{AWO}, that is, $\phi = 0$. This occurs around 7 Hz for normal persons. It has led to the modeling of the respiratory system, in the neighborhood of the natural frequency, as an overdamped, second-order system (see Section 1.9). However, Peslin *et al.* (1972a) indicate that when the normal respiratory impedance spectrum from dc to 60 or 70 Hz is considered, at least a fourth-order system is suggested. This could be produced by a single airway-alveolar compartment model with gas compression and inertance included.

At the natural frequency, the imaginary part of Z is zero and the magnitude of Z is equal to its real part, which represents the effective resistance of the system. In this way a total respiratory resistance, R_{TR}, has been evaluated for the respiratory system as a whole, as

$$R_{TR} \equiv \text{Re}(Z_{TR}) \quad \text{for } \omega = \omega_n \tag{9.40}$$

Total respiratory resistance and the natural frequency have been the only parameters routinely evaluated during this procedure. They provide some distinction between normals and obstructors, and are correlated highly with R_{AW}.

Mead (1960) demonstrated that high-frequency respiratory mechanical characteristics can be obtained while the subject is breathing if the frequency content of the imposed pressure difference, P_{AWO}, is sufficiently above the highest frequency component in the breathing pattern. This provides the basis for a clinically applicable procedure, since minimal cooperation from the patient is required. The patient simply breathes into an instrument such as that in Figure 9.11 and nearly insensible oscillations of pressure are imposed on his or her breathing movements. Computations are made from measured Q_{AWO} and P_{AWO} after each is passed through a high-pass filter with a corner frequency of about 1.5 to 2 Hz.

However, determining total respiratory impedance by superimposed forced oscillations during breathing presents several problems associated with the nonlinear nature of the respiratory system. As gas flow and lung volume change during breathing, the operating point of the system changes so that the representative (linearized) small-signal pressure-flow relation changes with time. Also, during breathing, the dimensions of the large extrathoracic airways, especially the cross-sectional area of the glottal region (Stanescu *et al.*, 1972), can vary, causing computed values of total respiratory mechanical properties to vary on the order of hundreds of percent during a breath. This large change can mask small changes in lung mechanics that can occur due to disease.

Several methods have been tried (and are under investigation) to establish methods of defining values of total respiratory mechanical properties that are primarily representative of the mechanical state of the lungs alone. These approaches include the selection of an arbitrary standard operating point, designated by direction and magnitude of flow (Hyatt *et al.*, 1970); the use of white noise and spectral analysis to obtain an impedance spectrum averaged over a number of breaths (Michaelson *et al.*, 1975); and the computation of the impedance spectrum for sequential discrete instants during a breath and selection of the spectrum that fits some reasonable criteria (Horowitz *et al.*, 1976). Note that during a panting maneuver, such as that used to determine R_{AW}, the glottis is held open by muscle reflex so that it does not greatly influence the value of the airway resistance obtained.

In the frequency range for which the breathing pattern has components, superimposed forced oscillations are not useful for evaluating total respiratory mechanics. Instead, for fundamental frequencies that can be voluntarily achieved (usually up to 4 Hz), we obtain the mechanical properties of the pulmonary system alone by measuring the difference in pressure between the thoracic esophagus and the airway opening and relating this to lung volume and gas flow. For tidal breathing at these low frequencies, normal lungs can be represented as a series combination of an effective resistance (the real part of the pulmonary acoustic impedance, Z_L) and an effective compliance, $C_{effL} = -1/\omega \, \text{Im} \, (Z_L)$, corresponding to a uniform, single-degree-of-freedom, viscoelastic system [Figure 9.2(b)].

The value of the effective pulmonary compliance computed for any frequency in this range should yield the same value as that for zero frequency; that is, the static pulmonary compliance C_{stL}. If the effective compliance computed for nonzero frequencies is sufficiently different from C_{stL}—in particular, if C_{effL} decreases as frequency increases—then a single-degree-of-freedom viscoelastic system can be ruled out.

A test—reported to be sensitive to the onset of small airways disease—that is based on an extension of this reasoning uses the pulmonary dynamic compliance C_{dynL} as an approximation of the effective compliance of the system. Based on a model of a normal pulmonary system, such as Figure 9.2(b) and Equations (9.3a) and (9.3b), pulmonary dynamic compliance is defined as

$$C_{dynL} \equiv \frac{V_L(t'') - V_L(t')}{\Delta P_L(t'') - \Delta P_L(t')}$$

evaluated for *any* breathing waveshape at successive instants t' and t'' at which $Q_{AWO}(t') = Q_{AWO}(t'') = 0$. In general, C_{dynL} is strictly equivalent to Ceff$_L$ only if the former is evaluated for a pure sinusoidal breathing pattern.

A decreasing dynamic compliance with increasing frequency (Cdyn$_L$ < 0.8 Cst$_L$ at fundamental breathing rates between 2 and 4 breaths per second) is considered abnormal. It has led to the representation of such lungs by a system composed of a number of viscoelastic mechanical units (multiple degrees of freedom) each with its own time constant $\tau_i = (R$AW$_i) \cdot (C$st$_i)$. Based on such multiunit mechanical models, the observation of a decreasing Cdyn$_L$ with increasing frequency coexistent with a normal RAW and a normal Cst$_L$ has been taken as an indication of small-airways disease (Woolcock *et al.*, 1969).

Large-amplitude volume and flow behavior of the ventilatory system

Several features of respiratory mechanics are exhibited for large changes in volume and flows. These characteristics arise because the airways that must distribute the gas within the thoracic cavity are subjected to essentially the same effective forces that the respiratory muscles exert to empty and fill the alveolar regions of the lung. The extrapulmonary intrathoracic airways are directly exposed to local interpleural pressure. The airways within the lungs are subjected to the increased and decreased tensile forces produced by the stretching of their parenchymal attachments as the lung regions in which they are embedded inflate and deflate. Consequently, as the alveolar regions are expanded and compressed, the length and cross-sectional area of each airway generation undergo corresponding changes.

One manifestation of this is the observation of an approximately inverse relationship between plethysmographically determined airway resistance and the lung volume at which it is measured (Briscoe and DuBois, 1958). The larger the volume of the lung the more expanded the airways and the lower the resistance to flows produced during a panting maneuver, and vice versa, so that

$$R\text{AW} \cong \frac{(SR\text{AW})}{V\text{TG}} \tag{9.42}$$

where SRAW is a constant of proportionality referred to as *specific airway resistance* (Bates *et al.*, 1971). SRAW represents a characteristic of a subject's airways normalized for his or her lung volume. VTG is volume of thoracic gas.

Another manifestation of the effects of changes in airway dimensions during ventilatory maneuvers is the *flow limitation* exhibited during forced expirations. If it were possible to keep the volume of the lung constant and vary the pressure drop and flow through the airways, characteristic *isovolume* pressure-flow curves would result, depending on the volume of the lung for which the curve was obtained.

Figure 9.12 gives idealized examples of such curves for normal lungs. In practice these curves are obtained by cycling the lungs through a succession of increasing volume amplitudes and flows. The pressure-flow curve for each cycle is plotted and points on each curve corresponding to the same volume are connected. Three features generally appear: (1) Inspiratory flow continually increases as the difference in pressure is increased at any lung volume. (2) For high lung volumes (near TLC), expiratory flow increases as the difference in pressure becomes more negative. (3) For lung volumes below about 80% of the TLC, the expiratory flow reaches a value that is never exceeded, even though the difference in pressure becomes more negative. This condition is referred to as *flow limitation* in which the flow is *effort-independent*. That is, expiratory flow cannot be increased, no matter how much expiratory efforts are increased (Fry and Hyatt, 1960). Flow limitation has been attributed to compressive dimensional changes of the membranous intrapulmonary airways occurring dynamically during expiratory maneuvers.

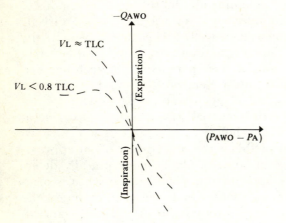

Figure 9.12 Idealized isovolume pressure-flow curves for two lung volumes for a normal respiratory system. Each curve represents a composite from numerous inspiratory-expiratory cycles, each with successively increased efforts. The pressure and flow values measured as the lungs passed through the respective volumes of interest are plotted and connected to yield the corresponding curves.

The maximum value of flow achieved at any given lung volume depends considerably on, among other things, the properties of the gas mixture that is breathed and the mechanical properties of these small, peripheral airways and the lung parenchyma (Mead *et al.*, 1967; Pride *et al.*, 1967). But it is not greatly affected by the properties of the airways larger than the ones that limit flow. Thus characteristics of the lung exhibited while the expiratory flow is effort-independent reflect the status of the peripheral parts of the lungs, i.e., the small airways in which obstructive disease is thought to produce its initial lesions and the alveolar parenchyma that provide tensile forces that tend to keep these airways expanded.

These phenomena can be displayed in two clinically useful ways, both based on measures of only volume flow of gas at the airway opening during a forced expiration from TLC to RV (referred to as a forced expiratory vital capacity maneuver). The equivalent volume of gas expired during this maneuver is the *forced vital capacity* (FVC). Two alternate (and equivalent) methods of displaying the events within a forced expiration involve the plotting of either (1) volume flow of gas at the airway opening against its integral (or volume change in a spirometer) subtracted from FVC, or (2) the integral of expired-gas volume flow (or spirometer volume change) subtracted from FVC versus time (Figure 9.13). The first method produces the *maximum expiratory flow volume* (MEFV) curve and the second corresponds to the spirogram of the *timed vital capacity* (TVC) routinely performed as part of standard spirometry tests.

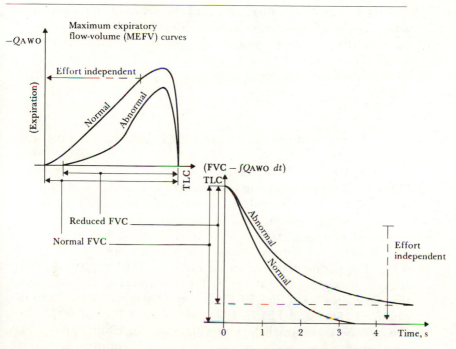

Figure 9.13 Alternative methods of displaying data produced during a forced vital capacity expiration. Equivalent information can be obtained from each type of curve; however, reductions in expiratory flow are subjectively more apparent on the MEFV curve than on the timed spirogram.

The normal MEFV curve reaches a maximum flow at a volume slightly below TLC; and as the forced expiration continues below about 25% of FVC (below TLC), the expired flow rate decreases nearly linearly with decreasing volume. This linear region corresponds to effort-independent flow; it is reproducible and characteristic of the state of the lungs. The MEFV curve represents the relation between a variable (FVC $-\int Q_{AWO}\, dt$) and its derivative (Q_{AWO}). When this relationship is a straight line through the origin, it represents a homogeneous linear first-order differential equation:

$$Q_{AWO} = -K(\text{FVC} - \int Q_{AWO}\, dt) \tag{9.43}$$

Since the coefficient (slope of the linear part of the MEFV curve, $-K$) is negative, it corresponds to an exponential decay from the initial value of FVC $-\int Q_{AWO}\, dt$ at which the relation became linear. Thus the latter part of the TVC spirogram for 25% FVC below TLC to RV is approximately exponential, corresponding to the effort-independent region in the MEFV curve, and is reproducible and unique for a given subject. The region of each curve between TLC and approximately 25% of the FVC below TLC is effort-dependent. It provides information about the larger, upper airways and extrapulmonary parts of the ventilatory system (chest wall, respiratory muscles, etc.). The effort-independent region reflects mechanics of the smaller airways and parenchyma of the lungs. We can make comparable inferences about the state of these various parts of the respiratory system from either the MEFV curve or the TVC spirogram.

Parameters of the forced expiratory vital capacity maneuver

The MEFV curve has gained popularity because it provides a dramatic display compatible with subjective evaluation of lung impairment by direct visual inspection. We can easily recognize decreases in maximum flows, or a characteristic concave effort-independent region, for even minimal small airways (obstructive) disease. This is harder to detect visually in a spirogram (Figure 9.13). The parameters used to describe the MEFV curve are basically the maximum flow at a given lung volume, e.g., forced expiratory flow after 50 or 75% of the forced vital capacity has been expired, FEF50% and FEF75%, respectively, or flow at 60% TLC, $Q_{MAX}60\%$. It is especially useful when studying children to normalize these flows to a measure of lung volume to compensate for size of the individual (Zapletal *et al.,* 1971). Therefore an MEFV display normalized by dividing both axes by FVC yields these data directly. Normalized flows such as FEF50%/FVC are related to the average slope of the effort-independent portion of the MEFV curve.

A number of parameters have been proposed and used to describe the forced expiratory spirogram. Besides the forced vital capacity FVC itself, only two others are described here: the *forced expiratory volume in one second*, FEV_1, and the *maximum midexpiratory flow* MMF, also referred to as the mean forced expiratory flow between 25 and 75% of the vital capacity below TLC, FEF25–75%.

One characteristic of advanced obstructive disease is a reduction of the maximum volume that can be expired forcefully as compared with that which can be expired slowly from TLC. Therefore, even though the (slow) VC may be reduced in both restrictive and obstructive diseases, the FVC of an obstructor can be smaller than his or her (slow) VC.

FEV_1 is the equivalent volume of gas expired during the initial 1 s of the forced expiratory maneuver. Its value depends partially on data from the effort-dependent part of the curve and is therefore not a good index of small-airways disease, being correlated more closely with R_{AW}. If the entire TVC spirogram were a perfect exponential, then FEV_1 would be related to the log decrement for the curve. FEV_1/FVC and equivalently FEV_1/VC have been found to be nearly independent of body size for normal individuals. A decreased FEV_1/FVC can suggest obstruction, and FEV_1/VC can be reduced even more than FEV_1/FVC in obstructive disease.

The MMF or FEF25–75% represents an average flow produced during the middle half of the forced vital capacity. It is computed as

$$MMF = \frac{0.5 \; FVC}{t_{25\%FVC} - t_{75\%FVC}} \tag{9.44}$$

where $t_{25\%FVC}$ and $t_{75\%FVC}$ are the times at which 25 and 75% of the forced vital capacity, respectively, have been exhaled. It is an estimate of the maximum flow at 50% of the FVC, called FEF50%, which is obtained from the MEFV curve. It is therefore no less valuable as an indicator of small-airways disease. Dividing MMF by FVC is a useful normalization for differences in size among individuals.

The patterns of obstruction and restriction

Figure 9.14 shows typical data for forced vital capacity maneuvers of obstructed, restricted, and normal individuals, displayed on an absolute-volume axis. We can see distinctive patterns that bear out the foregoing discussion of static mechanics. Note that the vital capacities of the restrictor and obstructor are less than those of normals. The obstructor exhibits increased TLC and RV; the restrictor exhibits decreased TLC, but RV that is approxi-

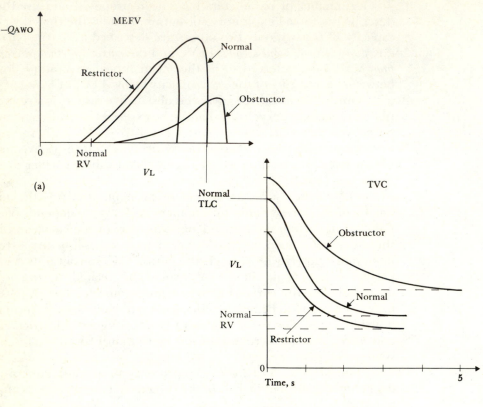

Figure 9.14 The corresponding flow-volume curve and timed spirogram for forced expiratory vital-capacity maneuvers plotted on an absolute-volume axis for comparison of classic restricted, obstructed, and normal subjects.

mately normal. The peak expiratory flows of both patients are reduced, but the slope of the restrictor's MEFV curve is approximately normal. Data for the obstructor display an exaggerated concavity over the latter part of the MEFV curve, whereas data for the restrictor are straighter. A normal individual and a restrictor expel their vital capacities in about the same time, whereas expiration for the obstructor is prolonged.

From this discussion it is clear that we need a minimum of four parameters to distinguish restrictors and advanced and early obstructors from normal subjects. These parameters include measures of absolute lung volume (for example, TLC); maximum volume change, FVC, or VC; a measure of the slope of the MEFV curve (for example, MMF/FVC); and a measure of the curvature of the MEFV curve or, equivalently, the shape of the TVC spirogram. Moment analysis has been suggested as a means of obtaining such curvature or shape parameters (Ligas *et al.*, 1977).

9.7 Measurement of gas concentration

Analysis of the composition of gas mixtures is one of the primary methods of obtaining information about lung function. In respiratory studies, the concentration of a component in a gas mixture is not routinely expressed as mass per volume, but is most frequently given in terms of partial pressure or molar fraction [which can be expressed as an equivalent volume fraction, as shown by (9.22)].

Discrete samples of gas or blood are all that are required in certain circumstances. However, as analytical devices with fast response times have been developed, continuous measurement of intrabreath events has become possible and desirable. At the present time, however, the sensor portion of most instruments is still too large to be placed at the site in the respiratory system occupied by the gas to be analyzed. Thus a gas sample must be transported from the respiratory system to the sensor within the instrument.

Input systems for continuous sampling usually consist of a thin (capillary) tube or catheter and an input connector (which may include a valve or a mixing chamber). Depending on the particular instrument and the application, the transport pathway can vary from centimeters to meters. This introduces transit delays and mixing within the sample and requires that the characteristics of the catheter and connector be matched to those of the instrument. Adjustment of the delay time, which depends on the mean velocity of the sample through the catheter, requires consideration of the following: the pressure drop along the catheter; the pressure within the instrument; the length and diameter of the catheter; geometry of the input connector; the sampled gas composition; and the volume flow of sample required by the instrument for accurate results. Some minimal time delay is always produced by catheter sampling systems, so that electrical or numerical signal processing is required if a gas analyzer's output is to be synchronized with the output from another, independent instrument, for example, a flowmeter.

Water vapor presents a major problem in sampling respiratory gas by catheter. Investigators have used thin, flexible, annealed stainless steel inlet tubing, carrying sufficient current through its length to heat its wall above body temperature, to prevent changes of gas composition and plugging of its lumen by water condensation. However, heating of the sample within the catheter increases axial diffusion, which can effectively filter out high-frequency components of fast-changing concentration waveshapes. An additional difficulty in measurement is introduced by the tendency of water vapor to be adsorbed and desorbed from surfaces within the system (Fowler, 1969). The establishment of an equilibrium between the water molecules on these surfaces and in the moving sample lags behind changes in partial pressures in the sample. Therefore the gas delivered to the sensor does not represent the gas entering the inlet tube until after that equilibrium is reached. For precision measurements in some applications, the sampled gas is passed through a tube filled with a drying agent. This effectively eliminates water vapor, but prolongs the overall response time of the measurement system.

At one time almost all analyses of gases performed in pulmonary laboratories involved techniques that employed a series of liquid chemical agents to sequentially separate particular species of gases from a mixture by selective chemical absorption or reaction. These include the classical procedures and devices developed by Haldane, Scholander, and Van Slyke (Bartels *et al.*, 1963). In recent years these have been replaced by electronic instruments that exploit phenomena associated with various physical properties of particular gases. Such instruments are reliable, accurate, easy to use, and compatible with automated pulmonary function testing systems. On the other hand, the classical wet chemical methods are time-consuming and tedious and consequently inefficient. However, if great care is taken, they provide extremely accurate measurements that represent the standards by which newly developed procedures are judged. Therefore they are used quite frequently to calibrate or back up other instruments.

Measurements of pH and partial pressures of O_2 and CO_2 dissolved in blood are routinely performed with specifically adapted electrode systems. These are discussed in Section 10.3. Devices for measurements in the gas phase vary in complexity and capabilities, from those that can continuously detect and analyze several gas species simultaneously (e.g., mass spectrometer) to those that can be modified to test for a few gases individually (e.g., infrared analyzer) to those sensitive to a particular property possessed by only one gas important to the respiratory system (e.g., polarographic O_2 sensor). There is a parallel between increasing versatility and increasing cost.

Mass spectroscopy

A *mass spectrometer* is an apparatus that separates a stream of charged particles (ions) into a spectrum according to their mass-to-charge ratios and determines the relative abundance of each type of ion present. Medical mass-spectrometer systems include the following elements: a sample-inlet assembly, an ionization chamber, a dispersion chamber, and an ion-detection (collector) system (Figure 9.15).

The sample-inlet assembly consists of a heated or unheated capillary tube (approximately 0.25 mm ID) and sample-inlet chamber. Gas is drawn through this system by a rotary pump that reduces the pressure in the inlet chamber to about 10–20 mm Hg

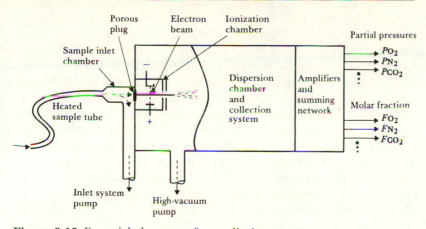

Figure 9.15 Essential elements of a medical mass spectrometer.

(1.3–1.7 kPa) absolute. A small amount of gas in the inlet chamber leaks by diffusion through a porous plug into the ionization chamber, which, along with the dispersion chamber, is evacuated to approximately 10^{-7} mm Hg (10^{-5} Pa) by a high-vacuum, high-capacity pump. A stream of electrons traveling between a heated filament and an anode bombard the gas entering the ionization chamber and cause the molecules to lose electrons, thereby producing positive ions. These are focused into a beam and accelerated by an electric field into the dispersion chamber, where the ion beam is sorted into its components on a molecular mass basis.

Dispersion techniques incorporated into commercially available systems involve a magnetic field or a quadrupole electric field or measurement of time of flight. The separated ion beams fall on the collector system that produces the output signal of the instrument. A mass spectrometer is of real value in respiratory applications only if it simultaneously produces separate continuous outputs for the several chemical species of interest. This has been achieved in two ways. One method uses a single collector that is swept sequentially by the component beams at a high rate of repetition. Individual sample-and-hold circuits, each corresponding to a particular species, register the ion current as the beam for their respective species falls on the collector. The second approach employs multiple collectors, the positions of which can be adjusted so that each continuously receives the ions of only one of the components of interest.

The ion current measured by the collector is proportional to the partial pressure of the corresponding component in the gas mixture. The inclusion of a circuit that sums over all components in conjunction with an appropriate calibration procedure makes it possible for the output to be expressed in terms of molar fractions.

The range of molecular weight that is adequate for most respiratory measurements extends from 4 (He) to 44 atomic mass units (CO_2). Expanded ranges make possible the monitoring of gases such as sulfur hexafluoride (146) and halothane (196). Several important gases produce outputs for the same atomic mass units. In particular, O_2 and CO_2 cannot be measured in the presence of ether or N_2O (Bartels *et al.*, 1963). Also CO interferes with N_2. CO and N_2O can be quickly and easily measured with infrared instruments, as described in the following discussion.

In an excellent review, Fowler (1969) discusses a number of problems and design criteria associated with the development of mass spectrometers for physiology and clinical laboratories. Such considerations include simplicity of operation, size, cost, sensitivity of the output to changes in sampled-gas temperature, water-vapor content and viscosity, characteristics of vacuum pumps, and various factors that affect the response time of the system as a whole.

In the years since that review appeared, many of the shortcomings cited have been satisfactorily resolved. Sensitivity, linearity, and SNR quoted by various manufacturers are appropriate for precision measurements. The response time (2 to 90%) for a step change in input is typically less than 100 ms (except for water vapor, which is longer). Transport delays associated with 1.3 to 1.6-m inlet catheters are on the order of 200 ms (with sample flowrates of 10 to 30 ml/min). Systems that can measure as many as eight component gases are now available, as are those that can sequentially sample from several different inlet catheters.

In vivo and *in vitro* measurements of gases dissolved in tissues and blood are possible with a nonthrombogenic catheter with a semipermeable membrane covering its tip. The catheter is inserted into the selected tissue or blood vessel. The inlet pump draws the gases out of solution through the membrane; no blood or liquid enters the catheter. Membranes of heparinized silicone rubber (Brantigan *et al.*, 1970) and Silastic have been used for blood gases, whereas Teflon has been found appropriate for measurements of gases in tissues (Brantigan *et al.*, 1972). Response times in these applications can range from 10 s to a number of minutes, depending on the catheter length, membrane material, and gas being measured.

Thermal-conductivity detectors

One of the properties of a gas mixture that changes with composition is its *thermal conductivity*. In general, the thermal conductivity of a gas is inversely related to its molecular weight. H_2 and He, for example, have thermal conductivities approximately 6.5 times greater than those of N_2 and O_2. As discussed in Section 9.3, heat transfer between a stationary heated body and a fluid moving past it is related to, among other factors, the velocity, the thermal conductivity, and the temperature of the fluid.

Thermal-conductivity detectors (TCD) have been developed for use in gas chromatography (Hamilton, 1975) and in instruments designed to analyze gas mixtures for He or H_2. In both applications, heated sensing elements operated in the constant-current mode (Section 8.5) are connected in a Wheatstone bridge. The heated elements can be either thermistors or coiled wires made of a metal with a high temperature coefficient of resistance (e.g., platinum, tungsten, or nickel). Thermal-conductivity detectors incorporating heated wires are called *katharometers*.

Gas chromatograph (GC) systems are discussed in detail in Section 10.4. Those that incorporate a TCD have two streams of a carrier gas moving at the same volume flow rate through the system. One stream, to which the gas mixture to be analyzed has been added, flows through a heated column that spatially (and temporally) separates the components of the mixture along the stream. Therefore the gas downstream of the column is composed of carrier gas mixed with only that component of the sample gas mixture that is currently being eluted from the column. The second, or reference, stream, which contains pure carrier gas only, bypasses the column but is heated to the same temperature as the sample stream.

Most gases of interest in the pulmonary laboratory can be detected on the basis of thermal conductivity. Since He is inert and has a thermal conductivity much different from these gases, it is used as the carrier gas. GC thermal-conductivity detectors consist of two matched cells, each containing a pair of sensing elements (Figure 9.16).

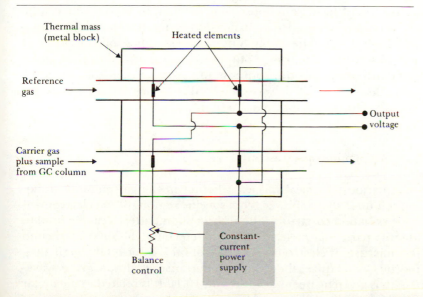

Figure 9.16 Thermal-conductivity detector for a gas chromatograph. Reference gas is the same as the carrier gas.

The reference gas (pure He) flows through one cell, while the carrier gas plus the sample passes through the other. The two streams of gas are at the same temperature and flow at the same velocity through their respective cells, causing the output of the bridge to depend on the difference in thermal conductivities of the gases in the two cells. This in turn is related to the mass concentration of the sample component in the carrier gas. For a constant flow rate through the system, the output of the bridge is approximately proportional to the mass flow rate of the sample component passing through the detector.

The response time of this detector system depends on the gas-flow rate. However, the overall dynamic behavior of the GC as a whole is limited by the processes in the column. Typically, a complete analysis of a gas sample requires minutes. In addition, only discrete samples can be analyzed, so that GC cannot be used for continuous or even on-line measurements. A GC does have advantages, however. An extremely accurate, complete analysis for most gas species of interest in pulmonary studies can usually be made with a single instrument from a single small (< 1 ml) sample. A GC is much less expensive (approximately one-tenth) than a mass spectrometer, which is the only laboratory instrument that can exceed its analytical versatility.

Instruments developed to measure He or H_2 in air have employed katharometers composed of four test cells operating at the same temperature. Each cell contains a single heated-filament wire that serves as one leg of a Wheatstone bridge. Two reference cells are sealed; both contain either air or O_2 (wet or dry). The remaining two cells are unsealed and can receive sample gas only by diffusion from a stream passing through the instrument. This minimizes loss of heat from the sensing element by forced convection. However, these so-called diffusion-fed filaments (McNair and Bonelli, 1969) have undesirably long response times, on the order of tens of seconds. The bridge output can be calibrated to yield molar fractions relative to the composition of the gas in the reference cells. Because of its slow response, this device is useful only for breath-averaged or discrete samples.

Absorption spectroscopy

Various chemical species, whether in the gas phase or in liquid solution, absorb power from specific regions of the electromagnetic radiation spectrum. These absorption patterns can be used to identify particular molecules and to determine their molar fraction in a mixture. If electromagnetic radiation is directed through a liquid or gas mixture, then the power transmitted at a given wavelength is given by Beer's law (Section 10.1). It is related to the molar density ρ of the substances that absorb that wavelength. The approach to absorption spectroscopy, which will be discussed in some detail here, uses a wide-band energy source, but selectively measures the power transmitted at only those wavelengths corresponding to the substances under study. Termed *nondispersive infrared* (NDIR) *analysis*, it is employed in instruments calibrated to measure the molar fraction of some gases important in respiration and anesthesia, such as CO_2, CO, water vapor, halothane, and N_2O.

The NDIR system, shown in Figure 9.17, is used to analyze a gas mixture for the presence of a single species of test gas. Two identical IR beams are intermittently interrupted (10 to 90 times per second, depending on the particular instrument) by a rotating chopper blade. The power pulses produced travel two parallel paths, one of which includes a test cell. A sample of the gas mixture to be analyzed is continuously drawn through the test cell from a sampling catheter. Since the sample is not contaminated, it can be returned to its original source if desired. The second path contains a reference cell which has windows exactly the same as the test cell, but which contains a gas mixture free of the test gas.

A detector (*Golay cell*) made up of two chambers separated by a diaphragm receives the power transmitted through the test and

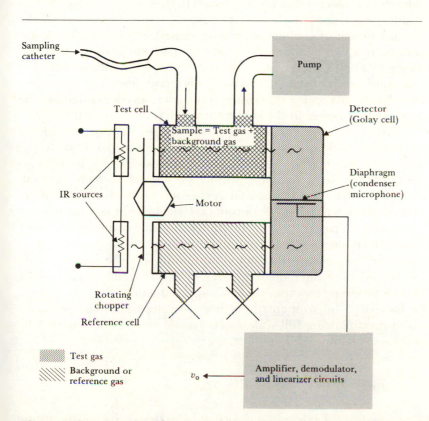

Figure 9.17 Infrared analyzer. This type of device is commonly used to measure gas-phase concentrations of gases such as CO_2, CO, N_2O, halothane and others.

reference pathways. Any difference in pressure between the two chambers produces a displacement of this diaphragm, causing a change (usually in capacitance) in a sensing circuit. The selectivity of the detector for the wavelengths absorbed by the test gas is achieved by filling both detector chambers with the pure test gas. Thus only IR energy of the wavelengths that can be absorbed by the test gas is absorbed in the detector, and this energy increases the temperature and pressure of the gas on each side of the detector diaphragm. Equation (10.1) indicates that the power of the transmitted IR radiation depends on the concentration (molar density) of the IR-absorbing gases in the pathways. The pulsed IR power reaching the detector produces corresponding pulsed changes in pressure in the detector chambers. The average difference in pressure between the two sides of the detector diaphragm is therefore related to the difference in test-gas concentration between the test and reference cells. The output of the detector circuit is demodulated and passed through a linearizing network that produces a signal proportional to the concentration of test gas in the gas sample in the test cell.

Possibly the gas mixture being analyzed contains gases with absorption spectra that partially overlap that of the test gas (for instance, N_2O and halothane; CO_2 and CO). The inaccuracy of the measurement of test-gas absorption caused by the interfering gas can be reduced by filling the reference pathway with the interfering gas. The IR power transmitted through this pathway at the absorption bands of the interfering gas is attenuated. The difference in pressure across the detector diaphragm is less dependent on the transmitted power in the overlapping parts of the spectra.

By Beer's law, the output voltage of the instrument is related to the molar density of the test gas. This output is related to the wet-gas molar fraction only if the total pressure and absolute temperature of the gas mixture within the test cell remain constant. Consequently, most IR gas analyzers require a warm-up period (on the order of 8 h) for stable output ($\pm 1\%$ change in zero setting and gain over at least 8 h). Also, the calibrated gain can vary whenever barometric pressure changes appreciably or if the inlet sampling catheter, viscosity of the gas mixture, or flow of the sample are altered. At flow rates on the order of 0.5 to 1 liter/min, a 90% full-scale step-response time of approximately 100 ms can be achieved. IR instruments have been developed to measure gases with the following full-scale molar fractions: 10% CO_2, 0.3% CO, 100% N_2O, and 3% halothane.

Emission spectroscopy

Figure 9.18 depicts a device used to detect the concentration of a single gas species in a mixture by measuring the intensity of the light in a given wavelength range produced when the gas mixture is ionized at very low pressures. The respiratory gas routinely measured using such a device is N_2. The system is evacuated by a high-capacity vacuum pump and the pressure (1 to 4 mm Hg) (150 to 550 Pa) is regulated by a needle valve that allows a small flow of gas to be drawn through the ionization chamber. Respiratory gases ionized by the voltage difference (600 to 1500 V dc) between the electrodes in the ionization chamber emit light in the range of 310 to 480 nm. Reflecting surfaces direct the light through a selective optical filter that absorbs unwanted wavelengths. A photoelectric tube produces a current proportional to the intensity of the light passed by the filter. For a fixed ionization-chamber geometry, vacuum, gas flow, and current, the amplified output of the phototube is a nonlinear function of the molar fraction of the gas species of interest. A linearizing circuit is used to produce an output voltage proportional to this molar fraction.

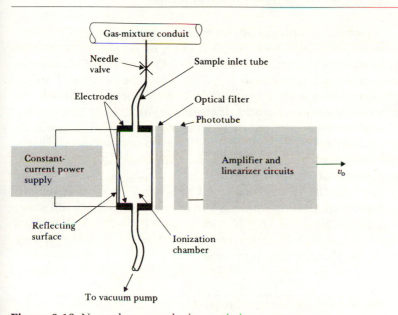

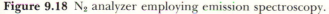

Figure 9.18 N_2 analyzer employing emission spectroscopy.

Spectroscopic N_2 analyzers yield the N_2 molar fraction in a gas mixture on a wet basis. Calibration procedures must take into account the humidity of the sample. The needle valve and conduit from which the sample is withdrawn may have to be heated to prevent plugging or loss of water vapor by condensation. The high vacuum within the system prevents condensation of water vapor in the transport tubing leading from the needle valve to the ionization chamber, but it may not prevent adsorption and desorption during changes of partial pressures of water vapor.

An evaluation of representative commercially available N_2 analyzers has been reported by Daniels *et al.* (1975). He found that high-quality linearization circuitry and proper calibration can produce a steady-state output that has as little as 0.5% rms error over the range of 0 to 80% N_2. In response to a step change in N_2 molar fraction, the transport delay and rise time (between 10% and 90% of the steady-state output) can each be on the order of 40 ms. Variation in output to a constant input can be less than 1.5% over 24 h. Deposition of electrode material on the glass walls of the ionization chamber over a long period of time eventually degrades the instrument's performance. O_2 and CO_2 do not interfere with the accuracy of N_2 determinations. However, He and Ar can produce errors. A mixture containing 40% N_2 and 5% He can produce an output corresponding to up to 43% N_2 from the analyzer.

Measurement of oxygen concentration

A number of approaches have been taken in the development of devices to measure concentration of O_2 in gas mixtures. A mass spectrometer can continuously measure O_2 easily and accurately, but the monetary investment involved cannot be justified if only a single gas species is to be measured. The emission and absorption spectroscopic devices already discussed are not useful for O_2. Instruments based on the paramagnetic properties of O_2 or on electrochemical (fuel) cells have met with mixed acceptance and have received limited clinical and laboratory application. At the present time instruments are available that use a disposable polarographic O_2 sensor (similar to that described in Section 10.3). This type of device provides an output that is linearly related ($\pm 0.3\%$ full scale) to P_{O_2} in a flowing gas sample containing 0 to 100% O_2. Reported accuracy is $\pm 0.7\%$ for continuous measurements. A 90% response time of less than 100 ms is possible.

9.8 Some tests of gas transport

The pulmonary function tests to be discussed in this section are concerned primarily with gas-phase transport between the airway opening and the alveoli, and interphase (or membrane) transport between alveolar gas and pulmonary capillary blood. Gas-transport tests are designed to achieve one or more of the following objectives. (1) Determine the homogeneity of the distribution of inspired gas (ventilation). (2) Determine the matching of ventilation to perfusion. (3) Evaluate the ability of the alveolar membrane to allow gas transfer. Because of the architecture of the respiratory system, it is usually impossible to isolate the processes involved or to make direct measurements at sites of interest. Access is available only at the boundaries of the system: the airway opening and the systemic circulation.

An overall evaluation of gas transport by the lungs can be obtained from a measurement of the partial pressures of O_2 and CO_2 in a sample of systemic arterial blood drawn while the subject is breathing air. If the gas-exchange ratio $\dot{V}_{CO_2}/\dot{V}_{O_2}$ is approximately 0.8, then the sum of the arterial partial pressures, PaO_2 and $PaCO_2$, should be approximately 140 mm Hg (18.7 kPa). If this sum is below 120 mm Hg (16 kPa), it is considered abnormal (Ayers et al., 1974). Because the acquisition of these data requires puncturing an artery, it is not used routinely as a pulmonary-function test, especially for children.

Further discussion of arterial blood gases is limited here to the observation that they can be used in a procedure to distinguish between two possible causes of abnormally low partial pressures: (a) the shunting of blood past the gas-exchange regions in the lung, (b) a mismatch between local alveolar ventilation and blood perfusion. Besides a sample of arterial blood gas, the procedure requires an estimate of the mean PO_2 in the alveoli. This is obtained from an end-expired gas sample collected as the subject exhales to RV. If the steady-state alveolar-arterial (A-a) O_2 difference in partial pressure does not appreciably change when the subject breathes 100% O_2 instead of air, then a shunt is assumed to be present. If the A-a difference decreases, then a ventilation-perfusion mismatch is implied.

Gas-phase transport

Tests of gas-phase transport are concerned with questions arising from two of the objectives mentioned above: (1) How is the inspired gas (ventilation) distributed in the lungs? (2) What is the equivalent volume of inspired gas not taking part in the exchange of gas with the blood; i.e., what is the effective dead space of the lung?

We can assess the distribution of gas in the lungs from multibreath and single-breath maneuvers by using a tracer gas that is insoluble in the pulmonary tissues and blood. The assumption can then be made that the tracer gas can enter or leave the lung only through the airway opening. Gases that fulfill this requirement are He, N_2, Ar, Ne, and Xe.

The multibreath He-dilution and N_2-washout procedures used to estimate lung volume (FRC) as described in Section 9.4 can also provide information about the efficiency of gas mixing in the lungs, i.e., whether the gas in all ventilated alveoli is diluted at the same rate by gas inspired during resting breathing.

As an example of this type of test, consider the washout of N_2

from the lungs during resting breathing of 100% O_2. A set of one-way valves, as shown in Fig. 9.7, is used to prevent mixing of the inspired O_2 with the expirate. If a pulmonary system were to act as a single, well-mixed compartment ventilated at a constant breathing rate and tidal volume, a time plot of the end-tidal expired-nitrogen molar fraction, F_{N_2}, would exhibit an exponential decay. Normal lungs exhibit a washout curve that can be approximated rather closely by a single exponential. The shape of the washout curve is not routinely used as a test of abnormal ventilation because it is difficult to compensate for the effects of variations in tidal volume and breathing frequency on the shape of the curve. However, abnormality is indicated if the F_{N_2} of a sample of gas obtained at the end of an expiration to RV after 7 min of O_2 breathing has not been reduced to 0.02. This procedure is obviously highly dependent on cooperation, since it is sensitive to changes in the tidal volume and frequency of breathing of the subject.

The single-breath N_2 washout can yield as many as three useful pieces of information: (1) An estimate of the anatomical dead space (approximately the volume of the conducting airways). (2) A measure of the distribution of ventilation, i.e., the relative local rates of filling and emptying the regions of the lungs. (3) An index of small-airway mechanical function, the closing volume CV.

The procedure requires that, after having reached a steady-state while breathing air, the subject then inspires 100% O_2 from RV to TLC. After a momentary pause, the individual is instructed to exhale very slowly to residual volume. The F_{N_2} in the expired gas, $F_{E_{N_2}}$, and the volume of the expired gas are continuously measured and displayed against each other on an x-y plotter. The interpretation of these plots requires a discussion of the events that occur in the lungs during both a vital-capacity inspiration and a slow vital-capacity expiration.

Consider the idealized normal upright lung (subject sitting or standing erect) (Figure 9.19). It has been found (Milic-Emili et al., 1966) that at residual volume, the *dependent,* or lowest with respect to gravity, parts of the lungs are less expanded than the upper regions. Thus there is a distribution of local alveolar volumes corresponding roughly to the distribution of the pressure on the interpleural surface of the lungs. That is, there is lower pressure at the top of the lungs (larger alveoli) and higher pressure at the base (smaller alveoli).

After the lung has been expanded to and held at TLC, the lung is more uniformly inflated, with all regions having the same relative local volume. This means that the top parts of the lungs must have changed their volumes less during a vital-capacity inspiration of 100% O_2 than did the lower, dependent parts in order for the two regions to reach approximately the same final volume at

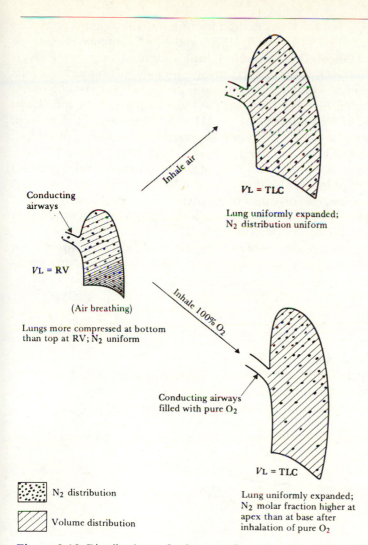

Conducting
airways

$V_L = TLC$

Lung uniformly expanded;
N_2 distribution uniform

Inhale air

$V_L = RV$

(Air breathing)

Lungs more compressed at bottom
than top at RV; N_2 uniform

Inhale 100% O_2

Conducting airways
filled with pure O_2

$V_L = TLC$

N_2 distribution

Volume distribution

Lung uniformly expanded;
N_2 molar fraction higher at
apex than at base after
inhalation of pure O_2

Figure 9.19 Distributions of volume and gas species at RV and TLC for a
vital-capacity inspiration of air or pure oxygen.

TLC. Consequently, less inspired O_2 was added to the upper
regions than the lower. If the subject had achieved steady state
while breathing air prior to performing this test, then it can be assumed that the F_{N_2} in the gas within the lungs was the same
throughout. Thus, since less diluting inspired O_2 is added to the
upper regions than the lower during a VC inspiration of pure O_2,
the F_{N_2} in the upper regions is higher than in the lower regions at
the end of this inspiration. Also at TLC, the conducting airways
(anatomical dead space) are filled with pure O_2.

For a slow vital-capacity expiration, following the inspiration of pure O_2, normal lungs exhibit four identifiable regions or phases (Fowler, 1949; Dolfuss *et al.*, 1967) on the F_{EN_2}-versus-volume plot [Figure 9.20(b)]. During phase I, lung volume changes but F_{EN_2} is zero as pure O_2 is emptied from the nonconducting airways past the N_2 sensor. Phase III is a (sloping) plateau corresponding to the emptying of the mixed alveolar gas from all parts of the lungs. Oscillations of F_{EN_2} during phase III have been attributed to local emptying of areas of different F_{N_2} caused by the changes in volume associated with the heartbeat (Fowler *et al.*, 1961). Phase II is the transition between the emptying of the anatomical dead space and the arrival of mixed alveolar gas at the N_2 sensor. Phase IV signifies a drastic change in the rates of emptying of the dependent parts of the lungs. It is dramatically evident if the lung is normal or has only minimal small-airways disease.

A system consisting of a single, perfectly mixed compartment and a transport dead space [Figure 9.20(a)] would exhibit a wash-

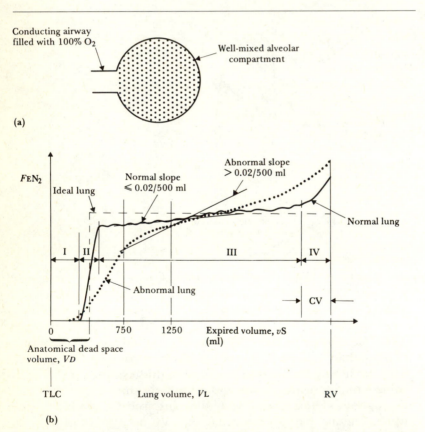

(a)

(b)

Figure 9.20 Single-breath nitrogen-washout maneuver. (a) An idealized model of a lung at the end of a vital-capacity inspiration of pure O_2, preceded by breathing of normal air. (b) Single-breath nitrogen-washout curves for idealized lung, normal lung, and abnormal lung. Parameters of these curves include anatomical dead space, slope of phase III, and closing volume.

out curve like that in Figure 9.20(b) (dashed line). By analogy, the anatomical dead space is taken as the volume emptied to the point at which the F_EN_2 reaches one-half of a representative mixed alveolar value. For conditions in the spirometer, we can compute

$$\text{Anatomical } V_D = VC - \frac{\int_0^{VC} F_EN_2 \, dv_S}{\hat{F}_EN_2(III)} \tag{9.45}$$

where

$$VC = \text{expired vital capacity}$$
$$v_S = \text{volume change of spirometer used to estimate integral of expired flow}$$
$$\hat{F}_EN_2(III) = \text{mean value for } F_EN_2 \text{ during phase III.}$$

Normal lungs exhibit an average slope during phase III that does not exceed the 0.02-increase in F_EN_2 per 500 ml of expired volume for an interval of expired volume between 750 and 1250 ml below TLC. A greater increase than this is taken to indicate a nonuniformity of local alveolar emptying rates.

The volume above RV at which phase IV begins is designated the *closing volume* CV. The absolute volume at which phase IV begins is the *closing capacity*, CC = RV + CV. As the lung volume approaches RV, the dependent gas spaces in the lung begin to cease emptying at the same rate at which they emptied during phase III. Therefore the expirate at the airway opening contains a higher proportion of gas from the superior parts of the lungs and less from the dependent portions. Since the upper parts of the lung had the higher F_{N_2} after the vital-capacity inspiration of pure O_2, the expirate passing the N_2 sensor at the airway opening has an increasing F_EN_2 as an increasing number of dependent lung units decrease their emptying rate as the lung approaches RV.

The small airways in the dependent parts of the lungs have been assigned a key role in this phenomenon. Even though some controversy exists (Knudson *et al.*, 1977), inferences about the mechanical state of the small airways have been made from the size of the CV relative to the VC (McCarthy *et al.*, 1972) and CC relative to TLC. Closing volume varies with body position, age, and disease. For normal, standing adolescents and young adults, CV/VC is on the order of 0.1. It may exceed 0.4 by age 60 years. Increases in CV are produced in the initial phases of small-airways disease. However, as the disease progresses, the slope of phase III increases and the transition between phases III and IV becomes less distinct [Figure 9.20(b)]. Therefore the ambiguity in the determination of the onset of phase IV associated with advanced obstructive diseases limits the use of the CV, except as an indicator of the beginnings of abnormalities of the small airways.

Effective (physiologic) dead space during alveolar-capillary gas exchange

When inspired gas cannot reach alveoli whose capillaries are perfused with blood and when blood cannot perfuse capillaries of alveoli that are ventilated with inspired gas, gas exchange is impaired. A tracer gas that is not diffusion-limited by the alveolar membrane can be used to evaluate the matching of ventilation and perfusion. The CO_2 added to the gas space in the lungs from the pulmonary capillary blood satisfies this requirement. It diffuses so freely that it can be assumed that the alveoli and capillaries are in equilibrium during the entire expiration, i.e., that their respective CO_2 partial pressures are equal.

In the absence of significant right-to-left heart shunt, systemic arterial CO_2 partial pressure provides an excellent estimate of an average pulmonary capillary P_{CO_2}. Consequently, a conceptual alveolar volume V_A can be defined as the equivalent volume of gas in the lung which communicates with the airway opening and which satisfies two conditions: (1) It contains all the CO_2 in the lungs at the end of inspiration. (2) This CO_2 exists at a partial pressure equal to that of systemic arterial blood. The *effective dead space, V_D,* sometimes called the *physiologic dead space,* is the remainder of the gas space in the lungs that is not alveolar space. If we consider that none of the CO_2 expired during a breath is contributed by the dead space—that all of it is coming from the alveolar space—then we can obtain an estimate of the volume of the effective dead space as a fraction of the expired tidal volume V_T from a mass balance of expired CO_2:

$$\frac{V_D}{V_T} = 1 - \frac{\hat{P}_{E}CO_2}{\hat{P}_{a}CO_2} \tag{9.46}$$

where $\hat{P}_{E}CO_2$ is the mean CO_2 partial pressure in the expirate and $\hat{P}_{a}CO_2$ is the mean partial pressure of systemic arterial CO_2, each determined over several breaths.

Even though V_D/V_T is important in inferring the etiology of diseases involving poor gas exchange, it is not routinely determined or used for mass screening because it requires taking a sample of the patient's arterial blood during a basal steady state. This is difficult to achieve, given the patient's excitement during testing and the patient's natural apprehension about sampling of arterial blood.

Diffusion processes

To complete the description of gas exchange in the lungs, we need to characterize the transport processes occurring between the alveolar gas space and the pulmonary capillary blood. Gas moves between these regions by diffusion. A parameter used to describe the diffusion processes in the vicinity of the alveolar membrane is the *diffusing capacity of the lung*, D. This is the constant of proportionality between the rate of uptake of tracer gas by the blood (obtained from measurements at the airway opening) and the difference of partial pressure of the tracer gas between the alveolar gas space and the capillary blood. Since it is impossible to measure alveolar partial pressures directly, and since they are affected by convective transport between the airway opening and the alveoli, diffusing capacity is not independent of the pattern of ventilation distribution in the lungs.

CO_2 diffuses across the alveolar membrane much more easily than O_2, so that a diffusion defect would affect O_2 transfer first. Because of this and the prime role O_2 plays in sustaining life, it is important to evaluate a diffusing capacity for O_2. However, obtaining the required PaO_2 requires a sample of arterial blood. To avoid this, clinicians use CO as the tracer gas because its properties are sufficiently close to those of O_2 for its diffusing capacity, D_{CO}, to provide a meaningful estimate of D_{O_2}. In addition, because of its affinity for hemoglobin, at low concentrations essentially all CO that enters the blood chemically combines with the hemoglobin in the red blood cells; P_{CO} exhibited by the blood is negligibly small and need not be measured.

One of the various methods that have been used to estimate D_{CO} involves a single-breath maneuver. The subject inspires a mixture of air, 0.3% CO (or less), and He (approximately 10%) from RV to TLC. He holds his breath at TLC for about 10 s and then forcefully exhales down to RV. Even though it necessitates subject cooperation, this procedure can be performed quickly and can be repeated easily. In addition, it does not require samples of arterial blood or an estimate of dead space before the clinician can obtain a value of alveolar $PACO$. The computation of D_{CO} from measurements made during this single-breath maneuver are based on a one-compartment model of the lung. If a well-mixed alveolar compartment is filled with a mixture of gases containing some initial $FACO$, then during breath-holding with the airway open, the CO diffuses into the blood in the pulmonary capillaries and the alveolar $FACO$ decreases exponentially with time:

$$\hat{F}ACO(t_2) = \hat{F}ACO(t_1) \exp\left[-\frac{D_{CO}(Patm - PAH_2O)(t_2 - t_1)}{VA} \right] \quad (9.47)$$

where VA is the equivalent volume of the alveolar gas space throughout which the inspired CO is assumed to be distributed; and t_1 and t_2 are the times corresponding to the end of the inspiration to TLC and the beginning of expiration to RV, respectively; that is, $t_2 - t_1$ is the duration of the breath-holding.

The mean fraction of alveolar CO at the end of the breath-holding, $\hat{F}_ACO(t_2)$, is taken as that of the gas expired at the end of the expiration to RV. The F_{HE} of this end-expiratory gas is also measured. Since the inspired He is insoluble in the lung tissues and blood, none of it should have left the lung during the breath-holding. It can be assumed that, during inspiration, both the He and CO were similarly distributed throughout the lungs, and that the dilution of the He in the alveoli at the end of inspiration is the same as that for the CO. The end-inspiratory F_{HE} should not change during breath-holding, so that it can be estimated from the measured end-expiratory $F_{EE}He$. The end-inspiratory alveolar F_ACO can be estimated from

$$\frac{\hat{F}_ACO(t_1)}{F_ICO(t_0)} = \frac{\hat{F}_AHe(t_1)}{F_IHe(t_0)} = \frac{F_{EE}He}{F_IHe(t_0)} \tag{9.48}$$

where $F_ICO(t_0)$ and $F_IHe(t_0)$ are the fractions of CO and He, respectively, in the inspired gas. In addition, the equivalent alveolar volume to which the gas is distributed can be estimated using a mass balance on the He:

$$V_A \cdot F_{EE}He = VC \cdot F_IHe(t_0) \tag{9.49}$$

Diffusing capacity depends on many factors besides the distribution of ventilation to the alveoli and the properties of the alveolar membrane. The distribution of pulmonary perfusion, cardiac output (flow rate), and volume of blood in the pulmonary capillaries also affect it. These, in turn, are related not only to disease processes but also to exertion during exercise or excitement and the patient's body position when the measurements are made. D_{CO} also varies with hematocrit and type of hemoglobin in the blood. Bates et al. (1971) describes the theory, history, and limitations of several methods of measuring D_{CO}.

Automated testing of pulmonary function

The instrumentation described in this chapter is the type that can be found in the modern, well-equipped pulmonary-function laboratory. A necessary adjunct to such a facility is an automated computing device. This can range from a programmable hand-held or desk-top calculator to a dedicated on-line analog and/or digital computer. Depending on the hardware, such systems can perform any or all of the following functions required for the operation of a pulmonary-function laboratory: control of valves in test apparatus, data acquisition, data reduction, display of intermediate results, computation of expected normal values for the subject being tested, record keeping, and generation of hard copies of results for distribution to the attending physician.

The current trend is toward inclusion of a microprocessor within a testing system so that results are computed on-line with the measurements. Such a system can be designed for the performance of a single test and the computation of its associated parameters, or it may be sufficiently versatile in instrumentation, apparatus, and computational power to accommodate a number of tests.

One of the simplest tests of pulmonary mechanics to computerize involves the forced vital capacity maneuver. The gas-transport test that is most easily automated is the single-breath N_2 washout. More elaborate systems attempt to provide for the determination of measures of gas exchange and distribution, static lung volumes, and D_{CO}. Automation of plethysmographically obtained measures of pulmonary function is in its embryonic stages.

The particular system configuration, the instrument employed for a given test, and the algorithms used for the pattern recognition required for data reduction vary among manufacturers. For instance, one system may be based on a spirometer, whereas another may have a hot-wire anemometer or a pneumotachometer, the output from which is integrated to yield a measure of volume.

One example of a commercially available system employs a 4-bit microprocessor to perform data acquisition and computations associated with the forced expiratory vital capacity maneuver and the single-breath N_2 washout (Anonymous, 1975). The system consists of a data processor/display unit, a transducer interface unit, and peripheral equipment including a vacuum pump for the nitrogen analyzer and an x-y plotter and ticket printer for hard copy of results. A Fleisch pneumotachometer is used to measure the volume flow of expired gas. Besides the microcomputer electronics and ADC, the system includes all amplifier, filter, and linearizer circuitry required by the flow, and N_2 analysis instruments. Patient morphometric data (standing height, weight, age, sex) are entered through a keyboard on the processor/display unit.

Two modes of operation are switch-selectable by the operator. In one, the patient performs an FVC maneuver and the system computes FVC, FEV_1, FEV_1/FVC, PEF, and FEF25–75%. In the second mode, the patient performs a single-breath N_2 washout. From simultaneously measured F_EN_2 and volume-flow-rate signals, the clinician obtains the closing volume CV, the slope of phase III of the F_EN_2-versus-expired-volume curve, and vital capacity VC. TLC is estimated from a static mass balance over the single-breath washout (Buist *et al.*, 1973; see Problem 9.19) so that the processor can compute RV (= TLC − VC), RV/TLC, closing capacity (CC = CV + RV), and CC/TLC. In addition, predicted values of FVC, FEV_1, FEF25–75%, CC/TLC, and slope of phase III are calculated from the patient's morphometric data.

The operator may observe the results of a test by selecting an output scanning mode in which the actual values are sequentially presented on a three-digit display on the processor/display unit, followed by the predicted values and finally the ratio of actual to predicted values. Or the operator may choose a hold mode, in which any one parameter is selected and displayed indefinitely. The results may be printed by the system's ticket printer for the patient's record.

This system has two features that are particularly helpful to the medical personnel conducting the tests. (1) The processor/display unit has a rectilinear voltmeter that sequentially illuminates a row of LEDs in proportion to the applied voltage. During the FVC maneuver, the number of lights on is proportional to the cumulative expired volume. For the N_2 washout, the display indicates the instantaneous expired flow rate. This device provides an incentive for patients who can use the information to control their performance. (2) The processor/display unit has the ability to display, on an x-y plotter, the sampled data from each experiment. Not only does this provide a graphical plot for patients' records and make possible hand calculation of additional parameters, but it also makes possible a subjective visual check of the patient's performance of the test maneuver. This feedback to the medical technician is of utmost importance, especially when untrained subjects are being screened.

Problems

9.1 For a single mechanical unit lung, assume that the relationship between pressure, volume, and number of moles of ideal gas in the lung is given by

$$P_A \left(\frac{V_L}{N_L}\right)^\alpha = K$$

in which $\alpha = 1$ and K is a constant. Derive the lowest-order (linear) approximation to the relationship between changes in pressure, changes in volume, and changes in moles of gas within the lung.

9.2 Define the acoustic compliance of a gas mixture as

$$Cg = -\frac{\partial V}{\partial P}$$

Using the relation in Problem 9.1, evaluate the acoustic compliance in liters per centimeter H_2O for a lung whose volume is 2 liters with an ideal-dry-gas alveolar pressure of 713 mm Hg (95 kPa).

9.3 Assuming zero net gas exchange with the blood and using (9.2), (9.3a, b, and c), and the results of Problems 9.1 and 9.2, draw an analogous equivalent circuit model for the lung represented by Figure 9.2(a) with gas compression included.

9.4 Assume that the chest-wall static compliance is 0.31 liter/cm H_2O and that the pulmonary static compliance is 0.19 liter/cm H_2O when the ventilatory system described by Figure 9.2 is at its resting volume (FRC). Evaluate the static compliance for the total respiratory system.

9.5 Discuss the effects (qualitative) of the placement of a container filled with 6-mm-diameter beads of soda lime in (a) the inlet side of a spirometer and (b) the outlet side of a spirometer, on the dynamics of the spirometer response and the accuracy of continuous measurements of lung volume changes (1) during very slow maneuvers (in the limit) from one static volume to another; and (2) for very fast maneuvers; for example, a forced-vital-capacity expiration, i.e., a maximum-effort exhalation from TLC down to RV.

9.6 Evaluate the effect on an estimate of FRC from (9.23), given that the experiment is terminated at a lung volume other than FRC. Evaluate the effect on an estimate of FRC from (9.24) if the final volume of the spirometer does not equal its original volume.

9.7 Design an analog circuit to solve (9.34) for v_L from continuous measurement of Q_2 and $(P_B - Patm)$.

9.8 Assume that an abnormal pulmonary system can be represented as two airway-alveolar-compartment units (negligible gas compression) connected in parallel. (Figure P9.1). Derive expressions for the effective compliance C_{effL} and effective resistance R_{effL} for voluntary breathing frequencies.

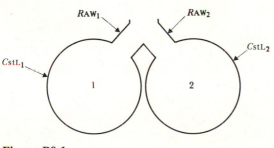

Figure P9.1

9.9 In a 1000-liter body plethysmograph, a 100-liter person blows into a pressure transducer, raising mouth pressure 30 cm H_2O (3 kPa). The pressure in the box drops 0.1 cm H_2O (10 Pa). Calculate the person's lung volume, assuming that $\alpha_B = 1.4$ and that atmospheric pressure is 760 mm Hg (101 kPa).

9.10 In Figure 9.17 the diaphragm bends to vary the capacitance in the condenser microphone. Design the first stage of a circuit that converts this variation in capacitance to an output voltage.

9.11 In an He-dilution experiment, a spirometer is preloaded with 10 liters of 5% He at room temperature, 25°C. After the patient has rebreathed, the He concentration in the spirometer is 4%. What is the FRC? [Assume $Ts(t_2) = 305$ K.]

9.12 Describe the experimental tests that yield a measure of the obstruction of the large airways.

9.13 Describe three tests that yield measures of obstruction in small airways.

9.14 Sketch a normal single-breath N_2-washout curve and explain why it has this shape.

9.15 Derive and discuss (9.45) and (9.46).

9.16 Derive (9.47) and describe how you could measure diffusing capacity of the lung.

9.17 An instrument requires 10 ml/min of flow to analyze a gas properly. Assuming a blunt flow profile, and given that the transit delay time of a sample is to be 200 ms, what is the relation between length and diameter for an inlet tube?

9.18 Discuss the merits of the automated system described in Section 9.8. In particular, address the subject of accuracy of measurement, especially of flow rate, by a single instrument over the wide range required for the FVC and N_2 washout experiments.

9.19 Derive an expression for TLC, using static mass balances on the lungs between the beginning and end of a slow inspiration of O_2 from RV to TLC, and between the subsequent TLC and the end of the slow expiration to RV at the finish of the N_2 washout test. Discuss the accuracy of this estimate.

(*Answer*):

$$TLC = \frac{VCI \; F_{A}N_2(t_0) - V_D \; F_{A}N_2(t_1)}{F_{A}N_2(t_0) - F_{A}N_2(t_1)}$$

in which

$$F_{A}N_2(t_1) = \frac{\int_{t_1}^{t_2} F_{E}N_2 Q_{AWO} \; dt}{VCE - V_D}$$

where VCI is the volume inspired from RV at t_0 to TLC at t_1 and VCE is the volume expired from TLC at t_1 to RV at t_2. $F_{E}N_2$ is the instantaneous expired N_2 molar fraction measured at the AWO between t_1 and t_2. $F_{A}N_2(t_0)$ is the N_2 molar fraction in the alveolar gas before the test began (t_0) and V_D is the anatomical dead space. Which terms must be estimated and which are accessible for measurement?

9.20 In an N_2-washout experiment, the subject's cumulative expired volume into a spirometer is 5 liters. At the beginning of the experiment, the spirometer has a volume of 7 liters but contains no N_2. At the end of the experiment, the molar fraction of N_2 in the spirometer is 0.026 and the $F_A N_2$ of the subject has decreased by 0.1. The final temperature of the spirometer is 303 K. What was the lung volume at which the subject was breathing?

9.21 Design an experiment requiring no surgery to measure the mechanical time constant ($\tau = RC$) of the lungs *in vivo* of an anesthetized, paralyzed animal (assume normal lungs).

9.22 A Fleisch pneumotachometer has 100 capillary tubes, each with a diameter of 1 mm and a length of 5 cm. What pressure drop occurs for a flow of 1 liter/s?

9.23 Show that the output of an instrument that is related to test-gas molar density will be related in the same way to test-gas molar fraction (on a wet-gas basis) only if the ratio of the pressure of the total gas mixture to its absolute temperature remains constant.

9.24 Derive the governing equation for the TBP for breathing within the box, including nonnegligible exchange of gases between the alveoli and pulmonary capillary blood.

9.25 Derive the governing equation for the TBP for breathing within the box for a lung characterized by two alveolar compartments (Figure P9.1). Assume that the net exchange of gases through the alveolar-capillary membrane is zero.

References

Anonymous, *Respiratory measurements and comparison system product specifications.* Kansas City, MO: Puritan-Bennett Corporation, 1975.

Ayers, L.N., B.J. Whipp, and I. Ziment, *A guide to the interpretation of pulmonary function tests.* New York: Projects in Health, Inc., 1974.

Bartels, H., E. Bucherl, C.W. Herty, G. Rodewald, and M. Schwab, *Methods in pulmonary physiology.* Translated by J.M. Workman. New York: Hafner, 1963.

Bates, D.V., P.T. Macklem, and R.V. Christie, *Respiratory function in disease.* Philadelphia: Saunders, 1971.

Blumenfeld, W., S.Z. Turney, and R.J. Denman, "A coaxial ultrasonic pneumotachometer." *Med. Biol. Eng.,* 1975, 13, 855–860.

Brantigan, J.W., V.L. Gott, M.L. Vestol, G.J. Fergusson, and W.H. Johnston, "A nonthrombogenic diffusion membrane for continuous *in vivo* measurement of blood gases by mass spectrometry." *J. Appl. Physiol.,* 1970, 28(3), 375–377.

Brantigan, J.W., V.L. Brantigan, and M.N. Martz, "A Teflon membrane for measurement of blood and intramyocardial gas tensions by mass spectroscopy." *J. Appl. Physiol.,* 1972, 32(2), 276–282.

Briscoe, W.A., and A.B. DuBois, "The relationship between airway resistance, airway conductance and lung volume in subjects of different age and body size." *J. Clin. Inv.,* 1958, 37, 1279–1285.

Buist, A.S., and B.B. Ross, "Predicted values for closing volumes using a modified single-breath nitrogen test." *Amer. Rev. Resp. Dis.,* 1973, 107, 744–752.

Clément, J., and K.P. van de Woestijne, "Pressure correction in volume and flow displacement body plethysmography." *J. Appl. Physiol.,* 1969, 27(6), 895–897.

Comroe, J.H., Jr., R.E. Forster, A.B. DuBois, W.A. Briscoe, and E. Carlsen, *The lung, clinical physiology and pulmonary function tests.* Chicago: Year Book, 1962.

Cotes, J.E., *Lung function.* 3rd ed. Oxford: Blackwell, 1975.

Daniels, A.U., L.A. Couvillon, and J.M. Lebrizzi, "Evaluation of N_2 analyzers." *Amer. Rev. Resp. Dis.,* 1975, 112(4), 571–575.

Dolfuss, R.E., J. Milic-Emili, and D.V. Bates, "Regional ventilation of the lung, studied with boluses of ^{133}Xe." *Respir. Physiol.,* 1967, 2, 235–246.

DuBois, A.B., S.Y. Botelho, G.N. Bedell, R. Marshall, and J.H. Comroe, Jr., "A rapid plethysmographic method for measuring thoracic gas volume. A comparison with a nitrogen washout method for measuring functional residual capacity in normal subjects." *J. Clin. Inv.,* 1956a, 35, 322–326.

DuBois, A.B., S.Y. Botelho, and J.H. Comroe, Jr., "A new method for measuring airway resistance in man using a body plethysmograph: Values in normal subjects and in patients with respiratory disease." *J. Clin. Inv.,* 1956b, 35, 327–336.

Finucane, K.E., B.A. Egan, and S.V. Dawson, "Linearity and frequency response of pneumotachographs." *J. Appl. Physiol.,* 1972, 10(2), 210–214.

Fleisch, A., "Der Pneumotachograph: ein Apparat zur Beischwindigkeitregstrierung der Atemluft." *Arch. Ges. Physiol.,* 1925, 209, 713–722.

Fowler, K.T., and J. Read, "Cardiac oscillations in expired gas tensions, and regional pulmonary blood flow." *J. Appl. Physiol.,* 1961, 16(5), 863–868.

Fowler, K.T., "The respiratory mass spectrometer." *Phys. Med. Biol.,* 1969, 14(2), 185–199.

Fowler, W.S., "Lung function studies III. Uneven pulmonary ventilation in normal subjects and in patients with pulmonary disease." *J. Appl. Physiol.,* 1949, 2, 283–299.

Fry, D.L., W.W. Stead, R.V. Ebert, R.I. Lubin, and H.S. Wells, "The measurement of intraesophageal pressure and its relationship to intrathoracic pressure." *J. Lab. Clin. Med.,* 1952, 40, 664–673.

Fry, D.L., R.E. Hyatt, C.B. McCall, and A.J. Mallos, "Evaluation of three types of respiratory flowmeters." *J. Appl. Physiol.,* 1957, 10(2), 210–214.

Fry, D.L., and R.E. Hyatt, "Pulmonary mechanics. A unified analysis of the relationship between pressure, volume and gas flow in the lungs of normal and diseased human subjects." *Amer. J. Med.,* 1960, 29, 672–689.

Hamilton, L.H., "Basic principles of gas chromatography, Part I and Part II." *J. Cardiovasc. Pulm. Tech.,* 1975, 3(2), 37; 3(3), 19.

Horowitz, J.G., F.P. Primiano, Jr., and C.F. Doershuk, "Variation in total respiratory impedance during breathing." *Proc. Ann. Conf. Eng. Med. Biol.,* 1976, 18, 362.

Hyatt, R.E., I.R. Zimmerman, G.M. Peters, and W.J. Sullivan, "Direct write-out of total respiratory resistance." *J. Appl. Physiol.,* 1970, 28(5), 675–678.

Knudson, R.J., M.D. Lebowitz, A.P. Burton, and D.E. Knudson, "The closing volume test: evaluation of nitrogen and bolus methods in a random population." *Am. Rev. Respir. Dis.,* 1977, 115, 423–434.

Leith, D.E., and J. Mead, *Principles of body plethysmography.* Bethesda, MD: NHLI, Division of Lung Diseases, 1974.

Ligas, J.R., F.P. Primiano, Jr., and G.M. Saidel, "A comparison of measures of forced expiration." *J. Appl. Physiol.,* 1977, 42(4), 607–613.

Lilly, J.C., "Flowmeter for recording respiratory flow of human subject," in J.H. Comroe, Jr. (ed.), *Methods in medical research,* Vol. 2. Chicago: Year Book, 1950, pp. 113–121.

Macklem, P.T., *Procedures for standardized measurements of lung mechanics.* Bethesda, MD: NHLI, Division of Lung Diseases, 1974.

Macklem, P.T., and J. Mead, "Resistance of central and peripheral airways measured by a retrograde catheter." *J. Appl. Physiol.,* 1967, 22(3), 395–401.

McCarthy, D.S., R. Spencer, R. Greene, and J. Milic-Emili, "Measurement of "Closing Volume" as a simple and sensitive test for early detection of small airway disease." *Amer. J. Med.,* 1972, 52, 747–753.

McNair, H.M., and E.J. Bonelli, *Basic gas chromatography.* Walnut Creek, CA: Varian Aerograph, 1969.

Mead, J., "Control of respiratory frequency." *J. Appl. Physiol.,* 1960, 15(3), 325–336.

Mead, J., J.M. Turner, P.T. Macklem, and J.B. Little, "Significance of the relationship between lung recoil and maximum expiratory flow." *J. Appl. Physiol.,* 1967, 22(1), 95–108.

Michaelson, E.D., E.D. Grassman, and W.R. Peters, "Pulmonary mechanics by spectral analyses of forced random noise." *J. Clin. Invest.,* 1975, 56(5), 1210–1230.

Milic-Emili, J., J. Mead, J.M. Turner, and E.M. Glauser, "Improved technique for estimating pleural pressure from esophageal balloons." *J. Appl. Physiol.,* 1964, 19(2), 207–211.

Milic-Emili, J., J.A.M. Henderson, M.B. Dolovich, D.Trop,

and K. Kaneko, "Regional distribution of inspired gas in the lung." *J. Appl. Physiol.*, 1966, 21(3), 749–759.

Peslin, R., C. Duvivier, and J. Morinet-Lambert, "Frequency response of the total respiratory system from 3 to 70 cps." *Bull. Physio-path. Resp.*, 1972a, 8, 267–279.

Peslin, R., J. Morinet-Lambert, and C. Duvivier, "Frequency response of pneumotachographs." *Bull. Physio-path. Resp.*, 1972b, 8, 1363–1376.

Pride, N.B., S. Permutt, R.L. Riley, and B. Bromberger-Barnae "Determinants of maximal expiratory flow from the lungs." *J. Appl. Physiol.*, 1967, 23, 646–662.

Primiano, F.P., Jr., and I. Greber, "Analysis of plethysmographic estimation of alveolar pressure." *IEEE Trans. Biomed. Eng.*, 1975, 22(5), 393–399.

Silverman, L., and J.L. Whittenberger, "Clinical pneumotachograph," in J.H. Comroe, Jr. (ed.) in *Methods in medical research*, Vol. 2. Chicago: Year Book, 1950, pp. 104–112.

Stanescu, D.C., J. Pattijn, J. Clément, and K.P. van de Woestijne, "Glottis opening and airway resistance." *J. Appl. Physiol.*, 1972, 32, 460–466.

Turney, S.Z., and W. Blumenfeld, "Heated Fleisch pneumotachometer: A calibration procedure." *J. Appl. Physiol.*, 1973, 34(1), 117–121.

Woolcock, A.J., N.J. Vincent, and P.T. Macklem, "Frequency dependence of compliance as a test for obstruction of the small airways." *J. Clin. Inv.*, 1969, 48, 1097–1106.

Zapletal, A., E.L. Motoyama, L.E. Gibson, and A. Bouhuys, "Pulmonary mechanics in asthma and cystic fibrosis." *Pediat.*, 1971, 48, 64–72.

Chapter ten

Clinical laboratory instrumentation

Lawrence A. Wheeler

The clinical laboratory is responsible for the analysis of patient specimens in order to provide information to aid in the diagnosis of disease and the effectiveness of therapy. The hospital department that performs these functions may also be called the department of clinical pathology or the department of laboratory medicine. The major sections of the clinical laboratory include *chemistry, hematology, microbiology,* and the *blood bank.*

The chemistry section performs analyses on blood, urine, cerebrospinal fluid (CSF), as well as other fluids, in order to determine how much of various clinically important substances they contain. Most applications of electronics in the clinical laboratory are in the chemistry section. The hematology section performs determinations of the number and characteristics of the formed elements in the blood (red blood cells, white blood cells, and platelets) as well as tests of the function of physiological systems in the blood (e.g., clotting studies). A number of the most frequently ordered of these tests have been automated on the Coulter Counter (see Section 10.6). The microbiology section performs studies on various body tissues and fluids to determine whether or not pathological microorganisms are present. Until recently, there was essentially no application of electronic instrumentation in microbiology. However, devices that automatically monitor the status of blood cultures (tests for the presence of microorganisms) are now being introduced into microbiology laboratories. The development of applications of electronic instrumentation for the blood bank is currently only beginning.

Since many critical patient-care decisions are based on test results supplied by the clinical laboratory, the accuracy and precision of these results is of paramount importance. Excellent design of equipment and effective quality-control programs are essential to achieve this aim. Although this topic is beyond the scope of this chapter, it is important for anyone involved in the design or use of clinical laboratory instrumentation to be continually aware of the potentially tragic outcome of erroneous test results.

A second important characteristic of many test procedures is fast response, since in many critical clinical situations the therapy selected by the physician depends on the test results. The application of electronics in the clinical laboratory has greatly decreased the time required to perform a wide variety of important tests.

10.1 Spectrophotometry

Spectrophotometry forms the basis for many of the instruments used in clinical chemistry. The primary reasons for this are ease of measurement, satisfactory accuracy and precision, and ability to utilize spectrophotometric techniques in automated instruments. In this section, the term *spectrophotometer* is used as a general term for a class of instruments. Photometers and colorimeters are members of this class.

Spectrophotometry is based on the property of substances of clinical interest to selectively absorb or emit electromagnetic energy at different wavelengths. For most laboratory applications, wavelengths in the ranges of the ultraviolet (200 to 400 nm), the visible (400 to 700 nm) and the near infrared (700 to 800 nm) are used, with the majority of the instruments operating in the visible range.

Figure 10.1 shows a general block diagram for a spectrophotometer-type instrument. The source supplies the radiant energy used to analyze the sample. The wavelength selector allows energy in a limited wavelength band to pass through. The cuvette holds the sample to be analyzed in the path of the energy. The detector produces an electrical output that is proportional to the amount of energy it receives, and the readout device indicates the received energy or some function of it (e.g., the concentration in the sample of a substance of interest).

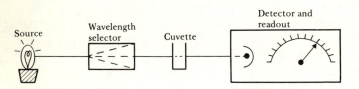

Figure 10.1 Block diagram of a spectrophotometer. (Based on R.J. Henry, D.C. Cannon, and J.W. Winkelman, eds. *Clinical Chemistry,* 2nd ed. Hagerstown, MD: Harper & Row, 1974.)

The basic principle of a spectrophotometer is that if we examine an appropriately chosen, sufficiently small portion of the electromagnetic spectrum, we can use the energy-absorption properties of a substance of interest to measure the concentration of the substance present. In the vast majority of cases, these substances, as normally found in a patient's samples (e.g., serum, urine, CSF), do not have the desired energy-absorption characteristics. In such cases, *reagents* are added to the sample, causing a reaction to occur. The reaction yields a product that does have the desired characteristics. The reaction products are then placed in the cuvette for analysis. The instrument-calibration procedures take into account the possible difference in concentration of the reaction product and of the original quantity of interest.

Let us discuss in detail the characteristics of each of the subsystems shown in Figure 10.1.

Power sources

Hydrogen or deuterium discharge lamps are used to provide power in the 200- to 360-nm range and tungsten filament lamps are used for the 360- to 800-nm range. Hydrogen and deuterium lamps produce both continuous and discrete spectra. Tungsten filament lamps produce a continuous spectrum. A problem with these power sources is that they produce about 90% of their power in the infrared range. The output in the ultraviolet and visible ranges can be increased by operating the lamp at voltages above the rated value, but this significantly reduces the expected life of the lamp. Another problem with tungsten lamps is that, during operation, the tungsten progressively vaporizes from the filament and condenses on the glass envelope. This coating, which is in general uneven, alters the spectral characteristics of the lamp and can cause errors in determinations.

The power supply used to supply the power source must be very well regulated. The output of the lamp below 800 nm varies as the fourth power of the filament voltage. Three basic types of power supplies have been used in spectrophotometers: batteries, constant-voltage transformers, and electronic power supplies. Batteries are primarily used in instruments that provide a high degree of portability. New nickel-cadmium batteries offer the advantages of dry cells along with being rechargeable. Their application is limited by their relatively small current output. Use of battery-operated equipment in the modern clinical laboratory is at present very limited.

Constant-voltage transformer power supplies are capable of providing adequate voltage regulation if the voltage supplied to them is reasonably well controlled. These devices, however, are particularly sensitive to variations in frequency. Constant-voltage transformer power supplies are very reliable suppliers of power because they do not include active elements.

When very close regulation of voltage is required, as is the case with most spectrophotometers, electronic power supplies are used. Modern instruments generally have solid-state components.

Wavelength selectors

A variety of devices are used to select portions of the power spectrum produced by the power source to be used to analyze the sample. These devices can be divided into two classes: filters and monochromators. There are two basic types of filters: glass and interference. *Glass filters* function by absorbing power. For example, a blue-colored filter absorbs in the higher wavelength visible range (red region) and transmits in the lower wavelength visible range (blue-green region). These filters (consisting of one or more layers of glass plates) are designed to be low-pass, high-pass, or bandpass (combination of low- and high-pass) ones, as shown in Figure 10.2.

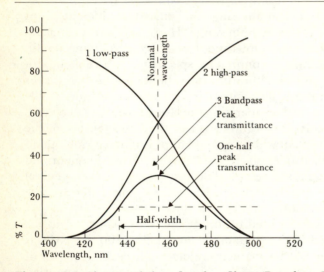

Figure 10.2 Characteristics of a glass filter. (Based on R.J. Henry, D.C. Cannon, and J.W. Winkelman, eds., *Clinical Chemistry,* 2nd ed. Hagerstown, MD: Harper & Row, 1974.)

In this figure, *%T* represents the percent *transmittance* of the incident light passed by the filter at any specified wavelength. Bandpass filters are designated by the wavelength at which they maximally pass power (i.e., their peak transmittance). For example, filter 480 has a peak transmittance at 480 nm. The usual bandwidth of glass filters is 50 nm. Figure 10.2 shows that as the bandwidth is reduced by "moving" the low-pass and high-pass filter characteristics closer together, the peak transmittance decreases. At a bandwidth of 30 nm, the peak transmittance is about 10%, which is too small for most applications.

Interference filters are made by spacing reflecting surfaces so that the incident light is reflected back and forth a short distance. The distance is selected so that light in the wavelength band of interest tends to be in phase and to be reinforced; light outside this band is out of phase and is canceled (interference effect). Harmonics of the frequencies in this band are also passed and must be eliminated by glass cutoff filters.

Several methods of constructing interference filters have been used. One commonly used type has two layers of half-silvered glass (with silvered sides facing each other) separated by a transparent dielectric spacer. This type of filter has a bandwidth of 10 to 15 nm with peak transmittance of 40 to 60%. They are available from 340 to 900 nm and provide very rapid symmetric roll-off with very high rejection of wavelengths more than 50 nm away from the nominal wavelength.

Another type, a multilayer interference filter, is similar except that it has successive layers of dielectric with high and low refractive indexes. This filter has excellent characteristics, with bandwidths as low as 4 nm and 90% peak transmittance. It can be designed to operate in most of the ultraviolet region. Two negative aspects of the multilayer interference filter are (a) relatively high cost and (b) the presence of harmonics within 50 to 100 nm of the filter's nominal wavelength.

Glass filters are used in applications in which only modest accuracy is required. Interference filters are used in many spectrophotometers, including the SMA 12/60 (Technicon Instrument Corporation) and CentrifiChem (Union Carbide) (see Section 10.2). Devices that use filters as their wavelength selectors are called *colorimeters* or *photometers*.

Monochromators are devices that utilize prisms and diffraction gratings. They provide very narrow bandwidths and have adjustable nominal wavelengths. The basic principle of these devices is to spatially disperse the input beam as a function of wavelength. A mechanical device is then used to allow wavelengths in the band of interest to pass through a slit.

Prisms are constructed from glass and quartz. Quartz is required for wavelengths below 350 nm. A convergent lens system is used to direct the light from the source through an entrance slit. The prism bends the light as a function of wavelength. The smaller wavelengths (ultraviolet) are bent the most. This produces an output beam in which the wavelength band of interest can be selectively passed by placing an opaque substance with a slit in it in the light path. The wavelength spectrum of the power passing through the slit is nominally triangle-shaped. In prisms, as in filters, the wavelength at which maximum transmittance occurs is the nominal central wavelength. Bandwidths of 0.5 nm can be obtained with this type of device. Prisms have been used over the wavelength range of 220 to 950 nm. The nonlinear spatial distribution of the power emergent from a prism requires relatively complex mechanical devices for slit-position control to select different nominal wavelengths.

Gratings are constructed by inscribing a large number of closely spaced parallel lines on glass or metal. A grating utilizes the principle that rays of light bend around sharp corners. The degree of bending is a function of wavelength. This results in a separation of the light into a spectrum at each line. As these wavefronts move and interact, the phenomenon of reinforcement and cancellation occurs. The light emerging from a grating is resolved spatially in a linear fashion, as opposed to the light from a prism, in which the separation of wavelengths is less at longer wavelengths. A grating uses a slit, as is the case with a prism, to select the desired bandwidth. The mechanics of the slit-positioning mechanism of a grating are less complicated than those of a prism, due to the linearity of the spatial separation of the wavelengths. Gratings can achieve bandwidths down to 0.5 nm and operate over the range of 200 to 800 nm.

An original grating is very expensive to produce. With the exception of extremely accurate research applications, replicas of the original grating are used. In the replication process, imperfections can occur. The number of imperfections is inversely related to the complexity of the replication process, and therefore to the cost of the grating. The imperfections cause the passage of light outside the bandwidth (other than harmonics, which always occur). This light is called *stray light*. In applications in which the effect of stray light causes significant errors—which is not the case in usual clinical laboratory applications—two diffraction monochromators operating in series essentially eliminate this problem. Of course this is an expensive approach.

Cuvette

The cuvette (Figure 10.1) holds the substance being analyzed. Its optical characteristics must be such that it does not significantly alter the spectral characteristics of the light as it enters or leaves the cuvette. The degree of care and expense involved in cuvette design is a function of the overall accuracy required of the spectrophotometer.

Sample

The sample (actually, in most cases, the substances resulting from the interaction of the patient specimen and appropriate reagents) selectively absorbs light according to the laws of Lambert, Bouguer, Bunsen, Roscoe, and Beer (Malinin and Yoe, 1961). The principles stated in these laws are usually grouped together and called *Beer's law*. The essence of the law was stated by Bouguer: "Equal thicknesses of an absorbing material will absorb a constant fraction of the energy incident upon it." This relationship can be stated formally as follows:

$$P = P_0 \, 10^{-aLC} \tag{10.1}$$

where

P_0 = radiant power arriving at cuvette
P = radiant power leaving cuvette
a = absorptivity of sample
L = length of the path through the sample
C = concentration of absorbing substance

Absorptivity is a function of the characteristics of the sample and the wavelength content of the incident light. This relationship is often rewritten in the form

$$\%T = 100 \, \frac{P}{P_0} = (100) 10^{-aLC} \tag{10.2}$$

where $\%T$ is the percent transmittance. The value of a is a constant for a particular unknown, and the cuvette and cuvette holder are designed to keep L as constant as possible. Therefore changes in P should reflect changes in the concentration in the sample of the absorbing substance.

Percent transmittance is often reported as the result of the determination; however, since the relation between concentration and percent transmittance is logarithmic, it has been found convenient to report absorbance. Absorbance A is defined as the log (P_0/P), so that

$$A = \log\left(\frac{P_0}{P}\right) = \log\left(\frac{100}{\%T}\right) = 2 - \log\,(\%T) \tag{10.3}$$

Note that the relationship

$$A = aLC \tag{10.4}$$

follows from (10.1) and (10.3). As previously stated, the spectrophotometer is designed to keep a and L as constant as possible so that a particular determination A ideally varies only with C. Therefore the concentration of an unknown could be determined as follows. The absorbance A_s of a standard with known concentration of the substance of interest C_s is determined. Next the absorbance of the unknown A_u is determined. Finally the concentration of the unknown C_u is computed, using the relationship

$$C_u = C_s\left(\frac{A_u}{A_s}\right) \tag{10.5}$$

If this relationship holds over the possible range of concentration of the unknown substance in patient samples, then the determination is said to obey Beer's law. This relationship may not hold because of absorption by the solvent or reflections at the cuvette. Then a relatively large number of standards with concentration values spanning the range of interest must be used to compute a calibration curve of concentration versus absorbance. This curve is then used to obtain a concentration value for the absorbance value of the unknown.

The amount of light absorbed by a compound is generally a function of wavelength, as shown by the solid line in Figure 10.3. The chemical reaction used in preparing the sample for spectrophotometry is designed to produce a compound whose concentration is proportional to the compound of interest and whose absorption spectrum's peak is separated from the absorption peaks of the other compounds in the sample.

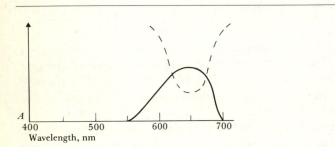

Figure 10.3 Example of absorption versus wavelength characteristics for a sample (solid line) and a bandpass filter (dashed line). (Based on R.J. Henry, D.C. Cannon, and J.W. Winkelman, eds.: *Clinical Chemistry,* 2nd ed. Hagerstown, MD: Harper & Row, 1974.)

The wavelength band of light allowed to pass through the wavelength selector is generally chosen to symmetrically cover the peak of the absorption curve. An example of this is shown by the dashed line in Figure 10.3. There are a number of other factors to consider, however. These include the absolute level of absorbance at the peak and its wavelength value. If the absorbance is too great ($A > 1.0$) or too small ($A < 0.11$), the errors of the photometric system become unacceptably large (Davidsohn and Henry, 1974). In the case in which the absorbance is very large, the sample can be diluted, but this procedure is time-consuming and can result in errors. The wavelength of the peak must be within the range of the spectrophotometer's capabilities.

Photometric system

A spectrophotometer's photometric system includes devices to measure the amount of power leaving the cuvette (detectors)

(Section 2.16), circuits for the amplification of the low currents developed by detectors (amplifiers) (Chapter 3), and devices to present the results of the determination to the technologist operating the instrument (meters or recorders). Commonly used detectors include barrier layer cells, phototubes, and photoconductive cells.

Design of meters for this application has been somewhat of a problem in the past years due to the need for precision and the nonlinear relationship between the detected quantity (power) and the quantity of interest (absorption). Now, with the development of low-cost digital electronics, the problems of computation and data presentation have been largely eliminated.

Flame photometers

Flame photometers differ in three important ways from the instruments previously discussed. First, the power source and the sample-holder function are combined in the flame. Second, in the primary utilization of flame photometry, the basic concept is the measurement of the emission of light by the sample rather than the absorption of light, although we shall also discuss atomic absorption-type flame photometers. Schematic representations of these two types of instruments are shown in Figure 10.4. Third, only determinations of the concentrations of pure metals can be accomplished.

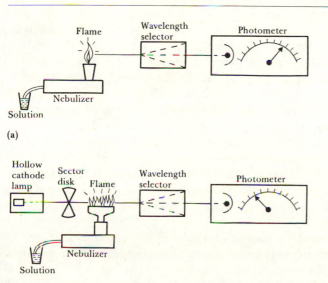

Figure 10.4 Block diagrams of instruments for (a) flame emission and (b) flame absorption. (Based on R.J. Henry, D.C. Cannon, and J.W. Winkelman, eds.: *Clinical Chemistry,* 2nd ed. Hagerstown, MD: Harper & Row, 1974.)

Atomic-emission instruments are based on the principle that when an atom in an excited state returns to the ground state, it emits power at a characteristic wavelength. The power required to raise the atoms to the excited state is supplied by the flame. The amount of radiation emitted at a particular wavelength is proportional to the concentration of the corresponding atom.

Atomic-absorption instruments use the same reaction, operating in the reverse direction. A source of radiant power at the characteristic wavelength of the atom to be analyzed is used to produce a beam that is passed through the flame. The atoms in the flame selectively absorb power at their characteristic wavelengths as they are raised to an excited state. The degree of power absorption at a particular wavelength is proportional to the concentration of the corresponding atom.

Atomic emission

At the normal levels of power used in flame photometers, only about 1% of the atoms are raised to the excited state. In addition, only a few elements produce relatively large amounts of power at a single wavelength as they move from higher-energy to lower-energy orbits. These two factors have essentially limited the use of atomic-emission flame photometry to determinations of Na^+, K^+, and Li^+. Instruments have been developed that can make determinations of other elements, such as Ca^{2+}, but relatively complicated optical systems are required.

As shown in Figure 10.4(a), the sample combined with a solvent is drawn into a nebulizer that converts the liquid into a fine aerosol that is injected into the flame. Several types of fuels have been used in flame photometers. Currently propane or natural gas mixed with compressed air is used. The solvent evaporates in the flame, leaving microscopic particles of the sample. These particles disintegrate to yield atoms. As mentioned previously, only a small portion of these atoms are in excited states. As the atoms fall to ground state, they release power at their characteristic wavelength.

A simple optical system—including only a filter and a lens to focus the filtered light on the detector—is normally used for determinations of Na^+ and K^+. If other determinations are being done, more sophisticated optical systems, including a monochromator, are required.

Many modern atomic-emission flame photometers are designed to include an internal standard to compensate for variations in the rate of solution uptake, aerosol production, and flame characteristics. Lithium (Li^+) is used for this purpose. It is not normally found in biologic samples, it has a high emission intensity, and its peak emission wavelength is well separated from those of sodium and potassium. A carefully controlled amount of Li^+ salt is added to the sample. An optical channel is provided to measure the power emitted by the Li^+, which, along with the known concentration of Li^+, is used to correct the determination of Na^+ or K^+ for variations in the instrument. Actually, in most applications, the determinations of Na^+, K^+, and Li^+ are done in parallel.

There are a few problems with the use of Li^+ as the internal standard. First, while it can correct for small variations in the characteristics of the instrument, it cannot correct for large variations. Second, Li^+ is being increasingly used for treatment of an important psychotic disorder—manic-depressive psychosis. If patients with this disorder were not identified to the clinical laboratory, significant errors in determinations of Na^+ and K^+ could occur. It is an unfortunate fact that the clinical laboratory is rarely given any clinical information to use in judging the accuracy of determinations.

Atomic absorption

This is a relatively new technique that has shown great promise for the very accurate determination of the concentration of a variety of elements, including calcium, lead, copper, zinc, iron, and magnesium. It is based on the fact that the vast majority of atoms in a flame absorb energy at a characteristic wavelength. A special power source is used that emits power at the characteristic wavelength of the atom whose concentration is being determined. This source is a hollow cathode lamp. These lamps are constructed from the metal to be determined or are lined with a coating of it. In most cases, a separate lamp is needed for each metal determination, but the special characteristics of a few metals make it possible to use one lamp for combinations of two or three of them. The cathode is placed in an atmosphere of an inert gas. When the cathode is heated, the atoms of the cathode leave the surface of the cathode and fill the cathode cavity with an atomic vapor. These atoms become excited due to collisions with electrons and ions. As these atoms return to the ground state, they release power at their characteristic wavelength, as previously discussed. This power is directed through the flame [see Figure 10.4(b)], and the amount of absorption is proportional to the amount of the atom present.

Atomic-absorption flame photometers normally require a monochromator and use a photomultiplier as the detector. One additional feature of these devices is that, since the atoms in the flame emit as well as absorb power at the characteristic wavelength, it is necessary to be able to differentiate between the two sources of power reaching the detector. This is accomplished by designing the source to produce pulses of power rather than a steady output level. This is usually done by placing a rotating-sector disk between the source and the flame. The detection electronics are designed using the phase-sensitive detector described in Section 3.15 to eliminate the dc component and analyze only the ac signal.

Fluorometry

This technique is based on the property of a number of molecules emitting light in a characteristic spectrum, the emission spectrum, essentially immediately after absorbing radiant energy and being raised to an excited state. The degree to which the molecules are excited depends on the amplitude and wavelength content of the radiant power in the excitation spectrum. Small amounts of power are lost in this process, which results in the emission spectrum being generally higher in wavelength content than the excitation spectrum.

The various options of power sources, wavelength selectors, and detection circuits just discussed are used in fluorometers of varying sensitivity. Mercury arc lamps are commonly used power sources. They produce major line spectra at 365, 405, 436, and 546 nm. Photomultipliers are normally used as detectors. A unique feature of these devices is the need to select operational bandwidths for two spectra, excitation and emission. Figure 10.5 shows a fluorometer block diagram. The detector is placed at a right angle to the power source to minimize the chance of direct transmission of light from the source to the detector. The wavelength characteristics of the wavelength selector are also chosen so that there is little or no overlap in the wavelengths they pass.

One advantage fluorometry has over spectrophotometric methods is its much greater sensitivity. This improvement may be as much as four orders of magnitude. This is due to the fact that in spectrophotometric methods, the difference between the absorption of a solution assumed to have a zero concentration ($\%T = 100$) of the unknown substance and the sample is used as a measure of the concentration of the unknown substance. With highly dilute samples (that is, $\%T = 98$), small errors in the process can cause large percent errors in the determination. In fluorometry, a direct measurement of the fluorescence of the sample is used to determine the concentration of the unknown substance.

A special advantage of fluorometry is its great specificity. A problem with spectrophotometric methods is that the light absorbed in the wavelength band is used by substances other than the unknown. In fluorometry, only a relatively small number of substances have the property of fluorescence. Thus many substances that might interfere with a spectrophotometric measurement cannot interfere with a determination of fluorescence. Also, substances that have similar excitation spectra may have different emission spectra, and vice versa. Therefore, appropriate selection

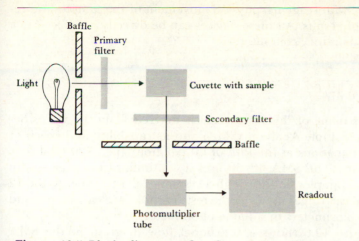

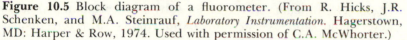

Figure 10.5 Block diagram of a fluorometer. (From R. Hicks, J.R. Schenken, and M.A. Steinrauf, *Laboratory Instrumentation*. Hagerstown, MD: Harper & Row, 1974. Used with permission of C.A. McWhorter.)

of the bandwidths of the two wavelength selectors can provide additional rejection of noise.

The combination of these characteristics makes fluorometry capable of detecting picogram amounts of unknown substances. Highly dilute samples are used to prevent the effect of the light produced by fluorescence from being absorbed by other molecules as it passes through the sample solution.

The principal disadvantage of fluorometry is the sensitivity of its determinations to temperature and pH of the sample (fluorescence in general is pH-sensitive).

10.2 Automated chemical analyzers

In this section, we shall describe three important examples of automated chemical analyzers. They are the SMA 12/60, the CentrifiChem, and the ACA (DuPont). Each of these devices offers great increases in productivity of the clinical laboratory and/or decreased response time for emergency requests (called STAT requests). The SMA 12/60 has been available for a number of years and is widely used in medium-size and large clinical laboratories. The CentrifiChem and the ACA have become available in the last few years, and their current utilization in clinical laboratories is much less than that of the SMA 12/60. Each of these devices utilizes spectrophotometric methods for making the actual measurements of the chemical quantity of interest. They differ in the way they perform the steps of sample aspiration, dilution, combination of sample with reagents, physical movement of the sample, and recording of results. All these devices can be directly interfaced to a central laboratory computer.

SMA 12/60

The name of this instrument is derived from the words Sequential Multiple Analyzer (SMA) and its capability to do each of 12 determinations at the rate of 60 per hour (i.e., 720 total tests each hour). The SMA 12/60 uses a continuous-flow concept, in which the samples flow through a system of plastic tubes to the 12 analytical cartridges in which the test reactions are carried out and then to colorimeters or a flame photometer.

Figure 10.6 shows a functional flow diagram of the SMA 12/60. The functions of the major subsystems are outlined below. Refer to the company's literature (Anonymous, 1974) for a detailed discussion.

Sampler

The sampler aspirates a portion of the patient's plasma from a sample cup. Forty of these sample cups are placed in a plastic ring-shaped holder that can be rotated automatically. After each sample aspiration, first air (to provide intersample segmentation), then wash solution, and finally air (to provide further intersample segmentation) are aspirated. The output of the aspirator goes into a plastic tube. The contents of the tube are propelled down it by the proportioning pump.

Proportioning pump

The proportioning pump performs two functions. It provides the pressure to move the samples through the instrument and it introduces air bubbles into the fluid passing through the plastic tubing. These bubbles clean the tubing by a wiping action on the wall and form additional barriers to intersample mixing by preventing laminar flow. The sample is then divided and delivered to the 12 analytical cartridges.

Analytical cartridge

The functions of heating and sampling and reagent combination (including dialysis when required) are performed in the analytical cartridges. There are two types of heating bath

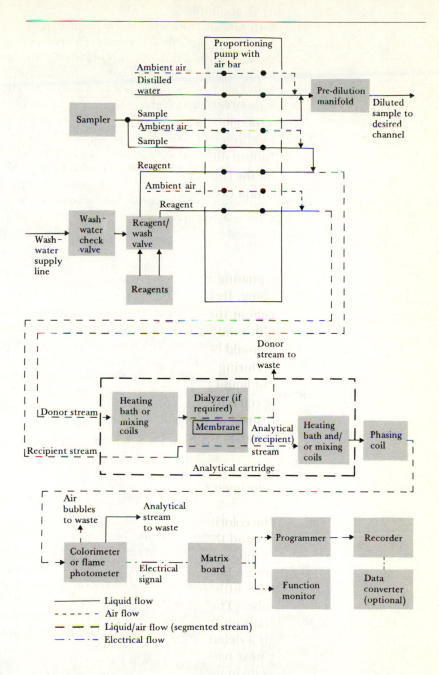

Figure 10.6 Block diagram of SMA 12/60. (From *Product Labeling for the Technicon 12/60 Multichannel Biochemical Analyzer*, Tech. Pub. UA4-0160-00, 4/74, volume 1, pages 6–7. Reproduced by courtesy of Technicon Instruments Corporation.)

assemblies. One provides fixed temperatures of 37.5 or 45°C. The other provides a variable temperature capability.

For many determinations, combining the sample and the reagents is accomplished by causing the sample stream and the reagent stream to pass on opposite sides of a dialysis membrane. The lower-molecular-weight substances of interest pass through to the reagent stream, whereas the higher-molecular-weight substances that cannot pass through (primarily protein) remain with the sample stream that goes to a waste container. Determinations of cholesterol, albumin, total bilirubin, direct bilirubin, lactate dehydrogenase, total protein, and fractionated lactate dehydrogenase do not utilize dialysis. In these determinations, a membrane is not used and the two streams are directly combined. In either case, the combination of sample and reagents is called the *analytical stream.*

Phasing coil

A phasing coil is constructed of a series of parallel loops of glass tubing. Its function is to adjust the arrival time of the analytical stream at the colorimeter (or flame photometer if sodium or potassium is one of the determinations being performed).

It should be stressed that the SMA 12/60 is a continuous-flow device. During operation of the instrument, there is always a stream of liquid passing through all the tubes. The function of the phasing coil is to control the time at which the portion of the analytical stream that contains the combination of the sample and the reagent passes through the colorimeter.

Colorimeter

The colorimeter has five optical channels arranged in a semicircle around the light source. There are four colorimeters in the SMA 12/60. Four of the channels each include two sets of lens, an interference filter, an adjustable aperture, a flowcell, and a phototube. The fifth channel, the reference channel, includes only a phototube. (The function of the reference channel is described in the discussion of the programmer.) The analytical stream passes through a debubbler as it enters the colorimeter. The debubbled stream next passes through the flowcell. The flowcell functions as the cuvette in the determination. The wavelength characteristics of the interference filter used depend on the determination being performed. The phototube provides an electrical signal that is proportional to the intensity of the light reaching it. Four different types of phototube are used, depending on the type of interference filter required for the determination. The outputs of the phototubes are connected to the programmer (via the matrix board).

For some determinations, the sample may contain substances

whose concentration is not being determined, but which absorb significant amounts of light in the wavelength range in which the determination is made. To eliminate the effect of these substances, a "blank channel" is used. The blank channel includes the sample and the reagents, but the reaction required for the determination is not allowed to occur. Each determination that requires a blank channel has both the corresponding analytical stream and the blank stream analyzed by the same colorimeter. In this way the output of the blank channel includes both the effect of the light-absorbing substances in the sample and variations in the intensity of the source lamp. Determinations that require blanks include lactate dehydrogenase (LDH), serum glutamic pyruvic transaminase (SGPT), total bilirubin, and total protein. A total of four blank channels is available.

Programmer

The programmer controls the operation of the SMA 12/60. Its primary functions include the overall synchronization of the instrument's operation, calibration of the instrument, and control of the sampling rate and sample-to-wash ratios. The primary timing signal of the system is produced by an optical device mounted on a constant-speed motor. The resulting timing pulses are routed to an electronic counter and a decoding network. The outputs of the decoder network are connected to inverter circuits that produce the current to select the appropriate relay on a relay switching board. The first channel is selected for 9 s, the next ten for 4.5 s each, and the last channel for 6 s to complete the processing of all channels in 60 s. The timing of the instrument is designed such that, when it is properly calibrated, a channel's relay is closed when the determination has reached steady state. Each sample channel produces a sequence of relatively flat periods (corresponding to the time the wash solution is passing through the colorimeter) and peaks (corresponding to the time the sample is passing through it). The outputs of the colorimeter, including the sample channel, blank channel (when used), and the reference channel, are connected to function boards via the matrix board. The function boards perform a signal-conditioning function. Their outputs are connected to preamplifiers via the appropriate relay board. The preamplifier outputs are connected to a log-ratio board that converts from transmittance to absorbance and subtracts either the corresponding reference or blank value from the sample value. This is done to remove the effects of variations in the light source and, in the case of the blank channel, the effects of absorption of light by substances other than the unknown quantity. The output of the log-ratio board is connected to a recorder and a CRT. The CRT is used by the technologist to select the phase coil during calibration and to monitor the operation of the instrument.

Recorder

A strip-chart recorder is used for recording the result on a preprinted form. This form includes numerical scales for each determination and, if desired, a gray zone denoting the corresponding normal range. In addition, the results may be fed to a laboratory computer that processes the data and prints out patient reports, thereby saving time spent on manual data logging and computation.

CentrifiChem

The CentrifiChem is based on a method developed at the Oak Ridge National Laboratory (Anderson, 1969). A block diagram of the system is shown in Figure 10.7. The CentrifiChem is composed of two major components, a pipettor and an analyzer. The function of the pipettor is to automatically load accurately measured quantities of specimen (1 to 50 μl) combined with diluent (10 to 50 μl) and the reagents used for the particular test being performed (250 or 350 μl) into separate wells in a transfer disk. There are 30 pairs of sample and reagent wells in the transfer disk. The same test is performed on all samples. The very small quantities of sample and

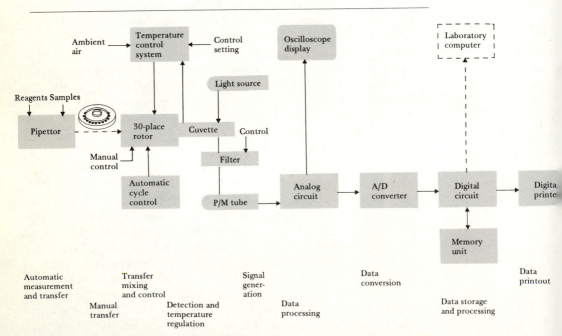

Figure 10.7 Block diagram of CentrifiChem. (From *CentrifiChem System Instruction Manual*, Union Carbide Corporation, Rye, New York.)

reagents required are a significant advantage of this instrument. In many cases, in particular with infants, it is very difficult to obtain the quantities of blood needed to run a large number of tests using other methods. CentrifiChem's requirement for small volumes of reagent leads to savings of tens of thousands of dollars per year in a laboratory serving a medium-sized hospital (300 to 500 beds). These savings should recover the cost of the machine in a few years.

The second major unit of the CentrifiChem is the analyzer. The transfer disk is placed in a rotor in the analyzer. The analyzer controls, which are set for the particular test being performed, include the following.

1 Filter selection This control operates a servomotor that positions a nine-position filter wheel. These filters are the interference type (see Section 10.1).

2 Temperature selection Reaction temperatures of 25, 30, and 37°C can be selected. The temperature is controlled by the temperature of a stream of air that is blown over the rotor.

3 Blank control The control allows a blank reading to be made and subsequently subtracted from all cuvette readings.

4 Terminal-rate switch This switch is used to select either the terminal or rate modes of data analysis. The characteristics of these types of operations are discussed in the following.

After the controls have been set, the rotor is spun up to a speed of 900 rev/min (rpm) in approximately 2 s. During this acceleration period, the sample and the reagents are moved by centrifugal force into their individual cuvettes. A bubble stream is drawn through them to ensure mixing. The rotor continues to rotate at 900 rpm until the entire measurement procedure is completed.

Each cuvette is constructed to allow light to pass through the reaction mixture. The light enters a quartz window, travels 1 cm through the reaction mixture, and exits through a glass base plate. There is one fixed set of light source, optics, filter, and photomultiplier (PM) tube. As the rotor spins, the cuvettes sequentially pass through the light beam and the percent transmittance is measured. The characteristics of colorimeter systems are described in Section 10.1. The emphasis in this discussion is on the CentrifiChem's electronic subsystem.

Timing signals derived from the position of the rotor are used to synchronize the operation of the system's electronics. A timing pulse is produced every 2 ms. The position of the rotor is also used to identify which cuvette is currently being read by the colorimeter. The PM output is passed through a log amplifier to convert the transmittance into absorbance. Next, the analog absorbance voltage enters a sample-and-hold circuit that detects and stores its peak value. The analog voltage representing the peak absorbance value is displayed on an oscilloscope for use by the technologist in monitoring the operation of the CentrifiChem. The timing on the display is designed such that the current level of absorbance in each cuvette is continuously displayed. The output of the sample-and-hold circuit is also connected to a 12-bit ADC.

The digital data from the ADC are fed to an eight-bit microprocessor, designated the "digital circuit" in Figure 10.7. The microprocessor is programmed to carry out the following functions: read test parameters from the front panel, process the absorbance data from the PM tube, print the results, and recognize special instructions that occur after printout of the data (Miranda and Hatziemmanuel, 1976). The special instructions to be processed include reading the contents of data gathered and stored in memory, updating the memory on command, recalculating the data and printing them, and restarting the test without slowing the rotor.

The system was designed around a microprocessor, the Intel 8008, because this approach provided greater reliability and flexibility than hard-wired digital circuits, and also lowered the total cost. In addition to the 8008 CPU, the digital circuit contains a clock used to determine terminal or rate-reaction times (controlled by the CPU) and an input multiplexer to route the data in the proper sequence. The block labeled memory unit in Figure 10.7 includes RAM for storage of data and control parameters such as rotor position, ROM for the storage of the test sequence and other instructions, and output registers for the storage of processed data to be printed.

The operation of the system depends on the use of the interrupt function (Section 3.16). The parameters required for the two types of reactions are: initial time (T_0 in Figure 10.8), ΔT, the position of the filter (determined by the test to be performed), selection of type of reaction, and units of concentration or absorbance. These parameters may be entered via front-panel thumbwheel

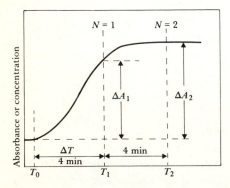

Figure 10.8 Measurements of terminal-reaction mode. (From *CentrifiChem System Instruction Manual*, Union Carbide Corporation, Rye, New York.)

switches or automatically selected from program memory by the CPU for a particular test selection.

Two interrupts control the processing of absorbance data: a *once-around* pulse from the rotor and a *data-ready* signal from the ADC. Each time a conversion of the analog signal to digital form is completed, the data-ready interrupt signal causes the CPU to transfer the data into memory and to subtract the control absorbance from the reading. When the once-around interrupt is received, the CPU checks to see that all 30 cells in the rotor were read and restarts the process. If all 30 cells were not read, the CPU discards the data and initiates a new run.

This and other self-checking routines are possible only with a microprocessor-based system. The results from eight revolutions of the rotor are averaged to reduce the effect of noise on the results. The T_0 and ΔT parameters are also handled by interrupts to the CPU. Output of data is initiated by an interrupt signal from the printer. When no interrupt signal is received, the CPU can process data, calculate averages, and update the output storage registers.

The microprocessor is programmed to perform one of two types of analyses, terminal reaction or rate reaction. These analyses are briefly discussed here. See the literature by Union Carbide (Anonymous, 1975) for a detailed discussion of the calculations that are performed.

The *terminal-reaction analysis* is used when the absorption of the cuvette after the chemical reaction has gone to completion is proportional to the concentration of the unknown substance. Figure 10.8 shows that three absorption readings are made in this mode. The first is 3 s after the rotor has begun to spin. This measurement is stored in track 1 (one of the two areas in memory in which averaged absorption readings are stored, as discussed above). The second set of readings is taken 4 min later, and is stored in track 2. The processor subtracts the values in track 1 from those in track 2 (removing the absorption reading of the non-reacted substances) and outputs these results on a small printer. This procedure is repeated in another 4 min.

If these two readings agree within a specified tolerance, the determination is completed; otherwise the process is allowed to continue for another 4 min, and another check is made. This procedure is continued until two consecutive values agree within the tolerance. This ensures the fact that the terminal level has been obtained.

The *rate reaction* is subdivided into two types: initial rate and standard rate (see Figure 10.9). In the initial-rate reactions, it is the initial rate of the reaction that is linearly related to the concentration of the quantity of interest. In the standard-rate reaction, it is the rate after the initial period of 2 min that is linearly related to concentration. These analyses differ only in the time delay from the beginning of spin to when the first measurement is made and

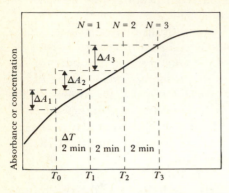

Figure 10.9 Measurements of rate-reaction mode. (From *CentrifiChem System Instruction Manual*, Union Carbide Corporation, Rye, New York.)

the spacing of the measurements. Since it is the rate of the reaction that is of interest, the slope of the absorption-versus-time curve is the quantity computed by the processor. Three slope values are computed and printed. The multiple readings are made to ensure that the rate of the reaction is constant at the point the determination is made.

The terminal-reaction method of analysis is used with determinations of substances such as albumin, bilirubin, and glucose. The initial-rate reaction is used in tests for creatinine, cholesterol, and blood urea nitrogen (BUN) among others. The standard-rate reaction is used primarily in determinations of enzymes. Enzyme tests are one of the strong points of the CentrifiChem. Enzyme concentrations of particular clinical importance that are evaluated by this device are alkaline phosphatase, creatinine phosphokinase (CPK), lactate dehydrogenase (LDH), serum glutamic oxaloacetic transaminase (SGOT), and serum glutamic pyruvic transaminase (SGPT).

ACA

The DuPont Automatic Clinical Analyzer (ACA) differs from the SMA 12/60 and the CentrifiChem in that it is oriented toward flexibility rather than maximizing throughput. It performs determinations in serial rather than in parallel, but it can select any of 40 tests for each sample. A functional block of the ACA is given in Figure 10.10 (Anonymous, 1975).

The ACA uses the unique concept of combining the sample with the reagents in the analytical test pack (ATP). There is a different ATP for each determination made by the ACA. During the operation of the ACA, the ATP moves from station to station on a conveyer. Any sequence of ATPs can be selected. The time re-

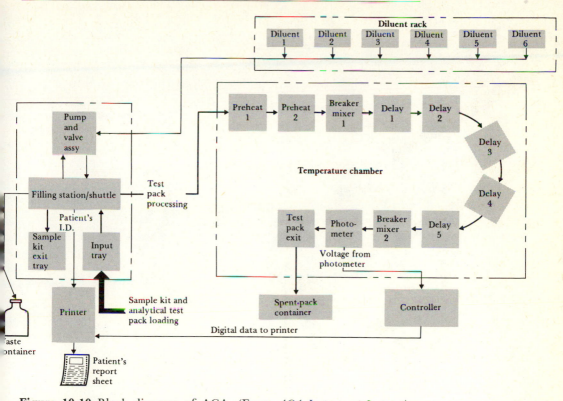

Figure 10.10 Block diagram of ACA. (From *ACA Instrument Instruction Manual,* DuPont Company, Automatic Clinical Analysis Division, Wilmington, DE 19898.)

quired to perform any of the ACA determinations is 7 min, with a 37 s spacing between completions of determinations. This means that the ACA can be used to perform any of its determinations as STAT requests. This feature gives the clinical laboratory an important new capability. As expected, this flexibility results in a higher cost per test than other automated methods. However, the details of these economic considerations are beyond the scope of this text. Let us now discuss the general characteristics of the ACA.

The patient sample is placed in a special holder called a sample kit, which has a patient-identification card attached to it. The ATPs corresponding to the determinations that are to be made on the sample are loaded behind the sample kit on the conveyer mechanism. Figure 10.11 shows the construction of the ATP. The last ATP is followed by a special end-of-run kit. The basic operations carried out by each subsystem are as follows.

Patient identification When the sample kit first enters the ACA, it passes through a station in which the patient-identification

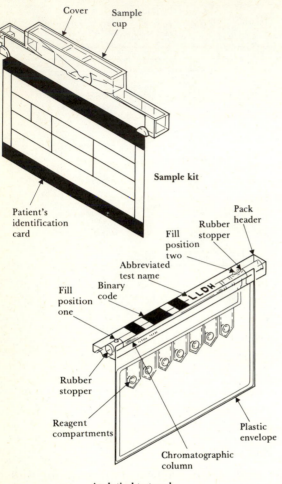

Cover

Sample cup

Sample kit

Patient's identification card

Pack header

Rubber stopper

Fill position two

Abbreviated test name

Fill position one

Binary code

Rubber stopper

Reagent compartments

Plastic envelope

Chromatographic column

Analytical test pack

Figure 10.11 Sample kit and analytical test pack of ACA. (From *ACA Instrument Instruction Manual,* DuPont Company, Automatic Clinical Analysis Division, Wilmington, DE 19898.)

information that has been entered manually on the patient-identification card on the side of the sample kit is transferred to the printer paper. This is accomplished by use of a system of an ultraviolet lamp and sensitized paper.

Filling station In the filling station, *aliquots* (measured liquid volumes) of the sample are withdrawn from the sample kit and mixed with a diluent (which may be different for different determinations). Then 5 ml of the combined solution is injected into each ATP. The ATP's binary code is read by electronic devices in the filling station to determine which diluent to use for that particular ATP. After the ATPs have been filled, they continue to the preheaters and the sample kits are placed in the sample-kit exit tray.

Preheaters In the preheaters, the ATP is heated to 37°C, and is maintained at this temperature for the remainder of the process.

Breaker-mixer 1 At this station, the reagents in four of the plastic compartments (see Figure 10.11) are crushed and mixed with the diluted sample.

Delay stations As the ATP successively passes through the five delay stations, the chemical reactions of the first four reagents, diluent, and sample occur.

Breaker-mixer 2 Here the last three reagent compartments are crushed and mixed with the reaction solution. For some determinations, a delay is included here to allow sufficient time for the reactions to go to completion before the ATP enters the photometer station. This delay is controlled by the binary code that was read in the filling station and that identified the type of test.

Photometer In the photometer, the plastic envelope of the ATP is formed into a cuvette by a unique pressure device. The pressure in the plastic pack is measured and used to determine whether an adequate amount of sample and diluent has been inserted in the ATP. If the pressure is too low, the test result is flagged with the letter P. The ATP binary code is again decoded, and this information is used by the photometer control board to select measurement method, filter type, and ADC constants. The control board uses an array of 21 ferrite cores for storage of data.

The ACA can use one of three measurement methods: rate, two-filter, and two-pack. In the rate method, the change in absorption of the cuvette during a fixed period is used as the measure of the concentration of the unknown. In the two-filter method, measurements of absorption are made with two different filters. The measurement of the concentration of the unknown is proportional to the difference between these absorption values. The two-pack method uses the difference between the absorption of the unknown combined with different reagents in the two ATPs at the same wavelength band as the determination. The output of the photometer is converted to digital form (as specified by the photometer controller) and sent to the printer.

Printer The printer prepares the ACA report, which includes the patient-identification information obtained in the filling station and the photometer results for all the ATPs filled with the patient's sample.

10.3 Blood-gas and acid-base measurements

The fast and accurate measurement of the blood levels of the partial pressure of oxygen (Po_2), the partial pressure of CO_2 (Pco_2), and the concentration of hydrogen ions (pH) are vital in the diagnosis and treatment of many pathological conditions. Significant abnormalities of these quantities can rapidly be fatal if not treated appropriately. These measurements are usually made on specimens of arterial blood, although "arterialized" venous samples are often obtained from infants.

The Po_2 level is a measure of the degree of O_2 content (in the absence of a significant decrease in the hemoglobin level or decrease in its O_2-carrying capacity, such as in carbon monoxide poisoning) of the arterial blood.

For young adults, normal ranges of Po_2 in arterial blood are from 90 to 100 mm Hg (12 to 13.3 kPa). Due to the sigmoid nature of the O_2 disassociation curve, a Po_2 of 60 mm Hg (8 kPa) still provides an O_2 saturation of 85%. Decreases in Po_2 are seen in a variety of settings. These can be divided into (1) decreased delivery of O_2 to the site of O_2 exchange between the inspired air and the blood (i.e., the lung alveoli) and (2) decreased delivery of blood to the alveoli to which O_2 is being supplied. Examples of the first group include decreased overall ventilation (e.g., narcotic overdose or paralysis of the respiratory muscles), obstruction of major airways (e.g., aspirated foreign objects such as food, or spasm of the airway muscles, such as that which occurs in an acute attack of asthma), or filling of the alveoli and small airways with fluid (e.g., pneumonia or aspiration of water in drowning). Examples of the second group include congenital cardiac abnormalities, in which blood is shunted past the lungs (e.g., the Tetralogy of Fallot), and obstruction of flow through the pulmonary blood vessels (e.g., pulmonary emboli). The important lung diseases of emphysema and chronic bronchitis usually display characteristics of both these types of abnormalities.

The Pco_2 level is an indicator of the adequacy of ventilation, and is therefore increased in the first group of disorders discussed above, but it is generally normal in the second group unless the defect is massive in nature. In young adults the normal range of Pco_2 in arterial blood is 35 to 40 mm Hg (4.7 to 5.3 kPa).

The acid-base status of the blood is assessed by measuring the hydrogen ion concentration [H^+]. It is conventional to use the negative logarithm to the base 10 (pH) to report this quantity, that is

$$pH = -\log_{10} [H^+] \tag{10.6}$$

The normal range of pH in arterial blood is 7.38 to 7.44. Decreases in pH (i.e., increased quantity of hydrogen ions) occur with a decreased rate of excretion of CO_2 (respiratory acidosis) and/or with increased production of fixed acid (e.g., diabetic ketoacidosis) or abnormal losses of bicarbonate (the principal hydrogen-ion buffer in the blood). Acidosis resulting from the last two processes is called metabolic acidosis. Increases in pH (i.e., decreased quantity of hydrogen ions) occur with an increased rate of excretion of CO_2 (respiratory alkalosis) and/or abnormal losses of acid (e.g., from prolonged vomiting), which is called metabolic alkalosis. Note that a measurement of P_{CO_2}, or the level of bicarbonate in the blood, along with a measurement of pH must be done to be able to classify the type of acid-base abnormality (Davenport, 1975).

The basic concepts of ions, electrochemical cells, and reference cells are discussed in Chapter 5. This section shows how these concepts are used to design electrodes for the measurement of pH, P_{CO_2}, and P_{O_2}.

Measurement of pH

The measurement of pH is accomplished by utilizing a glass electrode with the property of generating an electrical potential when solutions of differing pH are placed on the two sides of its membrane (Cremer, 1906). Figure 10.12 gives a block diagram of a pH electrode.

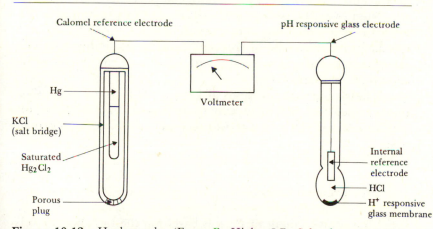

Figure 10.12 pH electrode. (From R. Hicks, J.R. Schenken, and M.A. Steinrauf, *Laboratory Instrumentation*. Hagerstown, MD: Harper & Row, 1974. Used with permission of C.A. McWhorter.)

The glass electrode is a member of the class of ion-specific electrodes that react to any extent only with the specific ion. The approach of a hydrogen ion to the outside of the membrane causes the silicate structure of the glass to conduct a positive charge (hole) into the ionic solution inside the electrode. The Nernst equation [Equation (4.1)] applies, so the voltage across the membrane changes by 60 mV/pH unit. Since the range of physiological pH is only 0.06 pH units, the pH meter must be capable of accurately measuring changes of 0.1 mV.

The basic approach is to place a solution of known pH on the inside of the membrane and the unknown solution on the outside. Hydrochloric acid is usually used as the solution of known pH. A reference electrode, usually an Ag-AgCl or a saturated calomel electrode, is placed in this solution. A second reference electrode is placed in the specimen chamber. A salt bridge is included within the reference to prevent the chemical constituents of the specimen from affecting the voltage of the reference electrode. The potential developed across the membrane of the glass electrode is read by a pH meter. This pH meter must have an extremely high input impedance, because the internal impedance of the pH electrode is in the 10- to 100-MΩ range.

The Nernst equation shows that the voltage produced by a pH electrode varies with the temperature of the specimen and the reference solution. Some pH electrodes include a water bath that allows the pH determination to be made at 37°C, while others require a temperature correction. This temperature correction can be made by changing the constant used to convert from the electrode voltage to the meter scale reading in pH units by setting a temperature-control knob to the temperature at which the pH measurement is being made. A more complex correction has been suggested (Adamsons et $al.$, 1964; Burton, 1965) that includes the effect on instrument output of temperature and the CO_2 content of the specimen. This type of correction can be made in modern devices that measure pH and P_{CO_2}, and in addition have memory and computational capabilities.

Calibration with solutions of known pH is performed before measurements of patient specimens are made. Two solutions, one with a pH near 6.8 and one with the pH near 7.9, are normally used.

Measurement of P_{CO_2}

The measurement of P_{CO_2} is based on the fact that the relation between log P_{CO_2} and pH is linear over the range of 10 to 90 mm Hg (1.3 to 12 kPa), which includes essentially all the values of clinical interest. This result can be established by an examination of some fundamental chemical relationships between H^+, H_2CO_3, HCO_3^-, and P_{CO_2}. The first three quantities are related by the equilibrium equation

$$H_2O + CO_2 \rightleftharpoons H_2CO_3 \rightleftharpoons H^+ + HCO_3^- \qquad (10.7)$$

In addition, the relationship between P_{CO_2} and the concentration of CO_2 dissolved in the blood, $[CO_2]$, is given by

$$[CO_2] = a(P_{CO_2}) \qquad (10.8)$$

where $a = 0.0301$ mmol/liter per mm Hg P_{CO_2}. The mass relationship corresponding to (10.7) can then be written as

$$k' = \frac{[H^+][HCO_3^-]}{[H_2CO_3]} \qquad (10.9)$$

Next we use the fact that the $[H_2CO_3]$ is proportional to $[CO_2]$ to obtain the result

$$k = \frac{[H^+][HCO_3^-]}{[CO_2]} \qquad (10.10)$$

where k represents the combined values of k' and the proportionality constant between $[H_2CO_3]$ and $[CO_2]$. Now, using (10.8), we obtain the following result:

$$k = \frac{[H^+][HCO_3^-]}{aP_{CO_2}} \qquad (10.11)$$

Next, taking the base-10 logarithm of (10.11) and rearranging, we obtain

$$\log [H^+] + \log [HCO_3^-] - \log k - \log a - \log P_{CO_2} = 0 \qquad (10.12)$$

Using the definition of pH results in

$$pH = \log [HCO_3^-] - \log k - \log a - \log P_{CO_2} \qquad (10.13)$$

This shows that pH has a linear dependence on the negative of log P_{CO_2}.

This result is used in the construction of the P_{CO_2} electrode shown in Figure 10.13 (Severinghaus, 1965). The assembly includes two chambers, one for the specimen and a second containing a pH electrode of the type discussed. In contrast to the basic pH measurement device in which the pH electrode is placed in the specimen, in this case the pH electrode is bathed by a buffer solution of bicarbonate and NaCl.

The two chambers are separated by a semipermeable membrane, usually made of Teflon. This membrane allows dissolved CO_2 to pass through, but blocks the passage of charged particles, in particular H^+ and HCO_3^-. When the specimen is placed in its chamber, CO_2 diffuses across the membrane to establish the same concentration in both chambers. If there is a net movement of CO_2 into or out of the chamber containing the buffer, $[H^+]$ increases or decreases, respectively, and the pH meter detects this change. Since the relationship between pH and the negative log P_{CO_2} is only

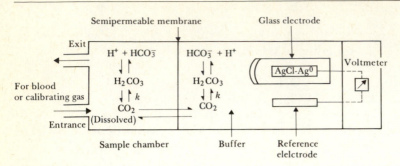

Figure 10.13 P_{CO_2} electrode. (From R. Hicks, J.R. Schenken, and M.A. Steinrauf, *Laboratory Instrumentation*. Hagerstown, MD: Harper & Row, 1974. Used with permission of C.A. McWhorter.)

a proportional one, it is necessary to calibrate the instrument before each use with two gases of known P_{CO_2}.

Using the values of pH obtained from processing these two standards, we obtain a calibration curve of P_{CO_2} versus pH. We then use the measured pH value to obtain the specimen's P_{CO_2} from this curve. With some instruments, the capability of calibrating the P_{CO_2} electrode is built into the instrument so that the calibration curve is set up in the electronics of the instrument by setting the values of two potentiometers.

The P_{O_2} electrode

Figure 10.14 shows the basic components of the Clark-type polarographic electrode (Fatt, 1976). The measurement of P_{O_2} is based on the following reactions. At the cathode, reduction occurs:

$$O_2 + 2H_2O + 4e^- \rightarrow 2H_2O_2 + 4e^- \rightarrow 4OH^-$$
$$4OH^- + 4KCl \rightarrow 4KOH + 4Cl^- \tag{10.14}$$

At the anode, which in this P_{O_2} electrode is the reference electrode, oxidation occurs.

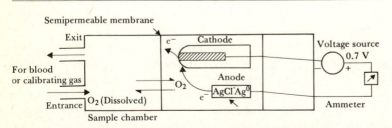

Figure 10.14 P_{O_2} electrode. (From R. Hicks, J.R. Schenken, and M.A. Steinrauf, *Laboratory Instrumentation*. Hagerstown, MD: Harper & Row, 1974. Used with permission of C.A. McWhorter.)

$$4Ag + 4Cl^- \rightarrow 4AgCl + 4e^- \qquad (10.15)$$

This produces the four electrons required for the reaction in (10.14). The cathode is constructed of glass-coated Pt and the reference electrode is made of Ag-AgCl. A polarizing voltage of 600 to 800 mV is required for these reactions to occur. This voltage is usually supplied by a mercury cell.

We determine the value of Po_2 by using the fact that the flow of current through the external circuit connecting the electrodes is proportional to Po_2. The presence of O_2 and the resulting chemical reaction can be thought of as producing a variable source of current in the circuit whose value is directly proportional to the Po_2 level. When the Po_2 level is zero, the current flowing through the circuit is called the background current. Part of the calibration sequence involves setting the Po_2 meter to zero when a CO_2/N_2 gas is bubbled through the specimen chamber.

Equation (10.14) shows that the reaction consumes O_2. This loss is a direct function of the area of the Pt electrode exposed to the reaction solution and the permeability of the semipermeable membrane to O_2. The exposed area of the Pt electrode usually has a diameter of 20 μm.

The polarizing voltage is selected to provide a sufficient potential to drive the reaction, without permitting other electrochemical reactions that would be driven by greater voltages to take place. The choice of the semipermeable membrane is based on a tradeoff between consumption of O_2 and the time required for the Po_2 values in the specimen and measurement chambers to equilibrate. The more permeable the membrane to O_2, the higher the consumption of O_2 and the faster the response. Polypropylene is less permeable than Teflon and is preferable in most applications. Polypropylene is also quite durable, and maintains its position over the electrode more reliably than other membrane materials. Since the electrode consumes O_2, it partially depletes the oxygen in the immediate vicinity of the membrane. If movement of the sample takes place, undepleted solution brought to the membrane causes a higher instrument reading—the "stirring" artifact. This is avoided by waiting for a stagnant equilibrium to occur.

The reaction is very sensitive to temperature. To maintain a linear relationship between Po_2 and current, the temperature of the electrode must be controlled to $\pm 0.1°C$. This has been traditionally accomplished by using a water jacket. However, new blood-gas analyzers are now available that use precision electronic heat sources. The current through the meter is approximately 10 nA/mm Hg (75 nA/kPa) O_2 at 37°C, so that the instruments must be designed to be accurate at very low current levels.

The system is calibrated by using two gases of known O_2 concentration. One gas with no O_2, typically a CO_2/N_2 mixture, and a second with a known O_2 content, usually an O_2-CO_2-N_2 mixture, are used. The specimen chamber is filled with water and the calibrating gas containing no O_2 is bubbled through it. The P_{O_2} meter output is set to zero after equilibrium of O_2 content is achieved, usually in about 90 s. Next, the second calibrating gas is used to determine the second point on the P_{O_2}-versus-electrode-current calibration scale (that is electrically set in the machine). Then the value of the specimen P_{O_2} can be measured. It should be noted that the time required to reach equilibrium is a function of the P_{O_2} of the specimen. It may take as long as 360 s for a specimen with a P_{O_2} of 430 mm Hg (57 kPa) (Moran *et al.*, 1966) to reach equilibrium.

10.4 Chromatography

Chromatography is basically a group of methods for separating a mixture of substances into component parts. Although the use of the term chromatography is firmly established, *chromatography* is really a misnomer, since the color of the mixture's components is not really used to identify substances in modern techniques. All chromatographic techniques involve the use of two phases. One phase is fixed—liquid or solid—and the other is mobile—gas or liquid. When a liquid stationary phase is used, the process is called *adsorption*. When a solid stationary phase is used, the process is called *partition*.

A common feature of these methods is that differences in the rate of movement of components of the mixture in the mobile phase caused by interaction of these components with the stationary phase are used to separate the components (Cawley, 1965). The four possible combinations of stationary and mobile phases have been used in chromatographic methods.

From the viewpoint of the clinical laboratory, these methods are primarily used for the detection of complex substances such as drugs and hormones. For example, *gas-liquid chromatographs* (GLC) and *thin-layer chromatographs* (TLC) have been useful in determining the drug or drugs used in overdoses. The availability of this information is vitally important to the clinician in selecting appropriate therapy. The characteristics of the GLC are presented here as an important example of the use of chromatographic methods in the clinical laboratory.

Gas-liquid chromatographs

The basic components of a GLC are shown in Figure 10.15. Prior to being injected into the GLC, the patient sample usually must undergo some initial purification, the extent of which depends on the particular determination that is being performed.

The functions of the major subsystem units are as follows.

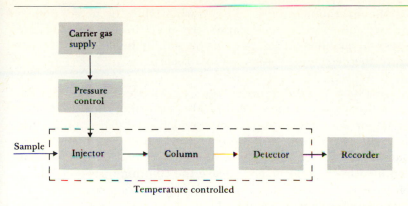

Figure 10.15 Block diagram of a gas-liquid chromatograph (GLC).

Injector The injector is used to introduce 1 to 5 ml of the patient sample contained in a solvent (usually a volatile organic solvent) into the GLC. The temperature of the injector is set to flash-evaporate the sample and solvent.

Carrier gas The inert carrier gas (usually N_2 or He) is the mobile phase of the chromatograph. It sweeps the evaporated sample and solvent gas down the column.

Column The column typically is less than 7 mm in diameter and 1 m long. It is packed with the solid support material (e.g., diatomaceous earth). The solid support is coated with the liquid phase. The small size of the solid beads produces a very large surface area for interaction of the mobile and stationary phases. This interaction produces the separation of the components. The column is enclosed in an oven whose temperature is carefully controlled. A temperature programmer gradually increases the temperature of the column in a sequence designed for maximum efficiency of separation for the particular type of substance being analyzed.

Detector The detector is located at the end of the column. Its function is to provide an electrical output proportional to the quantity of the compound in the effluent gas. A number of types of detectors are available for use with different types of samples. They include ionization detectors, thermal-conductivity detectors (Section 9.7), and electron-capture detectors. Ionization detectors are most commonly used in clinical laboratory applications. A discussion of the physical principles employed in these detectors is beyond the scope of this chapter. See Littlewood (1970).

All the detectors are sensitive to classes of compounds, not only to some particular component of interest. Therefore both the concentration of the detected compounds and the time during the operation of the column when they occurred (i.e., a concentration-versus-time graph) are used in determining the types and quantities of components present in the sample. The output of the detector is connected to a recorder.

Recorder   In the recorder, the x axis represents time and the y axis the output of the detector. The recording thus provides a display of the quantity of a component (i.e., the area under the peak) that was present and the time at which it was eluted off the column. From this information, the components present can be identified by the time taken to leave the column, or preferably by comparison with recordings obtained by analyzing compounds of known composition with the GLC.

Figure 10.16 shows a recording obtained from the analysis of a blood specimen for the levels of the important anticonvulsant drugs phenobarbital and phenytoin. A measured amount of heptabarbital was added to the specimen to serve as an internal standard. The area under the phenobarbital and phenytoin curve is compared with the area under the heptabarbital curve to compute the blood levels of these drugs.

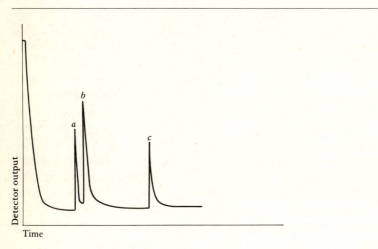

Figure 10.16 Example of a GLC recording for the analysis of blood levels of phenobarbital (peak *a*) and phenytoin (peak *c*). Peak *b* corresponds to the level of heptabarbital (the internal standard).

Gas-liquid chromatography provides a number of important capabilities in the analysis of complex compounds. They include speed, ability to operate with small amounts of sample, and great sensitivity. Most instruments can complete analyses of clinically important substances in less than 1 h, often 15 min or less. As mentioned previously, only milliliter amounts of the sample are needed. The sensitivity of the device depends on the detector used, but good-quality instruments can detect 1-ng quantities of a compound.

10.5 Electrophoresis

Devices based on electrophoretic principles are used in the clinical laboratory to measure quantities of the various types of protein in plasma, urine, and CSF; to separate enzymes into their component isoenzymes; to identify antibodies; and for a variety of other applications.

Basic principles

Electrophoresis may in general be defined as the movement of a solid phase with respect to a liquid (the buffer solution). The main functions of the buffer solution are to carry the current and to keep the pH of the solution constant during the migration. The buffer solution is supported by a solid substance called the *medium*.

The discussion in this section is limited to zone electrophoresis. In this technique, the sample is applied to the medium; and under the effect of the electric field, groups of particles with similar charge, size, and shape characteristics migrate at similar rates. This results in the separation of the particles into zones. The factors that affect the speed of migration of the particles in the field are discussed in the following paragraphs.

Magnitude of charge

The mobility of a given particle is directly related to the net magnitude of the particle's charge. Mobility is defined as "the distance in centimeters a particle moves in unit time per unit field strength, expressed as voltage drop per centimeter" [mobility = $cm^2/(V \cdot s)$] (Henry *et al.*, 1974).

Ionic strength of buffer

The more concentrated the buffer, the slower the rate of migration of the particles. This is because the greater the proportion of buffer ions present, the greater the proportion of the current they carry. It is also due to interaction between the buffer ions and the particles. Buffer ions such as the barbitals (Anonymous, 1975a) are monovalent and react minimally with the proteins. A relatively dilute buffer yields good separation of the components of the specimen, but the edges of the component areas are indistinct. A highly concentrated buffer results in less space between the components, but distinct area boundaries of the components. A potential problem with a concentrated buffer is the precipitation of certain types of proteins.

Temperature

Mobility is directly related to temperature. The flow of current through the resistance of the medium produces heat. This heat has two important effects on the electrophoresis. First, it causes the temperature of the medium to increase, which decreases its resistance and thereby causes the rate of migration to increase. Second, the heat causes water to evaporate from the surface of the medium. This increases the concentration of the particles and further increases the rate of migration. Due to these effects, either the applied voltage or the current must be held constant in order to maintain acceptable reproducibility of the procedures. For short runs at relatively low voltage levels, either can be held constant. But when a gel is used as the medium, heating is a significant problem. With this type of medium, constant-current sources are normally used to minimize production of heat.

Time

The distance of migration is directly related to the time it takes the electrophoresis to be carried out. Other factors that influence migration are electroendosmosis, chromatography, particle shape, "barrier" effect, "wick flow," and streaming potential. Henry *et al.* (1974) and Hicks *et al.* (1974) have discussions of these effects.

Types of support media

A large variety of support media have been used in various electrophoretic applications. They include paper, cellulose acetate, starch gel, agar gel, acrylamide gel, and sucrose. We discuss cellulose acetate electrophoresis here because it is used extensively in clinical laboratories and because the same general method is used with other media.

Cellulose acetate has a number of desirable properties compared with the paper that was the medium first used in electrophoresis. These include the following.

1 Very small quantities of sample required
2 Short time required for electrophoresis (15–20 min)

3 Improved resolution of component bands
4 Good mechanical strength when wet
5 No special preparation required
6 Easily cleared after staining
7 Regularity of pore sizes
8 Well suited for densitometry due to good transparency

Figure 10.17 shows the basic concepts of cellulose acetate electrophoresis. The cellulose acetate strip is saturated with the buffer solution and placed in the membrane holder (the "bridge"). The bridge is placed in the "cell," with both ends of the strip in the buffer wells.

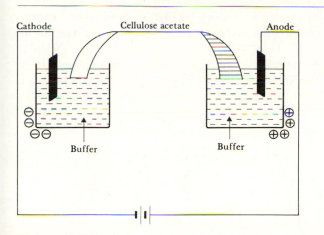

Figure 10.17 Cellulose acetate electrophoresis. (From R. Hicks, J.R. Schenken, and M.A. Steinrauf, *Laboratory Instrumentation*. Hagerstown, MD: Harper & Row, 1974. Used with permission of C.A. McWhorter.)

A number of electrophoreses (typically eight) can be done on one strip. The sample for each test is placed on the strip at a marked location. Next, the electrical potential is applied across the strip. With this type of electrophoresis, constant-voltage-source power supplies are often used. A typical voltage is 250 V, which results in an initial current of 4 to 6 mA. As discussed previously, this current increases slightly during the procedure. After 15 to 20 min, depending on the particular device used, the electrical voltage is removed. The next step is to fix the migrated protein bands to the buffer and to stain them so that they can be seen as well as subsequently quantitated. This may be done in separate or combined exposures to a fixative and a dye. The membrane is now "cleared" to make it transparent. The densities due to the dyed-specimen fractions are not affected. The membrane is dried in preparation for densitometry.

The *densitometer* is a device that consists of a light source, a filter, and a detector (typically a photodiode). The design and operation of this type of device was discussed in Section 10.1.

The membrane is placed in a holder in the densitometer. The path of migration of one of the specimens is then scanned. The low-voltage output of the detector is amplified by a very stable analog preamplifier. The output of the preamplifier is sent to an analog x-y recorder and to an analog integrator circuit. The x-y recorder produces a plot, with the x coordinate representing migration distance and the y coordinate representing membrane density (which is directly proportional to the amount of specimen component that has moved the corresponding migration distance). The integrator has circuitry that detects the beginning and end of a significant peak and computes the area under the peak. These numbers are printed on the analog recording next to the corresponding peak. This process is repeated for each of the specimens on the membrane.

Figure 10.18 presents examples of the types of plots which are obtained in performing electrophoresis. These plots are for serum protein electrophoresis.

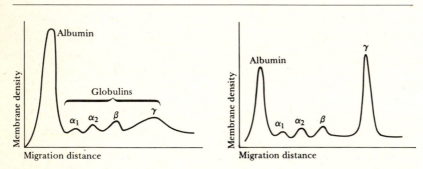

Figure 10.18 Examples of patterns of serum protein electrophoresis. The left-hand pattern is normal; the right-hand one is the pattern seen when there is an overproduction of a single type of gamma globulin.

10.6 Hematology

Basic concepts

The blood consists of formed elements, substances in solution, and water. This section covers only devices that measure characteristics of the formed elements. These formed elements consist of *red blood cells* (RBCs), *white blood cells* (WBCs), and *platelets*. The primary functions of the RBCs are to carry oxygen from the lungs to the various organs and to carry carbon dioxide back from these organs to the lungs for excretion. The primary function of the

WBCs is to help defend the body against infections. There are five normal types of WBCs. In order of decreasing numbers in the blood, they are: neutrophils, lymphocytes, monocytes, eosinophils, and basophils. In disease, the total number and relative proportions of these types of WBCs can change; in addition, abnormal types of WBCs appear. Platelets plug small breaks in the walls of blood vessels and also participate in the clotting mechanism.

The basic attribute of the formed elements in the blood that is measured is the number of elements of each type per microliter. The normal range of RBCs in an adult male is 4.6 to 6.2 $\times$ $10^6/\mu l$ and in an adult female, 4.2 to 5.4 $\times$ $10^6/\mu l$. The normal ranges of WBCs and platelet counts are the same for men and women. The normal range of the WBC count is 4,500 to 11,000/μl and that for the platelet count is 150,000 to 400,000/μl. The *hematocrit* (hct) is a determination of the ratio of the volume of all the formed elements in a sample of blood to the total volume of the blood sample. It is reported in percentage, with the normal range in adult men 40 to 54% and the normal range in adult women 35 to 47%. *Hemoglobin* (hgb) is a conjugated protein within the RBCs that transports most of the O_2 and a portion of the CO_2 that is carried in the blood. It is reported in grams per deciliter, with the normal range in adult men 13.5 to 18 g/dl and the normal range in adult women 12 to 16 g/dl.

A second group of measurements is made to characterize the RBC volume and hgb concentration. These measurements include the *mean corpuscular volume* (MCV) in cubic micrometers, the *mean corpuscular hemoglobin* (MCH) content in picograms, and the *mean corpuscular hemoglobin concentration* (MCHC) in percent. These values are called the RBC indexes. Normal ranges for these parameters are as follows.

MCV: 82–98 $(\mu m)^3$
MCH: 27–31 pg
MCHC: 32–36%

The RBC count (in millions per microliter), hct (in percent), MCV (in cubic micrometers), hgb (in grams per deciliter), MCH (in picograms) and MCHC (in percent) are related as follows.

$$MCV = 10 \text{ hct/RBC count} \qquad (10.16)$$

$$MCH = 10 \text{ hgb/RBC count} \qquad (10.17)$$

$$MCHC = 100 \text{ hgb/hct} \qquad (10.18)$$

The units for RBC count, hgb, and hct used in these calculations are such that the units for MCV, MCH, and MCHC are those given above.

Example 10.1 Calculate the RBC indexes from the following data.

RBC = 5 million/μl
hgb = 15 g/dl
hct = 45%

Answer

$$\text{MCV} = 10\,\frac{\text{hct}}{\text{RBC count}} = \frac{450}{5} = 90(\mu\text{m})^3$$

$$\text{MCH} = 10\,\frac{\text{hgb}}{\text{RBC count}} = \frac{150}{5} = 30 \text{ pg}$$

$$\text{MCHC} = 100\,\frac{\text{hgb}}{\text{hct}} = \frac{1500}{45} = 33.3\%$$

Electronic devices for measuring blood

There are two major classes of electronic devices for measuring blood. One type is based on changes in the electrical resistance of a solution when a formed blood element passes through an aperture. The Coulter Counter and Celloscope (Lors & Lundberg Co.) are examples of this type of device. The second type utilizes deflections of a light beam caused by a passage of formed blood elements to make its measurements. The Fisher Autocytometer and the Technicon Autoanalyzer are examples of this type. An excellent review of these types of devices is given in Brittin and Brecher (1971).

The series of types of Coulter Counters used in clinical laboratories include the models A, C, F, S, and Z. Let us review the characteristics of one of them—Model S—here. The analyzed sample is blood that has been anticoagulated, preferably with Versene or double oxalate. Anticoagulants are substances that interfere with the normal clot-forming mechanism of the blood. They keep the formed elements from being clumped together; clumping would prevent these elements from being accurately counted. The initial step in the analysis procedure is the automatic aspiration of a carefully measured portion of the specimen. Next, the specimen is diluted 1:224 with a solution of approximately the same osmolality as the plasma in Diluter I, Figure 10.19 (Pinkerton *et al.*, 1970). The diluted specimen is then split, with part going to the mixing and lyzing chamber and part to Diluter II.

The function of the diluting and lyzing chamber is to prepare the specimen for measurements of its hemoglobin content and WBC count. The lyzing agent causes the cell membranes of the RBCs to rupture and release their hemoglobin into the solution.

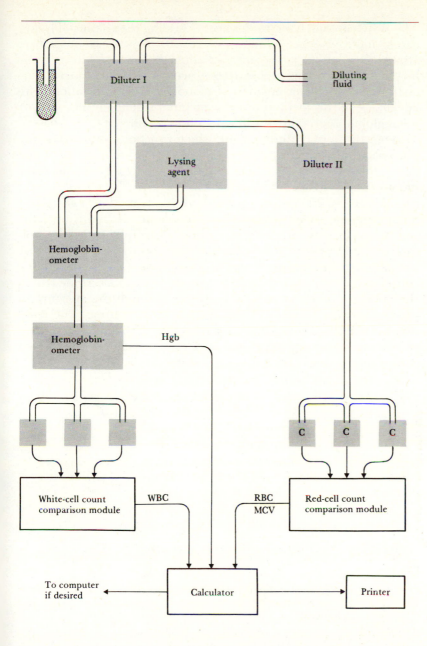

Figure 10.19 Block diagram of a Coulter Model S. (From I. Davidsohn and J.B. Henry, *Todd Sanford Clinical Diagnosis by Laboratory Methods,* 15th ed. Philadelphia: W.B. Saunders Co. Used with permission of W.B. Saunders Co.)

The WBCs are not lyzed by this agent. Adding the volume of lyzing agent increases the dilution to 1:250. A second substance, Drabkin's solution, is present that converts hemoglobin to cyanmethemoglobin. This is done to conform with the accepted standard method for determination of hemoglobin concentration. The advantage of this method is that it includes essentially all forms of hemoglobin found in the blood. The specimen is next passed through the WBC counting bath, which functions as a cuvette for the spectrophotometric determination (see Section 10.1) of the hemoglobin content. The final step in this process is the measurement of the WBC count.

Figure 10.20 outlines the method that is used in making this determination (Ackermann, 1972). This same method is used for counting RBCs. A vacuum pump draws a carefully controlled volume of fluid from the WBC-counting bath through the aperture. A constant current passes from one electrode (E_1) in the WBC-counting bath through the aperture to the second electrode (E_2) in the aperture tube. As each WBC passes through the aperture, it displaces a volume of the solution equal to its volume. The resistance of the WBC is much greater than that of the fluid, so that, in the circuit connecting the two electrodes, a voltage pulse is created whose magnitude is related to the volume of the WBC.

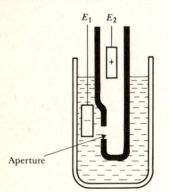

E_1 E_2

Aperture

Figure 10.20 Diagram of electrode placement for the Coulter Model S cell-counting circuit.

To increase the accuracy of the measurement, the system uses three parallel counting units. They share the common WBC-counting-bath electrode, and have individual aperture-tube electrodes. The output of each of these circuits is connected to a preamplifier. The amplified voltage pulses pass through a threshold circuit. (This threshold level is adjustable; the setting of it is discussed in the following.) Pulses that exceed the threshold enter a pulse-integrator circuit, which produces a dc voltage proportional to the WBC count. The outputs of the three pulse-integrator circuits are sent to a voting circuit. If the three outputs agree within a specified range, they are averaged. If one output disagrees with the other two by more than the specified range, it is not used in computing the average. If all three outputs disagree by more than the specified range, an error indicator is set and a zero value is produced.

The next step in the signal processing is to correct the average count signal for coincidence. Coincidence is the passage of two or more WBCs through the aperture at the same time. Statistical analysis is used to estimate the average level of coincidence for the aperture size and any uncorrected count level. An analog circuit makes this correction. The corrected count is now ready for analog-to-digital conversion. The digital value is displayed and also recorded on a printer.

We will now examine the right side of Figure 10.19. The first step is the further dilution of the specimen by $1:224$ in Diluter II. This second dilution is required because of the much greater concentration of RBC in the blood than WBC. A system identical to the one described for WBC count is used to obtain the RBC count. An additional RBC measurement is the MCV. This is made by averaging the magnitudes of the voltage pulses, since these values are proportional to the volume of the RBC.

The circuitry described to this point provides estimates of the RBC count, WBC count, hgb, and MCV of the specimen in digital form. These numbers are input to a special-purpose computer circuit that calculates the values of hct, MCH, and MCHC using the relationships given in (10.16), (10.17), and (10.18). The seven blood parameters are printed on a result report card. The printer includes a patient-identification number that is input to the Model S by the technologist. In computerized clinical laboratory systems, this identifying number and the seven blood parameters are directly transmitted to the central computer.

The threshold voltage is selected as part of the calibration procedure. Specimens with RBC and WBC count values determined by reference methods are processed and the threshold is set to give counts that agree with the reference values.

Automated differential counts

Determination of the proportion of the various types of WBCs (normal and abnormal) is called the *differential count*. It is given as the percent of each type of WBC present. Usually 100 or 200 WBCs are counted. The differential count has been traditionally done by having a technologist examine a smear of blood on a slide with a microscope. This is a time-consuming procedure, so an automated process would be very useful. In the past few years, several approaches to this problem have been developed. We shall briefly discuss one of these, the Hematrak (Geometric Data Corporation), to illustrate the direction of development of these new techniques.

The operation of the Hematrak is based on pattern-recognition techniques. The specimen that is evaluated is a blood smear stained with Wright's stain. Figure 10.21 shows the basic components of the system and the flow of information in the system (Levine, 1974). The smear is scanned by a color video scanner by means of microscope optics. The technologist selects the initial point for the scan. The device scans the smear until it finds a nucleated cell (mature RBCs of the type that are normally found in peripheral blood smears do not have nuclei). The digitized image of the cell is then transmitted into the image memory.

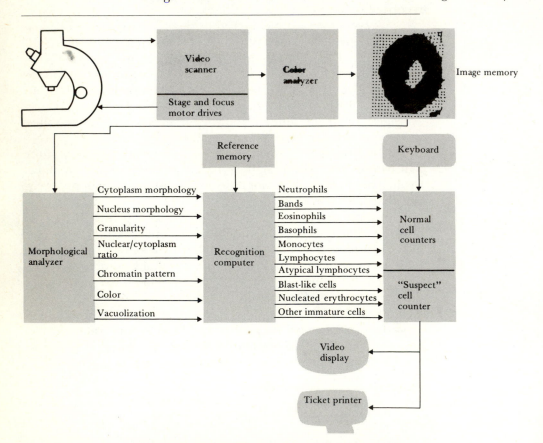

Figure 10.21 Block diagram of HEMATRAK. (From M. Levine, "Automated Differentials: Geometric Data's HEMATRAK," *Amer. J. Med. Tech.,* 40: 464, 1974.)

The morphological analyzer, a special-purpose digital device, then extracts important attributes of the cell, including nuclear morphology (shape), cytoplasmic morphology, nuclear/cytoplasm ratio, chromatin pattern, and cytoplasm characteristics. These attributes are transmitted to a recognition computer that compares these attributes to the stored attributes of various cell types (normal and abnormal) that can be found in the blood. The cell is classified as belonging to the group which its attributes most closely match. When a cell is classified as an abnormal form (e.g., an immature form such as those found in the blood in acute myelogenous leukemia), the scan is stopped and a signal is displayed to alert the technologist that a "suspicious" cell has been found. The technologist examines the cell and either accepts the Hematrak classification or enters a different classification on the keyboard.

The differential count is displayed on a CRT, printed on a test-result card similar to that used by the Coulter Counter, and, in a computerized clinical laboratory, sent directly to the central computer. The reader should see Dutcher *et al.* (1974) for further details on the system and the results of clinical trials of its effectiveness.

Problems

10.1 Discuss the differences between photometers or colorimeters and monochromators. What are the factors to be considered in selecting one or the other for a particular determination?

10.2 A filter photometer is being used to determine total concentration of serum protein (grams per deciliter). A technologist runs one standard with known total protein concentration of 8 g/dl and obtains a %T reading of 20%; processes a patient sample and gets a %T reading of 30%; assumes the instrument's operation satisfies Beer's law; and calculates the patient value. What value should be obtained? Would you agree with the methodology? If not, what would you do differently and why?

10.3 A spectrophotometer is being calibrated before being used to determine concentration of serum calcium. Four standards (i.e., samples of known calcium concentration) are analyzed, and given the following values.

Standards	% Transmittance	Calcium concentration, mg/dl
1	79.4	2
2	39.8	8
3	31.6	10
4	20.0	14

Does this determination follow Beer's law? If a patient sample were processed and a percentage of 35 were obtained, what would the calcium concentration be?

10.4 Sketch a double-beam spectrophotometer and explain its operation.

10.5 Discuss the reasons why fluorometers can be used to detect much smaller quantities of substances than absorption spectrophotometers.

10.6 Assume that you are the biomedical engineer at a 300-bed hospital. The clinical laboratory director plans to buy an automated chemical analyzer and wants your advice on which type to buy. What factors would you consider in your analysis? This is a broad question, but try to be as specific as possible in your response.

10.7 A blood specimen has a hydrogen-ion concentration of 40 nmole/liter and a P_{CO_2} of 60 mm Hg. What is the pH? What type of acid-base abnormality does the patient have?

10.8 Sketch a suitable design of an amplifier for the P_{O_2} electrode.

10.9 For normal changes in blood pH, how much will the pH meter voltage change?

10.10 The following values are obtained for a specimen of venous blood:

$$MCV = 90 \ (\mu m)^3$$
$$hct = 40\%$$
$$MCH = 30 \ pg$$

Compute the RBC count, the MCHC, and the hgb concentration.

10.11 Design a circuit to perform the RBC counting function in a Coulter Counter and include the voting logic.

References

Ackermann, P.G., *Electronic instrumentation in the clinical laboratory*. Boston: Little, Brown, 1972.

Adamsons, K., S.D. Salha, G. Gillian, and A. Games, "Influence of temperature on blood pH of the human adult and newborn." *J. Appl. Physiol.*, 1964, 19, 894.

Anderson, N.G., "Analytical techniques for cell fractions; XII, a multiple cuvet rotor for a new microanalytical system." *Anal. Biochem.*, 1969, 28, 545–562.

Anonymous, *Automatic clinical analyzer instruction manual*. Wilmington, Del.: DuPont, Automatic Clinical Analysis Division, 1975a.

Anonymous, *CentrifiChem instruction manual*. Rye, N.Y.: Union Carbide, 1975b.

Anonymous, *Microzone electrophoresis manual*. Fullerton, Calif.: Beckman Instruments, 1975c.

Anonymous, *Product labeling for the SMA 12/60 multichannel biochemical analyzer*, Tarrytown, N.Y.: Technicon Instruments Corporation, April 1974, Vols. I–III.

Brittin, G.M., and G. Brecher, "Instrumentation and automation in clinical hematology." *Prog. Hematol.*, 1971, 7, 299–341.

Burton, G.W., "Effects of the acid-base state upon the temperature coefficient of pH of blood." *Brit. J. Anesth.*, 1965, 37, 89.

Cawley, L.P., *Principles of chromatography.* In *Manual for workshop on chromatography.* Chicago: American Society of Clinical Pathologists, 1965.

Clark, L.C., "Monitor and control of blood and tissue oxygen tensions." *Trans. Amer. Soc. Artif. Intern. Organs*, 1956, 2, 41–47.

Cremer, M., "Zeitschrift fuer Biologie," *Z. Biol.*, 1906, 47, 562–611.

Davenport, H.W., *The ABC of acid-base chemistry*, 5th ed. Chicago: University of Chicago Press, 1975.

Davidsohn, I., and J.B. Henry, *Todd Sanford clinical diagnosis by laboratory methods*, 15th ed. Philadelphia: Saunders, 1974.

Dutcher, T.F., J.F. Benzel, J.J. Egan, D.F. Hart, and E.A. Christopher, "Evaluation of an automated differential leukocyte counting system." *Amer. J. Clin. Pathol.*, 1974, 62, 523–529.

Ellis, K.J., and J.F. Morrison, "Some sources of error and artifacts in spectrophotometric measurements." *Clin. Chem.*, 1975, 21, 776–779.

Fatt, I., *Polarographic oxygen sensors.* Cleveland: CRC Press, 1976.

Henry, R.J., D.C. Cannon, and J.W. Winkelman, *Clinical chemistry.* New York: Harper & Row, 1974.

Hicks, R., J.R. Schenken, and M.A. Steinrauf, *Laboratory instrumentation.* New York: Harper & Row, 1974.

Levine, M., "Automated differentials: Geometric Data's HEMATRAK." *Amer. J. Med. Tech.*, 1974, 40, 462–468.

Littlewood, A.B., *Gas chromatography.* New York: Academic, 1970.

Malinin, D.R., and J.H. Yoe, "Development of the laws of colorimetry." *J. Chem. Educ.*, 1961, 38, 129–131.

Miranda, H., and M. Hatziemmanuel, "Blood analyzer tests 30 samples simultaneously." *Electron.*, 1976, 49(8), 150–154.

Moran, F., L.J. Kettel, and D.W. Dugell, "Measurement of blood Po_2 with the microcathode electrode." *J. Appl. Physiol.*, 1966, 21, 725–728.

Pinkerton, P.H., I. Spence, J.C. Ogilvie, W.A. Ronald, P. Marchant, and P.K. Ray, "An assessment of Coulter counter model S.J." *Clin. Pathol.*, 1970, 23, 68–76.

Severinghaus, J.W., "Blood gas concentrations," in W.O. Fenn and H. Rahn (eds.), *Handbook of physiology.* Washington, D.C.: American Physiological Society, 1965, Vol. II, Sec. 3, Respiration, pp. 1475–1482.

Thomas, H.E., *Handbook of biomedical instrumentation and measurement*, Reston, Va.: Reston, 1974.

Chapter eleven

Medical imaging systems

Melvin P. Siedband and James E. Holden

Photographic, x-ray, ultrasonic, thermal, television and other imaging systems can be thought of as cameras. All camera images are limited by spatial resolution, amplitude scale, and noise content. The photographic image can be enlarged until it becomes quite "grainy"—the graininess is the bound on both spatial resolution and noise. The x-ray image is resolution-limited by the dimensions of the x-ray source and noise-limited by the beam intensity. The ultrasonic image is limited by the angular resolution of the transducer and the ability to separate true signals from false signals and noise. The thermal image is noise-limited by the equilibrium exchange of photons, and the television image by the electron-storage capacity of the camera tube.

All imaging systems, however, produce images, and the image can be studied without regard to the camera that produced it. Cameras can be considered as devices that map or transfer an image from one surface to another. They can be defined as if they incorporate an aperture through which signals related to all elements of the original image must pass to appear in the final image. A camera, whether TV, x-ray, or some other image-forming device, can be described in terms of its spatial transfer function. The first problem is to define some fundamental terms, which may then be used to describe the characteristics of medical imaging systems.

11.1 Information content of an image

In simplest terms, the total information content of an image is the product of the number of discrete picture elements (*pixels*) and the number of amplitude levels of each pixel. Since the pixels are seldom quantized or well separated into neat boxes, but tend to overlap each other, some arbitrary counting method is required. Noise, whether originating from photographic grain or from electrical charges, or fundamentally limited by the number of quanta (x-ray, gamma ray or light) limits the amplification permitted in a channel. For convenience, the number of amplitude steps within a channel is taken to be the same as the measured signal-to-noise ratio, SNR. The noise figure of a channel is the ratio of measured SNR to the theoretical or best SNR.

Resolution

An image can be considered as a surface of given dimension having a spatial resolution expressed in terms of line pairs per millimeter (lp/mm). Resolution is defined this way so that objects and the spaces between the objects are counted equally. If we examine copper mesh having 10 holes/cm or 100 holes/cm², the system must resolve 1 lp/mm and have 2 pixels/mm to display each mesh hole and mesh wire. A single countable object requires at least 1 line pair, 2 pixels, on each axis, so that the space between objects as well as the object itself may be resolved.

Figure 11.1 shows the image of a set of round objects for a television scanning system. The first problem is to determine how many television scanning lines are required to resolve these objects. We assume that the television scanner consists of a mechanically directed light sensor that can be swept one line at a time across the image, stepped down to the next line, and so on until the entire image is raster scanned. We assume that the output of the light sensor feeds a similarly scanning light projector that paints a beam

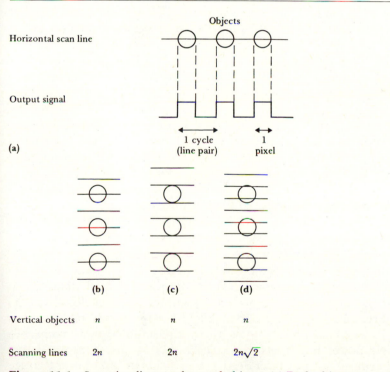

Figure 11.1   Scanning lines and round objects. (a) Each object represents 1 pixel, but each cycle of output signal represents 2 pixels. (b) n vertical objects require $2n$ scanning lines. (c) If objects are located between scanning lines, $2n$ lines are insufficient. (d) $2n\sqrt{2}$ lines are required for adequate resolution.

559

of light onto a photographic film to reproduce the original image as the beam of light is modulated by the output of the light sensor.

The first requirement of the scanning apparatus is to direct a scanning line through each of the round objects. If the round object is white, the output signal is positive; if the round object is dark, the output signal is negative. For a succession of light objects with dark spaces between them, each object represents the positive half-cycle of the signal, and each space between the objects represents the negative half-cycle of the signal. In general, each object requires one whole cycle of spatial frequency passband, the positive half-cycle for the object itself and the negative half-cycle for the space between the objects. If two objects touch, then this single-line scanning system cannot differentiate between them. It is necessary to have an additional scanning line between the two objects to determine whether or not there is a space between them.

In any real system, however, we do not know the location of the countable objects relative to the position of the scanning line before the scan. For a row of n objects arranged vertically, there must be $2n$ scanning lines. However, if we assume that the objects are vertically disposed in a random way, we must have an additional number of scanning lines to provide a reasonable probability of running at least one scanning line through each object and at least one scanning line through the space between such objects.

In general, the number of scanning lines is increased by $\sqrt{2}$ to allow for randomness. Thus, if there is a total of n^2 objects in a square field of view, randomly distributed, we assume that the vertical distribution is that of n objects. A system would have approximately $2n\sqrt{2}$ scanning lines to have a reasonable probability of detecting each of the objects and the spaces between the objects. For the n^2 objects within the field, a minimum of n cycles of passband would be required to resolve these objects for each scanning line. The total image passband is therefore $2n^2\sqrt{2}$ cycles per image.

In a real television system, an additional factor must be allowed for the time it takes for the camera tube and monitor tube scanning electron beams to be magnetically repositioned to the starting point following each horizontal scanning line and each vertical field. The blanking time (which is somewhat longer than the retrace time) of such systems is about 18% of the total horizontal time for each line. A typical 525-line standard United States television system has approximately 480 scanning lines visible, and a vertical resolution equivalent to about 180 or fewer countable objects. To reduce flicker and to make the image stationary with respect to 60-Hz power line interference, each 1/30-s image frame of 525 lines consists of two interlaced 1/60-s fields of $262\frac{1}{2}$ lines. Retrace and blanking take about 22 lines per field, 8% of the frame time. Because the aspect ratio of most television systems is $3:4$—that is, the height is three-fourths the width—the horizontal resolution corresponds to just under 240 countable objects. Thus the television chain looking at the output of a 15-cm x-ray image intensifier should be able to resolve 12 mesh/cm, since this corresponds to about 180 mesh holes across the field of view of the 15-cm intensifier tube. (It may see a slightly higher value mesh if the mesh is turned so that the diagonal axis of the mesh is the vertical axis of the television system.)

Since each object and the space between each object represent information, they should be given equal weight. We define a space on the surface of the image of dimensions equivalent to one-half cycle of bandwidth of horizontal axis and the same dimension in the vertical axis as a cell or pixel. We define the cell or pixel as having the smallest dimension of objects we wish to resolve in the image. This does not mean that, if we have objects smaller than the pixels, they will not be detected. Rather it defines the smallest size of an object for which amplitude information can be preserved. Objects smaller than that are spread over at least the pixel dimensions. For example, if a system has a pixel dimension of 0.5 mm and we examine tungsten-wire phantoms (objects) of 0.1 mm dimension, instead of appearing as high-contrast objects of 0.1 mm, they will appear as lower-contrast objects of 0.5-mm dimension.

The bandwidth Δf required for a television system is given by

$$\Delta f = \frac{n_h n_v 2\sqrt{2}}{F_h F_v T} \tag{11.1}$$

where

$$n_h = \text{maximum number of objects in a horizontal line}$$
$$n_v = \text{maximum number of objects in a vertical line}$$
$$F_h = \text{fraction of horizontal scan time spent on the picture (1.0}$$
$$\text{minus blanking fraction)}$$
$$F_v = \text{fraction of vertical scan time spent on the picture}$$
$$T = \text{total frame scanning time}$$

Example 11.1   A standard United States closed circuit TV system has 240 objects in the horizontal direction, 180 in the vertical, $F_h = 0.82$, $F_v = 0.92$, and $T = 1/30$ s. Calculate the bandwidth.

Answer

$$\Delta f = \frac{(240)(180)(2)(2)^{1/2}}{(0.82)(0.92)(1/30)} = 4.85 \text{ MHz}$$

The fly's eye consists of a mosaic of discrete detectors. If we assume that each eye is 800 μm in diameter and consists of 60 detectors across the spherical surface (about 3000 total), we discover some interesting things. The Rayleigh criterion for the resolution limit of a telescope is

$$\theta = \frac{1.22\lambda}{d} \qquad\qquad (11.2)$$

where

θ = angle between two just-resolved objects
λ = mean wavelength of light
d = diameter of lens

For light of $\lambda = 0.6$ μm, each detector of the fly's eye subtends:

$$\theta = \frac{(1.22)(0.6)(60)}{800} = 0.055 \text{ rad} \quad \text{or } 3.16° \qquad (11.3)$$

and the eye covers the full hemisphere with a small overlap between mosaic elements.

There are television image detectors that use large-scale integrated-circuit technology to select the output of photodiodes in a matrix of, say, 512×512 diodes. Each diode junction is charged during the scanning process and the action of the light is to partially discharge this junction. The scanning action causes the remaining charge of each detecting junction to be transferred to a storage part of the detector. Then, in a manner similar to that of a shift register, the charge is transferred from detector to detector and finally to an output bus, where it is amplified. The resolution limit is similar to that of the television scanning situation, in which fixed scan lines must detect randomly disposed objects. Thus a 512×512 matrix of detectors can resolve $512/(2\sqrt{2}) \times 512/(2\sqrt{2})$ or 181×181 line pairs.

Both mosaic detectors—the fly's eye and the charge-coupled device (CCD) television detector—use each element as an independent detector and map each element of the visual field into a corresponding element of the detector.

When the image sensor or retina consists of a mosaic of detectors, the limit to resolution is obvious. Continuous surfaces such as films, charge-storage surfaces of TV camera tubes, Xerox selenium plates, and light-emitting phosphor screens also have limits to resolution. When the detector has a finite thickness, as is the case with phosphor screens, the image is formed throughout the detector, but is observed at one surface. The light is scattered within the screen, which has the effect of spreading the images of point objects. For thick, diffusing detectors, the distance between centers of two just-resolved objects is about three times the thickness of the screen. This factor can be improved by adding dyes or light absorbers to reduce lateral spreading of light, as is done in TV tubes using a dark screen.

Television-camera tubes using electron-beam scanning have

spatial resolution limited by the thickness of the electron-storage surface and the dimensions of the electron beam. If the storage layer is thin, the resolution improves and the charge per unit area increases; but the beam current must increase and electron repulsion (space-charge) effects increase the width of the beam. One way to increase the resolution is to increase the area of the storage layer. The beam-scanning spacing between successive horizontal lines is such that the lines overlap just enough so that a uniform charge is deposited in the surface. Since the electron spread of the beam is almost a Gaussian distribution, the spacing limit is analogous to the Rayleigh limit for optical systems.

Optical systems are diffraction-limited by the lens and limited by other factors, such as multiple reflections within the film emulsion, the plastic substrate, and the lens elements. The emulsion is made with an *antihalation* (antiscatter) material, and the substrate often contains a dye to reduce lateral transfer of light.

Image noise

All images are limited by both noise and spatial resolution. If we attempt to dissect an image into smaller and smaller areas, we soon find that the image is limited to some smallest element, or that the lens or scanning aperture imposes a bound on how small an element we can resolve within the image. Further, within that smallest element, we can say that the image is either on or off. The on-off criterion certainly applies when we are considering silver grains of film. It also applies when we are considering a beam of electrons hitting a cathode-ray-tube phosphor: The beam is not continuous, but consists of discrete electrons. The phosphor particles vary in size and probability of being illuminated. For elements of larger size, we can say that the image has a gray, or amplitude, level, which can be defined by a digital number. This is another way of saying that the image is characterized by the number of on or off states of smaller elements.

If for each of a large number of trial measurements q, there is a small probability p of a certain type of event, the average number of this type of event is simply $m = qp$. For example, if we wait q seconds for randomly distributed raindrops to fall within a certain area, and for each second, the probability of observing a raindrop is p, then m is the average number observed in several observations of q seconds each. The relative probability of any *particular* number of drops K in a measurement having an average m is given by the Poisson probability density distribution:

$$p(K;m) = \frac{e^{-m}m^K}{K!} \tag{11.4}$$

We can check that this distribution really has the average m:

$$\sum_{K=0}^{\infty} Kp(K;m) = m \qquad (11.5)$$

The sum of $p(K;m)$ for all outcomes K from zero to infinity is, of course, equal to one. Finally, the variance of the distribution is also equal to m:

$$\sigma^2 = \sum_{K=0}^{\infty} (K - m)^2 p(K;m) = m \qquad (11.6)$$

Thus the rms fluctuation of outcomes around the average value m is just $\sqrt{m}$. If we were to examine a succession of measurements that have an average outcome of 100 events, we would find very few with *exactly* 100 events, but in fact they would be distributed about the average with a standard deviation of 10 events.

Independent raindrops falling on concrete squares and x-ray photons impinging on detector pixels have the same statistical properties. If the average number of raindrops per square is 100, the probability of finding exactly 100 is 0.040, even though the *average* is 100/square. If we made a scanning voltmeter that read N volts for N events, as we used the scanning voltmeter to sample the output of the individual pixel, we would find that there would be a fluctuation of $\sqrt{N}$ rms volts. See Figure 11.2.

Now we change from the steady signal N to a modulated signal $N(1 \pm \overline{M})$, where $0 \leq \overline{M} \leq 1$ is the modulation and $N\overline{M}$ is the incremental increase representing the information-containing signal S. The maximum signal exists when $\overline{M} = 1$, so that the maximum SNR equals $N/\sqrt{N} = \sqrt{N}$. Thus, for a time-average value of 100 events per pixel in 1 s, the maximum SNR equals 10. If the linear dimension of the cell is doubled, the area is multiplied by four, and, for the same time period, there are 400 events per larger pixel, for a maximum SNR of 20. Similarly, if only the integration time of the original cell is changed from 1 to 4 s, there is also the possibility of detecting 400 events per pixel and a maximum SNR of 20. For purely random signals having the same time average, time integration or spatial integration have the same effect. In other words, decreasing the resolution of an image (increasing the area of the pixel) either increases the SNR of the image or, for the same noise level, reduces the requirement for number of events. For those cases in which $\overline{M}$ is not equal to 1, the signal is $\overline{M}N$, but the noise level is still $\sqrt{N}$, so that the SNR is $\overline{M}\sqrt{N}$.

The detection of low-contrast signals in a noisy field requires a fairly high SNR. See Figure 11.3, in which events correspond to gamma-ray photons, which register as counts on an image. We ask the question: "What is the probability that the number of photons

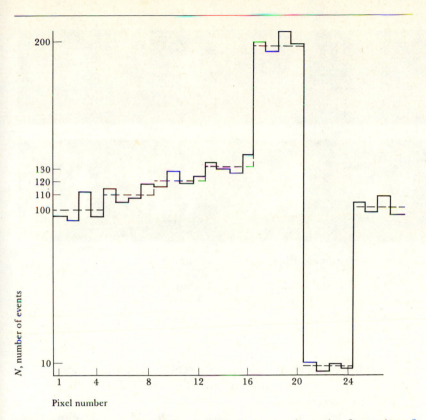

Figure 11.2 The number of events N that occur in each of a series of pixels. Pixels 1 to 4 show an average value of 100 events, with average fluctuations of 10 events. An average increment of 10 events per pixel is shown in pixels 5 to 8. Note that pixel 3 has more events than either 6 or 7, even though the average number has increased by a whole standard deviation. As the average increment gets larger, in pixels 9 to 16, there is less likelihood of such an ambiguity, that is, the SNR increases. Finally, pixels 17 to 24 show the original average signal of 100 events per pixel square-wave modulated with a period of 8 pixels and a modulation $\bar{M}$ of nearly 1. It is evident from this figure that the maximum value of $\bar{M}$ is 1.

per pixel randomly exceeds $N + J\sqrt{N}$ as a function of J units of standard deviation?"

We find that (in reference to a table of integral values of the standard deviation) where $J = 1$, 16% of the pixels exceed the bound; for $J = 2$, 2.3% of the pixels exceed the bound; for $J = 3$, 0.14% of the pixels exceed the bound; and for $J = 4$, 0.003% of the pixels exceed the bound. However, if we are looking at, say, the field of view of a typical television camera having 180×240 countable objects or $360 \times 480 = 1.7 \times 10^5$ pixels, then even for $J = 4$, each television frame randomly has 5 pixels exceeding the bound. In other words, the modulation of N must be greater than that

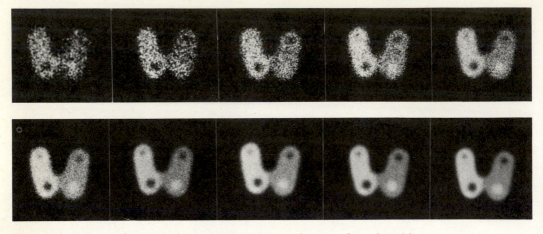

Figure 11.3 In each successive gamma-camera picture of a thyroid phantom, the number of counts is increased by a factor of 2. The number of counts ranges from 1563 to 800,000. The Polaroid camera aperture was reduced to avoid overexposure as the number of counts was increased.

required to produce the SNR $\overline{M}\sqrt{N}$ greater than 4 in order to simply detect the existence of a signal with fewer than five "false alarms" or random exceedances.

If we define C as the contrast of the $\overline{M}$ factor above, the number of photons required must be at least equal to bJ^2/C^2, where b is the total number of pixels. J must be at least 4, for reasons described earlier. If d is the linear dimension of the pixel and A is the area of the field, the total number of photons required equals $AJ^2/(d^2C^2)$. A good estimate for the number of photons of a grain-limited visual field would then be $N = 25A/(d^2C^2)$ (with the assumption that $J = 5$). However, this number must actually be greater at low light levels and with low-contrast signals because of the presence of television scanning lines, phosphor granularity and other factors. The number approximately doubles to almost $50A/(d^2C^2)$. If we assume that, at the limit of resolution, an absolute-minimum contrast of approximately 5% is required, then the number of photons required for detection is

$$N = A \left[\frac{7.2}{d(C - 0.05)} \right]^2 \tag{11.7}$$

Although (11.7) has been developed for the case in which d is the linear dimension of a single pixel, d can be extended to the dimension of any object. That is, as object size increases, the contrast required for the same detection probability decreases.

11.2 Modulation transfer function

The *modulation transfer function*, MTF, is a modified form of the spatial frequency response of an element or of the entire imaging system. The limiting resolution of a system, while defining a system in terms of the smallest resolution element that can be clearly seen, is not a sufficient indicator of system performance, because a system may resolve a 2.0 mesh/mm copper screen at high contrast and perform poorly when attempting to resolve the gall bladder of a patient who presents a low-contrast image. The MTF is plotted by measuring the amplitude response as a function of spatial frequency, assuming 100% response at zero frequency and ignoring phase shifts. See Figure 11.4. We assume that the amplitude is zero past the first phase rotation (crossover). The MTFs of each image transmission component may be combined as point-by-point products at each spatial frequency to obtain the MTF of the overall system.

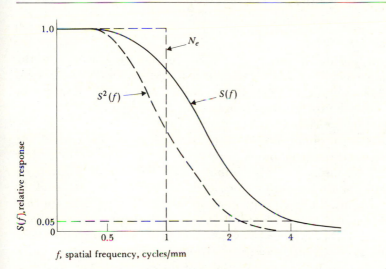

Figure 11.4 Modulation transfer function, $S(f)$, for a typical x-ray system. $S(f)$ is squared and integrated to yield N_e, the noise-equivalent bandwidth. The limiting resolution, 4 cycles/mm, is indicated at the 0.05 contrast level. The abscissa is plotted in cycles per millimeter, which is the same as line pairs per millimeter.

To measure MTF, we use a sinusoidal test object to modulate the input signal to cover the band of frequencies from zero to the maximum frequency. Sinusoidal test objects are hard to make, so the usual procedure is to use a square-bar pattern. In the case of x-ray systems, the bar pattern is usually made of lead or tungsten alloys, and consists of a series of bars and spaces starting at a low frequency and increasing in frequency (that is, decreasing in spacing). Such test objects are placed in front of the x-ray image detector and the system is irradiated. Similar photographic bar patterns can be imaged by the various lenses of the system, so that they may be tested independently by optical means. The detector consists of a microscope with a small slit in the focal plane of the microscope lens, behind which is mounted a photomultiplier tube. The output of the tube is fed to a recorder, which may record the square-wave amplitude as a function of frequency.

A square-wave function may be analyzed in terms of its sine-wave components by means of a Fourier-series expansion. A matrix inversion of the Fourier-series expansion of square-wave terms yields an equation defining sine-wave amplitudes in terms of square-wave amplitudes. In the following formula, $S(f)$ represents the amplitude of the sine wave at frequency f obtained by substituting measured values $M(f)$ of the square-wave amplitudes at f, $3f$, $5f$, and so forth,

$$S(f) = \frac{4}{\pi} \left[M(f) - \frac{M(3f)}{3} + \frac{M(5f)}{5} - \frac{M(7f)}{7} + \cdots \right]$$

(11.8)

It is thus possible to convert the measured square-wave data to the sine-wave data required for obtaining the MTF. Other means exist for obtaining the MTF, such as observation of the impulse or point-spread function or observation of the response to a single fine line to determine the line-spread function.

Once we obtain the MTF of the system or elements of the system, we can derive other numbers of great value from it. The limiting resolution of the component or the system is often assumed to be the resolution measured at the 5% contrast level. In x-ray systems, the low-frequency contrast is assumed to be the amplitude value of the MTF at 0.1 lp/mm. The amplitude of a signal is related to the number of events per pixel. By taking equivalent bandwidths or by integrating over unit bandwidths, we can obtain a measure of the information content of the cell. However, we know that SNR is related to $\sqrt{N}$, where N is the number of events per pixel. In order to obtain a measure of the visual equivalence of various systems as a function of amplitude, we must obtain an rms equivalence. This can be done by integrating over the square of the amplitudes for all frequencies.

11.3 Noise-equivalent bandwidth

Another way of looking at the information content is to note that N is related to area and that the square of the amplitude response is proportional to the number of events contained within an area defined by a given linear dimension. A noise-equivalent bandwidth N_e at a spatial frequency f is that of an equivalent system that has 100% amplitude response from zero frequency to N_e and zero response above N_e when compared with a system having an amplitude response as a function of spatial frequency, $S(f)$ = MTF. The N_e is obtained by integrating the square of the MTF amplitudes:

$$N_e = \int_0^\infty S^2(f) \, df \tag{11.9}$$

It is as if N_e defines a mosaic of detectors of resolution N_e, say N_e pixels/cm, having the same SNR properties as a continuum of detectors having the MTF from which the N_e is derived. The value of N_e is an excellent measure of the equivalent spatial resolution from the point of view of the noise performance of any system.

The system N_e may be estimated from elemental N_es.

$$\frac{1}{N_e} = \left[\left(\frac{1}{N_{e1}} \right)^2 + \left(\frac{1}{N_{e2}} \right)^2 + \cdots \right]^{1/2} \tag{11.10}$$

The N_e concept becomes an extremely handy way to express the spatial frequency response as a single number. N_e is a useful and practical means for describing systems, and ought to be used in preference to limiting resolution.

The eye is a noise-limited instrument. Since low-amplitude functions, such as the 5% contrast point at which limiting resolution occurs, are squared as they are integrated, they have little effect on overall performance of the system and the ability to perceive and detect real objects of moderate contrast. Plotting the MTF of each of the elements of the system in the same plane, preferably the plane of the detector, enables the designer of the system to visualize the contribution of each element to resolution of the system.

11.4 Photography

The common process of photography is based on the lattice properties of silver bromide crystals in the film emulsion. Light photons eject electrons from the bromine atoms. Some of these electrons are caught by the silver atoms and neutralize them. This frees them from the lattice to form metallic silver atoms. For a single silver atom, the neutralizing electron may be lost thermally and the silver atom bound again to the lattice. If, say, five or more contiguous silver atoms are freed at almost the same time, the probability is high that they will remain in the free, metallic state. Chemical processing (developer) causes adjacent silver ions in the grain to accumulate around this metallic silver atom to form a grain of about 10^9 metallic silver atoms, while the remaining silver bromide is carried away by the solution (fixer).

Let us assume that about 25 light photons are required to produce the first 5 silver atoms at a sensitivity site and to render a single grain capable of being developed without regard to effects of emulsion or development. What this means is that, for a given type of emulsion and development, the number of grains per unit area and the size of the grains can be varied, but the amount of light required per grain is constant. Thus fine-grained films require more light per unit area than coarse-grained films. Actually, the number of photons required to render a grain developable is not constant, but is distributed statistically about some mean value. Simple statistical averaging procedures can be used to show that the conclusion just drawn remains essentially true.

The energy required to free the electrons from the bromine is on the order of 2.4 eV, which corresponds to a wavelength of 520 nm (Figure 2.21)—i.e., blue light or shorter. To make the film sensitive to longer wavelengths, various electron-emitting dyes are absorbed onto the grain, where they are in close proximity to the silver atoms. The weak photons generate an electron in the dye that is then acquired by the silver. The sensitivity to short wavelengths can also be reduced by mixing into or preceding the emulsion with light-absorbing dyes. Thus it is possible to make emulsions of varying sensitivities (and grain size), and spectral responses: orthochromatic (blue and green), panchromatic (blue, green, and red), or infrared (red and infrared).

The image formed in the film prior to chemical development is called the *latent image*. It is still possible for some of the metallic silver atoms to return to their lattice coupling because of slow thermal effects. This is called *latent image fading*. It is important that the first five or so neighboring silver atoms be freed in a time that is not too short or too long. All films have some range of exposure times such that a constant light-intensity-time product will bring the emulsion to a particular value of density, where density is defined as $D = \log 1/T$, T being the light transmission of the film. Note that density D here is the same as absorbance A in (10.3). When this constant relationship of time and intensity fails to hold constant for longer or shorter exposures, it is called reciprocity law failure. Some films lose almost half their sensitivity for exposures of 10 min when compared with films exposed for 100 ms.

Figure 11.5 shows the characteristic curve of film as a plot of density versus log exposure (D–$\log E$). This is also often referred to as the *H and D curve*, after Hurter and Driffield, who used this description 80 years ago. The curve shows that a minimum exposure is needed before the film begins to respond, evidenced by the curvature at the toe of the curve. The saturation level above the shoulder is the level of maximum density for the processing conditions used. The minimum density is also called the *fog level*. The

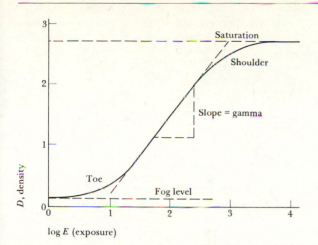

Figure 11.5 The characteristic curve of film is a plot of density versus log exposure. Higher gamma films have a higher contrast, but a poorer ability to record a wide range of exposure.

slope of the straight-line portion of the D–log E curve is called the *gamma,* a measure of the relative contrast of the film.

The effective speed of a film-developer combination is proportional to the reciprocal of the light-intensity-time product required to increase the density D over its zero-exposure value by an increment of 1.0. For most films, the speed can be increased by extending development, with the result that more grains are developed. Of course, if there are too few grains per unit area, the image is limited statistically in the expected way.

The N_e value for most photographic negative films is about 40 lp/mm. Since the resolving power of the eye is about one minute of arc, at a viewing distance of 36 cm, the resolution of the eye is about 5 lp/mm. Under those conditions, enlargement of the negative image by a factor of 8 (40/5) results in no significant loss of information. Slower, detailed films permit greater enlargement. If some loss of information or increase of grain or noise can be tolerated, then greater enlargement is possible.

When films are exposed to high-energy electrons (>1 keV), excitation of more than five silver atoms takes place. In fact, the use of electrons to expose film also reduces the effects of light scatter (no light!) and permits the film to be developed to a value of N_e several times greater than that of visible light exposure. *Electron-beam recording* (EBR) on film permits the use of 8-mm film to record about 30 times the information of light exposures.

Equation (11.7) gives an estimate for counting the N events necessary to produce a just-detectable image. The estimate also holds when $1/C$ represents the number of *gray levels*—discrete levels of intensity. We assume a rather grainy, low-resolution image of 100 × 100 mm, such that there are only three gray levels and a cell size of 3 mm. The number of events necessary (we assume that each event is a grain) is

$$
\begin{aligned}
N &= A\left[\frac{7.2}{d(C - 0.05)}\right]^2 \\
&= 100^2\left[\frac{7.2}{3(1/3 - 0.05)}\right]^2 \\
&= 7.3 \times 10^5 \text{ grains} \qquad \text{(poor picture)}
\end{aligned}
\qquad (11.11)
$$

Where the number of gray levels is increased to 10 and the cell size is 0.5 mm, the number of events must be greater than

$$
\begin{aligned}
N &= 100^2\left[\frac{7.2}{0.5(0.1 - 0.05)}\right]^2 \\
&= 8.3 \times 10^8 \text{ grains} \qquad \text{(good picture)}
\end{aligned}
\qquad (11.12)
$$

Since each grain requires about 25 photons captured, about 2×10^{10} photons are required to take a picture. A lesser exposure necessarily increases the noise or decreases the gray scale. Optical defocusing reduces the noise due to graininess, but has the effect of increasing the cell size, i.e., decreasing the resolution.

11.5 Television systems

Secondary emission

In order to understand the beam-scanning mechanism of television-camera tubes, storage tubes, display storage tubes, and kinescopes, it is necessary to understand secondary emission phenomena. When electrons are emitted from a hot cathode, they have a distribution of energies due to the cathode temperature and the resistance of the cathode coatings. The electrons cannot land on a surface if they do not have sufficient kinetic energy. If they reach the surface with excess energy, they may expel secondary electrons.

Figure 11.6 shows an experimental arrangement of a tube with an anode collecting plate covered with an electron shield. The electron shield may be biased negatively with respect to the anode to repel secondary electrons back to the anode, or biased positively to collect the secondary electrons. We assume here that it is biased positively, so that all secondary electrons that leave the anode do not return, but are gathered by this shield. A microammeter is in series with the shield.

The curve shows the *secondary emission ratio,* from which we

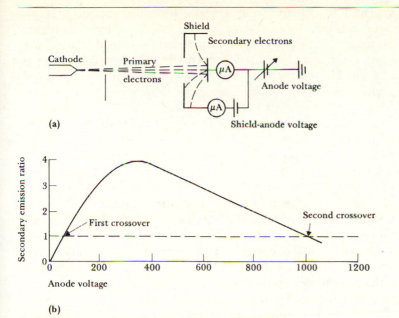

(a)

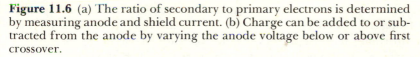

(b)

Figure 11.6 (a) The ratio of secondary to primary electrons is determined by measuring anode and shield current. (b) Charge can be added to or subtracted from the anode by varying the anode voltage below or above first crossover.

obtain the current as a function of anode voltage. The velocity distribution of the beam is such that all the beam electrons can be collected when the anode voltage is more than 5 V. As the voltage is increased, the excess energy of the beam electrons expels secondary electrons. We assume that the surface of the anode is of bright metal having a clean surface, such as bright silver. When the voltage is approximately 50 V, for each primary electron that arrives, one secondary electron leaves. This point is called *first crossover*.

As the voltage is increased, more secondary electrons leave the surface than primary electrons arrive. Depending on the material, it is possible for the secondary-emission ratio—the ratio of secondaries to primaries—to reach values of four or five or more. For most materials, such as untreated gold and silver, the secondary-emission ratio reaches a maximum of about two. For cesiated antimony over silver, the secondary-emission ratio may be as high as six, and for some of the newer secondary-emitting III-V compounds, the secondary-emission ratio may be as high as 25. The maximum secondary emission is reached at between 150 to 350 V. Then it begins to fall, until at about 1 kV, *second crossover* is reached. Then the arriving primary electrons penetrate the material, so that only one secondary electron per primary can escape.

If the collector surface is made of a dielectric material, such as

NaCl or KCl, at voltages in excess of 1 kV, one arriving primary electron can cause the release of many secondary electrons within the material, which can induce conductivity. For the lifetime of the secondary electrons, the material, normally a dielectric, behaves as a conductor. If charges were previously placed on the surface of the material, then these charges would be discharged by the *secondary electron conduction* (SEC) effect.

If a metal surface is coated with a dielectric material and wire mesh is placed just over the dielectric surface, then the potential of the mesh limits the potential of the dielectric. If the surface is at $+200$ V and the mesh at $+205$ V with respect to cathode, then arriving electrons remove surface electrons to cause the surface to move in a positive direction until the surface reaches $+205$ V. At this point the secondary electrons cannot be collected by the mesh, and they return to the surface. If the mesh is operated below the surface potential or if the surface is operated below first crossover, then beam electrons are deposited on the surface. Thus, when we adjust the operating potential, the beam either deposits or removes electrons from dielectric surfaces.

Electron tubes, similar in construction to small cathode-ray tubes, have been made using these principles. The beam of electrons is scanned over the surface and is modulated with TV picture information. It deposits electrons on a dielectric target or storage surface. On the next scan that covers the surface, the operating potentials are changed so that the *unmodulated* beam removes all the deposited electrons. The dielectric target can be made so that the front surface (insulator) faces the electron source, while the back surface (metallized) is connected to an amplifier. In this way, a single TV image can be stored and recalled for comparison. It can also be subtracted from later television images.

Some semiconductors exhibit a conduction process at lower accelerating voltages. This is called *electron-bombardment-induced conductivity*, EBIC. The secondary-electron-conduction (SEC) effect usually occurs well above 1 keV—typically 5 keV—electron energy. The EBIC effect in some semiconductors occurs at landing energies as low as 50 eV.

The nature of the anode surface is quite important. If the surface is rough, secondary electrons are less able to escape. It is analogous to a roughened mirror: if the reflected energy cannot escape, the surface behaves like a blackbody and the secondary electrons are trapped. Surfaces of vidicon-camera tubes are quite rough, so the secondary-emission ratio is fairly low.

Many camera tubes, such as the vidicon, Plumbicon, and silicon-target vidicons operate on the principle of photoconduction, or photoresistive action occurring within a thin layer. The scanning electron beam deposits charge on the surface and the light impinging on the opposite surface induces conductivity in the material, which discharges some of the deposited-beam electrons. The next time the beam comes by, it replaces that charge.

The voltage drop of a resistor in series with the target is sensed by an amplifier as the camera video signal.

If we wish to have high sensitivity in camera tubes, storage of charge is necessary. The beam serves as a means of interrogation. The beam places a charge on a pixel and then continues to scan the rest of the surface. During the frame time—the time between each complete scan—the surface is charged and the bulk material responds to the visible light. A simple switching process, unlike an interrogating process, would mean that the pixel was active only when the beam was impinging on it. Obviously, for camera tubes that have approximately 10^5 elements, an integrating type of sampling detector interrogating each frame has higher overall sensitivity. However, the capacity of the element must be sufficient to store charge between passages of the beam. A compromise must be reached between sensitivity (increasing the layer thickness) and resolution and charge storage (decreasing the layer thickness).

Example 11.2 Calculate the SNR for a charge-storage tube that has an active area of 1 cm², a layer thickness of 10 μm, a relative dielectric constant of 1.2, 10^5 pixels, and a 5-V change to produce reading action.

Answer Target capacitance is

$$C = \frac{\epsilon_0 \epsilon_r A}{x} = \frac{(8.8 \times 10^{-12} \text{ F/m})(1.2)(10^{-4} \text{ m}^2)}{(10^{-5} \text{ m})}$$
$$= 106 \times 10^{-12} \text{ F} = 106 \text{ pF}$$

The change in charge during reading action is

$$q = Cv = (106 \times 10^{-12})(5) = 530 \times 10^{-12} \text{ C}$$

The number of electrons in this charge is

$$n_e = \frac{530 \times 10^{-12}}{1.6 \times 10^{-19}} = 3.3 \times 10^9$$

The number of electrons per pixel is

$$n_p = \frac{3.3 \times 10^9}{10^5} = 33,000$$

The SNR $= (33,000)^{1/2} = 180$.

Camera tubes

The reading beam of the camera tube is usually adjusted to match the required dimensions for a standard 525-line scanning system, that is, 480 scanning lines across the active surface of the tube. The beam deposits electrons uniformly in one complete frame. To minimize flicker, television scanning systems use two interlaced fields. The first field of $262\frac{1}{2}$ lines scans the surface of the tube in one-sixtieth of a second and a second field of $262\frac{1}{2}$ lines is directed between the lines of the first frame. The overall effect of this is not to gather more information, but merely to increase the flicker rate of the images. A side benefit is that the vertical scanning frequency, the *field rate*, is the same as the power-line frequency, so that stray power-line magnetic fields produce stationary images. For this reason, 60-Hz vertical frame rates are chosen in the United States and 50-Hz frame rates are chosen in Europe.

Figure 11.7 shows the way the vidicon and the various types of lead-oxide camera tubes are constructed. The tube has a hot cathode which is the electron source and which operates at ground potential. A control grid G_1, which modulates the beam of electrons, surrounds the cathode. An accelerating electrode, G_2, provides an electric field attracting the cathode electrons and has a beam-forming aperture. A metal cylinder, G_3, may be combined with a mesh, G_4, to provide a field for the beam of electrons. An axial magnetic field provides further beam focusing. Two orthogonal magnetic coils (yokes) provide *x-y* deflection. The target or retina of the tube is mounted on the interior surface of the glass face plate. Light is imaged on one surface of the retina and the beam impinges on the other.

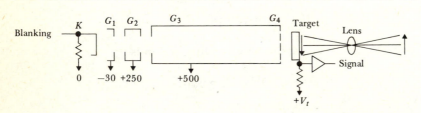

Figure 11.7 The vidicon has a cathode and a series of grids to form, shape, and control the electron beam. Magnetic deflection (not shown) scans the beam over the target, which is mounted on the interior of the glass face plate. From the target, light-modulated signal current flows through the load resistor and is amplified.

The principal difference between a vidicon and a lead-oxide vidicon is the material used for the target. In the vidicon, the material is usually antimony trisulfide, which functions as a light-modulated resistor. The sensitivity can be varied by adjustment of the supply voltage of the target. The lead-oxide tubes function as depleted junction photoconductors, and the sensitivity cannot be varied by adjustment of the supply voltage of the target.

The circuits of vidicon cameras can be designed to provide an increase in target voltage if the camera does not detect a large-enough video signal. Such automatic gain-control circuits make it possible for the vidicon camera to operate over a very wide range of light levels. This is more difficult when using lead-oxide tubes. Rather, the automatic gain control provides a signal to a motor driving the lens iris or an amplifier gain-control signal. The re-charging current provided by the scanning electron beam appears across the target load resistor and is detected by the signal ampli-fier, which amplifies it, mixes the necessary vertical-horizontal syn-chronizing signals with the video, and then feeds mixed video signal to the television monitors, as well as various tape recorders, disk recorders, etc.

Several signal-storage tubes have been made that use electron optics of vidicon camera tubes. One tube has a storage target in the form of a mosaic of dielectric islands formed on the surface of a single crystal of a conducting silicon substrate. If an island is charged negatively with respect to the cathode, its electric field repels the beam electrons. If the islands are slightly charged, the beam does not land on the island, but is deflected to the substrate spaces between islands, and a signal voltage appears across the target load resistor.

If an island is slightly positive, the beam lands (below first crossover) and neutralizes the positive charge by depositing elec-trons. If the substrate is made sufficiently positive (above first cross-over), the beam removes electrons. The operating conditions can be controlled and the beam modulated to deposit image charge in-formation on the islands. The charge pattern may be read nonde-structively for several minutes as a clear TV image.

Patient exposure

Image-storage techniques as a means of reducing exposure of patients to x rays are not always effective. The time constant of the eye is approximately 0.2 s, and pulsing fluoroscopic systems that operate at rates faster than this offer no net decrease in radiation exposure. When operating at slow rates, the system loses real-time capability and becomes analogous to a slide show. We can reduce patient exposure by using slide-show techniques or by remem-bering the last full frame of information when there is something to be seen. Several advantages accrue to image-storage systems when they are used for manipulation of images. The *sticky fluoro-scopic* approach is one way to use the image storage. In this case, the last full frame of information remains displayed after the x rays go off. The best way to achieve reduction of exposure is, of course, to turn off the x rays.

Another trick involving storage of images is called *harmoniza-tion*. In this technique, an out-of-focus image is stored and subtracted from the real-time, sharply focused picture. Since the out-of-focus image has lower spatial-resolution components in the image, subtracting it from the real-time image has the effect of canceling large-area objects and enhancing edges. This may make certain tumors, bone edges, or other boundaries more visible.

Other techniques in using image storage involve the use of x-ray filters to vary the energy content of the beam reaching the patient. These compare images as a function of distribution of x-ray energy. Energy-absorption analysis may be done in order to detect endogenous (normally occurring) or exogenous (added to the body) iodine to obtain contrast enhancement of soft tissues, cancel bony images, or observe rates of change of blood velocity or heart volume. With advances being made in storage of digital images and computer manipulation of images, these techniques will become even more popular and more widely used in departments of diagnostic radiology in the future.

11.6 Radiography

A simple x-ray system consists of a high-voltage generator, an x-ray tube, a collimator, the object or patient, a grid, an intensifying screen, and the film. (See Figure 11.8.) A simple x-ray generator has a line circuit breaker, a variable autotransformer, an exposure timer and contactor, a step-up transformer and rectifier, and a filament control for the tube. Medical x-ray exposures are of the order of 80 kVp (peak kilovolts), 300 mA, 0.1 s. Power levels range up to more than 100 kW.

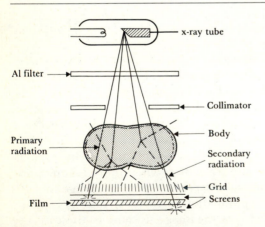

Figure 11.8 The x-ray tube generates x rays that are restricted by the aperture in the collimator. The Al filter removes low-energy x rays that would not penetrate the body. Scattered secondary radiation is trapped by the grid, while primary radiation strikes the screen phosphor. The resulting light exposes the film.

Generation of x rays

The x-ray tube is a temperature-limited diode. Emission current is the smaller of the values of currents defined by the Richardson-Dushman equation, $J_1 = aT^2 e^{-u/\kappa T}$ and that of the Langmuir equation, $J_2 = bV^{3/2}$, where J is the emission current density, T is the filament temperature, u is the work function of the filament, κ is Boltzmann's constant, a and b are constants, and V is the anode-cathode voltage. Since the filament cools primarily by radiation, the radiant power equals the power input: $\sigma T^4 = I^2 R$, where σ is the Stefan-Boltzmann constant and I and R are the current and resistance of the filament. Thus tube anode current is controlled by adjusting the filament current, with a compensation of filament current for variations of anode voltage. The fractional change of anode current is an order of magnitude greater than the change of filament current, so the circuits for filament control must be precisely regulated.

The electrons strike the anode and produce x rays through two mechanisms: *bremsstrahlung*, produced by the deflection of the arriving electrons by the nucleus of the anode atoms; and *characteristic radiation*, produced when the anode's innermost atomic electrons, knocked out of orbit by the arriving electrons, are replaced by outer-shell electrons. Because the deceleration is proportional to the density of the electrons, which is in turn proportional to Z (the atomic number of the anode material), the efficiency of x-ray production is proportional to ZV. A useful formula is

$$\text{eff} = 1.4 \times 10^{-4} \, ZV, \tag{11.13}$$

where eff is the efficiency of conversion of electron energy to x rays. Since the electron energy is also proportional to V, the total x-ray energy produced is proportional to ZV^2.

Operating an x-ray tube at a fixed voltage V produces x-ray photons having a distribution of energies. Transmission of x rays through thick body parts is roughly proportional to E^3, where E is the energy of the x-ray photon. Thus lower-energy x-ray photons are less able to penetrate the anode or the glass wall of the tube. For electrons of 100 keV energy impinging on a tungsten anode, the energy distribution of the exiting x-ray photons shows characteristic radiation peaks at 58 and 68 keV (K- and L-shell replacement electrons), the bremsstrahlung, and the absorption of the lower energies. See Figure 11.9.

The unit of x-ray exposure is the *roentgen* (R). One R is defined as the radiation that produces ionization of either sign of 2.58×10^{-4} C/kg in dry air. The energy required to form an ion pair in air averages 33.7 eV. The unit of absorbed dose (e.g., in tissue) is the rad, which is equal to 10^{-2} J/kg. Because a patient

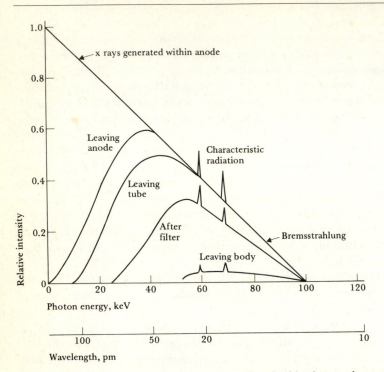

Figure 11.9 The lowest-energy x rays are absorbed in the anode metal and the tube glass envelope. An Al filter further reduces the low-energy x rays that do not pass through the body and would only increase the patient dose. Only the higher-energy x rays are capable of penetrating the body and contributing to the film darkening required for a picture. Note that the average energy increases with the amount of filtration.

absorbs 95 to 99% of the radiation from an incident beam, and because under these conditions the roentgen and the rad are close in value, the units are often interchanged.

Detection of x rays

As the radiation passes through the patient, a portion is scattered as secondary radiation, most is absorbed and 1 to 4% of the primary radiation is transmitted to the detector. A *grid* of fine lead strips, analogous to a miniature venetian blind, is often placed in front of the detector. The short axis of lead strips is aimed toward the focal spot of the x-ray tube, so that most of the primary radiation passes between the strips, while most of the secondary radiation is intercepted.

After passing through the grid, the radiation is detected. Film may be used as the detector, but, because of the low Z of the film and the thin emulsion, the film is relatively radiolucent. To improve the probability of detecting the x-ray photons, *intensifying screens* consisting of plastic sheets loaded or coated with high-Z scintillation powders (for example, $CaWO_4$) are placed against each surface of a *double-emulsion film*. The use of screen-film techniques increases the sensitivity and reduces the exposure by a factor of 20 to 100, depending on the screens used.

From consideration of the radiation-noise limit, we know that there is a minimum value for the number of x-ray quanta required to produce an image at a given resolution. The object is to choose a detector that has the required resolution, determine an acceptable noise limit, and operate the detector to meet those objectives.

The number of photons detected per square millimeter required to just see a fine object of dimension d and contrast C is found from (11.7). We assume that 1 R of typical radiation exposure is equivalent to about $3 \times 10^8 \ \phi_x/mm^2$, where ϕ_x/mm^2 is the number of x-ray photons per square millimeter when the x-ray beam is not filtered by much material. Then the radiation exposure required to produce an image can be estimated:

$$R/image = \frac{2 \times 10^{-7}}{(QDE)(RL)d^2(C - 0.05)^2} \tag{11.14}$$

where QDE is the *quantum detection efficiency* (the fraction of x-ray photons detected) and RL is the *radiolucency* (the average fraction of incident x-ray photons that exit the object or patient and contribute to the image). Operation at values of x-ray exposure below that estimated by the formula results in noisy images. Operation above these factors produces quieter images, but at the cost of unnecessary exposure of the patient to radiation.

In choosing an x-ray film-screen combination, we should choose a screen that will give the necessary resolution and choose a film that will provide adequate film density when sufficient radiation has been received to meet statistical requirements. If the film chosen is too sensitive, the film reaches maximum density before a sufficient number of photons have been detected to meet the statistical requirements. Thus, when the film is correctly exposed, it appears noisy. A better procedure is to use film of lower sensitivity, which permits the *increase* of the x radiation reaching the film. Then the statistical requirements are exceeded, and at correct exposure the film noise is acceptably low.

The more sensitive screens are thicker than the less sensitive ones. Screen thickness varies from 300 μm or more for very high sensitivity, low-resolution screens to less than 100 μm for detail screens. The value for N_e of the screens is a function of screen thickness. The N_e has a value of about 2.5 lp/mm for the most sensitive screens to about 7 lp/mm for detail screens. The film has an N_e of about 15 lp/mm for double-emulsion x-ray film to about 40 lp/mm for common photographic single-emulsion films. The screens obviously dominate the film when we are determining the MTF and N_e of a radiographic system.

The use of detail screens and high-resolution film to view low-resolution objects results in unnecessary exposure of the patient and may cause the image to reveal certain artifacts that may not be important for diagnosis. Certainly, high-resolution film-screen combinations are necessary for certain forms of arteriography, in which fine blood vessels must be seen, but not for discovering broad, soft-edge lesions of the lung. Measured in the plane of the film, there are very few body parts that have spatial resolutions in excess of 1 lp/mm. Seeking high resolution may not be the proper objective in the design of a system. Trying to achieve high-contrast performance and the proper relationship between contrast and SNR may be a more worthwhile goal. Of course, there are exceptions: mammography (radiography of the breast) requires resolution greater than 2 lp/mm.

Image intensifiers

X-ray image intensifiers are used in most fluoroscopic systems. They have replaced the old-fashioned fluoroscopic screens. The principal disadvantage of the fluoroscopic screen was that the radiologist's eyes had to become adapted to the dark in order to see low-contrast objects. Other disadvantages were difficulties associated with photographing the image, particularly when simultaneous viewing and recording were required.

It is possible to construct extremely fast reflective-refractive optical systems to collect the light of the fluoroscopic screen and to focus it on the input surface of the light-intensifier tube. The output of the light-intensifier tube is optically coupled to a television camera. Images may then be recorded by photographing the television monitor. It is particularly useful when a large field of view at moderate resolution and high contrast is to be studied, as in the case of examinations of the upper and lower gastrointestinal tract.

The x-ray image intensifier combines the functions of x-ray detection and light amplification in a single glass envelope. See Figure 11.10: x rays entering the tube strike the input phosphor, which emits light. The input phosphor is in close proximity to a photocathode, so that the light stimulates the emission of electrons. These are accelerated through the 25-kV electric field and focused by shaping the electric field. The electrons strike the output phosphor, which produces an image that is smaller but brighter than that produced at the input phosphor. The ratio of image brightness of the two phosphors is called the *brightness gain* of the intensifier tube. The brightness gain is the product of the geometric gain (the ratio of the areas of the input and output phosphors) and the electronic gain (the product of input quantum efficiency, photo-cathode efficiency, potential difference between input and output phosphor, and phosphor-output efficiency).

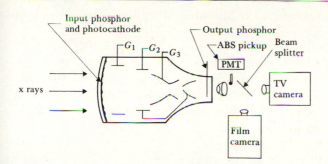

Figure 11.10 In the image intensifier, x rays strike the input phosphor screen, thus generating light. Light stimulates the photocathode to emit electrons, which are accelerated through 25 kV to strike the output phosphor screen. Brightness gain is due to both geometric gain and electronic gain.

A lens mounted on the image intensifier has the purpose of collimating or focusing the image of the output phosphor to infinity. A lens used as a collimator has maximum light-gathering power when compared with the same lens used as a single re-imaging element. The objective lens for each camera collects the light of the collimating lens and refocuses it on the film plane. The advantage of the two-lens system, in addition to its optical speed, is that the distance between the two lenses does not influence the focusing of the systems, and makes possible the use of a beam-splitting mirror, so that light may be directed to more than one output port at a time and proportioned appropriately.

For example, in a two-port fluoroscopic system, all the light may be directed to the television camera during fluoroscopy. During cineradiography, the individual cine frames require a brighter image than that needed for the television camera, so the beam splitter is positioned to direct 90% of the light to the cine camera and 10% of the light to the TV camera. Thus the radiologists may observe the images during the time motion pictures are being made.

Image noise

All radiographic images are noise-limited. Taking the image intensifier as an example, let us now calculate the x radiation required to produce a satisfactory SNR in moving images and then calculate the output of available light of the image intensifier.

We begin at the input phosphor, where the image is noise-limited by the number of absorbed x-ray photons. An input array of $316 \times 316 = 10^5$ pixels should have 10 gray levels, each equal to the fluctuation noise. Thus an average of 10^2 x-ray photons must be absorbed in each pixel. Moving images require about 10 frames/s, so the rate of x-ray photon absorption ϕ_x is

$$\phi_x = (10^5)(10^2)(10) = 10^8 \text{ photons/s}$$

Only 0.25 of the incident x-ray photons are absorbed by the phosphor, so the incident radiation is $10^8/0.25 = 4 \times 10^8$ photons/s. The input phosphor area is 10^4 mm^2, so the incident radiation per unit area is

$$4 \times 10^8/10^4 = 4 \times 10^4 \text{ photons/(s} \cdot \text{mm}^2)$$

The unit of radiation exposure is the roentgen (SI unit, C/kg). One R/s = 7.8×10^7 photons/(s · mm^2) for an x-ray tube operating at 80 kV and for the x-ray beam well filtered through 1 cm of Al. Thus the exposure required is

$$\text{Exposure} = (4 \times 10^4)/(7.8 \times 10^7) = 5.1 \times 10^{-4} \text{ R/s}$$
$$= 0.51 \text{ mR/s}.$$

To calculate the light output, we note that each x-ray photon absorbed in the input phosphor generates 2000 light photons ϕ_L, each having an energy of 2.2 eV. Thus

$$\phi_L = \phi_x(2000) = (10^8)(2000) = 2 \times 10^{11} \text{ photons/s}$$

The conversion efficiency of the photocathode is 15%. Thus the rate of electron emission is $(0.15)(2 \times 10^{11}) = 3 \times 10^{10}$ electrons/s.

These electrons are accelerated to become 25 keV electrons, which strike the output phosphor that has a 10% conversion efficiency. Thus the output power P_o is

$$P_o = (3 \times 10^{10})(0.1)(25000) = 7.5 \times 10^{13} \text{ eV/s}$$
$$= (7.5 \times 10^{13})(1.6 \times 10^{-19}) = 1.2 \times 10^{-5} \text{ W}$$

A typical conversion efficiency for visible light is 640 lumen/W. Thus the light flux is

$$P_o = (640)(1.2 \times 10^{-5}) = 7.7 \times 10^{-3} \text{ lumens}$$

The output area is 10^{-4} m^2, resulting in a luminous emittance of $(7.7 \times 10^{-3})/(10^{-4}) = 77$ lumens/m^2. We multiply by $1/\pi$ to achieve a luminance of $(77)(1/\pi) = 25$ cd/m^2. This luminance is many times that needed to darken film.

If we use a *fluorospot* filming technique (a film system that photographs the output phosphor) with the objective-lens aperture wide open, the film becomes too dark. An operator might reduce the dose of x radiation to achieve proper darkening of the film. However, this would be a mistake, because the image would be statistically limited at the photocathode, and noisy. The proper technique is to increase the dose of radiation to achieve satisfactory image quality and then stop down the film objective lens to achieve proper darkening of the film.

X-ray systems

A radiographic-fluoroscopic system comprises an x-ray table containing an x-ray tube coupled mechanically to the spot-film device. The spot-film device holds a cassette that contains a film and intensifying screens in a "parked" position in a lead-shielded enclosure. During fluoroscopy, the radiologist observes the televised output image of the x-ray image intensifier. When the object or event of interest is discovered, a motor drives the cassette to a position in front of the image intensifier and a radiographic exposure is made, the motor then returns the cassette to "park," and the system reverts to the fluoroscopic mode.

Tomographic systems are arranged so that the generator tube and cassette move about a pivot point or fulcrum during the exposure. The effect is to blur the image of objects outside the plane of the fulcrum. This procedure makes it possible to detect small lung or kidney tumors by blurring the images of overlying structures. There are today tomographic machines that move the tube and cassette in circular, spiral, or hypocycloidal trajectories of such precision that they resolve even the bones of the inner ear quite easily.

11.7 Thermography

The temperature of the skin varies as a function of the underlying circulation of the blood, the metabolism of local structures, the thermal conductivity, the difference in temperature between the skin and the environment, and the moisture of the skin. Defects of circulation, active tumors, changes in body structure, and other effects may affect the surface temperature and provide useful diagnostic information. While radiation thermometry and simple palpation can detect gross temperature differences or large-area changes, the small-area effects such as the temperature profile of blood vessels close to the skin or the temperatures of small areas on the face cannot be detected. Tumors may displace vessels (move them out of their normal locations) before they occlude them (stop their flow), so resulting temperature-profile changes are significant.

Errors in diagnosis

For many diagnostic procedures, an unambiguous diagnosis is not obtained. The image may contain an anomalous shadow rather than a high-contrast image of a tumor. The diagnostician gathers the hints, adds the probabilities, mixes well with past experience, and makes a diagnosis. In any given situation, an area of an image may provide the following combination of true or false readings.

1 Show an object, the object is really there—T_T
2 Show no object, the object is not really there—F_F
3 Show an object, the object is not really there—T_F
4 Show no object, the object is really there—F_T

The first two are correct choices; the third is called a false positive; and the fourth is called a false negative. The best diagnostic procedure is one that yields the lowest probability of false positives and false negatives.

If the probability of a particular disease is small, the error of a false positive should be even smaller. For example, if the probability of an actual case of hydrophobia in a mass screening of school children is 10^{-6}, then a false-positive rate of 0.01% would be intolerable, since 100 times as many children who actually have the disease would have to be treated (rather painfully). If a disease has a rather high incidence—e.g., breast cancer in women past 40 years of age—a high false-positive rate may be harmless if it merely triggers a second type of examination before a surgical decision. Also, if the procedure has a high false-negative rate, and if the disease has a high probability of occurrence, then there is the danger that a large number of real victims will be given false assurance that they are free of disease.

One problem of thermography as a mass-survey device for breast cancer is the high false-positive and false-negative rates, estimated to be over 20% in each case. For purposes of such screening, thermography must never be used without further tests of indicated positives, and the patients must be warned of the limitations of an indicated negative diagnosis.

Principles of detection

Thermal image detectors operate on two basic principles: thermal equilibrium or infrared photoconductivity. An early type of thermal-equilibrium detector was made by coating a thin film of cellulose nitrate with a heat-absorbing oil film. The surfaces of the oil and the object were in thermal equilibrium via the lens system.

That is, the heat radiated from each point of the film to each point of the object was exactly equal to the heat absorbed, so that the temperature pattern of the film represented the temperature pattern in the object. Because of properties of the oil, the thickness of the oil film was reduced where the oil was warmest. A monochromatic light source (sodium-vapor light) illuminated the film, and light interference effects permitted a clear display of the thermal profile.

Another type of thermal-equilibrium imaging device is the thermal vidicon, in which the semiconductor is deposited on a thermally insulated substrate and also comes to thermal equilibrium with the object via the optical system. Since the leakage resistance of semiconductors decreases rapidly with temperature, the electron beam of this camera tube charges the surface of the semiconductor, and the recharging currents are a measure of the temperature pattern.

Unfortunately, obtaining a uniform response over the surface of the detector is a formidable problem. An infrared lens transfers only a fraction of the energy $\Delta E/E$ between two surfaces:

$$\frac{\Delta E}{E} = \frac{C_1}{4f^2 + 1} \tag{11.15}$$

where f is the f number (ratio of focal length to diameter) of the lens and C_1 is a factor containing the infrared energy passband and the transmission of the lens. For a lens of $f/2.5$, and where $C_1 = 0.25$ due to the restricted infrared transmission of the lens, only $0.25/[(4)(2.5)^2 + 1] = 1\%$ of the energy can be transferred. If we assume that the lens is at almost the same temperature as the detector, we can use (2.45) to yield:

$$W_t = \epsilon\sigma T^4 \quad \text{and} \quad \Delta W_t = 4\epsilon\sigma T^3\,\Delta T \tag{11.16}$$

If T_1 and T_2 are the temperatures of two elements in the object space, T_1 is also the average temperature of the detector. And if 1% of the energy is coupled by the lens, then

$$0.01\epsilon\sigma(T_1^4 - T_2^4) = 4\epsilon\sigma T_1^3\,\Delta T$$

and

$$\Delta T = \frac{0.01(T_1^4 - T_2^4)}{4T_1^3} \tag{11.17}$$

For $T_1 = 300$ K and $T_2 = 301$ K, $\Delta T = 0.01$ K. This 0.01-K difference in temperature is that which would result from a 1-K scene difference and would require exceptional uniformity of the detecting surface and extremely low-noise signal amplifiers.

Scanners

For a practical reason—overcoming the problems of achieving uniformity of an imaging surface in thermal equilibrium—a single detector cell is most often used as a scanned detector. Since the same cell and optical system are used in a mechanically scanned arrangement, cell and optical inhomogeneities cancel out over the entire image.

The simplest mechanical scanner consists of a six-sided rotating mirror, which is gimballed to tilt as well as rotate. (See Figure 11.11.) The cell and optical system (lens or mirror) are focused on a small point in the scene via the mirror. Each 60° rotation of the mirror scans one horizontal line of scene, and each line is vertically displaced from the preceding one by the lower tilting of the mirror. One such system operates at 200 lines and 5 s per scene. The output of the cell is amplified and fed to a cathode-ray-tube display having a deflection circuit synchronized to the mechanical scanner. The output image is photographed so that the operator obtains a permanent record.

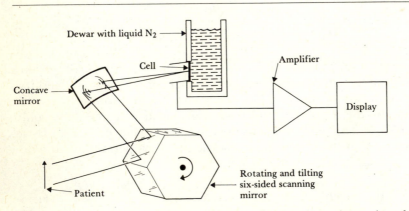

Figure 11.11 Reflecting system (mirrors). The rotating mirror aims the system to different points within the scene. The concave mirror is a front-surface mirror and is effective for all wavelengths. The optical efficiency is not very high because of the limited aperture of such mirror systems.

Variations of the mechanical scanner include components such as a solenoid (moving-coil) mirror, which is used for the vertical tilt, or a rotating prism, as shown in Figure 11.12, which is used in place of the rotating mirror. Figure 11.13 shows a typical arrangement of equipment. Figure 11.14 shows the use of such equipment in detecting breast cancer. Figure 11.15 demonstrates the use of such equipment in diagnosing vascular disorders.

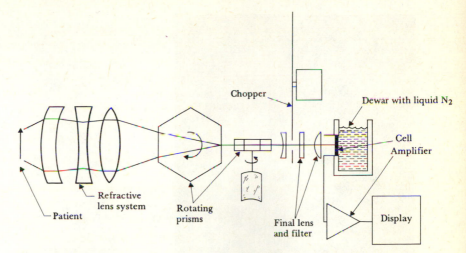

Figure 11.12 Refracting system (lenses). The two rotating prisms accept the infrared radiation from each element of the scene and send it to the final lens and filter. The refracting optical system is more efficient than the mirror system, but can be achromatized for only a limited band, the 3.0-to-5.25-μm band, and is used with InSb detectors.

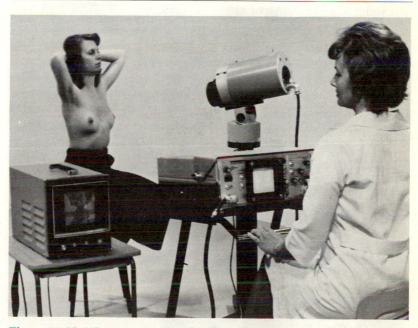

Figure 11.13 When one is using thermography equipment, the area of the patient to be scanned must be uncovered for a few minutes to allow thermal equilibrium with the environment. The room must be free of drafts. (Courtesy of AGA Corporation.)

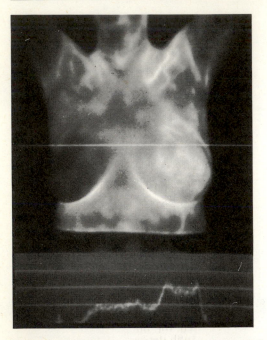

Figure 11.14 The light color on the right of the picture and the higher reading on the line scan show that the patient's left breast is warmer than her right. (Courtesy of General Electric Company.)

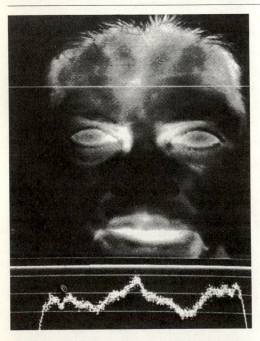

Figure 11.15 The patient's right supraorbital area is cooler than his left. This suggests blockage of the right internal carotid artery. (Courtesy of General Electric Company.)

Detection

Molecules of CO_2 and H_2O, as well as N_2 and O_2, absorb energy at particular values, causing absorption bands and transmission windows in the infrared wavelengths. (See Figure 11.16). The two main windows are the 3.25 to 5.25-μm and 8.25 to 14.00-μm bands. The shorter-wavelength windows (2.00 to 2.50 μm, 1.50 to 1.90 μm) are too close to the visible-light region, and the self-radiation of objects at 300 K is too deficient in energies in those bands for them to be of much utility.

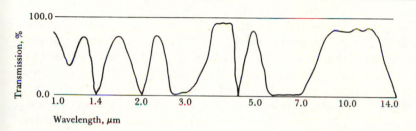

Figure 11.16 The transmission bands of the atmosphere are affected by the absorption characteristics of O_2, CO_2, H_2O, N_2, and other gases. The "windows" of 3.0 to 5.25 μm and 8.0 to 14.0 μm are used for thermal imaging. Near-infrared photography illuminates the patient with infrared radiation and uses photographic film as the detector for wavelengths below 1.4 μm. Thermal imaging is passive and uses only the self-radiation of the patient to form the image. Data shown are for 1-km distance.

While it is possible to focus the infrared energy onto a cell consisting of a temperature-sensitive resistor or bolometer, the thermal time constant of such a device would result in a time required to survey the entire scene, which might not be practical. A time constant of, say, 1 ms would dictate an extremely small thermal mass and it would require more than 1 min to scan the scene.

The detector cells are usually fast-time-constant photoconductors having a band gap or energy response for wavelengths just a bit longer than the window used. Indium antimonide, InSb, has a band gap of about 0.2 eV. This corresponds to a wavelength $\lambda = 1.239/0.2 = 6.2$ μm. That is, a cell with a band gap of 0.2 eV conducts charges when exposed to wavelengths shorter than 6.2 μm. The cell must be shielded from visible light, obviously. The light shield consists of a thin cover layer of, say, Ge or Si, which is opaque to visible but transmissive to infrared wavelengths.

If the cell is kept at room temperature, its own self-radiation would result in enough photons of energy greater than 0.2 eV so that it would conduct an extremely high background or dark current. Since the limit of signal detection is the ratio of signal current to the square root of dark current, it is important to reduce this dark current. A simple way to reduce it is to cool the cell at least to that point at which the dark current is, say, less than 10% of the average-scene signal current. Since the usual optical system is a mirror or lens that subtends a relatively small solid angle in front of the cell, perhaps no more than 0.1 steradian, this means that the dark current must be reduced to much less than 1% of the room-temperature value.

In other words, the cell must be cooled to that temperature at which the number of photons having energies greater than 0.2 eV (wavelengths shorter than 6.2 μm) is reduced to less than 1% of the number at 300 K for the same area.

From Planck's equation (2.43), we can determine the power contained in wavelengths longer than 6.2 μm of a 300-K blackbody. This power is about 2.3×10^{-3} W/cm^2. To have a radiation level below that required to produce 2×10^{-5} W/cm^2 requires that the temperature be reduced to less than 197 K, just above the temperature of dry ice (CO_2 boiling point $\cong$ 195 K). If a detector cell of smaller band gap is used, such as Hg:CdTe, 0.085 eV, to detect radiation out in the 8.25 to 14.00-μm window, cooling is required to near liquid N_2 temperatures, 78 K.

For detectors operating in the 3.25 to 5.25-μm window, it is possible to use refractors (lenses) and to achromatize the optical elements to maintain sharp focus over the required range of wavelengths. Special lens and faceplate materials include Si, Ge, ZnS, CaF_2, and NaCl, but not the common glasses, which are opaque at wavelengths greater than 3.25 μm. A rotating-prism scanner may be used in systems operating in this region, as shown in Figure 11.12.

For systems operating at the longer wavelengths (8.25 to 14.00 μm), the practical difficulties of achromatizing lenses dictate that the all-reflective system, shown in Figure 11.11, be used. Scanning is done by a rotating mirror. The general rules of image detection in noise apply to infrared detectors. However, the signal is that equivalent to a slight change of background. The detection of a breast tumor may mean sensing a 0.5-K change in a 37°C (310-K) background. If not deliberately dried, normal skin has an emissivity above 0.9. It is as if the image is of a light-gray object in a background just a bit less light. Images of objects near room temperature are never high contrast, black to white, in the infrared. If the range of temperature of the total scene is 5 K (34 to 39°C), a reasonable range for medical thermography, we can compute the maximum power contrast from (2.45):

$$W_t = \epsilon \sigma T^4$$

$$\frac{dW_t}{W_t} = \frac{4\epsilon\sigma T^3 \, dT}{\epsilon\sigma T^4}$$

$$= \frac{4\,dT}{T} \qquad\qquad (11.18)$$

Noise-equivalent power (NEP)

To enhance the contrast of the displayed image, the circuit biases out or subtracts the unmodulated portion of the signal current from the detector. However, this unmodulated portion of the signal plus the dark current of the cell contribute to the noise of the cell. In addition, not all input infrared photons are detected because of imperfections of the cell and the limited dimensions of the detector junction.

To measure the noise-equivalent power, NEP, of a detector, we add noise from a calibrated source of noise. Noise is injected at the input to just double the voltage of the output noise. For random-noise-limited systems, doubling the voltage of the output noise means that the voltage of the input injected noise is $\sqrt{3}$ times the noise voltage of the detector, since random signals add as functions of voltage squared,

$$v_t = (v_1^2 + v_2^2 + \cdots v_n^2)^{1/2} \tag{11.19}$$

If several cells are placed in parallel, the noise voltages add as above (random), but true signal voltages add directly (coherent). In general, the SNR improves in proportion to $\sqrt{A}$ and $1/\sqrt{\Delta f}$, where A is the area and Δf is the electrical-signal passband. The NEP may be normalized for passband and cell area to derive D^*, which is normalized for 1 cm^2 and 1 Hz:

$$D^* = (A \, \Delta f)^{1/2}(\text{NEP})^{-1} \qquad \text{cm} \cdot \text{Hz}^{1/2} \, \text{W}^{-1} \tag{11.20}$$

Low NEPs and high D^*s imply best sensitivity. Some typical detectors and their D^* values are as shown in the table.

Material	Operating T, K	λ_{max} μm	D^*, cm $\cdot$ Hz$^{1/2}$ W^{-1}
PbSe	78	6.5	3×10^{11}
PbTe	78	5.5	8×10^9
InSb	195	6.2	8×10^9
InSb	78	6.0	8×10^{10}
Ge:AuSb	78	8.5	1×10^{10}
Hg:CdTe	78	14.5	1×10^{11}

11.8 Nuclear medicine

Nuclear medicine is the branch of medicine that involves the use of radioactive material for the diagnosis of disease and for assessment of the patient. It therefore differs from radiography in that the source of gamma rays is not external to but rather *within* the patient. It differs in a second very important way: The radioactivity can be attached to materials that are biochemically active in the patient. Therefore nuclear medicine is said to image *organ function* as opposed to simple organ morphology. The basic imaging situation in nuclear medicine, then, is the measurement of a distribution of radioactivity inside the body of the patient. These distributions can be either static or changing in time.

Common to nearly all nuclear-medicine imaging instrumentation is the *sodium iodide detector,* shown in Figure 11.17. The detector consists of three main components: (a) the crystal itself, which scintillates with blue light in linear proportion to the energy a gamma ray loses in it; (b) a photomultiplier tube, which converts this light into a proportional electrical signal; and (c) the support electronics, which amplify and shape this electrical signal into a usable form. The simplest nuclear-medicine procedures do not involve images at all, but simply involve the placing of such a detector

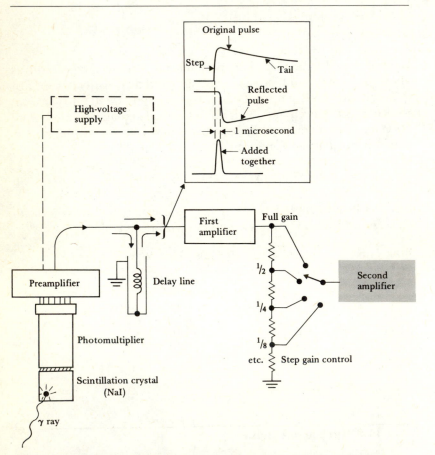

Figure 11.17 Basic implementation of a NaI scintillation detector, showing the scintillator, light-sensitive photomultiplier tube, and support electronics. (From H.N. Wagner, Jr., ed., *Principles of Nuclear Medicine*. Philadelphia: W.B. Saunders Co., 1968. Used with permission of W.B. Saunders Co.)

near the surface of the patient's skin and the counting of the gamma-ray flux.

The first nuclear-medicine imaging device involved the operator taking such a simple detector and moving it in rectilinear paths relative to the patient, in much the same way as we put together an aerial map of the earth. Any process that involves this rectilinear motion of the detector is called *scanning*.

Figure 11.18 shows how the sodium iodide detector must be

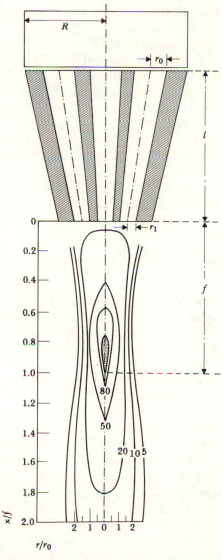

Figure 11.18 Cross section of a focusing collimator used in nuclear-medicine rectilinear scanning. Contour lines below correspond to contours of similar sensitivity to a point source of radiation, expressed as a percentage of the radiation at the focal point. (From G.J. Hine, ed., *Instrumentation in Nuclear Medicine.* New York: Academic Press, 1967.)

collimated in a scanning procedure in order to restrict its field of view, both along its longitudinal axis and transverse to it. The extension of the transverse field of view is the primary determinant of image resolution in a nuclear-medicine scan. If we know the approximate strength of the source, we can combine this information about strength with the basic resolution-element size determined by the collimator to calculate the scan speed necessary to provide the statistical accuracy desired in the image.

For example, consider the nuclear-medicine bone scan, in which an agent that seeks high metabolic turnover in the skeleton is used to locate sites of involvement of the bones by cancers originating elsewhere. A typical dose of such agents is 15 mCi (Ci is the symbol for the standard unit of radioactivity, 1 curie = 3.7×10^{10} nuclear decays/s). The total activity is distributed broadly over the skeleton. And this wide distribution, combined with the isotropic distribution of the gamma rays and the absorption of many of those gamma rays in the patient's own tissue, yields maximum count rates at the body surface of about 1000 cts/s. Typical dimensions of the pixel are 0.5×0.5 cm. If we demand a statistical fluctuation of 10% (100 cts) in this pixel for the position of greatest count rate, the speed is easily determined: counts in pixel = count rate/(horizontal speed $\times$ vertical dimension of pixel). Horizontal speed (cm/min) = count rate/(counts per pixel $\times$ vertical dimension of pixel):

$$1000 \, \frac{\text{cts}}{\text{s}} \, \frac{60 \text{ s}}{\text{min}} \, \frac{0.25 \text{ cm}^2}{100 \text{ cts}} \, \frac{1}{0.5 \text{ cm}} = \frac{300 \text{ cm}}{\text{min}}$$

In the basic stand-alone nuclear-medicine scanning instrument, a *pulse-height analyzer* selects events having the proper gamma-ray energy. These events are used to gate a light source that scans across a film in the same rectilinear fashion that the detector scans across the patient. The images are smoothed by integrating the rate of detector count in a simple rate-meter circuit. Alternatively events selected by the pulse-height analyzer may be scaled digitally as a function of position of the detector. The frequency of storage of scaled information is determined by the desire to have two to three picture elements within the basic resolution dimension determined by the detector collimator. The resulting digital image can be used in computerized image assessment, and can be presented for visual assessment on a storage oscilloscope or video-presentation device. Figure 11.19 shows examples of rectilinear scans that were acquired by these two basic methods.

A second type of nuclear-medicine imaging instrument, introduced about ten years after the rectilinear scanner, has since become the workhorse of the typical nuclear-medicine laboratory. This is the so-called *gamma camera*, sometimes called the Anger camera, after its original developer (Anger, 1958). The gamma

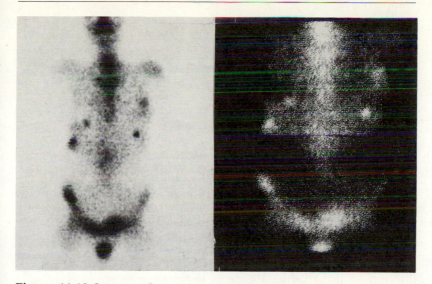

Figure 11.19 Images of a patient's skeleton obtained by a rectilinear scanner, in which a technetium-labeled phosphate compound demonstrates regions of abnormally high metabolism. The conventional analog image is on the left, the digitized version on the right.

camera is a stationary imaging system that is simultaneously sensitive to all the radioactivity in a large field of view. It does not depend on motion of the detector to piece together an image.

Figure 11.20 shows a simplified cross section of such an imaging system. The radiation detector is a single sodium iodide crystal 30 to 40 cm in diameter and 1.2 cm thick. This detector is viewed simultaneously by an array of photomultiplier tubes arranged in a hexagonal pattern at the rear of the detector. If a gamma ray enters the sodium iodide crystal, the resulting scintillation light spreads through the crystal, and thus each photomultiplier tube receives some portion of the total light. The fraction of the total light seen by each tube depends on the proximity of that tube to the original point of entry of the gamma ray.

The fundamental principle of operation of the gamma camera is that the relative fraction of the total light seen by each tube uniquely determines the position of the original point of entry of the gamma ray. Voltages corresponding to the x and y coordinates of the gamma-ray event are reconstructed from the signals of several photomultiplier tubes in an analog electronic circuit. In a modern instrument, this circuit employs operational amplifiers whose gain reflects the position of the given photomultiplier tube in the array. The center of the sodium iodide detector is conventionally assigned the position $x = 0$ and $y = 0$.

For example, a photomultiplier tube positioned far from the center in the conventional $+x$ direction but centered in the y direc-

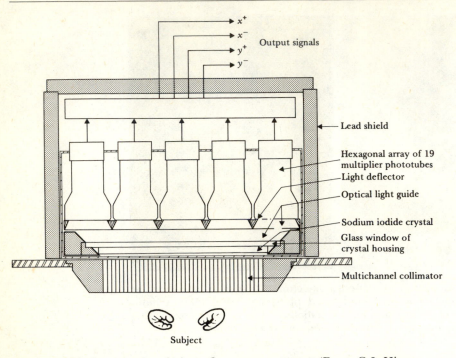

Figure 11.20 Cross-sectional view of a gamma camera. (From G.J. Hine, ed., *Instrumentation in Nuclear Medicine.* New York: Academic Press, 1967.)

tion would have amplifier gains such that the signal from that tube would provide a $+x$ signal disproportionately large relative to the $-x$ signal, but which would provide equal contribution to the total $+y$ and $-y$ signals. The image can be recorded in both analog and digital form. In the analog form, the $+x$, $-x$, $+y$, and $-y$ signals are used as deflection voltages on the plates of an oscilloscope.

Events that satisfy an energy-discrimination condition briefly unblank the oscilloscope and expose a film on which the composite image is formed. Alternatively, the signals can be digitized, and the resulting digitized x and y coordinates used to determine a computer address corresponding to the position of the event. A digital image is built up by incrementing the appropriate computer address at each event.

Figure 11.21 shows an example of gamma-camera images acquired using these two basic methods. One of the most important advantages of the gamma camera relative to the rectilinear scanner is its capability of measuring changes of the distribution of radioactivity as a function of time. Gamma cameras interfaced to computer systems can acquire data at frame rates in excess of 30 frames/s. In fact, even higher frame rates would be conceivable if it were not for the limitation imposed by safety rules regarding exposure of the patient to radiation.

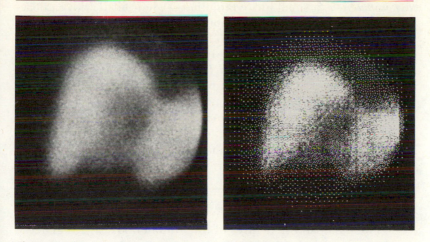

Figure 11.21 Gamma-camera images: anterior view of right lobe of a patient's liver. A colloid labeled with radioactive technetium was swept from the bloodstream by normal liver tissue. Left: conventional analog image. Right: digitized version of the same data.

Because nuclear-medicine images typically have a fundamental resolution distance that is roughly 1% of the image dimension and are composed of only 10^5 to 10^6 photons, they are simple to investigate quantitatively and provide a convenient way of studying the basic imaging concepts listed earlier in this chapter. Figure 11.22 shows the measurement of the response of a gamma camera to a line source of radioactivity. The line-spread function of the camera was easily generated by summing over one dimension of the digital image acquired in a nuclear-medicine computer. This line-response function was then Fourier-transformed to generate the modulation transfer function.

Figure 11.3 dramatizes the relationship between quality of image and number of photons. It shows images of a so-called

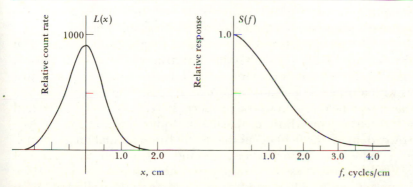

Figure 11.22 Line-spread response function obtained in a gamma camera under computer control, together with corresponding modulation transfer function.

thyroid phantom, a small lucite tank that—when filled with radioactive material—provides a distribution of radionuclides approximating that of a similarly labeled human thyroid. Resolution is demonstrated by the defects or holes intentionally placed in the radioactivity distribution pattern. Each phantom image shown represents an increase in number of photons by a multiplicative factor of 2 from the one before it.

The reference texts of Hine (1967) and of Wagner (1968) provide a complete survey of nuclear-medicine instrumentation for those desiring further information.

11.9 Ultrasonic scanning

The tissue and structures of the human body are, in general, good conductors of sound-wave energy. In particular, the absorption properties are such that a sound wave whose initial intensity is considered biologically safe is still easily detectable after having traversed 20 to 30 cm of human tissue. A sound wave of sufficiently high frequency is a useful probe of the internal structure of the human body. A measure of the size of the structure that can be probed using a wave is given by its wavelength, which is equal to the velocity of the wave divided by its frequency (Section 8.4). Structures of the order of 1 mm in size can thus be imaged by using sound waves in the megahertz frequency range. These high-frequency sound waves are called *ultrasonic waves.*

In a manner analogous to the situation in geometric optics, a sound wave crossing the boundary between two regions of different bulk properties, in particular of different bulk modulus and density, can undergo both reflection and refraction. The angle of refraction and the relative intensity of the reflected and refracted waves are strictly dependent on the bulk properties of the two regions involved. Of course, the simple analogy of geometric optics is useful only so far as the boundary between the two regions is smooth and uniform. It is reflection at just such boundaries that is utilized in the most common forms of ultrasonic imaging.

A piezoelectric transducer is placed in good sonic contact with the surface of the patient's skin. The transducer is then pulsed, causing it to vibrate for a short time at its resonant frequency. Just as with a transmitting radio antenna, the resulting sound radiation has a near-field region whose properties are quite complicated and a far-field region whose properties are quite simple. It is the narrowly defined far-field beam that is the fundamental imaging tool.

When this beam traverses a boundary between two regions of different properties, the boundary reflects some fraction of the beam's intensity. The same transducer detects this reflected radiation, the pulse rate of the transducer being such that the reflected waves from the most distant structures must be received before a new pulse is transmitted. Designers avoid problems due to the complex nature of the near field by making the receiver sensitive only after reflections from this near-field radiation have passed.

The time delay between a transducer pulse and a detected reflection is a measure of the depth of the boundary causing that reflection. The amplitude of the reflected wave is fundamentally a measure of the relative change in bulk modulus or density as the boundary is traversed. The pulse amplitudes are further modulated by the total attenuation suffered by the pulse on its passage to and from the boundary.

We can largely correct for this attenuation factor by using a simple correction scheme, assuming exponential attenuation and representative average values for the attenuation coefficient and velocity of sound in the scanned volume. A reflected pulse arriving after a delay t is increased in amplitude by a factor $\exp(kct)$, where k and c are the average attenuation coefficient and sound velocity, respectively. With a fixed transducer, then, the distribution of reflected intensity as a function of time can be considered to be a map of the discontinuity of tissues along the direction of the scan axis. This mode of ultrasound scanning is called *amplitude-mode*, or A-mode, scanning.

Figure 11.23 shows the application of A-mode scanning to the measurement of the position of the midline of the brain. This tissue discontinuity between the two hemispheres of the brain provides a readily visualized echo. The midline can be displaced from its normal central position by several pathological conditions, and the measurement of midline depth is thus an important diagnostic

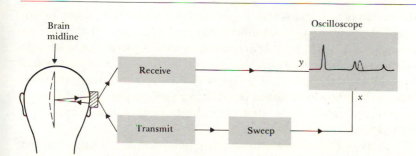

Figure 11.23 A-mode ultrasonic imaging shows the distance and reflectivity of objects along a single scan path.

tool. Figure 11.23 shows the relationship between this spatial position of the midline and its corresponding echo. The dashed midline position would yield the dashed echo time, displaced toward greater elapsed time by the greater total distance traversed by the sound pulse.

Figure 11.24 shows a *time-motion* ultrasound scan (TM scan), a simple extension of the A-mode concept. The depth (echo-delay)

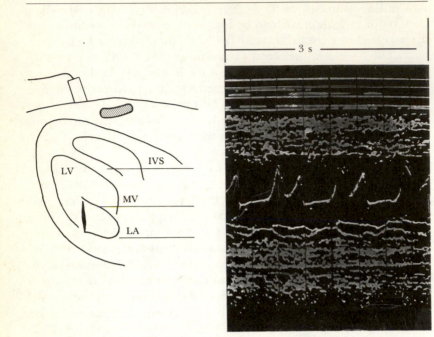

Figure 11.24 Time-motion ultrasound scan of the mitral valve of the heart. The central trace follows the motions of the mitral valve (MV) over a 3-s period, encompassing three cardiac cycles. The other traces correspond to other relatively static structures, such as the interventricular septum (IVS) and the walls of the left atrium (LA).

dimension is now the vertical axis, and the amplitude of the intensity of the returned signal modulates the brightness of the oscilloscope spot. A-mode signals are continuously recorded on a storage oscilloscope as time progresses on the horizontal axis. A vertical slice through the image thus corresponds to the information on A-mode amplitude versus delay at that given instant. Thus the variation of the depth of the structure along the transducer axis is recorded as a function of time.

A two-dimensional image can be made by combining the amplitude-mode information from many different directions. This imaging mode is called *brightness-mode,* or B-mode, scanning. (See Figure 11.25.) The amplitudes of the reflected signals can be used as unblanking signals in a storage-oscilloscope display system. The coordinates of the unblanked point are determined in a simple fashion. The transducer is suspended from a gantry arm such that its angle relative to some reference direction is available to the imaging electronics as a voltage signal. This angle determines a scan line across the image. The point on the scan line is determined by the elapsed echo-delay time.

The *x-y* position of the image that is intensified is thus deter-

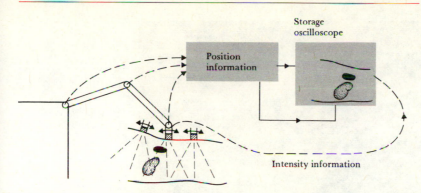

Figure 11.25 B-mode ultrasonic imaging shows two-dimensional shape and reflectivity of objects by using multiple-scan paths.

mined by both the position of the gantry and by the echo-delay time. This simultaneous requirement of both spatial and temporal information is signified by the four dashed lines feeding into the position-information and storage oscilloscope blocks in Figure 11.25. The brightness at any position is determined by the intensity of the echo, just as is the amplitude at any time in A-mode scanning.

The same analog image can of course be stored in a video storage tube, or even digitized for storage and manipulation in a digital computer. Figure 11.26 shows typical ultrasound data. The image can be considered to be a map of structural discontinuity. In a typical application, the clinician can differentiate between an abdominal cyst and a tumor, in that a fluid-filled cyst is free of reflections, while a tumor most likely has some internal structure.

The *resolution* of ultrasound scanning is very much dependent on the apparatus used. Moreover the resolution in the scan direction differs from the resolution transverse to the scan direction. Along the axis of the sound beam, the resolution is determined by the system's ability to measure the time delay between the transmitted and the received sound pulses, i.e., by the width of the temporal pulse of the original transmitted sound pulse. In the direction perpendicular to the axis of the sound wave, the resolution is primarily determined by the beam-focusing properties of the transmitting transducer. The design of a transducer that provides good resolution in this dimension, however, also extends the range of the near-field radiation. Thus improved resolution in this dimension carries with it the cost of decreased capability of imaging shallow structures.

There is an imaging consideration with respect to the contrast of an ultrasound image that is unique in medical imaging. It is possible during a scan to image the same boundary again and again, thus making the image brighter and brighter at that point. If all

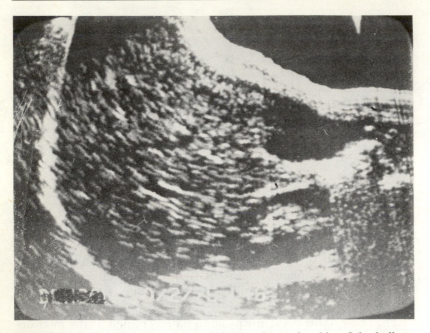

Figure 11.26 This B-mode ultrasonic image shows the skin of the belly at the top right, the liver at the left center, the gall bladder at the right above center, and the kidney at the right below center. The bright areas within the kidney are the collecting ducts. This image corresponds to that shown on the storage oscilloscope display of Figure 11.25.

boundaries are not imaged the same number of times, the final image does not give a true impression of structural discontinuity in the imaged volume. For this reason, sophisticated ultrasound equipment is capable of preventing such overwriting, despite multiple passes over the same anatomical region.

While the ultrasonic imaging techniques just described all require a pulsed system, a continuous-wave ultrasonic imaging system is also clinically useful (Spencer *et al.*, 1974). A focused ultrasonic transducer emits a pencil-like beam into the carotid artery. A direction-sensitive continuous-wave Doppler system detects the velocity of the blood. For those locations where the velocity exceeds a preset threshold, the beam of a storage oscilloscope is intensity-modulated to produce a spot or streak. As in the B-scan system, information is derived from the position-sensing arm, so the x-y position of the reflecting structures corresponds to the x-y position of the intensified point on the oscilloscope. The operator moves the transducer in the plane of the skin and builds up a two-dimensional image of the velocity of local blood. This ultrasonic angiography is like a radiographic image, in that it does not discriminate depth. It is useful in noninvasively identifying stenosis and calcified athero-sclerotic plaques.

Wells (1977b) presents a wealth of material on all aspects of ultrasonic imaging, and lists 1700 references!

11.10 Computer-assisted tomography

One of the most important limitations of the conventional transmission x-ray image is that it is a projection of information in a single direction. If there are, along the same beam path, regions of both small and large variations in electron density, then the small variations cannot be detected. An example of this is the conventional chest radiograph, in which the dense bony structures make it extremely difficult to derive any information about the less-dense region between the lungs.

The only way to be certain of preventing this obstruction of one structure by another is to expose radiographs from every possible direction. This is of course prohibited by limits on the dose of radiation the patient may safely receive. In recent years, however, technology has provided new ways of making each transmitted photon provide information on electron density more efficiently, and the idea of imaging otherwise-hidden structures by multi-directional measurements has become a practical one.

Computer-assisted tomography is the conventional name given to the diagnostic-imaging procedure in which anatomical information is *digitally reconstructed* from x-ray transmission data obtained by scanning an area from many directions. The ideas involved were originally developed for imaging of the brain. The dynamic range of densities in the brain is only a few percent, and yet it is encased in a bony structure so dense that most of the x rays absorbed in the head are absorbed by the bony structure. Thus imaging of the brain using conventional radiographic procedures is extremely difficult, even with enhancement by the use of artificial contrast material.

Figure 11.27 shows a schematic diagram of the scanning operation. A tightly collimated beam of x rays is passed through the patient's head in a direction transverse to his longitudinal axis. The emerging beam flux on the opposite side of the patient is constantly monitored in a scintillation detector. The x-ray source and detector are scanned together perpendicular to the beam direction, and roughly 160 distinct measurements of total attenuation of the x-ray beam are made at evenly spaced points along the scan path. The x-ray beam source and detector configuration is then rotated

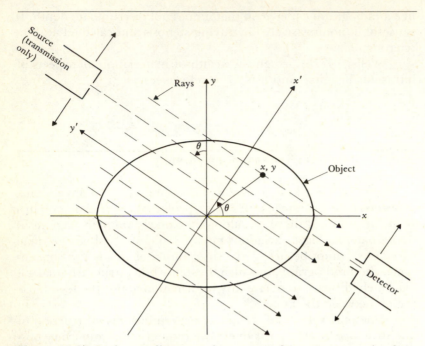

Figure 11.27 Basic coordinates and geometry for computer-assisted to-mography. The projection rays shown represent those measured at some angle θ. The source and detector pair are rotated together through a small angle and a new set of rays measured. The process is repeated through a total angle of 180°. (From R.A. Brooks and G. DiChiro, "Theory of Image Reconstruction in Computed Tomography," *Radiology, 117:* 561–572, Dec. 1975.)

through a small angle, usually 1°, and the procedure is repeated. The acquisition of absorption information by scanning is continued until an angle of 180° has been swept through.

The procedure is called tomography because only those structures lying in the narrow anatomical slice traversed by the beam are being imaged. The tightly collimated beam results in an imaging situation that is essentially scatter-free and that provides the efficiency necessary to make the procedure practical.

Fundamental to the procedure is the mathematical discovery that a two-dimensional function is determined by its *projections* in all directions. A sampling of projections at angles uniformly distributed about the origin can provide an approximate reconstruction of the function. The detail capable of being reconstructed has a straightforward dependence on the number of angles sampled and the sampling coarseness at each angle. If beam absorption is measured at 160 distinct points along each scanning path and a 1° angle increment is used, nearly 29,000 distinct pieces of x-ray absorption data are acquired. These are used to reconstruct a two-dimensional map of x-ray absorption as a function of position, presented as a 160×160 matrix of uniform square-picture elements.

Figure 11.28 shows a typical brain image taken using this procedure. We can see that it is possible to attain a striking image contrast for structures whose x-ray absorptions differ by only a few percent. This represents a significant breakthrough in the radiographic imaging of the head.

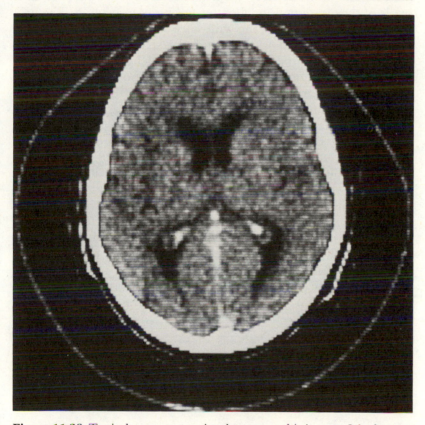

Figure 11.28 Typical computer-assisted tomographic image of the human head. Dark patches are ventricular spaces containing cerebrospinal fluid. The anatomical slice imaged here is located about 3 cm above the base of the brain.

A more recent development is the simultaneous use of several x-ray beams in a fan geometry. The geometry makes practical the scanning of the human chest and abdomen. Other aspects of whole-body scanning are similar to the scanning of the head, except that, in order to maintain the same spatial resolution, the images must have four times as many picture elements.

The reconstruction of images from the scanning data is performed using a small digital computer. The time required for reconstructing the picture is the same order of magnitude of that for acquiring the data. Some of the mathematical reconstruction algorithms allow reconstruction to begin as soon as the first projection data come in. These algorithms clearly provide a considerable saving in time by allowing the mathematical reconstruction to take place during the scan operation.

The mathematical algorithms fall into two general classes, the iterative and the analytic. In the *iterative* methods, an initial guess is made of the two-dimensional pattern of x-ray absorption. The projection data predicted by this guess are then calculated and these predictions compared with the measured results. Discrepancies between the measured values and the model predictions are employed in a continuous iterative improvement of the model array.

Figure 11.29 shows the scheme by which the model projections are generated and by which the discrepancies between model and measurement are used to best improve the model at each iteration. Each reconstructed picture element is represented by an average attenuation coefficient μ_{ij}, where the labels ij specify the position of the picture element in the image. The relative degree to which each element can remove x-ray flux from the ray at the kth beam position at scan angle θ is expressed by the four-labeled quantity $W_{ij}^{\theta k}$. These quantities are essentially determined by the geometric overlap between the finite-width x-ray beam at scan position θk and the square picture element at position ij. Clearly, the overwhelming majority of the more than 8×10^8 quantities $W_{ij}^{\theta k}$ are zero, because in most cases the ray θk does not pass through the element ij at all. The model array μ_{ij} determines the model projection data at each iteration according to

$$I^{\theta k} = I_0 \exp\left(-\sum_{ij} W_{ij}^{\theta k}\, \mu_{ij}\right) \tag{11.21}$$

$$P^{\theta k} = \ln\left(\frac{I_0}{I^{\theta k}}\right) = \sum_{ij} W_{ij}^{\theta k}\, \mu_{ij} \tag{11.22}$$

where I_0 is the constant intensity of the input beam and $I^{\theta k}$ is the intensity transmitted for position k at angle θ. The quantities $P^{\theta k}$, conventionally called the projection data for the position k at angle θ, are calculated in the manner shown in order to convert the observed measurements into quantities that are simple linear combinations of the unknown quantities μ_{ij}.

Just as the weights $W_{ij}^{\theta k}$ determine which picture elements are involved in the generation of the model projections, they also determine the manner in which the model array is changed at each iteration. In the simplest iterative reconstruction techniques, the discrepancy between the measured and model values of $P^{\theta k}$ is attributed equally to all the elements ij traversed by the ray θk, and each model-picture element is changed, according to the geometric

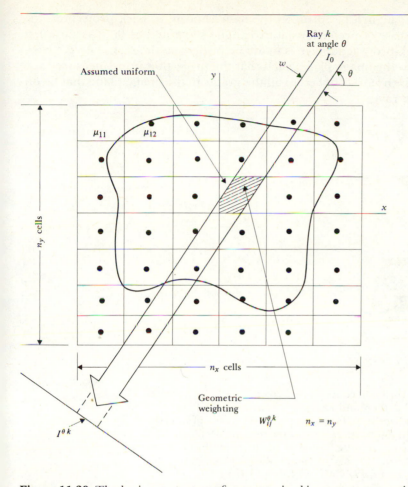

Figure 11.29 The basic parameters of computerized image reconstruction from projections. Shown are the picture element cells μ_{ij}, a typical projection ray $I^{\theta k}$, and their geometric overlap $W_{ij}^{\theta k}$. (From Ernest L. Hall, *Computer Picture Processing and Recognition*, to be published by Academic Press, 1978.)

weights $W_{ij}^{\theta k}$, so as to make the model and measured value for the scan line under consideration come into agreement. In actual practice, many time-saving variations of this fundamental idea have been successfully tried. Regardless of the exact way in which the model array is modified, the rays θk are cyclically iterated over until the model and measurement for *all* ray projections are in adequate agreement.

Analytic methods differ from iterative methods in a very important way. In analytic methods, the image is reconstructed directly from the projection data without any recourse to a comparison between the measured data and the reconstructed model. Fundamental to analytic methods is the concept of *back projection*.

Figure 11.30 shows the basic concept of back projection, for the case of projections at two angles separated by 90°. As shown, a back-projected image is made by projecting the scan data $P^{\theta k}$ back onto the image plane, such that the projection value measured for a given ray is applied to all the points in the image plane that lie on that ray.

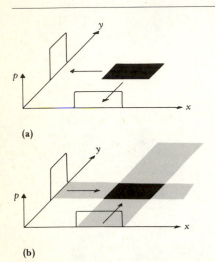

(a)

(b)

Figure 11.30 The back-projection concept. (a) Projections of this object in the two directions normal to the x and y axes are measured. (b) These projection data are projected back into the image plane. The area of intersection receives their summed intensities. One can see that the back-projected distribution is already a crude representation of the imaged object. (From R.A. Brooks and G. DiChiro, "Theory of Image Reconstruction in Computed Tomography," *Radiology, 117:* 561–572, Dec. 1975.)

The total back-projected image is made by summing the contributions from all the scan angles θ. The summing is carried out using the same geometric weights defined in the preceding paragraph. The back-projected image is already a crude reconstruction of the imaged object. More important, the exact relationship between the back-projected image and the desired actual array of attenuation is well understood; the latter can be calculated from the former using standard Fourier-analysis techniques. The back-projected image is Fourier-transformed into the frequency domain and filtered with a filter proportional to spatial frequency up to some frequency cutoff. The result is then transformed back into cartesian coordinates.

It can be shown by Fourier analysis that the same result is obtained if the projection data are filtered first. These filtered projections are used to construct the final back-projected image. The filtering operations can also be done in cartesian space, using convolution techniques (Bracewell, 1965). Analytic algorithms using this approach are sometimes given the general title of *convolution techniques*.

The iterative and analytic approaches to tomographic reconstruction of images are quite comparable in the important measures of speed, accuracy, and precision. Both approaches are in a high state of development and the relative merit of the two methods is still very much under discussion.

The review articles by Brooks and Di Chiro (1975, 1976) provide excellent further reading in the conceptual and mathematical aspects of computer-assisted tomography.

Emission computer-assisted tomography   The same principles just described for x-ray computer-assisted tomography can be applied in nuclear-medicine procedures. In fact, the first clinical applications of these principles were in a nuclear-medicine environment (Kuhl and Edwards, 1963). In the x-ray case, two-dimensional distributions of x-ray *attenuation* are reconstructed from the *summed attenuation* along a large number of straight lines through the imaged structures. In nuclear medicine, the goal is to image a distribution of *radioactivity*. Thus we must measure *sums* of *activity* along straight lines in a corresponding manner.

We can measure these sums in two distinct ways. In the first, the count rate recording instrumentation is made to be sensitive only to the activity lying on a line through the patient by means of detector collimation. The second takes advantage of a very special property of radioactive decay by positron emission. A positron, or anti-electron, emitted from a decaying nucleus stops after a few millimeters of travel in the patient's tissue and undergoes mutual annihilation with an atomic electron.

The most likely product of the annihilation event is two gamma rays. Conservation of energy and linear momentum dictates that they will have nearly equal energies and be nearly opposite in direction. These two gamma rays can be detected in temporal coincidence in a pair of opposed detectors. This coincidence count rate is proportional to the desired total activity along the line separating the two detectors. These two methods, which have come to be called *gamma-ray* and *positron-emission* computer-assisted tomography, respectively, both need to take into account the absorption of radiation between the decay event and the detector system. Corrections to the reconstruction based on both modeled and measured absorption have been successfully applied.

The review article of Brownell *et al.* (1978) provides background reading concerning emission tomographic methods.

Problems

11.1 How much time does it take to transmit a single television frame over telephone lines having a bandwidth of 3 kHz?

11.2 A student whose eyes have 3-mm-diameter pupils watches a television set that has a 48-cm vertical dimension. Using the Rayleigh criterion, how far could he sit from the set and still resolve adjacent lines?

11.3 A square 8 × 8 checkerboard is to be imaged using a raster scan system. The board is centered in this square image. When it is rotated 45° with respect to the image axes, its corners are just touching the centers of the image boundaries. Describe the horizontal and vertical characteristics of this raster scan and the total cycles/image required to detect all the checkerboard squares.

11.4 For the Poisson probability density distribution, calculate and plot $p(K;m)$ for $K = 0, 1, 2, 3, 4, 5$ and for $m = 3$.

11.5 A 100×100 pixel array has an average of 25 photons per pixel. How many picture elements will randomly exceed this average by more than 17 photons?

11.6 How many photons are required to produce a 200×200 cell picture having 6 gray levels?

11.7 Calculate N_e for $S(f) = 1/(1 + 2f)$, where f is in cycles per millimeter.

11.8 Three elements of an optical system have $N_e = 1, 2,$ and 4 cycles/mm. Calculate the system N_e.

11.9 A vidicon target has an active area of 2 cm², a layer thickness of 5 μm, and 10^4 pixels. Estimate the SNR.

11.10 For all other variables fixed, including probability of detection, plot the dimension d of an object versus contrast C for an x-ray image.

11.11 A thermographic system has an f number of $f/4$, $C_1 = 0.35$, and a scene temperature difference of 4 K. What is the resulting difference in detector temperature?

11.12 Explain why there is a requirement that thermographic detectors be cooled while they are being used to scan a patient.

11.13 In block-diagram form, show the design of a nuclear-medicine pulse-height analyzer. For each random pulse entering it that has an energy between two limits, it should output only one count. Note that for energies greater than both limits, the output pulse of the detector amplifier passes through both limits twice (rising and falling wave).

11.14 For the gamma camera describe the x- and y-signal contribution from a photomultiplier that is located in the lower left of the detector array.

11.15 A gamma camera has a line-source response function of $k \exp(-2|x|)$, where k is a constant and x is in centimeters. Calculate the transfer function $S(f)$ of the system.

11.16 Draw a block diagram for an A-scan ultrasonic signal amplifier that corrects for ultrasonic attenuation with distance.

11.17 For Figure 11.23, estimate the sweep speed required for a 10×10 cm display. Estimate the maximum rate of repetition.

11.18 For the ray θk shown in Figure 11.29, estimate and list the value for each nonzero $W_{ij}^{\theta k}$. For ease, assume that a complete overlap of beam and pixel corresponds to a $W_{ij}^{\theta k} = 1.0$.

11.19 Our measurement for the ray shown in Figure 11.29 yields $I_0/I^{\theta k} = 2.0$. Calculate our best guess for μ_{ij} using the $W_{ij}^{\theta k}$ values from Problem 11.18.

11.20 Assume that the object in Figure 11.30(a) occupies the center square of a 3×3 square array. Assume that it has a density of 1.0 and that all other squares have a density of 0. Sketch the resulting curves for $p(x)$ and $p(y)$, the projection data for the directions normal to the x and y axes. Sketch the square array shown in Figure 11.30(b) and assign a density for each square in the resulting back projection.

References

Anger, H.O., "Scintillation camera." *Rev. Sci. Instrum.* 1958, 29, 27.

Biberman, L.M., *Perception of displayed information.* New York: Plenum, 1973.

Bracewell, R., *The Fourier transform and its applications.* New York: McGraw-Hill, 1965.

Brooks, R.A., and G. Di Chiro, "Theory of image reconstruction in computed tomography." *Radiol.,* 1975, 117, 561–572.

Brooks, R.A., and G. Di Chiro, "Principles of computer assisted tomography (CAT) in radiographic and radioisotopic imaging." *Phys. Med. Biol.,* 1976, 21, 689–732.

Brown, F.M., H.J. Hall, and J. Kosar, *Photographic systems for engineers.* Washington: Society of Photographic Scientists and Engineers, 1966.

Brownell, G.L., J.A. Correia, and R.G. Zamenhof, "Positron instrumentation," in J.H. Lawrence and T.F. Budinger (eds.), *Recent advances in nuclear medicine,* vol. 5, New York: Grune and Stratton, 1978.

Coltman, J.W., "The specification of imaging properties by response to a sine wave input." *J. Opt. Soc. Amer.,* 1954, 44, 468–471.

Hall, E.L., *Computer picture processing and recognition.* New York: Academic, 1978.

Hine, G.J. (ed.), *Instrumentation in nuclear medicine.* New York: Academic, 1967.

Jacobson, B., and J.G. Webster, *Medicine and clinical engineering.* Englewood Cliffs, NJ: Prentice-Hall, 1977.

King, D.L., *Diagnostic ultrasound.* St. Louis: Mosby, 1974.

Kuhl, D.E. and R.Q. Edwards, "Image separation radioisotopic scanning," *Radiol.,* 1963, 80, 653–661.

Linfoot, E.H., *Fourier methods in optical image evaluation.* London: Focal, 1964.

Mees, C.E.K., and T.H. James, *The theory of the photographic process,* 3rd ed. New York: Macmillan, 1966.

Rose, A., *Vision—human and electronic.* New York: Plenum, 1973.

Schade, O.H., Sr., "An evaluation of photographic image quality and resolving power." *J. SMPTE,* 1964, 73, 81–119.

Siedband, M.P., *Electronic imaging devices. AAPM Summer School, 1971.* USDHEW Publication 74-8006, 1972.

Spencer, M.P., J.M. Reid, D.L. Davis, and P.S. Paulson, "Cervical carotid imaging with a continuous-wave Doppler flowmeter." *Stroke,* 1974, 5, 145–154.

Ter-Pogossian, M., *The Physics of Diagnostic Radiology.* New York: Harper & Row, 1971.

Wagner, H.N., Jr. (ed.), *Principles of nuclear medicine.* Philadelphia: Saunders, 1968.

Wallace, J.D., and C.M. Cade, "Clinical thermography." *Crit. Rev. Bioeng.,* 1974, 2, 39–94.

Wells, P.N.T., *Physical principles of ultrasonic diagnosis.* New York: Academic, 1969.

Wells, P.N.T. (ed.), *Ultrasonics in clinical diagnosis.* 2nd ed. Edinburgh: Churchill Livingstone, 1977a.

Wells, P.N.T. *Biomedical ultrasonics.* New York: Academic, 1977b.

Wolfe, W.L., *Handbook of military infrared technology.* Washington: GPO, 1965.

Chapter twelve

Therapeutic and prosthetic devices

Michael R. Neuman

As noted in earlier chapters of this book, the primary use of medical electronic instrumentation is in diagnostic medicine. Most instrumentation senses various physiologic signals, carries out some processing of these signals, and displays or records them. There is, however, a class of medical electronic devices that are useful therapeutically, or as prostheses. Electrical stimulators of one form or another represent an important subgroup in this area. Also available are other devices, such as incubators, ventilators, heart-lung machines, artificial kidneys, diathermy, and electrosurgical instruments. In this chapter we examine some of these devices and look briefly at their principles of operation.

12.1 Cardiac pacemakers and other electrical stimulators

There is a wide variety of electrical stimulators used in patient care and research. These range from very low-current, low-duty-cycle stimulators, such as the cardiac pacemaker, to high-current single-pulse stimulators, such as defibrillators. In this section, we examine the pacemaker in detail, and look at other applications of electrical stimulators.

Cardiac pacemakers

The cardiac pacemaker is an electrical stimulator that produces periodic electrical pulses that are conducted to electrodes located either on the surface of the heart, within the heart muscle (the myocardium), or within the cavity of the heart. The stimulus thus conducted to the heart causes it to contract; this can be used prosthetically in diseased states in which the heart is not stimulated at a proper rate on its own. The principal pathologic conditions in which cardiac pacemakers are applied are known collectively as *heart block*. These are reviewed by Furman and Escher (1970).

An *asynchronous* pacemaker is one that is free-running. Its electrical stimulus appears at a uniform rate regardless of what is going on in the heart or the rest of the body. It therefore gives a fixed heart rate.

Figure 12.1 shows a block diagram of an asynchronous pacemaker. The power supply is necessary to supply energy to the pacemaker circuit. In rare cases, for external pacemakers, this can be supplied through the power lines, but the risk of electric shock from leakage currents makes this technique very undesirable. A far more convenient method, and one that is usually used, involves deriving power from primary or secondary battery sources. In some implantable pacemakers, energy is transmitted to the implanted circuit by means of magnetic induction from an external coil located on the skin over the site of the implant.

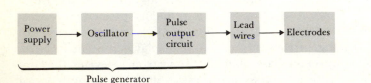
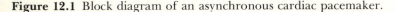

Pulse generator

Figure 12.1 Block diagram of an asynchronous cardiac pacemaker.

The oscillator establishes the pulse rate for the pacemaker; this, in turn, controls the pulse output circuit that provides the stimulating pulse to the heart. This pulse is conducted along lead wires to the cardiac electrodes.

Each of these blocks is important in the construction of the pacemaker; and each must be made highly reliable, since faulty operation of this device can cost a patient's life.

Another component of the overall construction of the pacemaker that is not included in Figure 12.1 is the package itself. Not only must the package of an implanted pacemaker be compatible and well tolerated by the body, but it must also provide the necessary protection to the circuit components in order to ensure their reliable operation. The body is a corrosive environment, so the package must be designed to operate well in this environment, while occupying minimal volume and mass. Implantable pacemakers are frequently encapsulated in a cast-epoxy resin, the external surface of which may or may not be coated with a layer of silicone rubber. This material is one of the best materials currently available in terms of biologic compatibility with soft tissues. The lead wires and electrodes are, therefore, also frequently molded in silicone rubber to provide maximum biocompatibility for the critical locations in which they are found.

Let us now examine each of the blocks in Figure 12.1 in more detail, and study some of the circuits involved.

Power supply

The most frequently used power supply for implantable pacemakers is a battery made up of primary cells. High-quality mercury cells are often used to obtain a 6- to 9-V source by connecting several cells in series. Modern pacemaker circuits exhibiting low-current drain characteristics give such cells a theoretical lifetime that approaches their shelf life. In practice, however, these cells are frequently discharged in about two years. This is generally due to a malfunction of the pacemaker electronics or early deterioration of the cells themselves, both cases often being related to internal defects or poor packaging practice. More recently developed lithium batteries are expected to last about 10 years.

Implantable pacemakers can also be powered from an external source. Figure 12.2 shows the power supply of a typical transcutaneous RF induction pacemaker. The patient wears, on a harness, a battery-powered RF oscillator and power amplifier connected to a pancake coil. The coil is placed close to the surface of the skin over a smaller internal subcutaneous coil, so that magnetic energy from the external coil induces a voltage in the internal coil. Thus a voltage transformer is formed. The induced voltage is then rectified and filtered to give a dc voltage. The magnitude of this voltage depends on the coupling coefficient between the two coils. Consequently, as the patient moves or changes the location of the external coil, the internally induced voltage changes. Since this affects the operation of the pacemaker, it is important that a voltage-regulator circuit be included in the implantable unit so that a constant voltage is provided to the pacemaker circuitry.

This transcutaneous power source has been demonstrated to

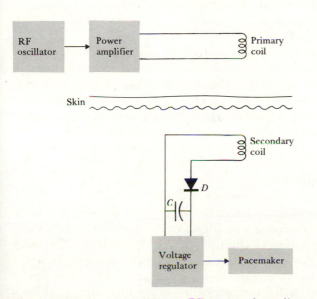

Figure 12.2 A transcutaneous RF-powered cardiac pacemaker system. The RF oscillator and power amplifier are located outside the body. Primary coil is placed on skin surface over implanted secondary coil that is located just beneath the skin. Remainder of circuitry is located at site of implanted pacemaker.

operate pacemakers successfully. One of its advantages is that it can use ordinary flashlight batteries as its source of power. These can be replaced in the external circuit when they begin to deteriorate. Such systems must provide continuous power to run the internal pacemaker. This can be achieved if the voltage regulator, instead of directly powering the pacemaker, charges a battery made up of secondary cells such as nickel-cadmium cells. These store a charge and operate the pacemaker for periods of time when external power is not being provided. Such systems have been arranged so that the external source need only be applied by patients to charge their internal batteries while they are sleeping by placing the external source in its harness before retiring.

A major limitation of this system is in the secondary battery itself. These batteries are not as efficient as the primary cells, and cannot store as much energy per unit mass. Furthermore, their properties deteriorate with frequent charge-discharge cycles so that their overall lifetime in the implanted unit is often no greater than that obtained from primary cells.

Nuclear energy sources for implantable pacemakers have been developed, and promise greater lifetimes through higher reliability. Several of these are reviewed by Schaldach and Furman (1975). These sources involve a decaying radioactive substance and absorber that becomes heated by the radiation from the source. This heat is then used to generate electrical energy through a thermopile, a series connection of high-efficiency thermocouples, that can provide an electrical output of 500 to 700 mV. This output is then raised to levels required by the pacemaker circuit by means of a dc-to-dc converter circuit. Figure 12.3 is a block diagram of this type of power supply.

A major problem is the protection of the patient and other individuals from ionizing radiation. Although the power source is well shielded, the source of radiation could be released when the patient suffers severe trauma, such as might happen in an automobile accident or fire. Units in use today are very sturdy and can withstand even this type of severe trauma.

Timing circuit

The asynchronous pacemaker represents the simplest form of a pacemaker because it provides a train of stimulus pulses at a constant rate regardless of the functioning of the heart. The oscillator in this case can be free-running: either a blocking oscillator or a multivibrator. In either case, to minimize demands on the power supply, it is desirable for the oscillator to operate under conditions requiring the least energy possible.

Figure 12.4(a) shows a blocking oscillator for a pacemaker. When power is initially applied to this circuit, the 3-μF capacitor is

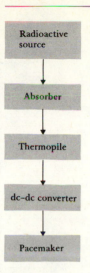

Figure 12.3 A cardiac pacemaker powered by a radioactive source. Heat from the source undergoing spontaneous decay generates electrical power in the thermopile which is at a voltage too low to operate the pacemaker circuitry, and so it must be converted to a higher voltage by the dc-to-dc converter.

charged through the 1-MΩ resistor. Once it is charged to a voltage that forward-biases the base-emitter junction of transistor Q_1, this element is turned on. This causes a collector current to pass through the transformer primary and an emitter current to flow through the 10-kΩ emitter resistance; in addition there is a small amount of current that goes to the output-circuit transistor base. The collector current in Q_1 causes a current to be induced in the secondary of the transformer that discharges the capacitor and turns off the transistor. The process then repeats itself to produce a pulse train. Thus, the pulse-repetition rate for this circuit depends on the time constant of the resistance and capacitance in the base circuit, as well as on the power-supply voltage and transistor turn-on voltage. The duration of each individual pulse is determined primarily by the characteristics of the transformer.

This circuit is simple and employs only a few components. Only two components are of key importance in determining the repetition rate; one determines the duration. The transistor itself acts only as a switch. The circuit is relatively insensitive to variations in transistor parameters.

Figure 12.4(b) shows a multivibrator timing circuit that contains several more components than the blocking oscillator. Multivibrators using complementary-pair transistors are used in pacemaker timing circuits so that both transistors are on only during the pulse interval itself. This conserves energy from the power

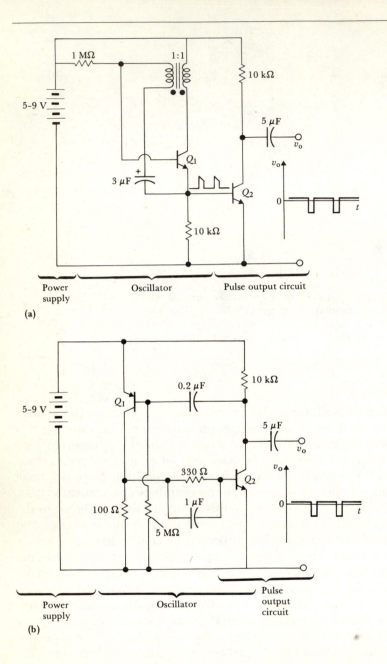

Figure 12.4 Two types of asynchronous cardiac pacemaker generator circuits. (a) A blocking oscillator circuit that is frequently used. (b) A complementary-pair multivibrator circuit designed for minimal consumption of power, so that it can be used with non-battery types of power supplies.

supply. The 0.2-μF base capacitor on transistor Q_1 is charged through the 5-MΩ resistor until the base voltage reaches approximately 600 mV, which turns on Q_1. Some of the collector current from this transistor passes to the base of transistor Q_2 and turns it on. This brings the base capacitor of transistor Q_1 to the negative supply voltage. The charge on the capacitor is discharged through Q_1, turning it off once sufficient charge has left the capacitor to lower its voltage below the turn-on voltage of the transistor. This, in turn, turns off transistor Q_2, and the process is repeated. The pulse repetition rate is determined by the 5-MΩ resistor and the 0.2-μF capacitor as well as by the voltage of the power supply. Although this particular circuit is designed to minimize the effects of power-supply voltage on its output, weakening batteries can change the pulse repetition rate.

Timing circuits in asynchronous cardiac pacemakers produce pulses at fixed rates, ranging from 70 to 90 beats per minute. Their width ranges from 0.5 to 2 ms and their amplitudes range from 5 to 9 V. Additional timing circuits are described by Hill (1973), Hill and Dolan (1976), and Schaldach and Furman (1975).

Output circuit

The pulse-output circuit of a pacemaker generator amplifies the electrical pulse to be applied to the stimulating electrodes to produce myocardial contraction. The output circuit consists of a transistor operated as a switch and an appropriate coupling circuit to the electrodes. In some cases in which monophasic pulses are applied directly to the electrodes, they are merely connected in series with the switch and power supply. Such unidirectional pulses, however, result in damage to the electrodes due to electrolytic corrosion, so biphasic pulses are more desirable.

In Figure 12.4(a) the output circuit consists of transistor Q_2, which is operated as an inverter and is coupled to the electrodes through the 5-μF coupling capacitor to give biphasic negative-going pulses. Because the net buildup of charge on the capacitor is zero in the steady state, between pulses the negative-going area of the pulse just equals the positive-going area. Thus the net current through the electrode over one pacemaker cycle is zero.

In Figure 12.4(b), transistor Q_2 of the multivibrator circuit also serves as the output circuit. In this way only the coupling capacitor of the electrode is required, in addition to those components already in the timing circuit. In some multivibrator pacemaker circuits, however, an additional output-circuit switch of the type described for the blocking oscillator is added to the circuit to isolate the load from the multivibrator to provide more stable operation. The stimulating current is dependent on the impedance of the electrode system. It will not be constant when constant-voltage pulses are used (Figure 5.27), but will have an average value (during the pulse) of the order of 1 mA.

Lead wires and electrodes

Since, in most pacemaker designs, the generator is located at some position remote from the heart itself, there must be an appropriate conduit to carry the electrical stimuli to the heart and to apply them in the appropriate place. The lead wires, in addition to being good electrical conductors, must be mechanically strong. Their distal ends must not only withstand the constant motion of the beating heart, but as the individual in whom the pacemaker is implanted moves about, these lead wires have to be able to withstand the stress of being flexed in various positions. A second requirement of the lead-wire system is that it must maintain good electrical insulation. If this is not the case, wherever faults in the insulation occur, there is effectively another stimulating electrode which, in addition to possibly stimulating the tissue in its vicinity, shunts important stimulating current away from its intended point of application on the heart.

To meet these requirements, lead wires presently used consist of interwound helical coils of spring-wire alloy molded in a silicone-rubber cylinder. The helical coiling of the wire minimizes stresses applied to it, while the multiple strands serve as insurance against failure of the pacemaker following rupture of a single wire. The soft silicone-rubber encapsulation both maintains flexibility of the lead-wire assembly and provides appropriate electrical insulation and biologic compatibility.

Cardiac pacemakers are either of the *unipolar* or *bipolar* type. In a unipolar one, a single electrode is in contact with the heart, and negative-going pulses are connected to it from the generator. A large indifferent electrode is located somewhere else in the body, usually mounted on the generator, to complete the circuit. In the bipolar system, two electrodes are placed on the heart, and the stimulus is applied across these electrodes. Both systems of electrodes require approximately the same stimulus for efficient cardiac pacing, as long as negative-going pulses are applied in the unipolar system.

There are clinically used pacemakers utilizing each system. The electrodes themselves can be placed on the external surface of the heart (epicardial electrodes), buried within the heart wall (intramyocardial electrodes), or pressed against the inside surface of the heart (endocardial or intraluminal electrodes). In the latter case, it is possible to introduce the electrodes into the heart through a shoulder or neck vein so that it is not necessary to surgically expose the heart during the implantation process.

As with the lead wires, the materials of which electrodes are made are important. The electrodes must be able to stand up to the repeated flexing they encounter due to the mechanical activity of the heart, and they must remain in place to provide effective pacing. They must also be made of materials that do not dissolve during long-term implantation, or cause undue irritation to the heart tissue adjacent to them. They must also be materials that do not undergo electrolytic reactions when the stimulus is applied. To avoid any junctional problems, these electrodes are often made of the same materials as the lead wires. Platinum is a very popular material for electrodes because it is chemically inert. Pacemakers today frequently use platinum electrodes that have been welded to special lead-wire alloys. In early pacemakers, the most common type of failure was associated with lead-wire breakage. Today, due to technological advances such as those just described, this problem has been greatly reduced.

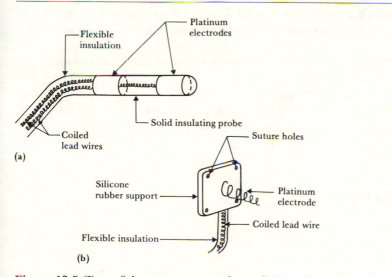

Figure 12.5 Two of the more commonly applied cardiac pacemaker electrodes. (a) Bipolar intraluminal electrode. (b) Intramyocardial electrode.

Figure 12.5 shows the basic structure of a typical bipolar intraluminal electrode and single intramyocardial electrode. The conducting bands around the circumference of the solid intraluminal probe contact the endocardium (internal surface of the heart wall) and electrically stimulate it. The intramyocardial electrode is placed on the exterior surface of the heart. A puncture wound is made into the wall of the heart and the helical spiral-shaped electrode is placed in this hole. To hold the electrode in place, the silicone-rubber supporting piece is then sutured to the epicardial (external) surface of the heart. This flexible back support provides a good mechanical match between the electrode and the heart wall.

For bipolar intramyocardial stimulation, a pair of these electrodes is attached to the myocardium.

Synchronous pacemakers

Often patients require cardiac pacing only intermittently, since they can establish a normal cardiac rhythm between periods of block. For these patients, it is not necessary to continuously stimulate the ventricles; in some cases continuous stimulation can even result in serious complications. For example, if an artificial stimulus falls in the repolarization period following a spontaneous ventricular contraction, ventricular fibrillation can result. Thus it is important in these cases that the artificial pacemaker does not compete with the heart's normal pacing action. Such a situation can be achieved with an asynchronous pacemaker by making the rate sufficiently high so that the heart does not have a chance to beat on its own between pacemaker stimuli. A better solution, however, involves the use of synchronous pacemakers.

There are two general forms of synchronous pacemakers: the demand pacemaker and the atrial-synchronous pacemaker. A diagram of the *demand* pacemaker is shown in Figure 12.6. It consists of a timing circuit, output circuit, and electrodes, just like those of the asynchronous pacemaker, but it has a feedback loop in addition. The timing circuit is set to run at a fixed rate, usually 60 to 80

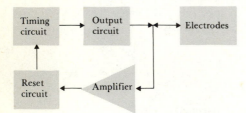

Figure 12.6 A demand-type synchronous pacemaker. Electrodes serve as a means of both applying the stimulus pulse and detecting the electrical signal from spontaneously occurring ventricular contractions that are used to inhibit the pacemaker's timing circuit.

beats/min. After each stimulus, the timing circuit resets itself, waits the appropriate interval to provide the next stimulus, and then generates the next pulse. However, if, during this interval, a natural beat occurs in the ventricle, the feedback circuit detects the QRS complex of the ECG signal from the electrodes and amplifies it. This is then used to reset the timing circuit. It awaits its assigned interval before producing the next stimulus. If the heart beats again before this stimulus is produced, the timing circuit is again reset and the process repeats itself. Thus we see that, if the heart's conduction system is operating normally and the heart has a natural rate that is greater than the rate set for the timing circuit, the pacemaker remains in a standby mode, and the heart operates under its own pacing control. In this way the heart can respond to changing demands of the organism by changing its rate in the usual physiologic manner. If, on the other hand, temporary heart block occurs, the pacemaker takes over and stimulates the heart at the fixed rate of the timing circuit.

The *atrial-synchronous* pacemaker is a more complicated circuit, as shown in Figure 12.7. In this case, the pacemaker is designed to replace the blocked conduction system of the heart. The heart's physiologic pacemaker located at the SA node initiates the cardiac cycle by stimulating the atria to contract and then providing a stimulus to the AV node which, after appropriate delay, stimulates the ventricles. If the SA node is able to stimulate the atria, the electrical signal corresponding to atrial contraction (P wave of the ECG) can be detected by an electrode implanted in the atrium and used to trigger the pacemaker in the same way that it triggers the AV node. Figure 12.7 shows the voltage v_1 that is detected by the atrial electrodes.

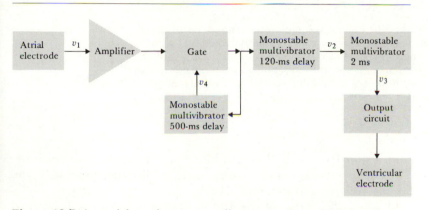

Figure 12.7 An atrial-synchronous cardiac pacemaker, which detects electrical signals corresponding to the contraction of the atria and uses appropriate delays to activate a stimulus pulse to the ventricles. Figure 12.8 shows the waveforms corresponding to the voltages noted.

This voltage is shown again in Figure 12.8 as a pulse that corresponds to each beat. The actual waveform detected by the atrial electrodes also shows some artifact during the ventricular contraction, but this has been omitted from Figure 12.8, for clarity. This atrial signal is then amplified and passed through a gate to a monostable multivibrator giving a pulse v_2 of 120-ms duration, the approximate delay of the AV node. Another monostable multivibrator giving a pulse duration of 500 ms is also triggered by the atrial pulse. It produces v_4, which causes the gate to block any signals from the atrial electrodes for a period of 500 ms following contraction. This eliminates any artifact caused by the ventricular

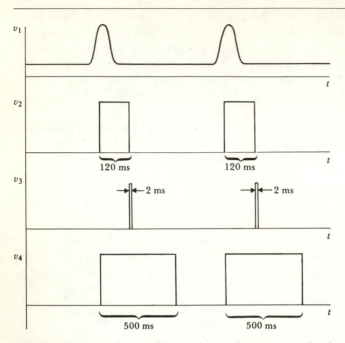

Figure 12.8 Waveforms of the various voltages appearing in the atrial synchronous pacemaker of Figure 12.7. v_1 is the signal detected by the atrial electrodes with the ventricular artifact removed. v_2 is the output of the 120-ms delay multivibrator. v_3 is the stimulus pulse to the output circuit and then to the myocardium. v_4 is the inhibit pulse that prevents the pacemaker from generating a ventricular pulse triggered by the artifact from a previous stimulus.

contraction from stimulating additional ventricular contractions. Thus the pacemaker is refractory to any additional stimulation for 500 ms following atrial contractions.

The falling edge of the 120-ms-duration pulse, v_2, is used to trigger a monostable multivibrator of 2-ms duration. Thus the pulse v_2 acts as a delay, allowing the ventricular stimulus pulse v_3 to be produced 120 ms following atrial contraction. v_3 then controls an output circuit that applies the stimulus to appropriate ventricular electrodes.

Often atrial-synchronous pacemakers have provisions to run at a fixed rate in case atrial stimulus is lost. This is achieved by combining the demand-pacemaker system with the atrial-stimulus pacemaker system so that an atrial stimulus disables a fixed-rate timing circuit. If the stimulus is absent, the fixed-rate timing circuit takes over and controls the output circuit in the same way as in the asynchronous pacemaker.

Example 12.1 An asynchronous cardiac pacemaker delivers 5-V pulses of 2-ms duration to bipolar electrodes, which can be approximated as being a 2-kΩ resistive load. The pulse rate of the pacemaker is 70 per minute. The pulses represent 25% of the energy consumed by the pacemaker. The pacemaker is powered by four mercury cells connected in series to give a voltage of 5.4 V. As the designer of this circuit, you are called on to specify a battery capable of operating the pacemaker for 5 years. What is the minimum acceptable capacity for each cell?

Answer The energy per stimulus pulse will be

$$E_p = \frac{v^2}{R} T = \frac{(5 \text{ V})^2}{2 \text{ k}\Omega} \times 2 \text{ ms} = 25 \text{ } \mu\text{J} \qquad \text{(E12.1)}$$

The number of pulses in 5 years (including one leap year) will be

$$N = 70 \text{ min}^{-1} \times 60 \text{ min/h} \times 24 \text{ h/d} \times 365.25 \text{ d/yr} \times 5 \text{ yr}$$
$$= 1.84 \times 10^8 \text{ pulses} \qquad \text{(E12.2)}$$

Thus the total energy in these pulses will be

$$E_t = NE_p = 1.84 \times 10^8 \times 25 \text{ } \mu\text{J} = 4.6 \text{ kJ} \qquad \text{(E12.3)}$$

The energy supplied by the battery must be four times as great:

$$E_b = 4E_t = 18.4 \text{ kJ} \qquad \text{(E12.4)}$$

If, for the sake of argument (since it would be unwise to draw such a large current from these cells due to polarization effects), we draw a current of 1 A from the battery, it would be supplying a power of 5.4 W. The period of time over which this power would have to be supplied to give an energy E_b would then be

$$t = \frac{E_b}{5.4 \text{ W}} = 3.41 \text{ ks} = 0.947 \text{ h} \qquad \text{(E12.5)}$$

Thus the battery capacity must be at least 0.947 A·h, or, rounding off, 1 A·h, to operate this pacemaker.

Bladder stimulators

Urinary incontinence and other neurologic bladder dysfunctions can, in some cases, be treated by electrical stimulation. In the case of incontinence, the sphincter muscles surrounding the urethra are unable to contract sufficiently to occlude the urethra, and increased pressure within the bladder due to coughing, laughing, or neurologically excited excessive contraction of the detrusor muscle of the bladder wall can result in the uncontrollable passage of urine. The individual with this problem is in a most unfortunate situation. Several investigators and manufacturers are looking for practical ways to control this problem through electrical stimulation. Some of these methods are reviewed by Hill (1973) and by Susset (1973). These involve placing stimulating electrodes in or near the muscles involved in sphincteric control of the urethra or on the nerves supplying these muscles. The electrodes stimulate electrically, with pulses of durations of from 0.5 to 5 ms at a repetition rate from 20 to 100 pulses/s, depending on the individual investigator.

When neural electrodes are used, pulse duration can be shortened to be in the range of 100 to 400 μs. Average stimulating currents (during the pulse) are of the order of 1 mA. Electrodes are frequently placed directly on sphincter muscles, and optimal locations are determined during the implantation surgery by placing a balloon attached to a pressure transducer within the urethra in the region of the sphincters and locating the electrodes so as to give a maximum increase in pressure within the balloon during stimulation.

Noninvasive stimulating electrodes have also been described. In the case of women, such electrodes can be placed on a vaginal pessary that is positioned so as to place the electrodes against the anterior vaginal wall, posterior to the urethra. In men, an anal plug containing electrodes can be used to stimulate the sphincter muscles of the urethra.

Some patients require continuous stimulation to avoid incontinence; and due to the high rate of stimulation, this requires greater capabilities of power supply over a period of time when compared with the cardiac pacemaker. For this reason, techniques of transcutaneous stimulation such as those shown in Figure 12.2 for the cardiac pacemaker are often used.

Another form of transcutaneous stimulator used in this application is the RF unit shown in Figure 12.9. The implanted circuit is entirely passive, with the internal secondary coil located just beneath the skin and coupled to an external primary coil placed over it. The primary coil is driven by a 1-MHz RF oscillator that is keyed by the timing circuit to produce the desired pulses. The power supply for this external circuitry is made up of replaceable or rechargeable batteries. The internal circuit consists of a capacitor C_1 to resonate the secondary coil to the oscillator frequency, a diode detector, and a filter capacitor C_2 to remove the RF component from the detected pulse waveform. The stimulus is then applied directly to the electrodes. Although the percutaneous transmission of energy is not very efficient, signal amplitudes of several volts can be obtained at the electrodes with primary-to-secondary coil spacings of approximately 1 cm.

Bladder stimulators are also used to help patients with incompetent bladders to void. Patients with certain neurologic injuries

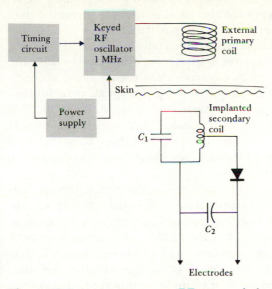

Figure 12.9 A transcutaneous RF-powered electric stimulator. Note that the implanted circuit of this stimulator is entirely passive and that the amplitude of the pulse supplied to the electrodes is dependent on the coupling coefficient between the internal and external coils.

find themselves unable to pass their urine because they cannot contract their detrusor muscle. Stimulators have been developed that can be controlled externally to cause the detrusor muscle to contract. This enables the patient to expel the contents of the bladder on command. Such stimulators require multiple electrodes on or within the bladder wall to effect complete emptying. Again the RF percutaneous technique can be used; this time it is necessary only to bring the transmitting unit over the secondary coil when the patient desires to void.

Suppression of pain

Electrical stimulation of tissues is sometimes used as a means of suppressing pain. Both battery-powered and transcutaneous RF-powered stimulators have been developed to alleviate severe intractable pain. Such devices have met with varying degrees of success. The success of the paraesthesia or anesthesia often depends on the selection of the patient. It is also known that in some cases the effectiveness of the stimulation decreases after periods of continuous stimulation.

Different types of stimulation systems have been developed. Cutaneous stimulators, operating through surface electrodes on the skin, have been shown to increase the pain threshold in the vicinity of the electrodes. This effect has been shown best when the stimulus is intermittent. Electrodes implanted in the immediate vicinity of peripheral nerves are also used to provide increased pain thresholds in areas innervated by the particular nerve distal to the point of stimulation. Implantable electrodes coupled to a subcutaneous inductive-type receiver system have been used in this case. Both bipolar and monopolar electrodes are used.

Stimulation of posterior portions of the spinal cord (dorsal-column stimulation) is another means of diminishing intractable pain. The technique of transcutaneous RF-transmission is usually used, with commercial units for carrying out these functions now on the market. Stimulus parameters for these devices are similar to those for the bladder stimulators.

Although the use of acupuncture is controversial, this method is used for the reduction of pain. The traditional methods of acupuncture, whereby the needles inserted into various locations in the body are twisted to provide appropriate stimulation, have been replaced by many modern practitioners of ancient art with electrical stimulation of the needles. External stimulators are connected to needles placed in the traditional manner, and because of the electrical stimulation it is no longer necessary to move the needles.

Muscle stimulators

There have been various applications of electrical stimulation to muscle. Stimulators can be used in physical therapy to determine whether muscle groups are able to contract by applying external stimuli to these muscles and observing the results. Stimulators are especially useful in cases in which temporary paralysis can result due to atrophy of the muscle caused by disuse, which significantly reduces the mass of the muscle. By periodic direct stimulation of the muscle, the clinician can exercise the muscle, even though the normal neurostimulation is not available. Electrical stimulation of muscle can also be used to regain function of paralyzed muscles when the paralysis is a result of neurologic injury. It has been demonstrated that patients with spinal-cord injury can regain some crude function of specific skeletal muscles by means of programmed electrical stimulation. One such example is an individual whose muscles controlling a hand are completely paralyzed; electrical stimulation can enable the person to gain a crude ability to grasp.

Another example of a stimulator that is commercially available is one concerned with problems of stroke victims. Often these patients encounter gait problems that are evidenced in a condition known as dropfoot. In this case, an individual picks up the paralyzed foot to walk, but is unable to lift the ball of the foot, so it drags along the ground. The person is thus particularly susceptible to tripping.

The *dropfoot* prosthesis shown in Figure 12.10 can help to minimize this problem. It consists of a switch in the heel of the patient's shoe. The contacts of the switch close when the patient takes weight off his foot. This switch controls a stimulator that continuously stimulates the muscles responsible for lifting the foot. When the individual again places weight on the foot, the switch contacts are opened and the stimulus is stopped. These devices are commercially available, but have had only limited acceptance in the United States. In Europe they have been in use for several years, however.

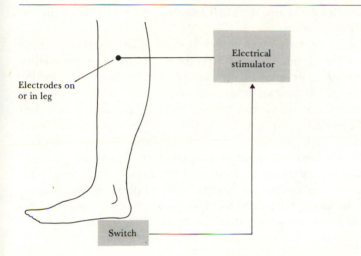

Electrical stimulator

Electrodes on or in leg

Switch

Figure 12.10 A stimulator system for use on stroke patients suffering from gait problems associated with dropfoot.

Stimulus parameters for skeletal-muscle stimulators vary widely according to the type of stimulation, the number of channels, the type of electrode used, and the factor of safety chosen by the designer. Constant-current stimulators are popular in this application, since the charge transferred per stimulus pulse is constant regardless of the electrode load impedance. Pulse currents are used which range from 2 to 20 mA at pulse durations of 1 ms. These constant-current pulses can produce voltage peaks (Figure 5.27) ranging from 3 to 30 V at the electrodes. Thus, if constant current is to be maintained, the power-supply voltage for the stimulator must exceed this.

12.2 Defibrillators and cardioverters

As we learned in Section 4.6, cardiac fibrillation is a condition wherein the individual myocardial cells contract asynchronously without any pattern relating the contraction of one cell and the next. This serious condition reduces the cardiac output to near zero, and must be corrected as soon as possible to avoid irreversible damage to the patient. It is one of the most serious medical emergencies of the cardiac patient. Hence resuscitative measures must be instituted within 5 min or less after the attack, or irreversible brain damage will occur.

Electric shock to the heart can be used to reestablish a more normal cardiac rhythm. Electrical machines that produce the energy to carry out this function are known as *defibrillators*. There are four basic types: the ac defibrillator, the capacitive-discharge defibrillator, the capacitive-discharge delay-line defibrillator, and the square-wave defibrillator. We shall examine each of these types in the following paragraphs.

Defibrillation by electric shock is carried out by passing current through electrodes placed directly on the heart or transthoracically, using large-area electrodes placed against the anterior thorax. The physician can achieve defibrillation of the heart with lower levels of current in the former than in the latter case, but electrodes can be placed directly on the heart only when the heart is exposed in a surgical procedure. Most defibrillators, however, have provisions for both types of defibrillation. They also incorporate appropriate safety features so that the high voltage used with surface electrodes cannot be accidentally applied when internal electrodes are being used, and the lower energy used with internal electrodes cannot be accidentally connected to the surface electrodes so that they fail to produce effective defibrillation.

The ac defibrillator

One of the earliest forms of electrical defibrillator was the ac defibrillator, which applies several cycles of alternating current to the heart from the power line through a step-up transformer. The circuit shown in Figure 12.11 is typical. To achieve defibrillation with internal electrodes requires voltages ranging from 80 to 300 V rms; external electrodes require nearly twice that value. Thus, to raise the power-line voltage to higher levels, there must be a tapped transformer which the operator can use to select the desired voltage. This transformer must be capable of supplying 4 to 6 A during the stimulus period.

The primary of the transformer is switched to provide the pulse. A switch activated by the operator starts a circuit that closes the primary switch for a predetermined interval of time and then opens it to reset the defibrillator for the next pulse. The interval used is usually of the order of 250 ms. Thus several positive and negative half-cycles of the 60-Hz secondary voltage appear at the electrodes.

Alternating-current defibrillators have largely been replaced

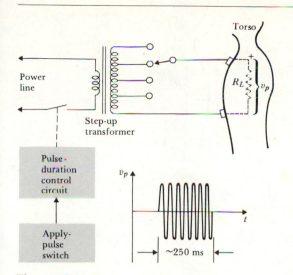

Figure 12.11 Basic arrangement for an ac defibrillator.

by various dc defibrillators. This is because it has been found that the dc signal has fewer deleterious effects on the heart than the ac pulse, and is less likely to produce ventricular fibrillation when applied at random during the cardiac cycle. The dc pulse is also found to have a diminished convulsive effect on skeletal muscles, and can be used in the conversion of supraventricular (atrial) arrhythmias as well.

Capacitive-discharge dc defibrillators

A shorter high-amplitude defibrillation pulse can be obtained using the capacitive-discharge circuit of Figure 12.12. In this case, a half-wave rectifier driven by a step-up transformer is used to charge the capacitor C. The voltage to which C is charged is determined by a variable autotransformer in the primary circuit. A series resistance R limits the charging current to protect the circuit components, and an ac voltmeter across the primary is calibrated to indicate the energy stored in the capacitor. The resistor also helps to determine the time necessary to achieve a full charge on the capacitor. Five times the RC time constant for the circuit is required to reach 99% of a full charge. A good rule of thumb is to keep this time under 10 s, which means that the time constant must be less than 2 s.

The clinician discharges the capacitor when the electrodes are firmly in place on the body by momentarily changing the switch S from position 1 to position 2. The capacitor is discharged through the electrodes and the patient's torso, which represent a primarily

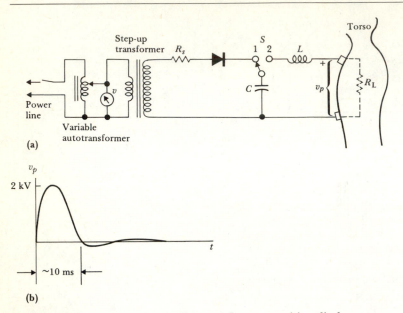

(a)

(b)

Figure 12.12 (a) Basic circuit diagram for a capacitive-discharge type of cardiac defibrillator. (b) A typical waveform of the discharge pulse. The actual waveshape is strongly dependent on the values of L, C, and the torso resistance R_L.

resistive load, and the inductor L. The inductor tends to lengthen the pulse, producing a waveshape of the type shown in Figure 12.12. The slightly underdamped case is illustrated here, but over-damping and critical damping can also occur, the latter being most desirable. The situation is determined entirely by the resistance between the electrodes, which can vary from patient to patient. Once the discharge is completed, the switch automatically returns to position 1 and the process can be repeated, if necessary.

With a circuit such as this, 50 to 100 J (W·s) is required for defibrillation, using electrodes applied directly to the heart. When external electrodes are used, energies as high as 400 J may be required.

The energy stored in the capacitor is given by the well-known equation

$$E = \frac{Cv^2}{2} \tag{12.1}$$

where C is the capacitance and v is the voltage to which the capacitor is charged. Capacitors used in defibrillators range from 10 to 50 μF in capacitance. Thus we see that the voltage for a maximum energy of 400 J ranges from 2 to 9 kV, depending on the size of the capacitor. This stored energy is not necessarily the same energy that is delivered to the patient. Losses in the discharge circuit and at the electrodes result in an actual delivered energy that is lower. Flynn (1972) tested 23 commercial defibrillators; the average delivered output to a standard load was only 60% of the indicated energy.

Example 12.2 A simplified version of the defibrillator shown in Figure 12.12 does not have the inductor L in the circuit, so it will give somewhat shorter pulses with higher initial peak voltages. If R_L, the torso resistance, is 100 Ω and a 300-J pulse is to be delivered to the patient, with 90% of the energy given in 8 ms, what value of C should be used, and to what voltage should it have been initially charged? What ac voltage must be available at the step-up transformer secondary, and what should be the value of R_s to allow the circuit to be at 99% of full charge within 10 s after it was turned on or discharged? What is the maximum current flowing through the patient? What is the maximum current that must be supplied by the step-up transformer secondary?

Answer When the switch is in position 2, the charged capacitor will be discharged through R_L. The energy dissipated by R_L will be

$$E = \frac{v^2}{R_L} \int_0^t \exp\left(\frac{-2t}{R_L C}\right) dt \qquad \text{(E12.6)}$$

where v is the voltage to which C was charged, and the switch was placed in position 2 at $t = 0$. Thus the total energy given to R_L when the capacitor is completely discharged will be

$$E_t = \tfrac{1}{2} C v^2 \qquad \text{(E12.7)}$$

90% of this energy will be dissipated by

$$\exp\left(\frac{-2t}{R_L C}\right) = 0.1$$

or

$$t = R_L C \frac{\ln (0.1)}{2} \qquad \text{(E12.8)}$$

Since t is required to be 8 ms,

$$C = -\frac{2t}{R_L [\ln (0.1)]} = \frac{-2 \times 8 \times 10^{-3} \text{ s}}{100 \ \Omega \times [-2.3]} = 69.6 \ \mu\text{F} \qquad \text{(E12.9)}$$

We now can determine the voltage to which the capacitor was charged from (E12.7).

$$v = \sqrt{\frac{2E_t}{C}} = \sqrt{\frac{2 \times 300 \text{ J}}{69.6 \times 10^{-6} \text{ F}}} = 2940 \text{ V} \qquad (\text{E}12.10)$$

The secondary of the step-up transformer must have a peak voltage of 2940 V or its rms voltage must be 2080 V.

To reach 99% of full charge in 10 s, the time constant of the charging circuit must be 2 s. Thus

$$R_s = \frac{2}{69.6 \ \mu\text{F}} = 28.7 \text{ k}\Omega \qquad (\text{E}12.11)$$

The maximum charging current will occur at the initiation of charging, and will be

$$i_{C,\max} = \frac{2940 \text{ V}}{28.7 \text{ k}\Omega} = 102 \text{ mA} \qquad (\text{E}12.12)$$

Thus R_s may dissipate as much as 300 W. The maximum current flowing through the patient will be

$$i_{p,\max} = 29.4 \text{ A}$$

Delay-line capacitive-discharge dc defibrillators

A superior output signal is obtained from a capacitive-discharge dc defibrillator if the pulse is formed from the circuit shown in Figure 12.13(a). In this case, the parallel combination of C_1 and C_2 stores the same energy as the single capacitor in Figure 12.12. However, its discharge characteristic is more rectangular in shape, as shown in Figure 12.13(b). This keeps the stimulus at peak voltage for a longer duration. Thus the same energy can be applied to the heart over approximately the same period of time without having to achieve currents as high as those seen with the single-capacitor circuit.

Square-wave defibrillators

Geddes (1976) presents a comprehensive review of defibrillators and includes a description of square-wave defibrillators. The capacitor is discharged through the subject by turning on a series *silicon-controlled rectifier* (SCR). When sufficient energy has been delivered to the subject, a shunt SCR short-circuits the capacitor and terminates the pulse. This eliminates the long discharge tail of the waveform. The output may be controlled by varying either the voltage on the capacitor or the duration of discharge. Advantages of this design include: (1) It requires less peak current, (2) it re-

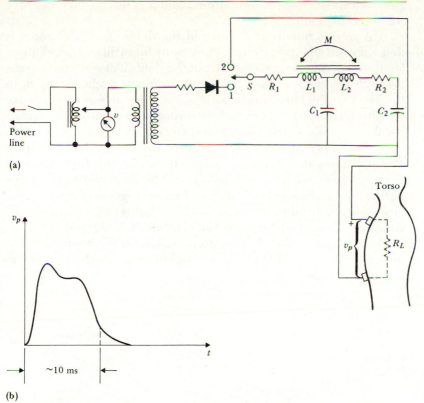

(a)

(b)

Figure 12.13 (a) Circuit diagram for the delay-line type of capacitive-discharge cardiac defibrillator. Addition of the delay line extends the duration of the discharge pulse near its peak value. (b) Waveform of actual pulse depends on values of circuit components. Dashed line indicates the tail of a trapezoidal defibrillator waveform.

quires no inductor, (3) it makes it possible to use physically smaller electrolytic capacitors, and (4) it requires no relay.

Defibrillator electrodes

An important aspect of any defibrillator system is the electrodes. It is essential that they maintain excellent contact with the body so that the energy from the defibrillator reaches the heart and is not dissipated at the electrode-skin interface. If energy is dissipated at this interface, it can cause serious burns to the patient, further complicating a very serious condition. To maintain good contact, the electrodes must be firmly placed against the patient. Often force-activated switches are contained within the electrode assembly, so that if firm-enough pressure is not applied to the electrodes, the circuit is interrupted and it is not possible to apply the defibrillation pulse.

A second important feature of the defibrillator electrodes is that they must be safe to use. They must be sufficiently well insulated so that they do not allow any of the defibrillator output to pass through the hands of the operator. It would be tragic indeed if, in the process of defibrillating a patient, the clinician's own heart were set into fibrillation. It is therefore important to consider the electrical safety of the defibrillator and electrodes.

Two types of electrodes are used for defibrillation. Figure 12.14(a) shows an internal type of electrode. It consists of the metal electrode itself, which is spoon-shaped. The electrode is placed in a well-insulated handle with protecting corrugation between the electrode and hand positions so that body fluids cannot accidentally complete the circuit between the operator's hand and the electrode. A control switch is also often located on the handle, so that once the electrodes are in place, the operator can push the switch to initiate the pulse.

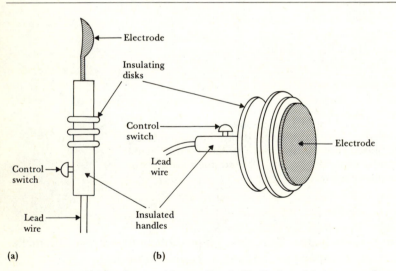

(a)   (b)

Figure 12.14 Electrodes used in cardiac defibrillation. (a) A spoon-shaped internal electrode that is applied directly to the heart. (b) A paddle-type electrode that is applied against the anterior chest wall.

Figure 12.14(b) shows the type of electrode used for external defibrillation. It consists of a large metal disk in an insulated housing that is approximately 100 mm in diameter. The rest of the handle is similar to that for the internal electrodes, with the exception that the insulating corrugation between the electrodes and the operator's hands are of greater diameter than the electrodes. The electrodes are sometimes called *paddles* because of their appearance. In operation, the electrodes (a pair must be used) are liberally coated with electrolyte gel of the type used with ECG-recording electrodes, and firmly pressed against the patient's chest. The operator then initiates the pulse with the control switch on the handle.

Cardioverters

If an operator applies an electric shock of the magnitude of that from a dc defibrillator to the patient's chest during the T wave of the ECG, there is a strong risk of producing ventricular fibrillation in the patient. Since the most frequent use of defibrillation is to terminate ventricular fibrillation, this problem does not occur, since there is no T wave. If, on the other hand, the patient suffers from an atrial arrhythmia, such as atrial tachycardia or flutter, which in turn causes the ventricles to contract at an elevated rate, this can be treated by dc defibrillation to help the patient revert to a normal sinus rhythm. In such a case, it is indeed possible to accidentally apply the defibrillator output during a T wave (ventricular repolarization) and cause ventricular fibrillation. To avoid this problem, special defibrillators are constructed that have synchronizing circuitry so that the output occurs immediately following an R wave, well before the T wave occurs.

Figure 12.15 is a block diagram of such a defibrillator, which is known as a *cardioverter*. Basically, the device is a combination of the cardiac monitor (Section 6.9) and the defibrillator. ECG electrodes are placed on the patient in the location that provides the highest R wave with respect to the T wave. The signal from these electrodes passes through a switch that is normally closed, connecting the electrodes to an appropriate amplifier. The output of the amplifier is displayed on a cardioscope so that the operator can observe the patient's ECG to see, among other things, whether the cardioversion was successful—or, in extreme cases, whether it produced more serious arrhythmias.

The output from the amplifier is also filtered and passed through a threshold detector that detects the R wave. This activates a delay circuit that delays the signal by 30 ms and then activates a trigger circuit that opens the switch connecting the ECG electrodes to the amplifier to protect the amplifier from the ensuing defibrillation pulse. At the same time, it closes a switch that discharges the defibrillator capacitor through the defibrillator electrodes to the patient. This R-wave-controlled switch discharges the defibrillator only once after the operator activates the defibrillator switch. Thus, when the operator closes the defibrillator switch, it is discharged immediately after the next QRS complex. After the discharge of the defibrillator, the switch connecting the ECG electrodes to the amplifier is again closed, so that the operator can observe the cardiac rhythm on the cardioscope to determine the effectiveness of the therapy.

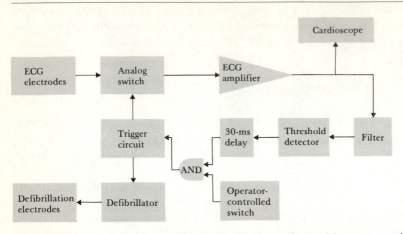

Figure 12.15 A cardioverter. The defibrillation pulse in this case must be synchronized with the R wave of the ECG so that it is applied to a patient shortly after the occurrence of the R wave.

12.3 Mechanical cardiovascular orthotic and prosthetic devices

Cardiovascular orthotic prosthetic devices are primarily mechanical in nature, but they are always associated with various pieces of electronic instrumentation that are necessary to control the devices and to monitor their operation.

Cardiac-assist devices

It has been the goal of cardiac surgeons and cardiologists to develop mechanical pumps that can be used to aid the failing heart after acute traumatic insults such as myocardial infarction. Devices ranging from pumps that can completely replace the heart to a device to reduce the load driven by the heart are being considered in the laboratory. In the latter case, physicians have developed an aortic-balloon system that is used clinically in some institutions. It consists of a long sausage-shaped balloon that can be introduced into the aorta through a femoral artery and connected to an external drive apparatus.

The operation of this balloon is quite simple. Let us consider the balloon as being in the aorta in its inflated state, occupying a major portion of the aortic lumen, but still allowing blood to flow past it. At the initiation of the next ventricular contraction, suction is applied to the balloon, causing it to collapse. The blood pumped by the left ventricle enters the aorta and replaces the volume previously occupied by the balloon. This requires only low pressure, and less effort from the left ventricle. After the contraction, the aortic valve closes, and pressurized CO_2 is applied to the balloon, causing it to expand. CO_2 is used because it is more soluble in blood than air is. If you are using CO_2, and if the balloon or its supply tubing should leak or rupture, there is less risk of fatal gas embolism.

As the balloon expands, it forces the blood surrounding it out of the aorta and into the rest of the body. Thus the balloon does most of the work normally done by the left ventricle, and causes the blood to circulate to the periphery. The process is then repeated after the next ventricular contraction.

This device must rely on a sophisticated system of electronic controls to detect ventricular contractions either from a pressure transducer at the arch of the aorta or, more commonly, from the ECG. The signal must then go through appropriate delay circuits to control the suction and pressurized CO_2 supplied to the balloon. Appropriate sensors must also be included in the system, to ensure that alarms are sounded if any leaks occur.

Example 12.3 An aortic-balloon cardiac-assist device is being applied to a patient in shock. Blood pressure is 80/60 and heart rate is 85 beats/min. Cardiac output has been determined by dye dilution to be 2.5 liter/min. Once the balloon has been started, the systolic pressure at the heart drops to 65 mm Hg and the heart rate and cardiac output remain the same. After several hours on the balloon, the systolic pressure is back at 80 mm Hg, the heart rate has dropped to 78 beats/min, and the cardiac output has risen to 3.4 liters/min.

Estimate the work done by the heart per beat and per minute before and after starting the balloon, as well as several hours later. If the balloon pumps against an average diastolic pressure of 60 mm Hg, how much work is it doing?

Answer For purposes of simplifying our analysis, to get an estimate of cardiac work, let us assume that the heart pumps against a constant pressure that is equal to the systolic pressure. The work per beat is then

$$W = \int_0^{V_s} P_s \, dV = P_s V_s \tag{E12.13}$$

where P_s is the systolic pressure and V_s is the stroke volume, which is related to cardiac output by

$$V_s = \frac{CO}{HR} \tag{E12.14}$$

where CO is cardiac output and HR is heart rate. Before the balloon is applied,

$$W = 80 \text{ mm Hg} \times \frac{2.5 \text{ liters/min}}{85 \text{ min}^{-1}}$$

$$= 2.35 \text{ mm Hg} \cdot \text{liters/beat} \qquad \text{(E12.15)}$$

The work per minute is

$$W = 2.35 \text{ mm Hg} \cdot \text{liters/beat} \times 85 \text{ beats/min}$$
$$= 200 \text{ mm Hg} \cdot \text{liters/min} \qquad \text{(E12.16)}$$

After the balloon has been started,

$$W = 65 \text{ mm Hg} \times \frac{2.5 \text{ liters/min}}{85 \text{ min}^{-1}}$$

$$= 1.91 \text{ mm Hg} \cdot \text{liters/beat} \qquad \text{(E12.17)}$$

or 162.5 mm Hg·liters/min. Thus the immediate effect of the assist device is to reduce the work done by the heart without affecting cardiac output. The balloon pump must now do work in pumping the blood after the aortic valve has closed. This work is given by

$$W = 60 \text{ mm Hg} \times \frac{2.5 \text{ liters/min}}{85 \text{ min}^{-1}}$$

$$= 1.76 \text{ mm Hg} \cdot \text{liters/beat} \qquad \text{(E12.18)}$$

or 150 mm Hg·liters/min. Note that the sum of this work and that of the heart is greater than the original work of the heart before the balloon was applied.

After the cardiac-assist device has been working several hours, cardiac output is improved and the heart can do more work. The work is now

$$W = 80 \text{ mm Hg} \times \frac{3.4 \text{ liters/min}}{78 \text{ min}^{-1}}$$

$$= 3.49 \text{ mm Hg} \cdot \text{liters/beat} \qquad \text{(E12.19)}$$

or 272 mm Hg·liters/min. This improvement in cardiac performance is due in part to the increased perfusion of the heart itself during diastole, due to the augmented diastolic pressure from the inflation of the balloon.

Pump oxygenators

In cardiac surgery it is often necessary to stop the heart from pumping during operative procedures. In this case, to keep the patient alive it is necessary to replace the heart's pumping action and also the oxygenation of the lungs, since they are usually not functioning as well. Machines, known as *pump oxygenators,* have been developed that can carry out these functions. They consist of pumps for maintaining arterial blood pressure connected in series with oxygenators that increase the blood O_2 content and remove CO_2. In surgery the pump oxygenator is usually connected between the superior and inferior vena cava or right atrium and a femoral artery, as shown in Figure 12.16. In some cases a femoral-artery-to-femoral-vein-bypass technique is used to keep all cannulae away from the heart.

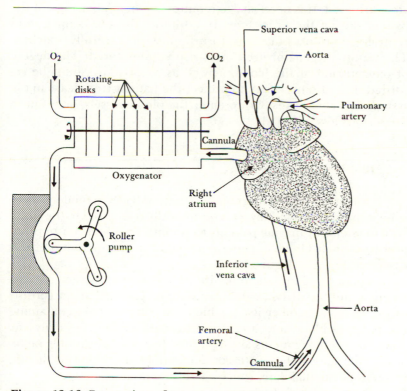

Figure 12.16 Connection of a pump oxygenator to bypass the heart. A disk-type oxygenator is used with a roller pump. Venous blood is taken from a cannula in the right atrium and oxygenated blood is returned through a cannula in the femoral artery.

Various types of pumps can be used. Roller pumps or multiple-finger pumps are often employed, since the pump itself does not come in contact with the blood. Disposable tubing can be used to contain the blood that is pinched between the propagating rollers or fingers. Pulsatile pumps—consisting of a chamber subjected to the reciprocating motion of a piston, membrane, or bladder—are also used, with appropriate check valves to direct the flow. Such pumps more closely follow the normal action of the heart and produce a pulsatile blood pressure.

There are two general types of oxygenators used with these prosthetic devices. One is the *film* type, in which a large surface-area film of blood is drawn into contact with a nearly 100% O_2 atmosphere by rotating disks (Figure 12.16). The second type is the *membrane* oxygenator, in which blood flows through fine tubes of a membrane permeable to gas. This device has a large exchange-surface area to allow the gas transfer to take place.

Electronic instrumentation is essential when pump oxygenators are used. It is necessary to monitor the hemodynamics of the patient during the procedure. In addition, the ECG, aortic, and central-venous pressure waveforms must be carefully watched. The pump oxygenator itself must also be monitored. The degree of oxygenation of the blood, as well as its pressure, must be recorded. It is also necessary to protect the patient from leaks in the system that could cause O_2 to enter the blood vessels, or result in the serious loss of blood.

12.4 Hemodialysis

One of the most important prosthetic devices in modern medicine is the artificial kidney. It is periodically connected to the circulatory systems of uremic patients to remove metabolic waste products from their blood. A general scheme for the operation of this device is shown in Figure 12.17.

There are two basic units in a hemodialysis system: the exchanger and the dialysate delivery system. The exchanger consists of the dialysis chamber itself, which is a compartment containing the patient's blood and a compartment containing the dialysate. These two compartments are separated by a semipermeable membrane that allows the waste components in the blood to diffuse through to the dialysate, which carries them away.

There are three basic types of exchangers in use. The *coil dialyzer* consists of a tube made of the semipermeable-membrane material wound into a coil, in such a way that the dialysate can be circulated between individual turns of it. This is the most commonly used type of dialyzer. It has the limitation that the coil must be fairly long to provide a large effective surface area for mass transport, and it thus imposes a relatively high resistance to the flow of blood. For this reason, and to maintain effective blood flow, it is necessary to put a pump in series with the arterial blood supply to increase the pressure. However, the increased pressure improves the ultrafiltration rate of the membrane. It is important in this unit that the dialysate also be forcibly circulated to ensure rapid mixing. Since fresh dialysate must be available to the surface

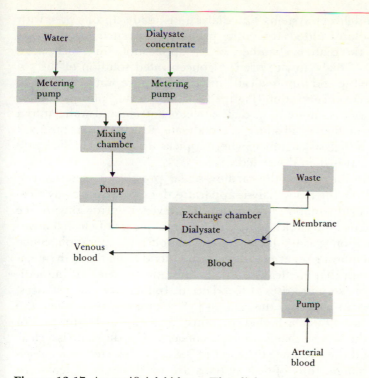

Figure 12.17 An artificial kidney. The dialysate delivery system in this unit mixes dialysate from a concentrate before pumping it through the exchange chamber.

of the membrane throughout the coil, a pump is necessary for the dialysate as well.

The second type of exchanger used in artificial-kidney systems is the *parallel-plate dialyzer*. It is constructed similar to a multilayer parallel-plate capacitor, with the plates made of semipermeable-membrane material. Blood is circulated between alternate pairs of plates, with the dialysate circulated between the other plates. Each plate thus serves as a membrane between dialysate and blood. The blood flows in thin sheets to maximize the surface-to-volume ratio for the dialyzer.

The third type of exchange apparatus is the *hollow-fiber kidney*. This consists of from 10,000 to 15,000 hollow fibers, with an internal diameter of approximately 0.2 mm and a length of approximately 150 mm, connected in parallel. The blood flows in the lumen of the fibers while the dialysate surrounds them. The walls of the fibers serve as the semipermeable membrane. The dialysate is pumped through the space surrounding the fibers to achieve the most efficient exchange.

The remainder of the artificial kidney consists of the

dialysate-delivery system. The dialysate is made up of water with various solutes added. It is either prepared in a batch and pumped through the dialysis chamber, or (in applications in which large amounts of dialysate are used) a concentrated solution of the solutes is made and automatically mixed with pure water to achieve the correct concentration (Figure 12.17). Metering pumps administer the correct amount of dialysate concentrate and water into a mixing chamber to produce the dialysate, which is then pumped through a dialysis chamber, where it picks up the metabolic waste products. It is then discarded.

As in the case of the cardiovascular prostheses, described in Section 12.3, the hemodialysis apparatus does not require any electronic instrumentation to function. However, in using this device with patients, the clinician finds that several pieces of electronic instrumentation greatly aid in its application and operation. Since only a membrane separates the patient's blood from the dialysate, it is important that any leaks in the membrane be detected immediately before serious losses of blood occur. In fact, in some instances, dialysate can leak into the patient's circulatory system. Since the blood is usually at a higher pressure than the dialysate, loss of blood is the hazard that is of major concern. The dialysate is a clear liquid, and the presence of blood in it can be detected as a colorimetric change, thus optical systems are used to detect leaks. In addition, instruments also monitor the pressure in the blood compartment to rapidly detect abnormalities, such as major leaks or clotting phenomena, that change the pressure.

The gross concentration of electrolytes of the dialysate is also monitored by electronic instrumentation. Since the solute is made up of electrolytes, the overall concentration of these in the dialysate is determined by impedance techniques. Thus, by measuring the conductivity of the dialysate in the mixing chamber, instruments can detect any major abnormalities in concentration before the dialysate enters the dialysis chamber.

Another problem common to both hemodialysis units and the pump oxygenator is that air bubbles cannot be tolerated in the blood that reenters the patient, since this produces air emboli that may be life-threatening. Thus it is important that some type of bubble detector be included in the path of the blood before it reenters the body. If bubbles are detected, the blood pump is turned off until the technician operating the dialyzer alleviates the problem.

Figure 12.18 shows a simple form of noninvasive bubble detector. A probe containing two metallic plates is clipped over the blood-return tubing so that the plates are firmly placed against the tubing wall. The tubing and the blood contained therein form the dielectric of a capacitor that is placed in a bridge circuit driven by a 2-MHz oscillator. The bridge is adjusted so that it is balanced when an aqueous solution is in the tube between the plates. When an air bubble is between the plates, the bridge is no longer balanced, since part of the dielectric of the capacitor is now air, which has a dielectric constant approximately one-eighteenth that of blood. This unbalance of the bridge increases its output to a threshold detector circuit, which in turn activates an alarm. Such devices have been demonstrated in the laboratory to be able to detect air bubbles as small as 0.1 ml.

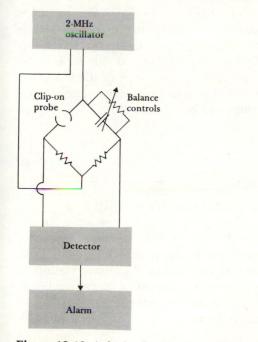

Figure 12.18 A device for detecting air bubbles in lines that reinfuse blood into a patient after the blood passes through a pump oxygenator or artificial kidney.

Example 12.4 The conductance of an electrolytic solution such as dialysate can be approximated by

$$\sigma = \sum_i N_i q_i \mu_i \tag{E12.20}$$

where

σ = equivalent conductance, S/cm
N_i = number of ions of i per cm³
q_i = charge, on ions of i, C
μ = mobility of ions of i in solution, cm²/(V · s)

The equation is summed for all ionic species present in the solution. Assume that dialysate is made up of the equivalent of 0.9 g equivalents of cations having a single electronic charge per ion and a mean mobility of 0.623 cm²/(V·s), and the same amount of oppositely charged anions having a mobility of 0.986 cm²/(V·s). Design a conductivity sensor that can detect increases of 0.05 g equivalents of anions in the dialysate. A threshold detector with a very high input impedance and a 1-mV threshold is available for your design.

Answer Let us use a bridge circuit such as that in Figure 12.18. The dialysate will be made to flow through a cuvette that has parallel 0.001 cm² Pt electrodes 5 cm apart. If we excite the electrodes with a low-voltage (under 500 mV, to minimize nonlinear effects) 50-kHz signal so that the polarization capacitance of the electrode effectively shunts the polarization resistance, the resistance of the solution between the electrodes will be

$$R = \frac{L}{\sigma A} \tag{E12.21}$$

$$= \frac{5 \text{ cm}}{\begin{aligned}&0.9 \times 6.023 \times 10^{23} \text{ liter}^{-1} \times 10^{-3} \text{ liter/cm}^3 \\ &\times 1.6 \times 10^{-19} \text{ C}(0.623 + 0.986) \text{ cm}^2/(\text{V·s}) \times 10^{-3} \text{ cm}^2\end{aligned}}$$

$$= 35.8 \ \Omega$$

If we use an equal-arm bridge, then for balance each resistor in the bridge should have that value. If we increase the concentration of anions by 0.05 g equivalents, the concentration of cations must change by the same amount, to maintain charge neutrality in the solution. Thus the resistance between the electrodes will decrease to

$$R' = R \times \frac{0.9}{0.95} = 33.9 \ \Omega \tag{E12.22}$$

The output at the bridge null detector will now be

$$v_0 = \left[\frac{1}{2} - \frac{33.9 \ \Omega}{(35.8 + 33.9) \ \Omega} \right] E = 0.0136 \ E \tag{E12.23}$$

where E is the bridge excitation. For the given threshold detector, we want this output to be at least 1 mV. Thus the lowest voltage we can use to excite the bridge will be 73.4 mV. This is well within the limits of 500 mV across the electrodes.

12.5 Ventilators

An important factor in respiratory therapy is being able to assist a patient in ventilating his lungs. Various mechanical devices have been developed over the years to carry out this function. These devices, known as ventilators or respirators, can be separated into two general categories: the *controller* and the *assister*.

When a patient is connected to a controller type of ventilator, his or her respiratory ventilation is determined by the machine. The device sets the respiratory cycle, and any tendency toward spontaneous respiration on the patient's part does not affect the machine, and can even oppose it. The assister, on the other hand, is controlled by the patient and used to augment his or her own ventilation activities. The assister detects the patient's attempt at respiration and augments it mechanically. Thus it assists rather than controls the patient in ventilation.

We can further classify ventilators as negative- or positive-pressure devices. *Negative-pressure* ventilators are more physiologic, in that the body of the patient is contained in a sealed chamber in which the pressure can be reduced. This negative pressure is transferred to the space within the thorax, producing a pressure gradient along the trachea that results in air entering the lungs. Pressure is then returned to atmospheric, allowing the lungs to recoil to their original shape and to expel some of their air. *Positive-pressure* ventilators, on the other hand, blow air into the lungs by increasing the pressure in the trachea. This causes the lungs to expand due to internal pressure and then to naturally recoil, expelling a portion of the air once the positive pressure is removed.

Ventilators can be time-cycled, volume-cycled, or pressure-cycled. Negative-pressure ventilators are usually time-cycled. This means that the negative pressure is applied to the body for a given period of time and then released for another given period of time, before the process is once again repeated. Modern time-cycled ventilators are electronically controlled. Astable-multivibrator circuits are used to establish the cycling or the rate of ventilation, as well as the ratio between inspiration and expiration times. These electronic circuits activate solenoid valves that regulate the airflow.

In the *volume-controlled* ventilator, the progression of the cycles of the ventilator is controlled by the volume of air administered to the patient. Thus, if a machine is set to cycle on a given volume, it does not cycle until that volume of air has been administered to the patient. It also has a pressure-override valve, so that if, while the machine is in the process of administering the set volume, the pressure exceeds a predetermined maximum value, the ventilator will cycle whether or not the appropriate volume has been administered. This is an important safety consideration, since uncontrolled pressures could cause serious damage. In the *pressure-cycled* ventilator, air is administered to the patient until the pressure reaches a predetermined limit, at which time the ventilator switches to its expiratory portion of the cycle, and the process is then repeated.

Most modern ventilators can be operated in any of these

modes; they may use electric or pneumatic control. Further details can be found in Hill and Dolan (1976).

In some instances, respiratory-assist devices are being developed with electronic instrumentation to evaluate their function as an integral part of the system. Figure 12.19 is a block diagram of an instrumentation system for a continuous-positive-airway-pressure device for use with newborns. The system consists of monitors for temperature, pressure, and O_2 fraction, including transducers located near the exit port of the device to sense the properties of the inspired air. The transducers are connected to electronic processing circuits that then make the parameters available for digital readouts. The signals are also compared with preset alarm levels, so that if they fall outside a predetermined normal range, alarms are sounded.

The device senses pressure by means of a semiconductor strain-gage pressure transducer in a bridge configuration. The out-

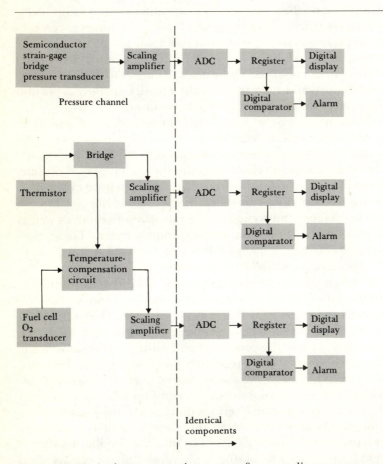

Figure 12.19 An instrumentation system for recording pressure, temperature, and percentage of O_2 in inspired air coming from a continuous-positive-airway-pressure apparatus.

put from the bridge is amplified by a scaling amplifier to yield an appropriate level for digital conversion by the ADC. The eight-bit converter operates at a slow strobe rate. Digital signals are then stored in a register connected to the digital display. The contents of the register are also compared with preset high- and low-alarm limits in the digital-comparator circuit. If it is found that the signal is out of its acceptable range, the comparator sets off the alarm, which flashes the digital display and produces an audible beep.

The temperature-measurement channel uses a thermistor as its sensor. A bridge circuit converts the resistance signal to a voltage, which is then amplified through a scaling amplifier; the remainder of this channel is identical to the pressure channel.

The final channel on the monitor is used for sensing the fraction of oxygen in the inspired air. It uses a fuel-cell type of O_2 transducer that generates a current proportional to the P_{O_2}. It is loaded with a resistance in order to produce an output voltage that is a function of the P_{O_2} in the air. Since this sensor is temperature-sensitive, compensation for its operating temperature must be included, as shown in Figure 12.19. The circuit could also use an independent thermistor to carry out the same function. The remainder of the channel is identical to that of the other channels.

This system has several redundant circuit elements. Everything to the right of the scaling amplifier is identical for each channel. An alternative design could multiplex the output from each scaling amplifier through a single ADC and associated circuitry, and then demultiplex it at the output to operate the respective digital displays and alarms. This approach was not taken because it did not have any economic advantages for three channels and the manufacturer desired to have three independent modular channels that could be operated separately if desired. While these factors are not necessarily important in the circuit design itself, they are very important with respect to the design of the entire product.

Monitoring of ventilators may also be done with a microcomputer as an alternative to the hard-wired system shown in Figure 12.19. One such system is shown in Figure 12.20 (Hathaway et al., 1976), which uses a four-bit microprocessor (Intel 4004). There are three analog input signals, multiplexed and converted from analog to digital form. Since the monitor is an integral part of a ventilator system, information on tidal volume is obtained from a sensor (LVDT) attached to the air-delivery piston/cylinder combination. Information on pressure is provided by a solid-state transducer; information on flow by a pneumotachometer and differential-pressure transducer (Section 9.3). A fourth input is a logic signal that tells the microcomputer whether the ventilator is in the inspiration or expiration phase.

There are also four system outputs provided by the microcomputer. These are: (1) inspired tidal volume from the LVDT, (2)

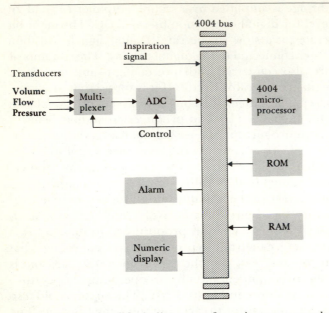

Figure 12.20 Simplified diagram of a microprocessor-based ventilator-monitoring system.

expired minute volume from integration of the flow signal, (3) minute leak (the difference between the inspired and expired volumes, accumulated over 1 min), and (4) peak pressure during inspiration.

The system's programming utilizes a series of subroutines that are used over and over to obtain the necessary information for display. Branchings to these subroutines are determined at decision points in the main microcomputer program. These branchings are caused by external logic signals that identify the inspiration or expiration phase, by internal signals that identify the peak pressure value, or by front-panel controls that enable the operator to select whether to display inspiration or expiration volumes.

A sample subroutine sends control signals to the multiplexer to select the desired channel (pressure and volume of air during inspiration and flow of air during expiration) and to start an analog-to-digital conversion. The converted data are then stored in the CPU for further processing. A comparison subroutine is employed to determine peak pressure, and a summation subroutine is utilized to accumulate data for minute-volume and minute-leak determinations. This same subroutine is used to integrate the flow signal to obtain expired volume. Finally a display subroutine provides for output of data to front-panel LEDs.

For this system, alarms are implemented in a manner similar to those shown in Figure 12.19. One input of the digital comparator is connected to front-panel thumbwheel switches and the other to the microcomputer output for each parameter. When the value on the data bus exceeds (peak pressure, minute leak) or falls below (minute volume) the desired setting, the alarm is triggered. The use of the microcomputer for this application has provided decreased complexity of this system compared with a previous hard-wired version, and also provides for the future inclusion of other parameters, such as compliance and resistance to flow.

12.6 Infant incubators

The care of premature newborns often requires that they be in an environment in which temperature is elevated and controlled, because they are unable to regulate their own temperatures. When infants are kept in a chamber maintained within a specific temperature range, O_2 requirements are minimized. This is especially important for premature newborns, who are more susceptible to respiratory problems than full-term infants, because their lungs may be unable to supply enough oxygen to meet elevated demands. Such controlled-temperature environments are maintained in infant incubators.

Temperature-controlled air is passed through the chamber in which the baby is located to maintain it at a set temperature. The temperature is controlled in modern units by means of the proportional control system shown in Figure 12.21. The temperature in the air-supply line varies a thermistor resistance that is compared with a fixed resistance that corresponds to the set temperature. If the temperature of the air entering the infant's chamber is lower than the set temperature, power is applied to the heater to correct for this difference. In the proportional-controller system, the amount of power applied to the heater is proportional to the difference in temperature between the actual air temperature and the set point. This means that the amount of power decreases as the temperature approaches the set point, an important feature to effect more precise control and to minimize overshoot of the set point.

The control system shown in Figure 12.21 uses the thermistor in a bridge circuit, with the set-point resistance as another arm of the bridge. The bridge output is amplified, giving the voltage v_1 at the output, which is proportional to the difference in temperature between the thermistor and the set point. A 1-Hz low-frequency sawtooth generator produces voltage v_2 having an amplitude equal to the maximum value of v_1 over which proportional control is desired. Then v_1 and v_2 are compared in a comparator circuit that produces an output voltage v_3 during that period of time when v_1 is greater than v_2. This voltage, in turn, controls a gate-pulse generator that produces turn-on pulses for the silicon-controlled switch while v_3 is high. The silicon-controlled switch allows the power-line voltage to be applied to the heater of the incubator during the period of time that v_1 is greater than v_2. Thus, as the temperature approaches the set point, as we can see by moving from left to right in the waveforms of Figure 12.21, v_1 decreases toward zero. This reduces the interval over the sawtooth cycle during which heater power is applied, thereby reducing the output of the heater.

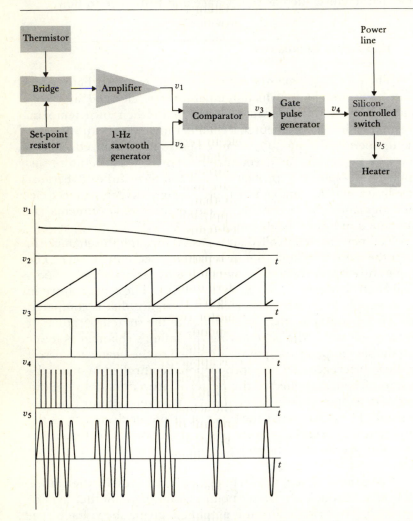

Figure 12.21 Block diagram and waveform diagram of a proportional temperature controller used to maintain temperature of air inside an infant incubator.

Some incubators, instead of controlling the air temperature directly, use the skin temperature of the infant as a control parameter. The thermistor is placed against the skin of the infant, and the controller is set to maintain the infant's skin at a given temperature. If the infant is cooler than the set point, the air entering the chamber of the incubator is heated an amount proportional to the difference in temperature between the set temperature and the baby's actual temperature.

Incubators also have a simple alarm system to alert the clinical staff if there is any dangerous overheating of the device. The system embodies a temperature-controlled switch that carries power to an audible alarm once the temperature exceeds the safe limit. Often there is a buzzer connected in series with a switch that is activated by a bimetallic strip. This keeps the system simple and reliable. In some cases, this circuit also immediately reduces power to the heater to stop the overheating.

Premature and, in some cases, full-term infants often develop respiratory distress or other anomalies. These infants frequently "forget" to breathe, and such apnea is life-threatening. A tap on the incubator wall or a slap on the foot is usually all such infants need to remind them to take another breath. Thus it is important to detect when apnea has occurred for a given period of time (10 to 20 s) and to alert the clinical personnel so that they can immediately attend to the infant. Various types of apnea monitors have been developed to carry out this function. They detect ventilation by one of the following methods (Chapter 9): transthoracic impedance, movement of the baby on a displacement detecting pad, or movement of the baby's chest wall. An alarm is sounded when respiratory activity ceases for periods of greater than a preset time, in the range of 10 to 20 s.

12.7 Surgical instruments

There are many devices that can be classified as surgical instruments; to consider all of them would require several volumes. There are, however, electrical and electronic devices that are important in the surgical care of patients, in addition to those used for monitoring patients in the operating and recovery rooms. In the next two sections, we examine two of these: the electrosurgical unit and the laser.

Electrosurgical unit

Electrical devices to assist in surgical procedures by providing cutting and hemostasis (stopping bleeding) are widely applied in the operating room. These devices, which in the United Kingdom are referred to as surgical diathermy apparatus, can be used to incise tissue, to destroy tissue through desiccation, and to stop bleeding by causing coagulation of blood. The process involves the application of an RF spark between a probe and tissue to cause localized heating and damage to tissue.

The basic electrosurgical unit is shown in Figure 12.22(a). The high-frequency power needed to produce the spark comes from a high-power, high-frequency generator, of either the spark-gap or the vacuum-tube type. The power to operate the generator comes from a power supply, the output of which may in some cases be modulated to produce a waveform more appropriate for particular actions. In this case, a modulator circuit controls the

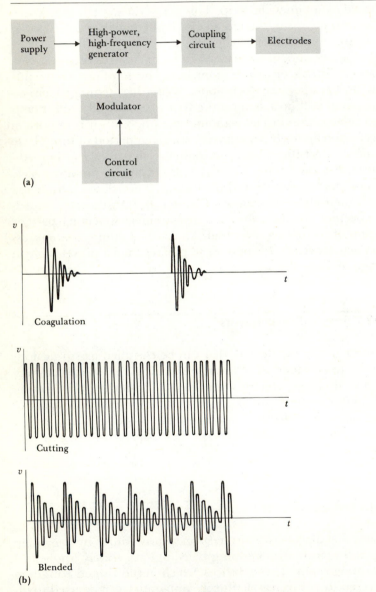

(a)

Coagulation

Cutting

Blended

(b)

Figure 12.22 (a) An electrosurgical unit. High-power, high-frequency oscillating currents are generated and coupled to electrodes to incise and coagulate tissue. (b) Three different electrical voltage waveforms available at the output of electrosurgical units for carrying out different functions.

output of the generator. The application of high-frequency power from the generator is ultimately controlled by the surgeon through a control circuit, which determines when power is applied to the electrodes to carry out a particular action. Often the output of energy from the high-frequency generator needs to be at various levels for various jobs. For this reason, a coupling circuit is inserted between the generator output and the electrodes to control this energy transfer.

The electrical waveforms generated by the electrosurgical unit differ for its different modes of action. To bring about desiccation and coagulation, the device uses damped sinusoidal pulses, as shown in Figure 12.22(b). The RF sine waves have a nominal frequency of 250 to 2000 kHz and are usually pulsed at a rate of 120 per second. Open-circuit voltages range from 300 to 2000 V and power into a 500-Ω load ranges from 80 to 200 W. The magnitude of both voltage and power depends on the particular application.

Cutting is achieved with a CW RF source, as shown in Figure 12.22(b). Often units cannot produce truly continuous waves, as shown in Figure 12.22(b), and amplitude modulation is present. Cutting is done at higher-frequency voltage and power, since the intense heat at the spark destroys tissue rather than just desiccating it, as is the case with coagulation. Frequencies range from 500 kHz to 2.5 MHz, with open-circuit voltages as high as 9 kV. Power levels range from 100 to 750 W, depending on the application.

The cutting current usually results in bleeding at the site of incision, and the surgeon frequently requires "bloodless" cutting. Electrosurgical units can achieve this by combining the two waveforms, as shown in Figure 12.22(b). This is known as the *blended* waveform; its frequency is generally the same as the frequency for the cutting current. For best results, surgeons prefer to operate at a higher voltage and power when they want bloodless cutting than they do when they want cutting alone.

Rioux (1975) reviewed the merits of various types of electrosurgical units and evaluated the operating characteristics of several commercially available units.

The *spark-gap* type of electrosurgical unit has been widely used, although the modern *vacuum-tube* type is far more desirable from an engineering point of view. Surprisingly enough, however, the spark-gap unit provides better cutting or coagulation action than its vacuum-tube counterpart. Sturdy, reliable spark-gap units continue to meet the surgeon's needs. They are available for the operating room and, in low-power versions, for office procedures.

Figure 12.23 shows the basic circuit, as described by Hill (1973). A step-up transformer that produces 1500 to 2000 V rms on the transformer secondary is connected across two spark gaps in series. The reason two are used is that, if one is accidentally shorted, the device can still obtain a spark from the other. The spark causes the resonant circuit, consisting of the tapped 40-μH coil and the two 0.005-μF capacitors, to have damped oscillations. These oscillations are coupled capacitively to the electrodes, using capacitors that are sufficiently small to minimize any possible leakage current at the power-line frequency.

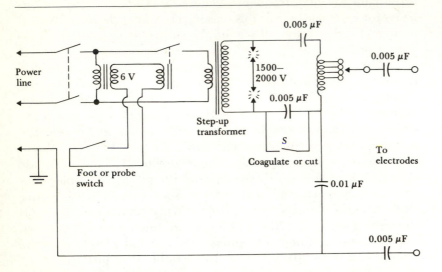

Figure 12.23 A spark-gap type of electrosurgical generator. The switch S is closed for cutting. (From D.W. Hill, *Electronic Techniques in Anesthesia and Surgery.* London: Butterworths, 1973.)

The device produces intermittent signals and is controlled by a low-voltage switch that can be located directly on the electrosurgical probe, or operated as a foot switch. Switch S selects either cutting current or coagulation current. Note that this switch adds another 0.005-μF capacitor in series with the other capacitor in the tuned circuit; this raises the frequency of the tuned circuit. The ac power source for the spark gap requires the waveform to still be pulsatile and damped, and thus not a true cutting waveform, as defined in Figure 12.22(b). Nevertheless, the increased frequency does improve the cutting action of the spark.

Figure 12.24 shows a vacuum-tube high-power generator that produces less electrical interference than the spark-gap type. The circuit is that of a Hartley oscillator, using a high-power vacuum triode as the active element. The coupling of power to the electrodes is done through the tuned transformer. The operator can vary the power supplied to the electrodes by adjusting the coupling coefficient of the transformer by moving one coil with respect to the other. Fine adjustments in power supplied to the electrodes are accomplished by tuning of the secondary by means of the variable capacitor.

Like the spark-gap unit, this generator circuit can be controlled through the high-voltage power supply. It is possible to

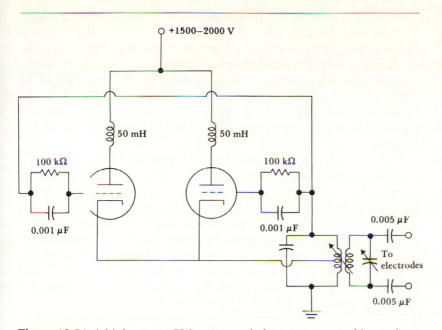

Figure 12.24 A high-power CW vacuum triode generator used in modern electrosurgical units. The inductance-capacitance tank circuit determines the frequency of oscillation of the circuit.

have an interrupted pulsatile type of RF signal appear on the electrodes by modulating the output of the generator by imposing a modulation signal on top of the power-supply voltage. This can be achieved more simply by placing raw ac from the step-up transformer at the plates and letting the triodes serve as the rectifiers as well. In this case, the modulation is at the power-line frequency. In either of these modulated schemes, there is a much greater chance of coupling interference into other electronic apparatus used in the operating room, such as patient-monitoring devices, because the modulation signal falls within the signal passband of the instrument.

In application, the indifferent or ground electrode is placed on the patient either as a large-area electrode applied to the thigh or as a large-area stainless steel plate placed under the patient's back or buttocks to establish contact. The probe itself is a pencillike structure with either a point for cutting or a flattened tip for coagulation. If the indifferent or ground electrode does not make good contact over most of its surface with the patient, hot spots can develop and produce burns on the patient's back or thigh.

Another problem that can produce burns is a bad connection between the indifferent electrode and its lead wire. If the lead wire breaks, it can come in contact with the patient. In this case, the lead wire can serve as an electrode similar to the surgeon's probe and cause serious burns on the patient's back or thigh.

In the use of the electrosurgical unit in the operating room, we must pay special attention when flammable anesthetics are used. In the spark-gap type of unit, care must be taken to ensure that the spark gap is within a sealed chamber, and that there is no opportunity for the anesthetic agent to enter that chamber and be ignited by the spark. Even in the case of the vacuum-tube oscillator circuit, high voltages are present in the circuit, and can result in sparks that could ignite anesthetic-air mixtures. Thus this unit also should be protected.

These safety precautions do not completely eliminate the risk of explosion when electrosurgical units are in use. The mechanism of action of these devices requires the production of a spark between the probe and the patient. This can easily ignite flammable anesthetics. Thus it is important that, if flammable anesthesia is necessary, surgeons make sure that the area in which they plan to use the electrosurgical unit is well ventilated with fresh air. Some electrosurgical probes come complete with a fresh-air jet blowing over the region in which the spark occurs, to sweep away the anesthetic.

12.8 Therapeutic applications of the laser

As we saw in Section 2.13, the laser makes available coherent light at high intensities that can be focused to a very fine point. When this focal point is projected on tissue and the tissue absorbs the radiation, the power may be great enough to immediately vaporize the tissue illuminated by the point, resulting in a coagulated incision. Thus the laser can be used as a surgical instrument in much the same way as the electrosurgical unit described in Section 12.7. The laser beam requires powers of from 25 to 100 W to cut various tissues of the body, ranging from skin through bone.

An important problem to be overcome before lasers can be widely used in this application is quick and easy manipulation of the laser beam to the point where the surgeon wants it. Unlike the electrosurgical probe that can be connected to its generator by a flexible insulated lead wire, the laser must be coupled to its point of application through a system of mirrors and a lens. Since the powers required are high enough to make the laser too large to be manipulated itself, this coupling scheme becomes important but cumbersome.

The laser has some important applications in other aspects of medicine. Since the laser can be used in the control of bleeding through photocoagulation and heating, it has been applied through a fiberoptic endoscope in the coagulation of bleeding gastric ulcers. In some cases, the power is sufficiently great to stop bleeding in experimentally induced lesions in dogs.

In ophthalmology, the laser has found an important therapeutic application. Laser photocoagulators are able to repair detached retinas much more quickly than conventional photocoagulators, thereby minimizing the risk of damage to the retina of the patient due to movement of the eyes. Such systems are now commercially available and in use at several institutions. Lasers have also been investigated as diagnostic and therapeutic instruments in many centers. This work ranges from dentistry to oncology (study and treatment of tumors). Laser radiation is even being investigated in the clinical laboratory for analysis problems. This is an important area to watch for future developments. Rockwell (1971) reviews the various applications of the laser in medicine; this reference is recommended for further details.

12.9 Speculation on the future

The other chapters of this text have shown many applications of medical electronics to diagnostic instrumentation. By contrast, the application of medical electronics to prosthetics and therapeutics is relatively small. Considerable possibilities exist, however, for expansion in this area, once electronic technology and reliability are improved. For example, many of the prosthetic devices described in this chapter that are based on mechanical devices require extensive electronic-control circuitry. The devices themselves are bulky, and when combined with the electronic instrumentation necessary for efficient operation, they constitute large, complex, and expensive systems. Further developments in microelectronics and highly reliable techniques for circuits, along with similar advances in micromechanics, should make it possible to develop totally implantable prosthetic devices. Some investigators are looking toward a future in which surgeons will be able to implant permanent cardiac-assist devices or, for that matter, artificial kidneys, that will function as well as the normal organ.

The development of new sensors, such as glucose or insulin sensors, might make possible the implantation of a prosthetic pancreas in patients suffering from diabetes. Stimulators for the control of neurological disease such as epilepsy, or musculoskeletal problems such as scoliosis (curvature of the spine) are being investigated today and may lead to devices for the control of these diseases. Clearly, it appears that as technology improves, along with our understanding of the mechanisms of the various diseases, there will be vast possibilities for new corrective devices that will open a wide new frontier.

Problems

12.1 An asynchronous cardiac pacemaker operates at a rate of 70 pulses/min. These pulses are of 2-ms duration and have an amplitude of 5 V when driving a 500-Ω load.

    a　What is the total energy supplied to this load over a 5-year period?

    b　Suppose that 35% of the energy from the power supply goes into the output pulses. What must be the capabilities of the power supply to operate the pacemaker for 5 years?

    c　Assume that the power supply is five 1.35-V mercury cells. What must the milliampere-hour capacity of each cell be to operate this pacemaker for 5 years?

    d　Even though a pacemaker such as this would have a 5-year capacity in its power supply, it is found that when it is implanted, the power supply becomes exhausted in a little over 2 years. Can you suggest some of the reasons why this theoretical calculation disagrees with actual practice?

    12.2　A transcutaneous RF-powered cardiac pacemaker has an externally positioned primary coil that is placed on the skin over the implanted secondary coil. The two coils have the same number of turns, and their coupling coefficient depends on the relative position. Depending on how the patient adjusts to the external coil, the coupling coefficient can vary from 0.3 to 0.65. What is the percentage difference in voltage at the secondary coil between conditions providing maximum and minimum coupling coefficients?

    12.3　A radioactive power source for a cardiac pacemaker has an unloaded output voltage of 0.7 V. It consists of a thermopile made up of 40 semiconductor thermocouples. One leg of each thermocouple has a Seebeck coefficient of $+200\ \mu V/°C$, while the other leg has a Seebeck coefficient of $-225\ \mu V/°C$. The cold junctions of the thermopile are operating at body temperature (37°C). What is the temperature of the hot junctions?

    12.4　Will there be any effect on the output of the timing circuit for the blocking-oscillator type of pacemaker generator shown in Figure 12.4(a) when the battery voltage diminishes and the battery internal impedance increases, as occurs with failing batteries? Describe any effects this might have on circuit performance.

    12.5　Repeat Problem 12.4 for the multivibrator type of pacemaker generator shown in Figure 12.4(b).

    12.6　Can a change in the load resistance across the electrode terminals of the output circuit of the blocking-oscillator type of pacemaker shown in Figure 12.4(a) affect the output? Base your answer on an analysis of this circuit.

    12.7　Repeat Problem 12.6 for the multivibrator pacemaker circuit shown in Figure 12.4(b).

    12.8　An important problem in the clinical application of pacemakers is to determine when a given pacemaker is about to fail. Then surgeons may replace it before there is a failure that puts the patient at extreme risk. Describe a technique that could be used to determine the status of the battery of an implanted pacemaker that cannot be directly contacted with electrical probes connected to test instruments. It is possible to place electrodes on the surface of the patient's body to observe signals from the pacemaker. Assume that you can use any of the test equipment available to the medical electronics engineer.

12.9 There are some limitations on the use of synchronous cardiac pacemakers, especially when the patient is in the vicinity of strong electromagnetic fields, such as those produced by nearby microwave ovens, powerful radio transmitters, or radar stations. Discuss these limitations and describe the mechanisms involved.

12.10 For the demand type of synchronous pacemaker shown in Figure 12.6, draw an appropriate waveform diagram, like the one in Figure 12.8, that describes the operation of this pacemaker with and without spontaneous ventricular beats.

12.11 How might the atrial-synchronous pacemaker in Figure 12.7 be modified to allow it to operate asynchronously in the absence of atrial contractions? Draw a block diagram for the modified circuit and explain its operation.

12.12 Compare the power requirements for a bladder stimulator that produces 5-V pulses—each having a duration of 2 ms, at a frequency of 100 pulses/s—with that of the cardiac pacemaker in Problem 12.1. Do you think that the power requirements of this stimulator make battery operation possible?

12.13 The circuit of the RF-powered bladder stimulator of Figure 12.9 produces pulses of RF energy having a voltage of 10 V rms as seen across the primary coil. The source impedance of the generator may be considered to be very low. The secondary coil has 1.2 times the number of turns of the primary and is coupled to the primary with a coupling coefficient of 0.5. What is the pulse amplitude seen across the electrodes when the tissue appears as a 500-Ω resistive load? What is the load impedance that the RF oscillator sees?

12.14 The effective load resistance seen by the electrodes of an electrical stimulator used for pain suppression can increase with time following the implantation and healing of the site of the stimulator. Discuss the way this affects the efficacy of the stimulator. List the precautions that can be taken in the design of the circuit to minimize these problems.

12.15 It was stated in the text that there is often a discrepancy between the stored energy in a capacitive-discharge cardiac defibrillator and the energy that is actually given to the patient during a discharge. Explain what you believe to be reasons for this discrepancy and what can be done to minimize it.

12.16 Capacitor-discharge types of cardiac defibrillators can be constructed with relatively small capacitances charged to high voltages or comparatively large capacitances charged to lower voltages. Contrast the two types of defibrillators. List and discuss the advantages and disadvantages of each.

12.17 If a capacitive-discharge type of cardiac defibrillator is discharged on a patient when the electrodes are not firmly in contact with the patient's chest wall, serious complications can develop. Describe what these are from the standpoint of what happens to the patient and the waveform produced by the defibrillator.

12.18 What precautions should a clinician take when it is necessary to defibrillate a patient who has an implanted pacemaker of either the synchronous or asynchronous types?

12.19 The 20-μF capacitor of the defibrillator circuit in Figure 12.12 is charged to an energy of 200 J. When the electrodes are attached to the patient, a 50-Ω resistive load is seen.

    a What value of inductance L is required for critical damping?

    b What is the peak current passing through the patient during the discharge under these conditions?

12.20 When it is necessary to defibrillate a patient, the clinician must be assured that the defibrillator will operate properly. Therefore it is necessary for the clinical engineer to have an aggressive program of testing and preventive maintenance of all cardiac defibrillators in the hospital. The key to this program is a method of evaluating the performance of each defibrillator. Design an instrument that is capable of measuring what you believe to be the key parameters of a cardiac defibrillator to assure the clinician that it is operating properly.

12.21 Instrumentation is needed to control a balloon-type cardiac-assist device. It must detect the R wave of the ECG and use this to control the mechanism for deflation of the balloon, followed by reinflation. Design the necessary instrumentation and control system in block-diagram form.

12.22 Design an instrumentation system for use with a pump-oxygenator system such as that shown in Figure 12.16. This system should monitor the oxygen saturation and pressure of the blood being reinfused into the body, as well as the pressure of the venous-return blood. Specify the transducers to be used in the instrumentation system and explain why your choice is the most desirable. Show the electronics in block-diagram form and include alarm circuitry to detect elevated arterial and venous pressures as well as reduced oxygen saturation.

12.23 An artificial-kidney system must be protected from leaks across the dialyzing membrane. Design an instrumentation system that can provide this protection, and describe its operation.

12.24 Redesign the electronics for the continuous-positive-airway-pressure monitor shown in Figure 12.19 so that only a single ADC and associated circuitry is required.

12.25 A proportional temperature controller based on the skin temperature of the infant, is used to regulate the temperature in an infant incubator. Several safety precautions must be taken to ensure proper control. Describe what you think these are, and modify the block diagram of Figure 12.21 to include them. Explain the operation of your new system.

12.26 As mentioned in the text, a broken lead wire on the back-plate or thigh-plate electrode of an electrosurgical unit can produce serious burns. Can you describe a way to eliminate this problem using an ancillary electronic circuit?

References

Burton, C.V., "Pain suppression through peripheral nerve stimulation," in W.S. Fields and L.A. Leavitt (eds.), *Neural organization and its relevance to prosthetics.* New York: Intercontinental, 1973, pp. 241–250.

Cook, K.J., and N.H. Horwitz, "An instrument for the evaluation of defibrillator performance." *J. Assoc. Adv. Med. Instrum.,* 1972, 6, 325.

Cromwell, L., F.J. Weibell, E.A. Pfeiffer, and L.B. Usselman, *Biomedical instrumentation and measurements.* Englewood Cliffs: Prentice-Hall, 1973.

Egan, D.F., *Fundamentals of inhalation therapy.* St. Louis: Mosby, 1969. Chapter 9, "Mechanical ventilation."

Flynn, D.J., F.W. Fox, and J.D. Bourland, "Indicated and delivered energy by dc defibrillators." *J. Assoc. Adv. Med. Instrum.,* 1972, 6, 323.

Furman, S., and D.J.W. Escher, *Principles and techniques of cardiac pacing.* New York: Harper & Row, 1970.

Geddes, L.A., "Electrical ventricular defibrillation." In D.W. Hill and B.W. Watson (eds.), *IEE Medical Electronics Monographs, 18–22,* Stevenage, Eng.: Peter Peregrinus, 1976, pp. 42–72.

Geddes, L.A., W.A. Tacker, J. Rosborough, P. Cabler, R. Chapman, and R. Rivers, "The increased efficacy of high-energy defibrillation." *Med. Biol. Eng.,* 1976, 14, 330–333.

Gill, C., W. Jakobi, T. Morton, and A. Wechsler, "The cardiovascular system as it relates to heart pacing," in *Medtronic currents,* Minneapolis: Medtronic, Inc., 1975, Vol. 1, ed. II.

Hampers, C.L., E. Schubak, E.G. Lowrie, and J.M. Lazarus, "Clinical engineering in hemodialysis and anatomy of an artificial kidney unit," in *Long-term hemodialysis.* New York: Grune & Stratton, 1973.

Hathaway, J.C., D.R. Asche, A.M. Cook, and R.R. Zumstein, "Microprocessor implementation of ventilator-patient monitoring." *Med. Instrum.,* 1976, 10(1), 69.

Hill, D.W., "Defibrillators, cardiac pacemakers and bladder and anal stimulators, and surgical diathermy apparatus and electrical safety precautions in the operating room," in *Electronic techniques in anaesthesia and surgery.* London: Butterworth, 1973.

Hill, D.W., and A.M. Dolan, *Intensive care instrumentation.* New York: Grune & Stratton, 1976.

Norman, J.C. (ed.), "The mechanics of cardiopulmonary

bypass and cardiac assist," in *Cardiac surgery,* 2nd ed. New York: Appleton-Century-Crofts, 1972.

Reswick, J.B., "A brief history of functional electrical stimulation," in W.S. Fields and L.A. Leavitt (eds.), *Neural organization and its relevance to prosthetics.* New York: Intercontinental, 1973, 3–16.

Rioux, J.E., and A.A. Yuzpe, "Know thy generator!" *Contemp. OB/GYN,* 1975, 6, 52–64.

Rockwell, R.J., "The current status of laser applications in medicine and biology." *Crit. Rev. Bioeng.,* 1971, 1, 49–68.

Roy, O.Z., "The current status of cardiac pacing." *Crit. Rev. Bioeng.,* 1974, 2, 259–327.

Sances, A., Jr., T.J. Swiontek, S.J. Larson, J.F. Cusick, G.A. Meyer, E.A. Millar, D.C. Hemmy, and J. Mkylebust, "Innovations in neurologic implant systems (electrostimulation)." *Med. Instrum.,* 1975, 9, 213–216.

Schaldach, M., and S. Furman, *Advances in pacemaker technology.* New York: Springer Verlag, 1975.

Scott, F.B., W.E. Bradley, and G.W. Timm, "Electro mechanical restoration of micturition," in W.S. Fields and L.A. Leavitt (eds.), *Neural organization and its relevance to prosthetics.* New York: Intercontinental, 1973, pp. 311–318.

Shealy, C.N., "Pain suppression through posterior column stimulation," in W.S. Fields and L.A. Leavitt (eds.), *Neural organization and its relevance to prosthetics.* New York: Intercontinental, 1973, pp. 251–260.

Susset, J.G., "The electrical drive of the urinary bladder and sphincter," in W.S. Fields and L.A. Leavitt (eds.), *Neural organization and its relevance to prosthetics.* New York: Intercontinental, 1973.

Sweet, W.H., and J.G. Wepsic, "Electrical stimulation for suppression of pain in man," in W.S. Fields and L.A. Leavitt (eds.), *Neural organization and its relevance to prosthetics.* New York: Intercontinental, 1973.

Young, J.A., and D. Crocker, *Principles and practice of inhalation therapy.* Chicago: Yearbook, 1970. Chapter 10, "Mechanical ventilation."

Watanabe, Y. (ed.), *Cardiac pacing.* New York: Elsevier, 1977.

Chapter thirteen

Electrical safety

Walter H. Olson

It is not surprising that incidents of accidental electric shock have been on the increase, since the number and variety of household and industrial electrical devices have proliferated. In perspective, however, we can see that the safety record for users of electrical energy is undoubtedly better than for users of fossil fuels.

Electronic instrumentation for medical practice has also increased greatly in quantity and complexity during the past few decades. Unfortunately, we encounter some special shock hazards because some of these instruments are connected to patients in ways that bypass the body's normal defenses. Early in 1969 there were reports that some catheterized patients could be electrocuted by currents well below normal perceptual levels. The safety scare that followed reached a peak in about 1971, when Ralph Nader (1971) and Carl Walter (1970) claimed that each year 1200 Americans were electrocuted during routine diagnostic and therapeutic procedures. This figure was not and cannot be documented, because there is seldom pathological evidence for these alleged electrocutions.

Although the furor caused some unnecessary actions to be taken, the knowledge of electrical hazards gained and the protection now incorporated into electronic instruments have eliminated many of the hazards and reduced the fears. Now, with proper training for personnel, modern equipment, and regular testing procedures, hospitals can minimize the risk of accidental electric shock. As new instruments and medical procedures are introduced, we must consider potential electrical safety hazards.

In this final chapter we shall discuss the physiological effects of electric current, shock hazards, methods of protection, and electrical testing procedures. One objective is to learn how to incorporate safety features into the design of medical instruments studied in previous chapters.

Electrical safety in the broadest sense involves more than electric shock. For example, lead breakage on cardiac monitors or electrocautery units is detrimental to patient care. Line-voltage variations can cause some infant apnea monitors to erroneously indicate proper respiration. Electrical interference can cause incorrect cardiotachometer readings. Slight leakage of electrical insulation in thermistors can cause errors in temperature measurements.

667

13.1 Physiological effects of electricity

For a physiological effect to occur, the body must become part of an electric circuit. Current must enter the body at one point and leave at some other point. The magnitude of the current is equal to the applied voltage divided by the impedance of the body and contact interfaces between the two areas of contact. Three general effects can occur when electric current flows through biological tissue: (1) resistive heating of tissue, (2) electrical stimulation of excitable tissue (nerve and muscle), and (3) electrochemical burns (for direct current).

Let us now discuss psychophysical and physiological effects in humans in the order that these effects occur for increasing current. The chart in Figure 13.1 summarizes the approximate range of currents that produce each effect in a 70-kg man for 1- to 3-s exposure to 60-Hz current applied to the hands. Susceptibility parameters for variations in these conditions are considered in Section 13.2.

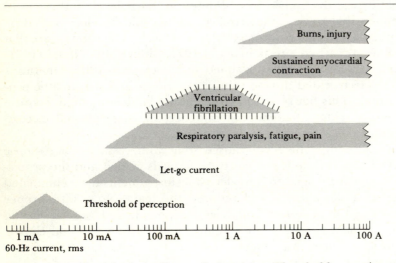

Figure 13.1 Physiological effects of electricity. Threshold or estimated mean values are given for each effect in a 70-kg male for 1- to 3-s exposure to 60-Hz current applied to copper wires grasped by the hands.

Threshold of perception

For the conditions just stated, when the local current density is large enough to excite nerve endings in the skin, the subject feels a tingling sensation. The *threshold of perception* is the minimum current that an individual can detect. This threshold varies considerably among individuals, and according to the measurement conditions. When someone with moistened hands grasps small copper wires, the lowest thresholds are about 0.5 mA at 60 Hz. Thresholds for dc current are 2 to 10 mA, and slight warming of the skin is perceived.

Let-go current

For higher levels of current, nerves and muscles are vigorously stimulated, eventually resulting in pain and fatigue. Involuntary contractions of muscles or reflex withdrawals by a subject experiencing any current above threshold may cause secondary physical injuries, such as falling from a ladder. As the current increases further, the involuntary contractions of the muscles can prevent the subject from voluntarily withdrawing. The *let-go current* is defined as the maximum current for which the subject can withdraw voluntarily. For men, the $\frac{1}{2}$ percentile for the let-go current threshold is 9.5 mA.

Respiratory paralysis, pain, and fatigue

Still higher currents cause involuntary contraction of respiratory muscles severe enough to cause asphyxiation if the current is not interrupted. During let-go experiments, Dalziel (1973) observed respiratory arrest at 18 to 22 mA. Strong involuntary contractions of the muscles and stimulation of the nerves can be painful and cause fatigue if there is long exposure.

Ventricular fibrillation

The heart is susceptible to electric current in a special way that is particularly dangerous. Part of the current passing through the chest flows through the heart. If the magnitude of the current is sufficient to excite only part of the heart muscle, then the normal propagation of electrical activity in the heart muscle is disrupted. Once the activity in the ventricles is desynchronized, the pumping action of the heart ceases and death occurs within minutes.

This desynchronization of cardiac muscle tissue is called *fibrillation*. Unfortunately it does not stop when the current that triggered it is removed. Ventricular fibrillation is the major cause of death due to electric shock. The threshold for ventricular fibrillation for an average-sized man varies from about 75 to 400 mA. Normal rhythmic activity will return only if a brief high-current pulse from a defibrillator is applied to simultaneously depolarize all the cells of the heart muscle. After all the cells relax together, a normal rhythm usually returns.

Sustained myocardial contraction

When the current is high enough, the entire heart muscle contracts. Although the heart stops beating while the current is applied, the normal rhythm ensues when the current is interrupted, just as in defibrillation. Data from ac-defibrillation experiments on animals show that minimum currents for complete myocardial contraction are in the range from 1 to 6 A. No irreversible damage to the heart is known to result from these currents.

Burns and physical injury

Very little is known of the effects of currents in excess of 10 A, particularly for currents of short duration. Resistive heating causes burns, usually on the skin at the entry points, because skin resistance is high. Voltages greater than 240 V can puncture the skin. The brain and other nervous tissue lose all functional excitability when high currents are passed through them. Also, excessive currents may force muscular contractions that are strong enough to pull the muscle attachment away from the bone.

13.2 Important susceptibility parameters

The physiological effects previously described are for an average 70-kg man and for 60-Hz current applied for 1 to 3 s to moistened hands grasping a No. 8 copper wire. The current needed to produce each effect depends on all these conditions, as explained below. Minimal rather than average values are often most important for safety considerations.

Threshold and let-go variability

Figure 13.2 shows the variability of the threshold of perception and the let-go current for men and women (Dalziel, 1973). On this plot of percentile rank versus rms current in milliamperes, the data are close to the straight lines shown, so a Gaussian distribution may be assumed. For men, the mean value for the threshold of perception is 1.1 mA; for women, the estimated mean is 0.7 mA. The minimum threshold of perception is 500 μA.

Let-go currents also appear to follow Gaussian distributions, with mean let-go currents of 16 mA for men and 10.5 mA for women. The minimum threshold let-go current is 9.5 mA for men and 6 mA for women. Note that the standard deviation for let-go current is much greater than the standard deviation for threshold-of-perception currents.

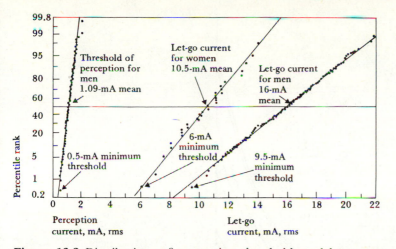

Figure 13.2 Distributions of perception thresholds and let-go currents. These data depend on surface area of contact (moistened hand grasping AWG No. 8 copper wire). (Replotted from C.F. Dalziel, "Electric Shock," *Advances in Biomedical Engineering*, edited by J.H.V. Brown and J.F Dickson III, 1973, *3*, 223–248.)

Frequency

Figure 13.3 shows a plot of let-go currents versus the frequency of the current. Unfortunately, the minimum let-go currents occur for commercial power-line frequencies of 50 to 60 Hz. For frequencies below 10 Hz, let-go currents rise, probably because the muscles can partially relax during part of each cycle. And at frequencies above several hundred hertz, the let-go currents rise, perhaps because of the well-known strength-duration tradeoff, and the refractoriness of excitable tissue.

Duration

Fibrillating-current thresholds for animals increase sharply for shocks that last less than about 1 s, as shown in Figure 13.4. The heart is known to be more vulnerable to fibrillation during about 100 ms of the heart cycle that corresponds approximately to the T wave in the ECG. Shocks of short duration, applied during other parts of the heart cycle, have much higher fibrillation thresholds.

Body weight

Several studies using various sizes of animals show that the fibrillation threshold increases with body weight. As Figure 13.5

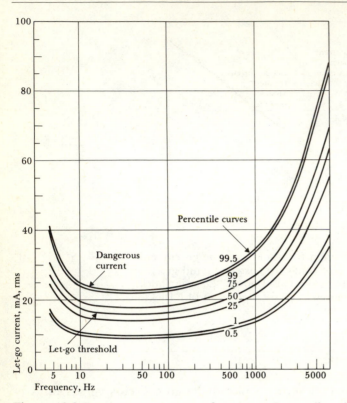

Figure 13.3 Let-go current versus frequency. Percentile values indicate variability of let-go current among individuals. Let-go currents for women are about two-thirds the values for men. (Reproduced, with permission, from C.F. Dalziel, "Electric Shock," *Advances in Biomedical Engineering,* edited by J.H.V. Brown and J.F. Dickson III, 1973, *3,* 223–248.)

shows, however, there is considerable scatter in the data, even for dogs only. Figure 13.4 also demonstrates the dependence of fibrillating current on body weight. These findings deserve more study because they are used to extrapolate fibrillating currents for humans.

Points of entry

When current is applied at two points on the surface of the body, only a small fraction of the total current flows through the heart, as shown in Figure 13.6(a). These large externally applied currents are called *macroshocks*. The magnitude of current needed to fibrillate the heart is far greater when the current is applied on the surface of the body than it would be if the current were applied directly to the heart. The importance of the location for the two

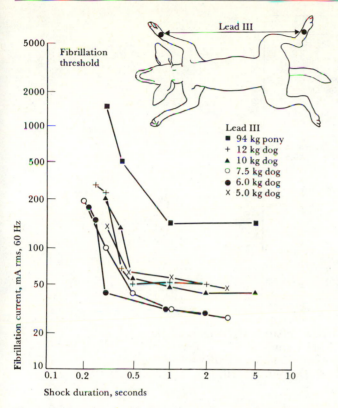

Figure 13.4 Thresholds for ventricular fibrillation in animals for 60-Hz ac current. Duration of current (0.2 to 5 s) and weight of animal body were varied. (From L.A. Geddes, *IEEE Trans. Biomed. Eng.*, 1973, *20*, 465–468. Copyright 1973 by the Institute of Electrical and Electronics Engineers. Reproduced with permission.)

macroshock entry points is often overlooked. If the two points are both on the same extremity, the risk of fibrillation is small, even for high currents. Geddes *et al.* (1973) showed that for dogs, the current needed for fibrillation is greater for ECG lead I (LA-RA) electrodes than for ECG leads II and III (LL-RA, LL-LA). Protection afforded by the skin resistance (15 kΩ to 1 MΩ/cm^2) is eliminated by many medical procedures that require insertion of conductive devices into natural openings or incisions in the skin. If the skin resistance is bypassed, less voltage is required to produce sufficient current for each physiological effect.

Patients are particularly susceptible when devices are placed into or near the heart. A device is especially hazardous if it provides a conductive path from outside the body to a point on or within the heart, and if this conductor is insulated from the body except at the tip near the heart. As Figure 13.6(b) shows, all the current flowing through such a conductive device flows through

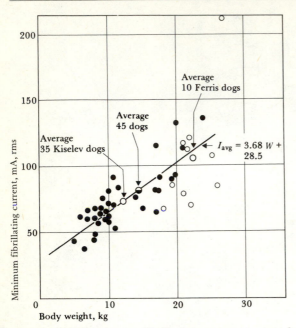

Figure 13.5 Minimum fibrillating current versus body weight. 60-Hz ac shocks for 3.0-s duration in dogs. ● Kiselev study (1963), ○ Ferris study (1936). (From C.F. Dalziel, "Electric Shock," in *Advances in Biomedical Engineering*, edited by J.H.V. Brown and J.F. Dickson III, 1973, *3*: 223–248.)

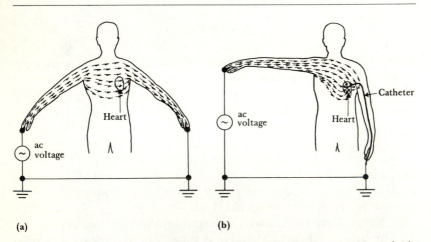

Figure 13.6 Effect of entry points on current distribution. (a) *Macroshock*, externally applied current spreads throughout the body. (b) *Microshock*, all the current applied through an intracardiac catheter flows through the heart. (From F.J. Weibell, "Electrical Safety in the Hospital," *Annals of Biomedical Engineering*, 2, 126–148 New York: Academic Press, 1974.)

the heart. The current density at the point of contact can be quite high, and fibrillation in dogs can be induced by total currents as low as 20 μA! (See Roy, 1976.) The sparse data we have for human-heart fibrillation with an intracardiac catheter indicate that currents ranging from 80 to 600 μA can cause fibrillation. The other connection can be at any point on the body. Internally applied currents that enter the body at the heart, as depicted in Figure 13.6(b), are called *microshocks*. The generally accepted safety limit for microshock is 10 μA. Patients that have such direct electrical connections to their heart are called *electrically susceptible patients*.

13.3 Distribution of electric power

Electric power is needed in health-care facilities not only to operate medical instruments, but also for lighting, maintenance appliances, patient conveniences (such as TV, hair curlers, and electric toothbrushes), clocks, nurse call buttons, and an endless list of other electrical devices. A first step in providing electrical safety is to control the availability of electric power and grounds in the patients' environment. This section is concerned with methods for safe distribution of power in health-care facilities. Let us consider this material before we discuss various macroshock and microshock hazards in the following sections.

A simplified diagram of an electric-power-distribution system is shown in Figure 13.7. High voltage (4800 V) enters the

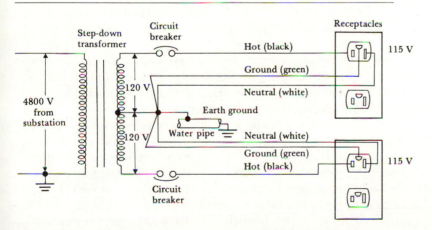

Figure 13.7 Simplified electric-power distribution for 115-V circuits. Power frequency is 60 Hz.

building—usually via underground cables. The secondary of a stepdown transformer develops 240 V. This secondary has a grounded center tap to provide two 120-V circuits between ground and each side of the secondary winding. Some heavy-duty devices (such as air conditioners, electric dryers, and x-ray machines) that require 240 V are placed across the entire secondary winding; electricians do this by making connections to the two ungrounded terminals. Ordinary wall receptacles and lights operate on 120 V, obtained from either one of the ungrounded hot (black) transformer terminals and the neutral (white) grounded center tap. In addition, for health-care facilities, the National Electric Code (NEC) for 1978 requires that all receptacles be grounded by a separate insulated (green) copper conductor (Article 517-11). Some older installations used metal conduit as a ground conductor. This type of ground is generally unsatisfactory, because corrosion and loose conduit connections are unreliable.

Patients' electrical environment

Of course, a shock hazard exists between the two conductors supplying either a 240-V or a 120-V appliance. Since the neutral wire on a 120-V circuit is connected to ground, a connection between the hot conductor and *any* grounded object poses a shock hazard. Shocks can also occur if sufficient potentials exist between exposed conductive surfaces in the patients' environment. Maximum potentials permitted between any two exposed conductive surfaces in the vicinity of the patient are specified by the 1978 NEC, Article 517-80 and 517-81 (frequency < 1000 Hz measured across 1000-Ω resistance):

1 *General-care areas* 500 mV under normal operation
2 *Critical-care areas* 100 mV under normal operation

In general-care areas, patients have only incidental contact with electrical devices. For critical-care areas, hospital patients are intentionally exposed to electrical devices, and insulation of externalized cardiac conductors from conductive surfaces is required. In critical-care areas, all exposed conductive surfaces in the vicinity of the patient must be grounded at a single patient-grounding point (Section 13.8). Also, frequent periodic testing for continuity between the patient ground and all grounded surfaces is required.

Each patient-bed location in general-care areas must have at least four single or two duplex receptacles. Each receptacle must be grounded. At least two branch circuits with separate automatic overcurrent devices must supply the location of each patient bed. For critical-care areas, at least six single or three duplex receptacles are required for each location of a patient bed. Two branch circuits are also required, at least one being an individual branch circuit from a single panelboard. An equipotential grounding system (Section 13.8) is also required for critical-care areas. (For details, see NEC 70–1978, Article 517.)

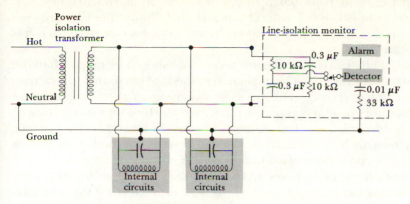

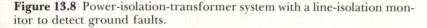

Electrical instruments

Figure 13.8 Power-isolation-transformer system with a line-isolation monitor to detect ground faults.

Isolated-power systems

Even installing a good separate grounding system for each patient cannot prevent possibly hazardous voltages that can result from ground faults. A ground fault is a short circuit between the hot conductor and ground that injects large currents into the grounding system. These high-current ground faults are rare, and often the circuit breakers open quickly. If the center tap of the stepdown transformer were not grounded, then very little current could flow, even if a short circuit to ground developed. So long as both power conductors are isolated from ground, a single ground fault will not allow the large currents that cause potentials between conductive surfaces.

Isolation of both conductors from ground is commonly achieved with an *isolation transformer*. A typical isolated-power system is shown in Figure 13.8. In an isolated system such as this, a single ground fault from either conductor to ground simply reverts the system to a normal grounded system. A second fault from the other conductor to ground is then required to get large ground current.

A continually operating *line-isolation monitor*, LIM (also called a dynamic ground detector) must be used with isolation transformers to detect the occurrence of the first fault from either conductor to ground. This monitor alternately measures the total possible resistive and capacitive leakage current (*total hazard current*) that would flow through a low impedance *if it were connected* between either isolated conductor and ground. When the total hazard current exceeds 1.7 to 2.0 mA for normal line voltage, a red light and an audible alarm are activated. The LIM itself has a monitor hazard current from 0.025 to 0.5 mA, and an alarm-current band-width of 0.1 to 0.3 mA. This makes the allowed fault hazard cur-rent for all appliances served by the transformer somewhat less than 2 mA.

The kinds of corrective action that should be taken when the alarm goes off must be explained to medical personnel so that they do not overreact. The periodic switching in some line-isolation monitors produces transients that can interfere with monitoring of low-level physiological signals (ECG and EEG) and give erroneous automatic heart rates. Or it can trigger synchronized defibrillators and aortic-balloon assist pumps during the wrong phase of the pa-tient's heart cycle. Some LIMs avoid these problems by using con-tinuous two-channel circuitry, instead of measuring the total haz-ard current by switching alternately between each line and ground.

Isolated-power systems were originally introduced to prevent sparks from coming into contact with flammable anesthetics such as ether. The NEC requires isolated-power systems in all those oper-ating rooms and all other locations in which flammable anesthetics are used or stored. The high cost (about $2000 per bed) of isolated-power systems must be weighed against the limited degree of protection they provide.

Emergency-power systems

Article 517 of the National Electrical Code (1978) specifies the emergency electrical system required for health-care facilities. An emergency system is required that automatically restores power to specified areas within 10 s after interruption of the normal source. The emergency system may consist of two parts: (1) the life-safety branch (illumination, alarm, and alerting equipment), and (2) the critical branch (lighting and receptacles in critical patient-care areas). (For additional details, see Article 517–61, 62, 63.)

13.4 Macroshock hazards

The high resistance of dry skin and the spatial distribution of current throughout the body when a person receives an electric shock are two factors that reduce the danger of ventricular fibrilla-tion. Also electrical equipment is designed to minimize the possibil-ity of humans coming into contact with dangerous voltages.

Skin and body resistance

The resistance of the skin limits the current that can flow through a person's body when the person comes into contact with a source of voltage. The resistance of the skin varies widely according to the amount of water and natural oil present. It is inversely proportional to the area of contact.

Most of the resistance of the skin is in the outer horny layer of the epidermis. For one square centimeter of electrical contact with dry intact skin, resistance may range from 15 kΩ to almost 1 MΩ, depending on the part of the body and the moisture or sweat present. If skin is wet or broken, resistance drops to as low as 1% of the value for dry skin. In contrast, the internal resistance of the body is about 200 Ω for each limb and about 100 Ω for the trunk. Thus internal body resistance between any two limbs is about 500 Ω. These values are probably higher for obese patients, because the specific resistivity of fat is high. Actually, the distribution of current in various tissues in the body is poorly understood.

Any medical procedure that reduces or eliminates the resistance of the skin increases possible current flow and makes the patient more vulnerable to macroshocks. For example, biopotential electrode paste reduces skin resistance. Also electronic thermometers placed in the mouth or rectum bypass the skin resistance, as do intravenous catheters containing fluid that can act as a conductor. Thus patients in a medical-care facility are much more susceptible to macroshock than the general population.

Electrical faults in equipment

All electrical devices are of course designed to minimize exposure of humans to hazardous voltages. However, many devices have a metal chassis and cabinet that can be touched by medical personnel and patients. If the chassis and cabinet are not grounded, as shown in Figure 13.9(a), then an insulation failure or shorted capacitor between the black hot power lead and the chassis results in a 115-V potential between the chassis and any grounded object. If a person simultaneously touches the chassis and any grounded object, a macroshock results.

The chassis and cabinet can be grounded via a third green wire in the power cord and electrical system, as shown in Figure 13.9(b). This ground wire is connected to the neutral wire and ground at the power-distribution panel. Then, when a fault occurs between the hot conductor and the chassis, the current flows safely to ground on the green conductor. If the ground-wire resistance is very low, the voltage between the chassis and other grounded objects is negligible. If enough current flows through the ground wire to trip the circuit breaker, this will call people's attention to the fault.

Note that direct faults between the hot conductor or any high voltage in the device and ground are not common. Little or no current flows through the ground conductor during normal operation

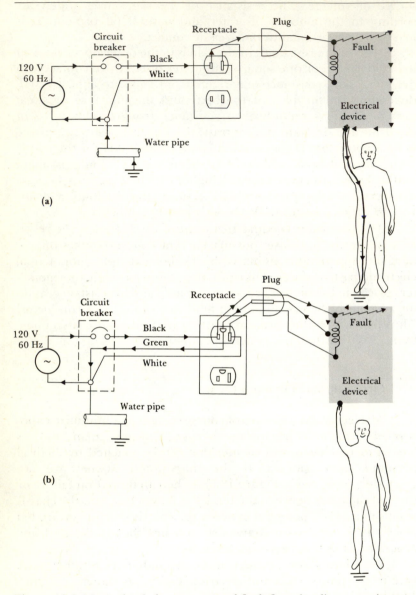

Figure 13.9 Macroshock due to a ground fault from hot line to equipment cases for (a) ungrounded cases and (b) grounded cases.

of electrical devices. The ground conductor is not needed for protection against macroshock until a hazardous fault develops. Thus a broken ground wire or a poor connection of a receptacle ground is not detected during normal operation of the device. Consequently, continuity of the ground wire in the device and the receptacle must be periodically tested.

Faults inside electrical devices may result from failures of insulation, shorted capacitors, or mechanical failures that cause shorts. Power cords are particularly susceptible to strain and physical abuse, as are plugs and receptacles. Ironically, it is possible for a device's chassis and cabinet to become hot because a ground wire is in the power cord. If the ground wire is open anywhere between the power cord and ground, then a frayed cord could permit contact between the hot conductor and the broken ground wire leading to the chassis. Often, macroshock accidents result from carelessness and failure to correct known deficiencies in the power-distribution system and in electrical devices.

Fluids—such as blood, urine, IV solutions, and even baby formulas—can conduct enough electricity to cause temporary short circuits if accidentally spilled into normally safe equipment. This hazard is particularly real in hospital areas that are subject to wet conditions, such as hemodialysis areas. Cabinets of many electrical devices have holes and vents for cooling that provide access for spilled conductive fluids. Designers of devices should protect patient electrical connections from this hazard.

13.5 Microshock hazards

Microshock accidents in electrically susceptible patients having direct electrical connections to the heart are usually caused by circumstances unrelated to macroshock hazards. Microshocks usually result from *leakage currents* in line-operated equipment or differences in voltage between grounded conductive surfaces due to large currents in the grounding system. The microshock current can flow either into or out of the electrical connection to the heart.

Leakage currents

Small currents (usually on the order of microamperes) that inevitably flow between any adjacent insulated conductors that are at different potentials are called *leakage currents*. Although most of the leakage current in line-operated equipment flows through the capacitance between the two conductors, some resistive leakage current flows through insulation, dust, and moisture.

The most important source of leakage currents is the currents that flow from all conductors in the electrical device to leads connected either to the chassis or to the patient. Leakage current flowing to the chassis flows safely to ground if a low-resistance ground wire is available, as shown in Figure 13.10(a). If the ground wire is broken, then the chassis potential will rise above ground, and a patient who touches the chassis *and* has a grounded electrical connection to the heart may receive a microshock [Figure 13.10(b)]. If there is a connection from the chassis to the patient's

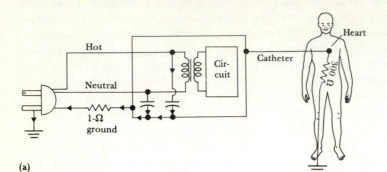

(a)

(b)

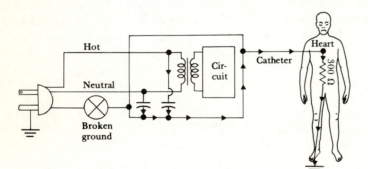

(c)

Figure 13.10 Leakage-current pathways. Assume 100 μA of leakage current from the power line to the instrument case. (a) Intact ground and 99.8 μA flows through the ground. (b) Broken ground and 100 μA flows through the heart. (c) Broken ground and 100 μA flows through the heart in the opposite direction.

heart *and* a connection to ground anywhere on the body, this could also cause a microshock [Figure 13.10(c)].

Conductive surfaces

The source that produces the microshock current need not be leakage current from line-operated equipment. Small potentials between any two conductive surfaces near the patient can cause a microshock if either surface makes contact to the heart and the other surface contacts any part of the body. Some examples are given later in this section.

Conductive paths to the heart

Specific types of electrical connections to the heart can be identified. The following clinical devices make patients electrically susceptible to microshock.

1 Electrodes of externalized cardiac pacemakers
2 Electrodes for intracardiac ECG measuring devices
3 Liquid-filled catheters placed in the heart to:
  a Measure blood pressure
  b Withdraw blood samples
  c Inject substances such as dye or drugs into the heart

It should be emphasized that an electrically susceptible patient is in danger of microshock only if there is some electrical connection to the heart. The internal resistance of liquid-filled catheters is much greater (50 kΩ to 1 MΩ) than the resistance of metallic conductors in pacemaker and ECG electrode leads. Internal resistance of the body to microshock is about 300 Ω, and the resistance of the skin can be quite variable, as discussed previously.

Roy (1976) showed that in dogs the surface area of the intracardiac electrode is an important determinant of minimum fibrillating current. Figure 13.11 shows that as catheters get smaller, so does the total current needed to fibrillate. This means that current density at the tip of the intracardiac electrode is the important microshock parameter. Smaller catheters tend to offer larger internal resistance.

Let us now discuss three examples of possible microshock incidents, to illustrate how subtle microshock hazards can be. These examples are illustrative only. They are certainly not the only ways that microshock can occur; they are not even necessarily the most probable.

Example 13.1 A patient with a transvenous pacing catheter connected to an external pacemaker powered by batteries is lying on a hospital bed that can be adjusted by an electric motor. The ground wire on the power cord of the motor is broken (a common defect that requires periodic testing to detect). Figure 13.12(a) and (b) depict two possible paths that could be followed by microshock current. Equivalent electric circuits are given in Figure 13.12(c) and (d), respectively. In both possibilities, 120 V is capacitively coupled (via the 2500 pF capacitance) from the wiring of the motor to

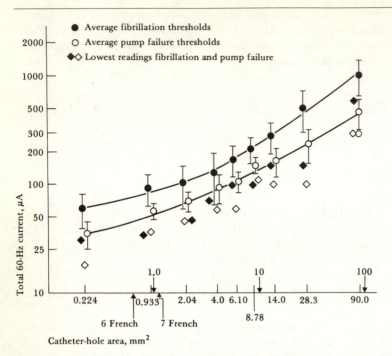

Figure 13.11 Thresholds of ventricular fibrillation and pump failure versus catheter area in dogs. (From O.Z. Roy, J.R. Scott, and G.C. Park, "Ventricular Fibrillation and Pump Failure Thresholds Versus Electrode Area," *IEEE Transactions in Biomedical Engineering, 1976, 23,* 45–48. Reprinted with permission.)

the frame of the bed. If the ground wire were intact, a leakage current of about 113 μA would flow harmlessly to ground. Since the ground wire is broken, this leakage current can flow in paths that may involve the patient. If the patient or an attendant touches both the bed frame and any grounded surface, the current flowing to ground will be below perceivable levels. However, as shown in Figure 13.12(a) and (c), if an attendant touches both the bed rail and the electrode terminals of the pacemaker, and if any part of the patient is touching a grounded object, the patient can receive a microshock. If each skin resistance involved were 100 kΩ, the microshock current would be

$$I = \frac{120}{[(1/\omega C)^2 + (R_{\text{total}})^2]^{1/2}}$$

$$= \frac{120}{[(1.06 \times 10^6)^2 + (3.0 \times 10^5)^2]^{1/2}}$$

$$\cong 109 \ \mu A$$

which is an order of magnitude above the controversial safety limit of 10 μA.

The same microshock current can flow in the opposite direction through the patient if the patient happens to be touching the bed rail and the attendant touches both the terminals of the pacemaker and some grounded object [Figure 13.12(b) and (d)]. Both these circuit paths are quite plausible. Either insulated pacemaker terminals *or* a properly grounded bed motor would prevent the microshock. The first solution is probably the most important, although both should be required.

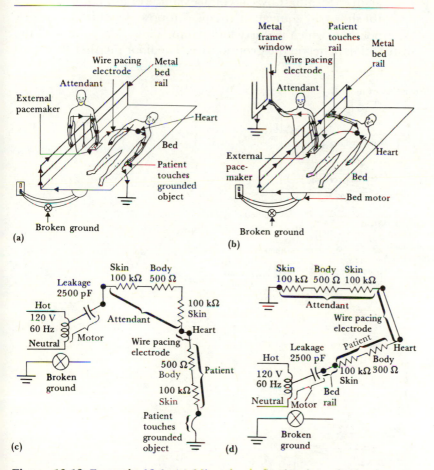

Figure 13.12 Example 13.1. (a) Microshock flowing into the heart on a pacing catheter. (b) Microshock flowing away from the heart on a pacing catheter. (c) Equivalent circuit for (a). (d) Equivalent circuit for (b).

Example 13.2 The following example illustrates the need for a single reference ground point for each patient in critical-care areas and also the need for 100-mV potential limits between conductive surfaces in these areas.

A patient in the intensive-care unit (ICU) is connected to an ECG monitor that grounds the right-leg electrode to reduce 60-Hz interference. Also the patient's left-ventricular blood pressure is being monitored by an intracardiac saline-filled catheter connected to a metallic pressure transducer that is grounded. Assume that these two monitors are connected to grounded three-wire wall receptacles that are on separate circuits which come from a central power-distribution panel many feet away. A microshock can occur if any device with very high leakage current, or with a fault, is operated on *either* circuit.

Figure 13.13(a) shows a typical example of this hazard; Figure 13.13(b) shows an equivalent circuit. Suppose that a faulty electric floor polisher, which is dusty and damp, allows 5 A to flow to the distribution panel on the ground wire. The floor polisher functions

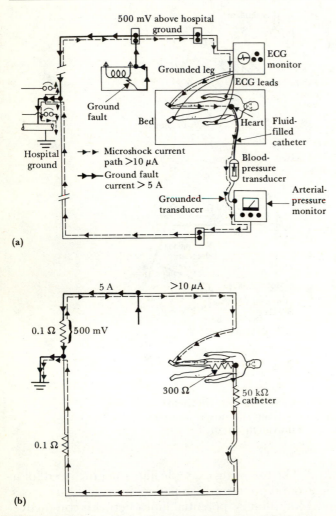

(a)

(b)

Figure 13.13 Example 13.2. (a) Large ground-fault current raises the potential of *one* ground connection to the patient. The microshock current can then flow out through a catheter connected to a different ground. (b) Equivalent circuit. Only power-system grounds are shown.

properly, so the fault is not noticed by the operator. The ground wire could easily have a 0.1-Ω resistance, so that 500 mV could appear across the patient between the ECG-monitor ground and the pressure-monitor ground. If the resistance of the patient's body and of the liquid-filled catheter is less than 50 kΩ, a current in excess of the 10-μA safe limit will flow. Of course, more current would flow if the ground resistance or fault current were higher. If a grounded pacing catheter were to be used instead of the liquid-filled catheter in this example, then much smaller differences in ground potential would be dangerous.

Most low-voltage hazards can be avoided if the grounds of all devices used in the vicinity of each patient are connected to a single patient-grounding point. Also, this prevents faults at one patient's bedside from affecting the safety of other patients. Modern pressure transducers and ECG monitors provide electrical isolation for all patient leads.

Example 13.3 Our final example illustrates the importance of grounds in isolated power systems. When the grounds on instruments powered by isolated systems are intact, only a few milliamperes of current flow to ground, even if a short-circuit fault from hot to ground occurs (Figure 13.8). If the ground wire of an electrical instrument fails, however, a particularly subtle hazard can develop in isolated systems, even without a short-circuit fault.

Figure 13.14 shows how a patient can be in danger if the chassis of two electrical instruments are connected to the patient, with either connection being an in-dwelling cardiac electrode. If the ground wire breaks on either instrument in Figure 13.14(a), then the patient can become the sensing element of the capacitance bridge shown in Figure 13.14(b). The capacitances C_A and C_B represent all the capacitance from the power lines to ground, and actually may be large capacitors that filter RF interference. Stray capacitance C_S between the isolated power lines and ground in the isolation transformer and wiring may not be large enough to trigger the line-isolation monitor.

For example, suppose that the patient resistance is 500 Ω. The sum of $C_A + C_S$ is 3000 pF and the two capacitors labeled C_{B1} and C_{B2} differ by 1500 pF. Then currents of about 50 μA can flow through the patient.

These conditions that produce possibly hazardous current are reasonable, because interference capacitors in instruments are usually connected only between the black hot power line and ground. Frequent testing of the integrity of ground wires minimizes this hazard. Electrical isolation of the leads that go to the patient from both instruments is the obvious solution, if it is feasible. Of course, the other safety measures are also important, because accidental connections between patients and some potentially hazardous source of current can never be eliminated entirely.

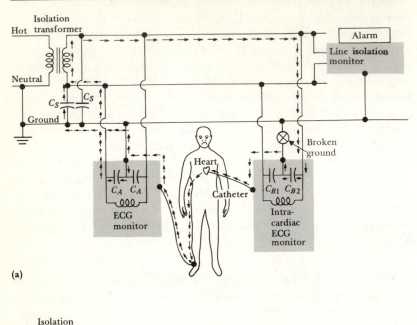

(a)

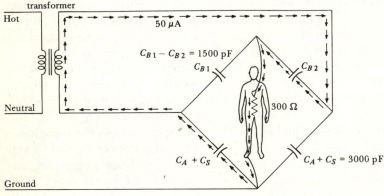

(b)

Figure 13.14 Example 13.3. (a) Ground-wire failure in an isolated-power system can place electrically susceptible patients in the sensing arm of a capacitance bridge. (b) Equivalent circuit. The line-isolation monitor may also add capacitance in parallel with C_A and C_B.

13.6 Electrical safety standards

Many organizations are continually developing and revising codes, standards, and regulations that affect health-care facilities. However, clear and widely accepted codes and standards for electrical safety have not yet emerged. Several tentative standards have yet to be accepted because major controversies have raged regarding the significance of the hazards and the effectiveness of various proposed safety measures.

The National Fire Protection Association (NFPA) is the most prominent electrical safety organization. Its published standards are widely adopted and enforced by state, county, and municipal authorities. The NFPA does not enforce standards, it only develops and publishes those that are drafted by 23 specialized panels of knowledgeable persons. After the NFPA has published them, they invite the public to comment. The most recent revisions of the NFPA documents that pertain to electrical safety in health-care facilities are as follows.

1 NFPA 70–1978 National Electrical Code (NEC), Articles 517, 660, 665

2 NFPA 76A–1978 Essential Electrical Systems for Health-Care Facilities

3 NFPA 76B–1977 Electricity in Patient Care Areas of Hospitals

4 NFPA 76C–1975 Use of High-Frequency Electricity in Health Care Facilities

5 NFPA 56A–1973 Safe Use of Inhalation Anesthetics

Section 13.3 gave some discussions of the first two standards. Although the NEC specifies requirements for distribution of electric power, the only special standards for health-care electrical equipment are for x-ray equipment and induction and dielectric-heating equipment. However, NFPA 76B does cover all medical electrical appliances by designating three classes of patient-care areas (*G*, general patient areas, *H*, heavily instrumented patient areas, and *W*, wet areas). Voltage and resistance limits for grounds and conductive surfaces in each area are given. Design goals for minimizing leakage current in chassis and in patient leads are a major concern. Table 13.1 presents the maximum limits for leakage currents in medical electrical appliances.

Actually, NFPA 76B is much more than a standard for safe use of electricity in hospitals. It describes shock hazards, systems of power distribution, methods of protection against electrical hazards, and procedures for testing the safety of electrical equipment.

Underwriters' Laboratories have developed a standard for medical and dental equipment (UL 544). UL standards for "hospital grade" receptacles and plug caps, explosion-proof connectors, isolated power systems, and conductive flooring are all useful.

Electrical appliance	Chassis leakage, μA	Patient lead leakage, μA
Appliances not intended to contact patients	500	NA
Appliances likely to contact patients (With or without patient leads)	100	50
Appliances with *isolated* patient leads	100	10

Table 13.1 Leakage current limits for electrical appliances

The Association for the Advancement of Medical Instrumentation (AAMI) has developed safety and performance standards for medical devices. One such standard deals primarily with electrical-leakage currents from medical devices (AAMI SCL-P 10.75).

Voluntary safety standards have also been developed by manufacturing associations, such as the National Electrical Manufacturers Association (NEMA) and the Electronics Industries Association (EIA). Industry and government agencies have developed internal standards and specifications (FDA-MDS-201-0035; IEEE 711-2; ISA E. S62.3; VA SPEC X-1432). The American National Standards Institute (ANSI) coordinates the dissemination of standards of safety developed by all public and private organizations. The International Electrotechnical Commission (IEC) has a technical committee (No. 62) that deals with electrical equipment in medical practice.

13.7 Basic approaches to protection against shock

There seem to be two fundamental methods of protecting patients against shock. First, the patient can be completely isolated and insulated from all grounded objects and all sources of electric current. Second, all conductive surfaces within reach of the patient can be maintained at the same potential, which is not necessarily ground potential. Neither of these approaches can be achieved in most practical environments, so some combination of the two methods is usually sufficient for each type of patient.

Not only must all hospital patients be protected from macroshocks, but all visitors and staff must be protected as well. Patients with reduced skin resistance (perhaps coupled to electrodes), invasive connections (such as intravenous catheters), or exposure to wet conditions (as happens during dialysis) need extra protection. The small number of electrically susceptible patients with accessible electrical connections to the heart need additional protection from microshock currents. Many of the specific methods of protection described here can be used in combination to provide redundant safeguards. We must also consider cost-benefit ratios with respect to both the purchase cost of safety equipment and periodic maintenance costs of such equipment.

13.8 Protection: power distribution

Equipotential grounding

Low-resistance grounds that can carry currents of up to circuit-breaker ratings are clearly essential for protecting patients against both macroshock and microshock, even if an isolated power system is used. Figure 13.9 shows the importance of adequate grounds for protection against macroshock. Grounding is equally significant in preventing microshock (see Figures 13.12, 13.13, and 13.14). An *equipotential grounding system* protects electrically susceptible patients by keeping all conductive surfaces and receptacle grounds in the patient's environment at the same potential. It also protects the patient from ground faults at other locations.

The equipotential grounding system has a *patient grounding point,* a *reference grounding point,* and connections, as shown in Figure 13.15. The patient grounding point is connected individually to all receptacle grounds, metal beds, metal door and window frames, water pipes, and any other conductive surfaces. These connections should not exceed 0.1 Ω. Also the potential difference between receptacle grounds should not exceed 20 mV (regardless of whether or not the system is energized). The potential difference between receptacle grounds and conductive surfaces should not exceed 100 mV. Each patient grounding point must be connected individually to a reference grounding point that is in turn connected to the building service ground.

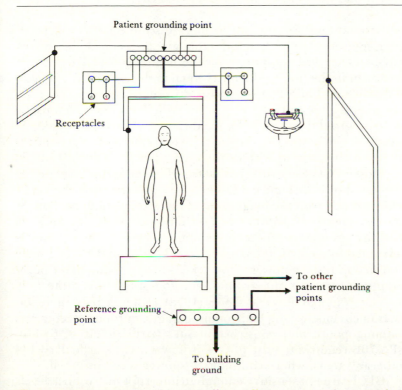

Figure 13.15 Equipotential grounding. All the receptacle grounds and conductive surfaces in the vicinity of the patient are connected to the patient grounding point near the head of the bed. Each patient grounding point is connected to the reference grounding point that makes a single connection to building ground.

Isolated power-distribution system

Unfortunately, even a good equipotential grounding system cannot eliminate voltages produced between grounds by large ground faults that cause large ground currents. However, these ground faults are rare in high-quality and properly maintained equipment. The isolation transformers discussed in Section 13.3 and shown in Figure 13.8 prevent this unlikely hazard. The isolated system also reduces leakage current somewhat, but not below the proposed 10-μA safe limit for electrically susceptible patients. There is usually enough capacitance between the transformer secondary circuit and ground to preclude protection against microshocks with isolation transformers. Isolated power systems provide considerable protection against macroshocks, particularly in areas subject to wet conditions. Such systems are absolutely necessary in situations in which flammable anesthetics are used. The additional protection against microshocks provided by isolation transformers does not generally justify the high cost of these systems.

Ground-fault circuit interrupters (GFCI)

Ground-fault circuit interrupters disconnect the source of electric power when a ground fault greater than about 6 mA occurs. In electrical equipment having negligible leakage current, the current in the hot conductor is equal to the current in the neutral conductor. The GFCI senses the difference between these two currents and interrupts power when this difference, which must be flowing to ground, exceeds the fixed rating. The devices make no distinction with respect to the path the current takes to ground: It may be via the ground wire or through a person (Figure 13.9).

Most GFCIs use a differential transformer and solid-state circuitry, as shown in Figure 13.16(a). The trip time for the GFCI varies inversely with the magnitude of the ground-fault current, as shown in Figure 13.16(b). The GFCI is used with conventional three-wire grounded power-distribution systems. When power is interrupted by a GFCI, the manual reset button on the GFCI must be pushed to restore power. Most GFCIs have a momentary pushbutton that creates a safe ground fault to test the interrupter.

The National Electric Code (1978) requires that there be GFCIs in circuits serving bathrooms, garages, outdoor receptacles, swimming pools, and construction sites (Articles 210-8, 680-6). NFPA 76B requires the use of GFCIs in wet areas, particularly hydrotherapy areas, where continuity of power is not essential.

GFCIs are not sensitive enough to interrupt microshock levels of leakage current, so they are primarily macroshock-protection devices. They can prevent some microshocks by interrupting the source of large ground-fault currents that cause potential dif-

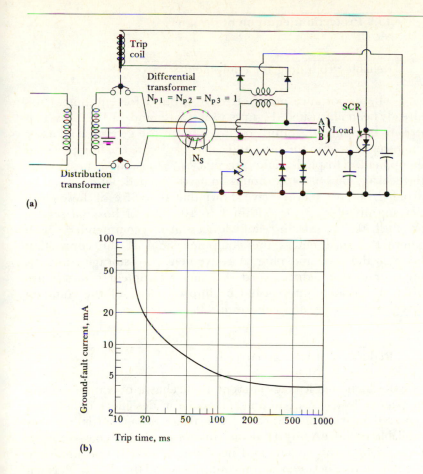

(a)

(b)

Figure 13.16 Ground-fault circuit interrupters. (a) Schematic diagram of a solid-state GFCI (three wire, two pole, 6 mA). (b) Ground-fault current versus trip time for a GFCI. [Part (a) is from C.F. Dalziel, "Electric Shock," in *Advances in Biomedical Engineering*, edited by J.H.V. Brown and J.F. Dickson III, 1973, *3*: 223–248.]

ferences in grounding systems which might be hazardous to electrically susceptible patients.

However, circuits in patient areas generally should not include GFCIs, because the loss of power to life-support equipment due to GFCI tripping is probably more hazardous to the patient than most small ground faults would be. Where brief power interruptions can be tolerated, the low cost of the GFCI ($45) is an attractive alternative to isolated-power-distribution systems ($2000).

13.9 Protection: equipment design

Reliable grounding for equipment

The importance of an effective ground for equipment has already been illustrated (Figures 13.9, 13.12, and 13.14). Most failures of equipment grounds occur either at the ground contact of the receptacle or in the plug and cable leading to the line-powered equipment. Hospital-grade receptacles, plugs, and heavy-duty low-leakage power cords should be used. Molded plugs should be avoided, because surveys have shown that 40 to 85% of these plugs develop invisible breaks within 1 to 10 years of hospital service (Weibell, 1974). Strain-relief devices are recommended, both where the cord enters the equipment and at the connection between the cord and plug. A convenient cord-storage compartment or device reduces cord damage. Equipment grounds are often deliberately interrupted by improper use of the common three-to-two prong adapters (*cheater adapter*).

Reduction of leakage current

Reduction of leakage current in the chassis of equipment and in patient leads is an important goal for designers of all line-powered instruments. Special low-leakage power cords are now available (< 1.0 μA/m). Leakage current inside the chassis can be reduced by using layouts and insulating materials that minimize the capacitance between all hot conductors and the chassis. Particular attention must be given to maximizing the impedance from patient leads to hot conductors and from patient leads to chassis ground. Most modern equipment meets the leakage-current limits given in Section 13.6. Old equipment with higher leakage should not be used with electrically susceptible patients unless proper grounding is assured.

Double-insulated equipment

The objective of grounding is to eliminate hazardous potentials by interconnecting all conductive surfaces. The other approach is to use a separate layer of insulation to prevent contact of any person with the chassis or any exposed conductive surface. Primary insulation is the normal functional insulation between energized conductors and the chassis. A separate secondary layer of insulation between the chassis and the outer case protects personnel even if a ground fault to the chassis occurs. The outer case, if it is made of insulating material, may serve as the secondary insulation. All switch levers and control shafts must also be double insulated (for example, plastic knobs may have recessed set screws). Double insulation generally reduces leakage current. For medical instruments, both layers of insulation should remain effective, even when there are spillages of conductive fluids. Double insulation protects against both macroshock and microshock.

Operation at low voltages

Most solid-state electronic diagnostic equipment can be powered by low-voltage batteries (<8 V) or low-voltage isolation transformers. Macroshock is avoided if the voltage is low enough to be safe even when the device is applied directly to wet skin. Low-voltage ac-powered equipment can still cause microshock if the current is applied directly to the heart. However, low-voltage ac equipment is generally safer than high-voltage ac equipment. See Section 105 in Article 517 of the National Electrical Code (1978) for requirements for low-voltage equipment used in inhalation-anesthetizing locations.

Driven right-leg circuit

Designers of low-level biopotential monitors (ECG, EEG) must eliminate interference from capacitively coupled ac-power lines. As we have seen, for safety reasons, grounding the patient is unacceptable. One solution, which was illustrated in Figure 6.19, is to sample the interference at the output of the biopotential amplifier and feed back to the patient a signal that minimizes the interference. The current fed back never exceeds the current already flowing in the patient due to capacitive coupling of the ac-power line. Interference is reduced, and as far as the hazards of low-voltage microshock are concerned, good isolation of the patient is provided. Current is typically less than 1 μA under normal operating conditions.

Current limiters

Semiconductor current limiters can be placed in series with patient leads on old ECG monitors to restrict the current to a few microamperes. Biopotential currents are below the microampere range because most biopotentials are less than 1 mV, and amplifier input impedances are very high. The reason that limiters are not widely used is that they short out or open circuit when they are subjected to the high voltages that defibrillators produce.

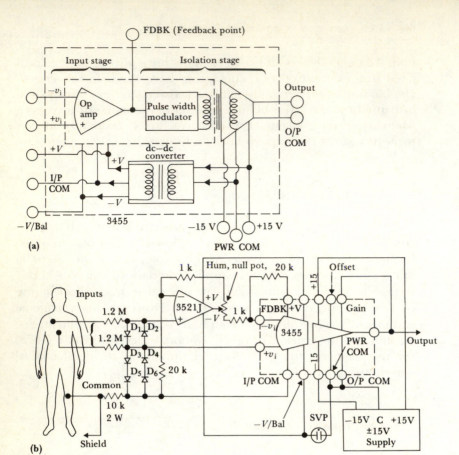

(a)

(b)

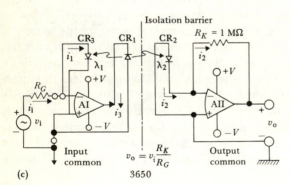

Isolation barrier

$$v_o = v_i \frac{R_K}{R_G}$$

3650

(c)

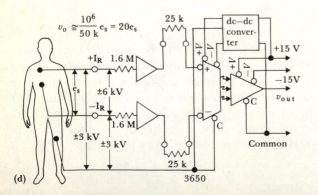

$$v_o \cong \frac{10^6}{50\text{ k}} e_s = 20e_s$$

3650

(d)

Electrical isolation

Optical isolation or transformer isolation of the electrical leads connected to patients is probably the best way to protect patients from most macroshock and microshock hazards. As Figure 13.17 shows, there is no direct electrical connection between isolated-input circuitry and line-powered circuits. Power for isolated-input circuits and the desired signal are transferred via separate optical or transformer links that have low coupling capacitance.

The transformer-isolation amplifier shown in Figure 13.17(a) is basically an operational amplifier, followed by a very accurate isolation stage. The output of the pulse-width modulator is transformer-coupled to the demodulator. The pulse-width modulation, the filtering (not shown), and the circuit shielding keep peak output noise to less than 1 mV. Additional external circuitry, shown in Figure 13.17(b), is necessary to limit leakage current in the patient leads and to protect the amplifier against defibrillator voltages. If components in the input amplifier fail, the input resistors limit leakage current. The diodes protect the input amplifier from large voltages and currents. The surge-voltage protection (SVP) prevents breakdown of the isolation barrier. It must have a rating higher than $120(2)^{-1/2}$ V peak, and is typically a 500-V spark gap.

Figure 3.17(c) shows an equivalent circuit for a single-ended linear optical isolation amplifier. The input amplifier AI, the LED CR_1, and the photodiode CR_3 give negative feedback, so that $i_1 = v_i/R_G$. The two photodiodes, CR_2 and CR_3, are matched; they receive equal light from the LED, so that $i_2 = i_1 = i_i$. Amplifier AII is a current-to-voltage converter, so $v_o = i_2 R_K$. Thus $v_o = v_i R_K/R_G$. Linearity depends primarily on the matching of photodiodes, and only full-scale output swing is affected by decreased LED output. Input buffer amplifiers and a dc-dc converter must be added, as shown in Figure 13.17(d). Circuitry designed to protect the amplifier from defibrillators, shown in Figure 13.17(b), should also be added.

Isolated heart connections

Undoubtedly the best way to minimize the hazards of microshock is to isolate or eliminate electrical connections to the heart.

◀ **Figure 13.17** Electrical isolation of patient leads to biopotential amplifiers. (a) A transformer isolation amplifier (Burr-Brown 3455). (b) Complete biopotential amplifier that uses a transformer isolation amplifier. (c) Equivalent circuit for a linear optical isolation amplifier (Burr-Brown 3650). (d) Complete biopotential amplifier that uses an optical isolation amplifier. (Reproduced with permission of Burr-Brown Research Corporation, Tucson, Arizona.)

Fully insulated connectors for external heart pacemakers powered by batteries (illustrated in Figure 13.12) have greatly reduced this hazard. Modern blood-pressure transducers have been designed with triple insulation between the column of liquid, the transducer case, and the electrical connections (Figure 13.18). Catheters with conductive walls have been developed (Ream *et al.*, 1977) that provide electrical contact all along that part of the catheter that is inside the patient, so that microshock current is distributed throughout the body, and is not concentrated at the heart. Conductivity of the catheter wall does not affect measurements of pressure made with liquid-filled catheters. Catheters that contain transducers in the tip for measuring blood pressure and flow should have low leakage currents.

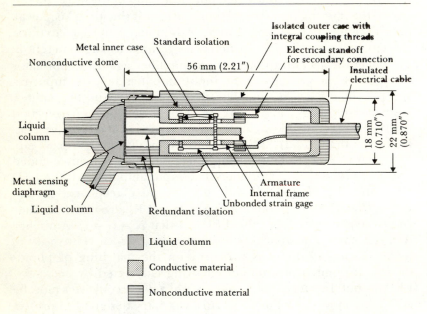

Liquid column

Conductive material

Nonconductive material

Figure 13.18 Redundant electrical isolation of a blood-pressure transducer. Three modes of isolation are provided: (1) External isolation of the case with a plastic sheath which provides protection from extraneous voltages; (2) standard internal isolation of the sensing (bridge) elements from the inside of the transducer case and from the frame; and (3) additional internal isolation of the frame from the case and the diaphragm in case of wire breakage. Thus isolation of the patient/fluid column from electrical excitation voltages is assured, even in the event of failure of the standard internal isolation. (Reproduced with permission of Statham Medical Instruments, a division of Gould, Inc.)

13.10 Testing the electrical system

When we test systems of electrical distribution and also line-powered equipment, we must consider the safety of both the pa-

tients and the personnel conducting the tests. We shall give only a
brief description and comment on the common tests.

Tests of receptacles

Receptacles should be tested for proper wiring, adequate line
voltage, low ground resistance, and mechanical tension. The
common three-light receptacle testers shown in Figure 13.19 are
deficient in several respects. These devices were designed to check
only the wiring, yet they can theoretically indicate only 8 (2^3) of 64
(4^3) possible states for an outlet. The three lights have only two
states (2^3), whereas each of the three outlet contacts has four states
(4^3) (hot, neutral, ground, and open).

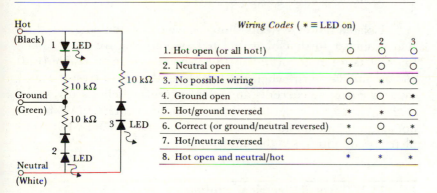

Wiring Codes (* ≡ LED on)	1	2	3
1. Hot open (or all hot!)	O	O	O
2. Neutral open	*	O	O
3. No possible wiring	O	*	O
4. Ground open	O	O	*
5. Hot/ground reversed	*	*	O
6. Correct (or ground/neutral reversed)	*	O	*
7. Hot/neutral reversed	O	*	*
8. Hot open and neutral/hot	*	*	*

Figure 13.19 Three-LED receptacle tester. Ordinary silicon diodes prevent damaging reverse-LED currents, and resistors limit current. The
LEDs are ON for line voltages from about 20 V rms to greater than 240 V
rms, so these devices should not be used to measure line voltage.

These testers give an OK reading when the ground and neutral wires are transposed, or when the green and white wires are
hot and the black wire is grounded. Tripping of the circuit breaker
would probably call attention to the latter miswiring, and of several
others as well.

Ground resistance can be measured by passing up to one am-
pere through the ground wire and measuring the voltage between
ground and neutral. Anyone doing these ground-wire tests should
take care that the microshock hazards described in Section 13.5
(and in Figure 13.13) are not incurred. The resistance of neutral
wiring can be tested similarly, by passing the current through the
neutral conductor. Ground or neutral resistance should not exceed
0.2 Ω for a 15-A circuit. Minimal mechanical retaining force for
each of the three contacts is about 113 g (4 oz).

Tests of interground voltage and resistance

The NFPA 76B requires the following potential and resistance limits for general patient-grounding systems. The voltage between any two receptacle grounds shall not exceed 20 mV, and the resistance shall not exceed $0.1\ \Omega$ (or $0.5\ \Omega$, if the branch circuits are different; or $1.0\ \Omega$, if the distribution panels are different). The voltage between any receptacle ground and any exposed conductive surface in the vicinity of the patient shall not exceed 0.5 V, and the resistance shall not exceed $0.5\ \Omega$ (or $1.0\ \Omega$, if the branch circuits are different). For complete specifications, refer to the test standards.

Tests of isolated power systems

Isolated power systems should have equipotential grounding that is similar to that of unisolated systems (Figure 13.15). The line-isolation monitor (Figure 13.8) should trigger a visible (red) and an audible alarm when the total hazard current (resistive and capacitive leakage currents and LIM current) reaches a threshold of 2 mA under normal line-voltage conditions. The LIM should not alarm for a total hazard current of less than 1.7 mA. For complete specifications, see the latest standard.

13.11 Tests of electrical appliances

Ground-pin-to-chassis resistance

The resistance between the ground pin of the plug and the equipment chassis and exposed metal objects should not exceed $0.15\ \Omega$ during the life of the appliance (Figure 13.20).

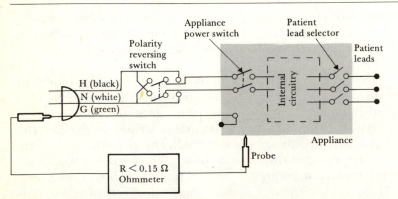

Figure 13.20 Ground-pin-to-chassis resistance test.

Chassis leakage current

Leakage current emanating from the chassis, as measured in Figure 13.21(a), should not exceed 500 μA for appliances not intended to contact patients, and 100 μA for appliances that *are* likely to contact patients. These are limits on rms current for sinusoids from dc to 1 kHz, and should be obtained with a current-measuring device of 1000 Ω or less. Figure 13.21(b) shows a suitable circuit. The limits on leakage current apply regardless of whether the polarity of the power line is correct or reversed, or

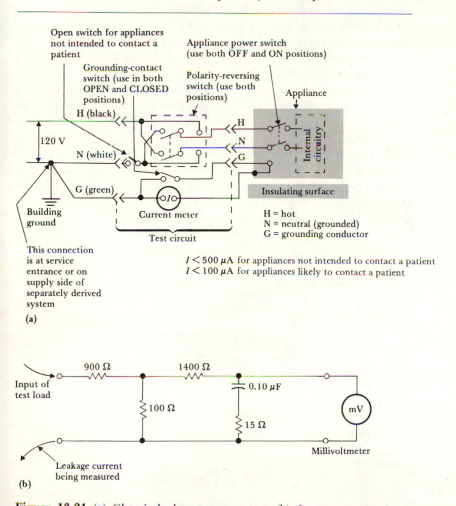

(a)

$I < 500\ \mu$A for appliances not intended to contact a patient
$I < 100\ \mu$A for appliances likely to contact a patient

(b)

Figure 13.21 (a) Chassis leakage-current test. (b) Current-meter circuit to be used for measuring leakage current. It has an input impedance of 1 kΩ and a frequency characteristic that is flat to 1 kHz, drops at the rate of 20 dB/decade to 100 kHz, and then remains flat to 1 MHz or higher. (Reproduced with permission from NFPA 76B, 1977, "Safe Use of Electricity in Patient Care Areas of Hospitals," copyright 1977, National Fire Protection Association, Boston, MA 02210; *proposed for adoption by the NFPA.*)

whether the power switch of the appliance is in the on or off position or whether all the control switches happen to be in the most disadvantageous position at the time of testing.

Leakage current in patient leads

Leakage current in patient leads is particularly important because these leads are the most common low-impedance patient contact. Limits on leakage current in patient leads should be 50 μA. *Isolated* patient leads must have leakage current that is less than 10 μA. Only *isolated* patient leads should be connected to intracardiac catheters or electrodes. Leakage current between individual or interconnected patient leads and ground should be measured with the patient leads active, as shown in Figure 13.22.

In addition, leakage current between any pair of leads or between any single lead and all the other patient leads should be measured, as indicated in Figure 13.23.

Finally, the leakage current that would flow through patient leads to ground if line voltage were to appear on the patient should be tested. Application of power-line voltage and frequency to the isolated patient leads should produce a leakage current to ground that is less than 20 μA (Figure 13.24).

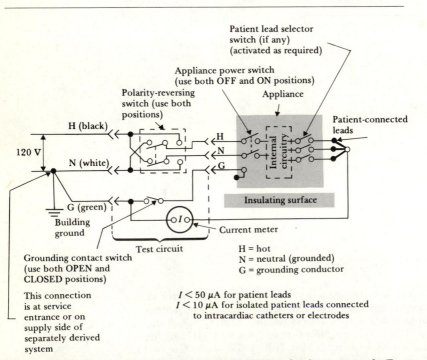

Figure 13.22 Test for leakage current from patient leads to ground. (Reproduced with permission from NFPA 76B, 1977, "Safe Use of Electricity in Patient Care Areas of Hospitals," copyright 1977, National Fire Protection Association, Boston, MA 02210; *proposed for adoption by the NFPA.*)

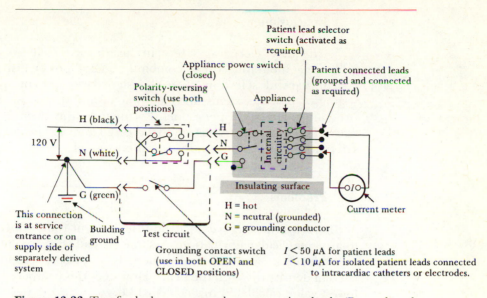

Figure 13.23 Test for leakage current between patient leads. (Reproduced with permission from NFPA 76B, 1977, "Safe Use of Electricity in Patient Care Areas of Hospitals," copyright 1977, National Fire Protection Association, Boston, MA 02210; *proposed for adoption by the NFPA.*)

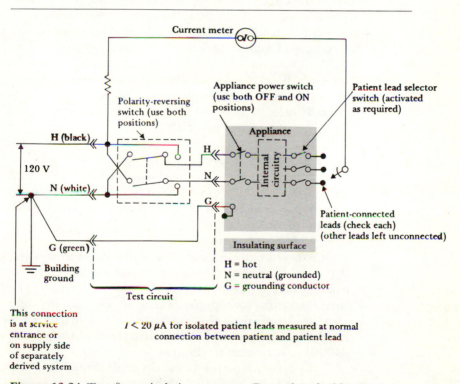

Figure 13.24 Test for ac isolation current. (Reproduced with permission from NFPA 76B, 1977, "Safe Use of Electricity in Patient Care Areas of Hospitals," copyright 1977, National Fire Protection Association, Boston, MA 02210; *proposed for adoption by the NFPA.*)

Conclusion

Adequate electrical safety in health-care facilities can be achieved at moderate cost by combining a good power-distribution system, careful selection of well-designed equipment, periodic testing of power systems and equipment, and a modest training program for medical personnel. Fortunately, the electrical-safety scare of the early 1970s has led to increased knowledge and greater safety for both patients and medical personnel.

Problems

13.1 From Figure 13.1, find the current required for arm-to-arm ventricular fibrillation. Assume that all this current passes through the area of the heart (about 10×10 cm). Calculate the current density through the heart. How does this compare with the lowest value calculated in Problem 13.6?

13.2 Assume that the cell membranes of a very large number of cells in parallel can be modeled by a 1-Ω resistor in parallel with a 100-μF capacitor. Determine the rms sinusoidal current versus frequency necessary to depolarize the cells. Assume that the peak potential of the cell membrane must be raised 20 mV above its resting potential to exceed threshold. Plot your results together with those of Figure 13.3 and compare.

13.3 From your knowledge of cardiac electrophysiology (Section 4.6) explain what rhythm would result from an intense 100-ms shock that occurred during (a) the P wave, (b) the R wave, (c) the T wave, (d) diastole. From these results, explain the shape of the curves shown in Figure 13.4.

13.4 Resketch Figure 13.6(b) for the case in which a catheter made of conductive plastic is used.

13.5 If the secondary earth ground in Figure 13.7 were not connected, would this prevent electrocution under no-fault conditions? What would be the result in case of a primary-to-secondary fault in the transformer?

13.6 Some authors hypothesize that it is current density flowing through the cell membrane that raises the resting potential of the cell to exceed threshold. Replot Figure 13.11 to show the average current density of the fibrillation threshold versus area of the catheter. Is the hypothesis correct? Explain any discrepancies.

13.7 Calculate the maximum safe capacitance between a liquid-filled catheter and dc-isolated pressure-transducer leads for a 120-V, 60-Hz fault in the transducer leads.

13.8 Compute the resistivity of the liquid necessary for safe operation of a liquid-filled catheter that is 1 m long and has a radius of 1.13 mm. (Use the data of Roy *et al.*, 1976, shown in Figure 13.11.) Assume that the patient is grounded and that a 120-V fault develops at the transducer.

13.9 Draw a complete equivalent circuit and compute the rms current through the patient's heart for the following situation. The patient's hand touches a faulty metal lamp that is 120 V rms above ground. A saline-filled catheter ($R = 50$ kΩ) for measuring blood pressure is connected to the patient's heart. Some of the pressure-transducer strain-gage wiring is grounded, and the transducer is somewhat isolated electrically. However, there is 20 MΩ of leakage resistance in the insulation between the ground and the saline in the transducer. There is also 100 pF of capacitance between the ground and the saline. Assume that the skin resistance of the patient is 1 MΩ. Is there a microshock hazard?

13.10 Show how a single electrical instrument can be the path for microshock current flowing both to and from the patient at the same time. Use complete diagrams and do a sample calculation.

13.11 Devise your own hospital-patient microshock situation. Give complete details, including a diagram and equivalent circuit. Describe all tests and acceptable test results necessary to ensure safety of the patient.

13.12 Design a tester for an electrical receptacle that will indicate as many states as possible, including those not detected by the common three-LED receptacle testers (Figure 13.19).

13.13 Recall the microshock hazard shown in Figure 13.12. An electrically operated hospital bed (120 V rms) has a broken ground wire and 300 pF of capacitance between the power line and the bed frame. An attendant simultaneously touches the bed with one hand and a terminal of an external cardiac pacemaker with the other hand. Assume that the patient's right leg is grounded. What is the minimum safe contact resistance/cm^2 for the attendant's skin? (Assume that the attendant has purely resistive skin and a contact area of 1 cm^2.) Neglect all other resistances.

13.14 A power engineer receives a lethal macroshock while standing in water and simultaneously touching the ungrounded metal casing on a high-voltage 60-Hz power transformer. Assume that the resistance of the skin of the engineer's hand is 100 kΩ and that the resistance of the skin on the engineer's feet is negligible. A capacitance of 25 nF is measured between the transformer casing and the high-voltage conductors. Find the minimal value of the high voltage, assuming that 75 mA is the minimal fibrillating macroshock. Draw an equivalent circuit.

References

Anonymous, "Patient safety," Application Note AN 718. Waltham, Mass.: Hewlett-Packard Co., 1971.

Anonymous, "Electrical safety test procedures for hospitals." Publication no. TP-371. Annapolis, Md.: Instrutek, Inc., 1973.

Anonymous, "Electrical safety." Special issue of *health devices*. Philadelphia: Emergency Care Research Institute, January 1974.

Cromwell, L., F.J. Weibell, F.A. Pfeiffer, and L.B. Usselman, *Biomedical instrumentation and measurements*. Englewood Cliffs, N.J.: Prentice-Hall, 1973.

Dalziel, C.F., and W.R. Lee, "Lethal electric currents." *IEEE Spectrum,* February 1969, 6, 44–50.

Dalziel, C.F., "Electric shock," in *Advances in biomedical engineering*. New York: Academic, 1973, 3, 223–248.

Dalziel, C. F., "The transistorized ground fault interrupter, its invention, development, recognition and mandatory application." Berkeley: University of California, 1977.

Friauf, W.S., "Test equipment for hospital safety programs." *Proc. Ann. Conf. Eng. Med. Biol.,* 1974, 16, 496.

Friedlander, G.D., "Electricity in hospitals: elimination of hazards." *IEEE Spectrum,* 1971, 8, 40–51.

Geddes, L.E., P. Cabler, A.G. Moore, J. Rosborough, and W.A. Tacker, "Threshold 60-Hz current required for ventricular fibrillation in subjects of various body weights." *IEEE Trans. Biomed. Eng.,* 1973, 20, 465–468.

Kilpatrick, D.G., and L.B. Kilpatrick, "Electrical safety standards in the health care delivery system." *Crit. Rev. Bioeng.,* 1971, 1, 289–332.

Nader, R., "Ralph Nader's most shocking exposé." *Ladies' Home Journal,* March 1971, 98–179.

National Electrical Code, NFPA No. 70-1978. Boston: National Fire Protection Association, 1978.

NFPA 56A–1973, "Inhalation anesthetics." Boston: National Fire Protection Association, 1973.

NFPA 76A–1978, "Essential electrical systems for health care facilities." Boston: National Fire Protection Association, 1978.

NFPA 76B–1977, "Standard for the safe use of electricity in patient care areas of hospitals." Boston: National Fire Protection Association, 1977.

NFPA 76C–1975, "High-frequency electrical equipment in hospitals." Boston: National Fire Protection Association, 1975.

Ream, A.K., M.J. Lipton, and B. H. Hyndman, "Reduced risk of cardiac fibrillation with use of a conductive catheter." *Ann. Biomed. Eng.,* 1977, 5, 287–301.

Roth, R.R., and E.S. Teltscher, and I.M. Kane, *Electrical safety in health care facilities*. New York: Academic, 1975.

Roy, O.Z., J.R. Scott, and G.C. Park, "60-Hz ventricular fibrillation and pump failure thresholds versus electrode area." *IEEE Trans. Biomed. Eng.,* 1976, 23, 45–48.

Starmer, C.F., and R.E. Whalen, "Current density and electrically induced ventricular fibrillation." *Med. Instrum.*, 1973, 7, 158–161.

Walter, C.W., "Electrical hazards in hospitals: Proceedings of a workshop." *Nat. Acad. Sci.*, 1970, 66.

Weibell, F.J., "Electrical safety in the hospital—1974." *Ann. Biomed. Eng.*, 1974, 2, 126–148.

Appendix A.1

Physical constants

$g = 9.8 \text{ m/s}^2$	Acceleration due to gravity
$c = 3 \times 10^8 \text{ m/s}$	Velocity of light
$\sigma = 5.67 \times 10^{-12} \text{ W/(cm}^2 \cdot \text{K}^4)$	Stefan-Boltzmann constant
$\kappa = 1.38 \times 10^{-23} \text{ J/K}$	Boltzmann's constant
$h = 6.63 \times 10^{-34} \text{ J} \cdot \text{s}$	Planck's constant
$R = 8.31 \text{ J/(mol} \cdot \text{K)}$	Gas constant
$F = 96{,}500 \text{ C/equivalent}$	Faraday's constant (equivalent = mole/valence)
$q = -1.602 \times 10^{-19} \text{ C}$	Charge on the electron
$\epsilon_0 = 8.8 \times 10^{-12} \text{ F/m}$	Dielectric constant of free space
$N = 6.02 \times 10^{23} \text{ molecules/mol}$	Avogadro's number

Appendix A.2

SI prefixes

Multiplication factor	Prefix	Symbol
10^9	giga	G
10^6	mega	M
10^3	kilo	k
10^{-1}	deci	d
10^{-2}	centi	c
10^{-3}	milli	m
10^{-6}	micro	μ
10^{-9}	nano	n
10^{-12}	pico	p

Appendix A.3

SI units

To convert from	To	Multiply by
degree	radian (rad)	0.0175
inch	meter (m)	0.0254
gallon	liter (l)	3.79
cycle/second	hertz (Hz)	1.0
minute	second (s)	60
hour	minute (min)	60
day	hour (h)	24
pound	kilogram (kg)	0.454
0.012 kg of carbon-12	mole (mol)	1.0
pound-force	newton (N)	4.45
degree Rankine	kelvin (K)	$t_K = t_R^\circ/1.8$
calorie	joule (J)	4.186
British thermal unit	joule (J)	1055
horsepower	watt (W)	745
cm H_2O	pascal (Pa)	98.1
mm Hg (torr)	pascal (Pa)	133.3
psi	pascal (Pa)	6895
atmosphere	pascal (Pa)	101325
poise	pascal · second (Pa · s)	0.1
	volt (V)	
	ampere (A)	
	ohm (Ω)	
mho	siemens (S)	1.0
gauss	tesla (T)	0.0001
maxwell	weber (Wb)	10^{-8}
	farad (F)	
	decibel (dB)	
	candela (cd)	
roentgen (R)	coulomb per kilogram (C/kg)	0.000258
rad	gray (Gy)	0.01
curie (Ci)	becquerel (Bq)	3.7×10^{10}

References

Anonymous. *Standard for metric practice.* ASTM E380-76, American Society for Testing and Materials, 1916 Race St., Philadelphia, PA, 19103. Also IEEE standard 268-1976, Institute of Electrical and Electronics Engineers, 345 East 47th Street, New York, NY 10017. February 1976.

Appendix A.4

Abbreviations

Abbreviation	Term
AAP	axon action potential
ac	alternating current
ACA	Automatic Clinical Analyzer
ADC	analog-to-digital converter
AF	audiofrequency
AM	amplitude modulation
ANSI	American National Standards Institute
ATP	analytical test pack
AV	atrioventricular
AWG	American wire gage
CC	closing capacity
CCD	charge-coupled device
CMG	common-mode gain
CMRR	common-mode rejection ratio
CMV	common-mode voltage
CNS	central nervous system
CPAP	continuous positive airway pressure
CPU	central processing unit
CSF	cerebro-spinal fluid
CV	closing volume
CW	continuous wave
D	d/dt
dc	direct current
DG	differential gain
EBR	electron beam recording
ECG	electrocardiogram
ECoG	electrocorticogram
EEG	electroencephalogram
EIA	Electronics Industries Association
emf	electromotive force
EMG	electromyogram
ENG	electroneurogram
EOG	electro-oculogram
EPROM	erasable programmable read-only memory
ERG	electroretinogram
ERP	early-receptor potential
ERV	expiratory reserve volume
FDA	Food and Drug Administration
FEF	forced expiratory flow
FET	field-effect transistor
FEV	forced expiratory volume
FM	frequency modulation
FRC	functional residual capacity
FVC	forced vital capacity
GC	gas chromatograph
GFCI	ground-fault circuit interrupter
GLC	gas-liquid chromatograph

Abbreviations (*Continued*)

Abbreviation	Term
GSR	galvanic skin response
hct	hematocrit
hgb	hemoglobin
IC	inspiratory capacity
ICU	intensive-care unit
ID	inside diameter
IR	infrared
IV	intravenous
j	$+\sqrt{-1}$
LED	light-emitting diode
LIM	line isolation monitor
lps	liters per second
LRP	late-receptor potential
MBC	maximum breathing capacity
MEFV	maximum expiratory flow volume
MMF	maximum mid-expiratory flow
MTBF	mean time between failures
MTF	modulation transfer function
NDIR	nondispersive infrared analysis
NEC	National Electric Code
NEMA	National Electrical Manufacturers Association
NEP	noise-equivalent power
NFPA	National Fire Protection Association
NREM	nonrapid eye movement
OD	outside diameter
PEEP	positive end expiratory pressure
PEF	peak expiratory flow
PEP	pre-ejection period
PFT	pulmonary function tests
PM	photomultiplier
p–p	peak-to-peak
PROM	programmable read-only memory
PSP	post-synaptic potential
PT	phototransistor
PVC	premature ventricular contraction
RAM	random-access memory
RAS	reticular activating system
RBC	red blood cell
REM	rapid eye movement
RF	radiofrequency
rms	root-mean-square
ROM	read-only memory
RV	residual volume
SA	sinoatrial
SCR	silicon-controlled rectifier
SEC	secondary electron conduction
SHR	signal-to-hysteresis ratio
SMA	Sequential Multiple Analyzer
SMU	single motor unit
SNR	signal-to-noise ratio
SVP	surge-voltage protection
TBP	total-body plethysmograph
TCD	thermal-conductivity detector

Abbreviations (*Continued*)

Abbreviation	Term
TLC	total lung capacity
TV	television
TVC	timed vital capacity
UL	Underwriters' Laboratory
VC	vital capacity
VCVS	voltage-controlled voltage source
WBC	white blood cell
WPW	Wolff-Parkinson-White

Appendix A.5

Chemical elements

Element and symbol	Atomic number	Atomic weight (C = 12)	Element and symbol	Atomic number	Atomic weight (C = 12)
actinium (Ac)	89		mercury (Hg)	80	200.59
aluminum (Al)	13	26.9815	molybdenum (Mo)	42	95.94
americium (Am)	95		neodymium (Nd)	60	144.24
antimony (Sb)	51	121.75	neon (Ne)	10	20.179
argon (Ar)	18	39.948	neptunium (Np)	93	237.0482
arsenic (As)	33	74.9216	nickel (Ni)	28	58.71
astatine (At)	85		niobium (Nb)	41	92.9064
barium (Ba)	56	137.34	nitrogen (N)	7	14.0067
berkelium (Bk)	97		nobelium (No)	102	
beryllium (Be)	4	9.01218	osmium (Os)	76	190.2
bismuth (Bi)	83	208.9806	oxygen (O)	8	15.9994
boron (B)	5	10.81	palladium (Pd)	46	106.4
bromine (Br)	35	79.904	phosphorus (P)	15	30.9738
cadmium (Cd)	48	112.40	platinum (Pt)	78	195.09
calcium (Ca)	20	40.08	plutonium (Pu)	94	
californium (Cf)	98		polonium (Po)	84	
carbon (C)	6	12.011	potassium (K)	19	39.102
cerium (Ce)	58	140.12	praseodymium (Pr)	59	140.9077
cesium (Cs)	55	132.9055	promethium (Pm)	61	
chlorine (Cl)	17	35.453	protactinium (Pa)	91	231.0359
chromium (Cr)	24	51.996	radium (Ra)	88	226.0254
cobalt (Co)	27	58.9332	radon (Rn)	86	
columbium (Cb)	(see niobium)		rhenium (Re)	75	186.2
copper (Cu)	29	63.546	rhodium (Rh)	45	102.9055
curium (Cm)	96		rubidium (Rb)	37	85.4678
dysprosium (Dy)	66	162.50	ruthenium (Ru)	44	101.07
einsteinium (Es)	99		samarium (Sm)	62	150.4
erbium (Er)	68	167.26	scandium (Sc)	21	44.9559
europium (Eu)	63	151.96	selenium (Se)	34	78.96
fermium (Fm)	100		silicon (Si)	14	28.086
fluorine (F)	9	18.9984	silver (Ag)	47	107.868
francium (Fr)	87		sodium (Na)	11	22.9898
gadolinium (Gd)	64	157.25	strontium (Sr)	38	87.62
gallium (Ga)	31	69.72	sulfur (S)	16	32.06
germanium (Ge)	32	72.59	tantalum (Ta)	73	180.9479
gold (Au)	79	196.9665	technetium (Tc)	43	98.9062
hafnium (Hf)	72	178.49	tellurium (Te)	52	127.60
helium (He)	2	4.00260	terbium (Tb)	65	158.9254
holmium (Ho)	67	164.9303	thallium (Tl)	81	204.37
hydrogen (H)	1	1.0080	thorium (Th)	90	232.0381
indium (In)	49	114.82	thulium (Tm)	69	168.9342
iodine (I)	53	126.9045	tin (Sn)	50	118.69
iridium (Ir)	77	192.22	titanium (Ti)	22	47.90
iron (Fe)	26	55.847	tungsten (W)	74	183.85
krypton (Kr)	36	83.80	uranium (U)	92	238.029
lanthanum (La)	57	138.9055	vanadium (V)	23	50.9414
lawrencium (Lr)	103		wolfram (W)	(see tungsten)	
lead (Pb)	82	207.2	xenon (Xe)	54	131.30
lithium (Li)	3	6.941	ytterbium (Yb)	70	173.04
lutetium (Lu)	71	174.97	yttrium (Y)	39	88.9059
magnesium (Mg)	12	24.305	zinc (Zn)	30	65.37
manganese (Mn)	25	54.9380	zirconium (Zr)	40	91.22
mendelevium (Md)	101				

Index

Page numbers in boldface type indicate the location of an illustration.